T0337974

Dellmann's

Textbook of
Veterinary Histology

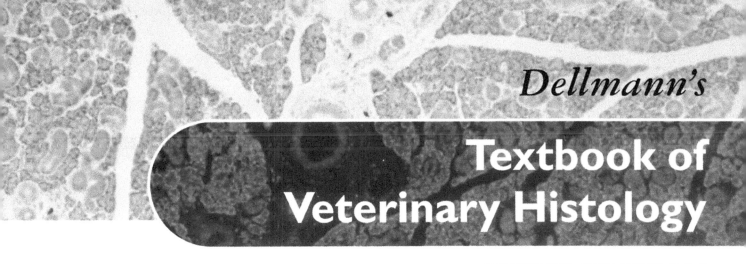

Dellmann's

Textbook of Veterinary Histology

SIXTH EDITION

JO ANN EURELL, DVM, PHD

Department of Veterinary Biosciences
University of Illinois
Urbana, Illinois

BRIAN L. FRAPPIER, DVM, PHD

Department of Biomedical Sciences
University of Missouri—Columbia
Columbia, Missouri

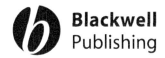

Blackwell
Publishing

©2006 Blackwell Publishing
All rights reserved

Blackwell Publishing Professional
2121 State Avenue, Ames, Iowa 50014, USA

Orders:	1-800-862-6657
Office:	1-515-292-0140
Fax:	1-515-292-3348
Web site:	www.blackwellprofessional.com

Blackwell Publishing Ltd
9600 Garsington Road, Oxford OX4 2DQ, UK
Tel.: +44 (0)1865 776868

Blackwell Publishing Asia
550 Swanston Street, Carlton, Victoria 3053, Australia
Tel.: +61 (0)3 8359 1011

Authorization to photocopy items for internal or personal use, or the internal or personal use of specific clients, is granted by Blackwell Publishing, provided that the base fee is paid directly to the Copyright Clearance Center, 222 Rosewood Drive, Danvers, MA 01923. For those organizations that have been granted a photocopy license by CCC, a separate system of payments has been arranged. The fee code for users of the Transactional Reporting Service is ISBN-13: 978-0-7817-4148-4/2006.

Sixth edition, 2006

Library of Congress Cataloging-in-Publication Data

Dellmann's textbook of veterinary histology / [edited by] Jo Ann Eurell, Brian L. Frappier.—6th ed.
    p. ; cm.
  Rev. ed. of: Textbook of veterinary histology / [edited by] H. Dieter Dellmann, Jo Ann Eurell. 5th ed. c1998.
  Includes bibliographical references.
  ISBN-13: 978-0-7817-4148-4
  ISBN-10: 0-7817-4148-3
  1. Veterinary histology. I. Eurell, Jo Ann Coers. II. Frappier, Brian L. III. Dellmann, Horst-Dieter. IV. Title. V. Title:
Textbook of veterinary histology.
  [DNLM: 1. Histology. 2. Anatomy, Veterinary. SF 757.3 D3575 2006]
SF757.3T49 2006
636.089'10189—dc22

                                                                                          2005008748

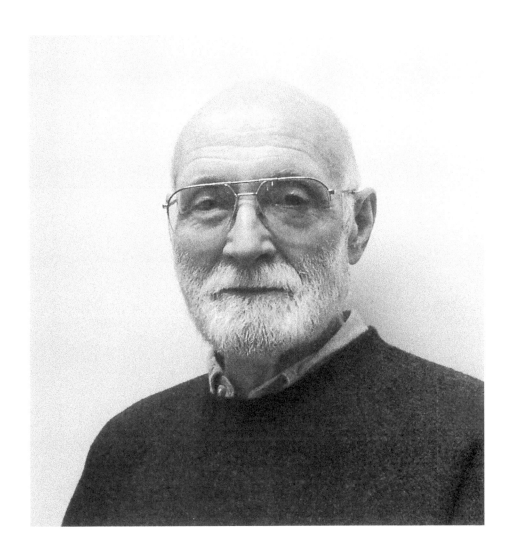

Dedicated to H.-Dieter Dellmann, Docteur-Vétérinaire, Habil.

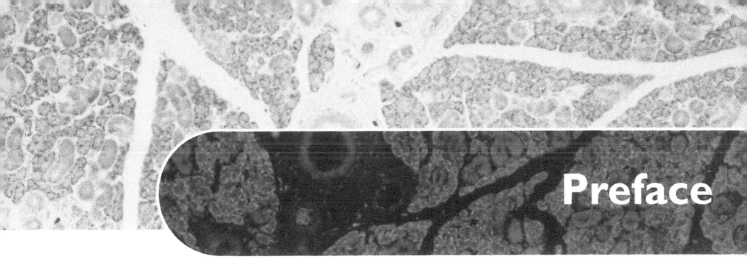

Preface

The publication of the sixth edition of the *Textbook of Veterinary Histology* marks the 30th year since H.-Dieter Dellmann and Esther M. Brown first brought this book to veterinary students, histology instructors, and other biologists in 1976. Dr. Dellmann continued this book through five English editions. The textbook has also been reprinted in Spanish, Japanese, Italian, Indonesian, Portuguese, and Korean editions for international veterinary students. We have attempted to recognize and honor Dr. Dellmann's dedication and contribution to veterinary histology by including his name in the title of this edition.

In the beginning, this textbook was conceived as a teaching tool for veterinary students rather than for graduate students or other histologists. We have attempted to continue this tradition. The text and images for this edition have been updated with the most current information available at the time of publication.

With the retirement of Dr. Dellmann, J. A. Eurell and B. Frappier have taken over the editorial role for this edition. We would like to thank contributors to the fifth edition who did not participate in this edition: A. Deldar, H.-Dieter Dellmann, G. Flottorp, I. Foss, and C. Henrikson. We would also like to thank D. Biechler for illustrations in the previous edition. New contributors for the sixth edition include: O. M. Andrisani, A. Beitz, M. Bergmann, E. J. Ehrhart, R. Hamor, R. Hullinger, L.-I. Larsson, J. Messick, J. Plendl, C. Plopper, and J. Verlander. M. Chansky has produced several new illustrations for this edition. Their expertise and participation has made this project possible.

At the University of Illinois, Jo Ann Eurell would like to recognize Joan Thompson for excellent technical histology support, and Dr. Thomas E. Eurell as a constant source of inspiration and encouragement. At the University of Missouri, Brian Frappier offers appreciation and thanks to Howard A. Wilson for years of expert advice, technical assistance, and attention to detail.

This edition of the textbook is accompanied by a CD-ROM containing a histology atlas with many images contributed by chapter authors. In addition, the family of W. E. Haensly has generously donated many images from his extensive collection. Dr. Haensly was a dedicated veterinary histologist, mentor, and friend, and we are pleased to present his work for the benefit of veterinary students for years to come. We thank his wife, Patricia, and his family for their generosity.

Jo Ann Eurell
Urbana, Illinois
Brian Frappier
Columbia, Missouri

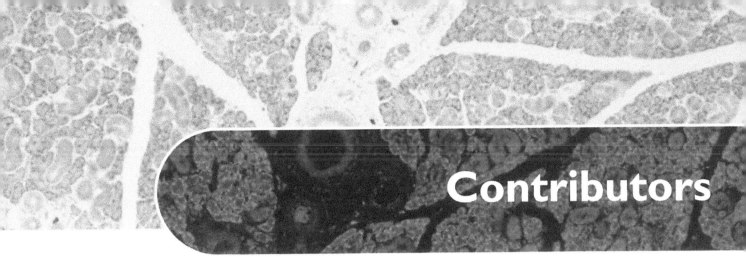

Contributors

Donald R. Adams, PhD
  University Professor Emeritus
  Department of Biomedical Sciences
  Iowa State University
  College of Veterinary Medicine
  Ames, Iowa

Ourania M. Andrisani, PhD
  Professor
  Department of Basic Medical Sciences
  School of Veterinary Medicine
  Purdue University
  West Lafayette, Indiana

Alvin Beitz, PhD
  Department of Veterinary and Biomedical Sciences
  College of Veterinary Medicine
  University of Minnesota
  St. Paul, Minnesota

Martin Bergmann, Dr. med. vet.
  Professor
  Institute of Veterinary Anatomy, Histology, and
  Embryology
  Justus-Liebig-University
  Giessen, Germany

Vibeke Dantzer, DVM, Dr. Vet. Sci.
  Associate Professor
  Department of Basic Animal and Veterinary Sciences
  Royal Veterinary and Agricultural University
  Copenhagen, Denmark

E. J. Ehrhart, DVM, PhD
  Associate Professor
  Colorado State University
  College of Veterinary Medicine and Biomedical Sciences
  Department of Microbiology, Immunology, and Pathology
  Fort Collins, Colorado

Jo Ann Eurell, DVM, PhD
  Associate Professor of Morphology
  Department of Veterinary Biosciences
  College of Veterinary Medicine
  University of Illinois
  Urbana, Illinois

Thomas F. Fletcher, DVM, PhD
  Department of Veterinary and Biomedical Sciences
  College of Veterinary Medicine
  University of Minnesota
  St. Paul, Minnesota

Brian L. Frappier, DVM, PhD
  Clinical Associate Professor
  Department of Biomedical Sciences
  College of Veterinary Medicine
  University of Missouri—Columbia
  Columbia, Missouri

Ralph E. Hamor, DVM
  Clinical Associate Professor
  Department of Veterinary Clinical Medicine
  College of Veterinary Medicine
  University of Illinois
  Urbana, Illinois

Ronald L. Hullinger, DVM, PhD
    Professor
    Department of Basic Medical Sciences
    School of Veterinary Medicine
    Purdue University
    West Lafayette, Indiana

Thor Landsverk, Dr. med. vet.
    Professor, Department of Basic Sciences and Aquatic
    Medicine
    Norwegian School of Veterinary Science
    Oslo, Norway

Lars-Inge Larsson, D. Sc.
    Professor, Division of Cell Biology
    Department of Anatomy and Physiology
    The Royal Veterinary and Agricultural University
    Frederiksberg, Denmark

Rudolf Leiser, Dr. med. vet., Dr. h.c.
    Professor
    Institute of Veterinary Anatomy, Histology, and
    Embryology
    Justus-Liebig-University
    Giessen, Germany

Joanne B. Messick, DVM, PhD
    Associate Professor
    Population Medicine and Diagnostic Sciences
    College of Veterinary Medicine
    Cornell University
    Ithaca, New York

Nancy A. Monteiro-Riviere, PhD
    Professor of Investigative Dermatology and Toxicology
    Center for Chemical Toxicology and Research
    Pharmacokinetics
    Department of Clinical Sciences
    College of Veterinary Medicine
    North Carolina State University
    Raleigh, North Carolina

Johanna Plendl, Dr. med. vet.
    Professor of Veterinary Anatomy
    Institute for Veterinary Anatomy
    Free University of Berlin
    Berlin, Germany

Charles G. Plopper, DVM, PhD
    Professor and Chair, Department of Anatomy, Physiology,
    and Cell Biology
    School of Veterinary Medicine
    University of California, Davis
    Davis, California

Charles McLean Press, BSc (Vet.), BVSc, PhD
    Professor, Department of Basic Sciences and Aquatic
    Medicine
    Norwegian School of Veterinary Science
    Oslo, Norway

Jānis Priedkalns, BVSc, MA, PhD
    Emeritus Elder Professor of Anatomy and Histology
    Faculty of Medicine
    University of Adelaide
    Adelaide, South Australia
    Professor, Faculty of Medicine
    University of Latvia
    Riga, Latvia

David C. Van Sickle, DVM, PhD
    Professor Emeritus, Department of Basic Medical Sciences
    School of Veterinary Medicine
    Purdue University
    West Lafayette, Indiana

Jill W. Verlander, DVM
    Director, Electron Microscopy Core Facility
    College of Medicine
    University of Florida

Karl-Heinz Wrobel, Dr. med. vet., Dr. rer. nat.
    Professor
    Institute of Anatomy
    University of Regensburg
    Regensburg, Germany

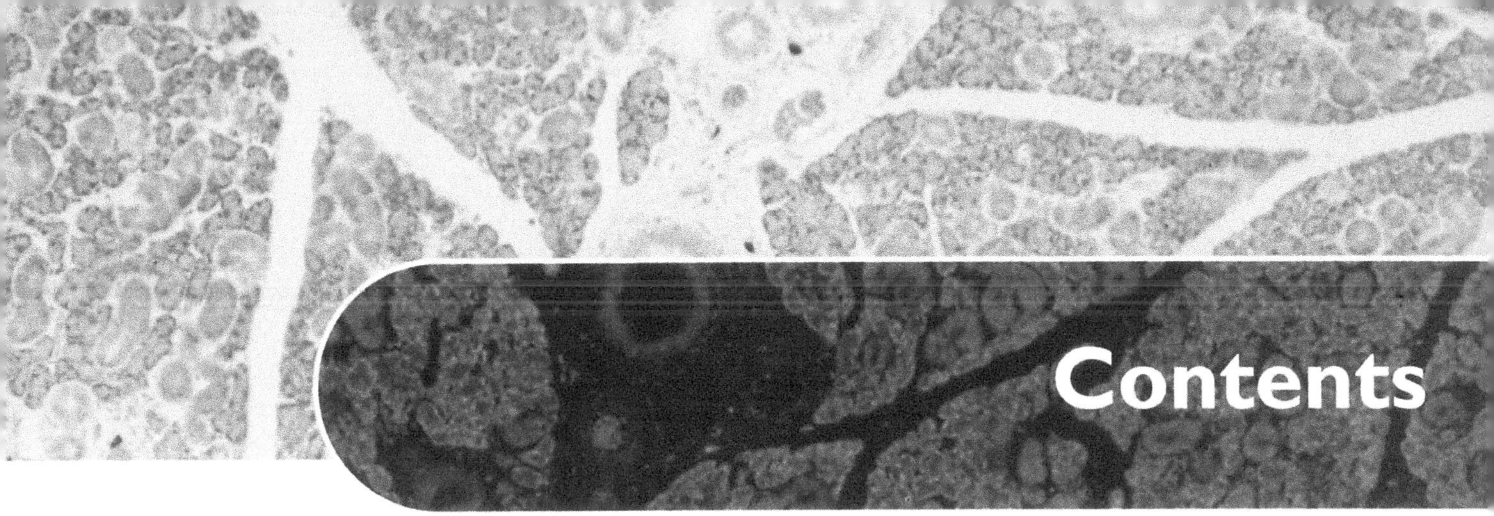

Contents

1 Cytology 1
Lars-Inge Larsson

2 Epithelium 17
Brian L. Frappier

3 Connective and Supportive Tissues 31
Jo Ann Eurell
David C. Van Sickle

4 Blood and Bone Marrow 61
Joanne Messick

5 Muscle 79
Jo Ann Eurell

6 Nervous Tissue 91
Alvin J. Beitz
Thomas F. Fletcher

7 Cardiovascular System 117
Johanna Plendl

8 Immune System 134
Charles McL. Press
Thor Landsverk

9 Respiratory System 153
Charles G. Plopper
Donald R. Adams

10 Digestive System 170
Brian L. Frappier

11 Urinary System 212
Jill W. Verlander

12 Male Reproductive System 233
Karl-Heinz Wrobel
Martin Bergmann

13 Female Reproductive System 256
Jānis Priedkalns
Rudolf Leiser

14 Placentation 279
Vibeke Dantzer
Rudolf Leiser

15 Endocrine System 298
Ron Hullinger
Ourania M. Andrisani

16 Integument 320
Nancy A. Monteiro-Riviere

17 Eye 350
Ralph E. Hamor
E. J. Ehrhart

18 Ear 364
Jo Ann Eurell

Index 377

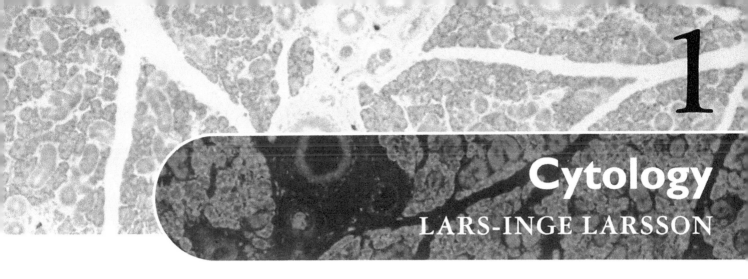

Cytology

LARS-INGE LARSSON

General Overview
Cell Membrane
Nucleus
    Nuclear Envelope
    Nucleoplasm
    Nucleoli
Cytosol
Organelles
    Rough and Smooth Endoplasmic Reticulum and
        Ribosomes
    Golgi Complex and Vesicular Transport
    Mitochondria
    Peroxisomes

Cytoskeleton
    Microtubules
    Microfilaments
    Intermediate Filaments
Inclusions
Cell Surface Modifications
Cell Cycle, Cell Division, and Apoptosis
From Cells to Tissues
    Intercellular Junctions
    Cell Communication

GENERAL OVERVIEW

The cell is the smallest unit of life, and all living matter (**protoplasm**) is composed of cells. Cells possess the unique abilities to replicate and to create energy from inanimate matter, which are qualities that characterize life itself. Many living creatures are unicellular (i.e., consist of a single cell), but higher organisms are comprised of a multiplicity of cells that specialize in different functions including absorption, digestion, and excretion.

In primitive **prokaryotic** cells, like bacteria, there is little organization of the many molecules that are needed for the life processes. In contrast, in **eukaryotic** organisms, the genetic material is organized in a nucleus (karyon) and many other processes have become restricted to membrane-bounded **organelles**. Such **compartmentation** prevents unordered mixing of different biochemical pathways, thus allowing for more sophisticated functions. The compartmentation also allows the cells to increase in size by ordered delivery of membrane-delimited molecules to their appropriate destinations. Thus, bacteria only reach 1 to 5 μm in size, while most eukaryotic cells are 5 to 50 μm.

Eukaryotic cell structure and function thus depend upon membranes and membrane-enclosed structures. The cell itself is delimited by the **cell membrane**. The **cytoplasm** consists of organelles, inclusions, and cytoskeletal components enclosed in a semiviscous liquid, the **cytosol** (Fig. 1-1). The study of the structural components of the cell is referred to as **cytology**, while the study of the integration of cells to form tissues and organs is referred to as **histology**. Such integration involves three different components: the cells themselves, the **extracellular matrix** (**ECM**), and **tissue fluids**. The ECM components are synthesized by cells and are present in different proportions in different tissues. Tissue fluids transport nutrients, hormones, gases, and waste products to and from the cells.

Many parts of the cell can be studied in the light microscope, which allows maximal resolution of structures down to 0.2 μm in diameter at magnifications up to 1000 to 1500 times. However, many cellular structures are smaller and the electron microscope, offering much better resolution (down to 0.1 nm) and higher magnifications (up to ×400,000), has to be used for their study.

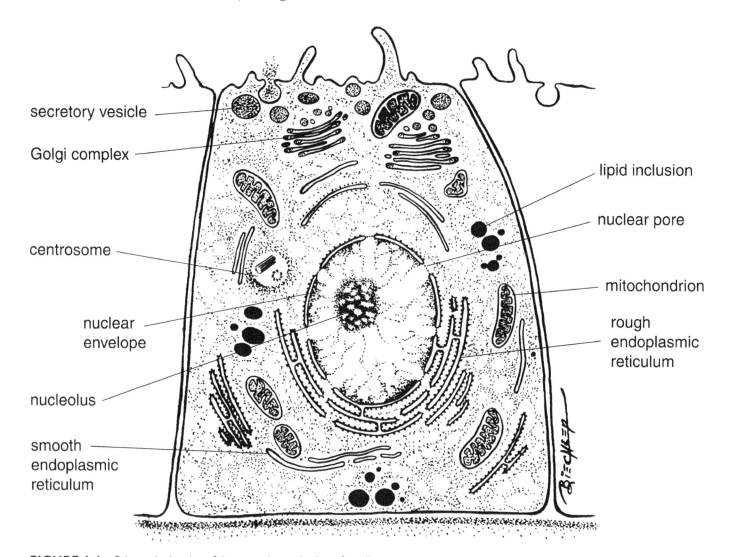

secretory vesicle

Golgi complex

centrosome

nuclear
envelope

nucleolus

smooth
endoplasmic
reticulum

lipid inclusion

nuclear pore

mitochondrion

rough
endoplasmic
reticulum

FIGURE 1-1   Schematic drawing of the general organization of a cell.

In most cases, it is necessary to stain cells and tissues to increase their contrast in the light or electron microscope. A common light microscopy stain is a combination of the dyes, hematoxylin and eosin, which stain nuclei blue and cytoplasm pink, respectively. When negative molecular groups bind positively charged (basic) dyes (such as derivatives of hematoxylin), the stained structures are described as **basophilic**. In contrast, basic components (hemoglobin in mature red blood cells) attract positively charged (acidic) dyes such as eosin and are termed **acidophilic**. Electron-absorbing heavy metal ions are used as stains for electron microscopy. These stains show little chemical specificity, but impart contrast to cellular structures. In contrast, histochemistry allows the localization of specific molecules by use of antibodies tagged with labels that are detectable in the light or electron microscope (immunohistochemistry). Often, antibodies are labeled with fluorescent dyes that can be observed in special fluorescence microscopes. Enzyme histochemistry makes use of enzyme substrates that produce colored or electron-dense reaction products that precipitate at the site of enzyme activity. The study of living cells requires the use of special optical methods (phase contrast or interference contrast microscopy), which impart contrast to different cell components. Additionally, living cells can be stained with vital dyes that make it possible to follow fluorescent proteins expressed by genetically manipulated living cells.

CELL MEMBRANE

The **cell membrane** (plasmalemma) encloses the cell and forms its area of contact with the surrounding environment. The internal milieu of the cell must be kept constant, so the cell membrane is involved in the active and passive transport of ions, water, oxygen, carbon dioxide, nutrients, and secretory and excretory products. The cell membrane is also involved in anchoring the cell to surrounding structures, as well as participating in signaling and recognition events. This structure is sometimes referred to as a **unit membrane,** which follows the theory that all biologic membranes share the same structure.

The cell membrane is 8 to 10 nm thick and has a characteristic trilaminar structure in electron micrographs (Fig. 1-2). The trilaminar structure consists of an outer and inner electron-dense lamina separated by an electron-lucent layer. Biochemically, the

ciated proteins making up the electron-dense laminae and the hydrophobic tails forming the electron-lucent layer. The bilayer also contains other lipids, such as cholesterol and carbohydrate-containing glycolipids.

Proteins associated with the cell membrane are either inserted into the phospholipid bilayer (**integral proteins**) or attached to its inner or outer surfaces (**peripheral proteins**). **Transmembrane proteins** are integral proteins that span the entire thickness of the lipid bilayer. A fluid mosaic is created by transmembrane proteins, which can diffuse laterally in the lipid bilayer. Protein diffusion is restricted by cytoskeletal components, cell junctions, and peculiar membrane substructures known as **lipid rafts**. Lipid rafts contain high concentrations of cholesterol and sphingolipids, which decrease the fluidity of the lipid bilayer. Some rafts contain proteins called caveolins, which reorganize the membrane into pear-shaped invaginations known as **caveolae**. These invaginations are believed to participate in signaling events and the cellular uptake of certain proteins such as albumin.

Some integral membrane proteins attach to oligosaccharides, forming glycoproteins, while others attach to larger polysaccharides (glycosaminoglycans), forming proteoglycans. Both oligosaccharides and glycosaminoglycans are present on the outside of the cell membrane. Together with the carbohydrate portion of the glycolipids, they form a carbohydrate-rich external cell coat, the **glycocalyx,** which is involved in many important functions relating to cell recognition, signaling, and mechanical protection. Blood group antigens form part of the glycocalyx of blood cells. The glycocalyx can be demonstrated by histochemical staining using the periodic-acid-Schiff method or with labeled lectins, which are proteins that bind to specific carbohydrate structures. The cell membrane is asymmetrical with respect to membrane proteins, the glycocalyx, and phospholipids.

Some **transmembrane proteins** are involved in cell-to-cell or cell-to-matrix interactions, while others form carriers or channels that transport substances such as ions and glucose through the membrane. Still other transmembrane proteins form **receptors** that transmit signals from outside the cell to inside. Certain hormones, including steroid hormones, can pass through the plasmalemma and bind directly to intracellular receptors. Most

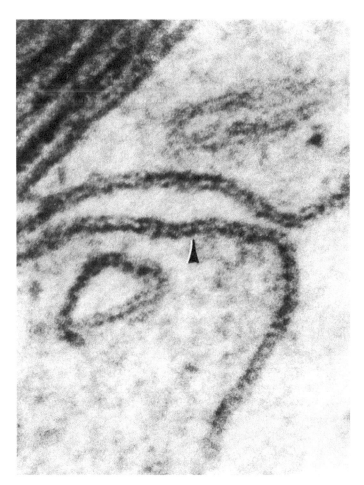

FIGURE 1-2 Trilaminar plasma membrane (arrowhead) of a neurolemmocyte (×415,000).

cell membrane is composed of **phospholipids,** which have a hydrophilic head and hydrophobic tails. The phospholipids form a bilayer in the membrane with the hydrophobic tails facing each other. Thus, the hydrophilic heads of the outer layer face the outside of the cell, while the heads of the inner layer face the cytosol (Fig. 1-3). Such arrangement of the phospholipids has been correlated to the trilaminar structure with the polar heads and asso-

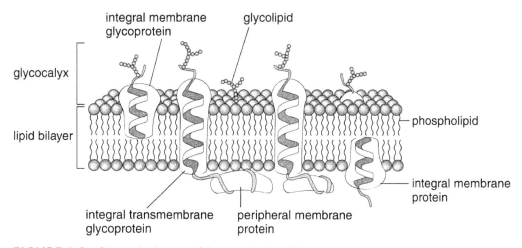

FIGURE 1-3 Schematic drawing of the organization of the cell membrane.

hormones, growth factors, and neurotransmitters are either too large or too hydrophilic to pass through the cell membrane, and therefore use transmembrane proteins as receptors. Binding to the extracellular region of such receptors evokes intracellular activation of so-called **second messengers,** such as cyclic adenosine monophosphate (cAMP). Second messengers are intracellular molecules that convey the extracellular message into the interior of the cell.

NUCLEUS

The shape, structure, and position of the nucleus vary considerably between cell types, and these characteristics are useful for cell identification. For example, lymphocytes have a round nucleus while granulocytes have a lobulated nucleus. The **nucleus** is centrally located in many cell types, but it is displaced to the periphery in others (e.g., fat cells and skeletal muscle cells). Most cells have a single nucleus, but some, like osteoclasts, possess multiple nuclei. Multinucleated cells may originate either from fusion of mononuclear cells or from incomplete division. Mature, mammalian red blood cells lack a nucleus altogether.

Nuclear Envelope

The nucleus is enclosed by a **nuclear envelope,** which contains nuclear pores that control the flow of materials between the nucleus and the cytoplasm. The nuclear envelope is comprised of two concentric unit membranes that are separated by a narrow (25 to 70 nm) space (Fig. 1-4). The outer membrane is often studded with ribosomes and may be continuous with the rough endoplasmic reticulum. On the inside of the inner membrane, the **nuclear lamina** is present. The nuclear lamina is a fibrous sheath, composed of specialized intermediate filaments called **lamins** that provide the nucleus with mechanical strength. At intervals, circular **nuclear pores** interrupt the nuclear envelope.

Materials pass through these pores in a manner that is strictly controlled by proteins of the nuclear pore complex. In this way, protein synthesis is restricted to the cytoplasm, permitting the nucleus to process and refine messenger ribonucleic acids (RNAs) without risking their translation into proteins during processing. This refinement is not possible in prokaryotes and provides eukaryotic organisms with possibilities for more complex exploitation of the genome (e.g., through alternative splicing of primary messenger RNAs).

Nucleoplasm

Chromatin refers to deoxyribonucleic acid (DNA) complexed with proteins, of which the basic **histones** form the quantitatively most important part and are involved in chromatin packing. Nonhistone proteins refer to proteins that are also involved in chromatin packing and protection or that participate in regulation of DNA duplication, transcription, and repair.

In specimens stained with hematoxylin or other basic dyes, the nucleus has areas of intense staining referred to as **heterochromatin.** Heterochromatin often occurs at the periphery of the nucleus attached to the nuclear lamina and consists of condensed DNA. Additionally, the nucleus contains lightly stained **euchromatin** that represents uncoiled DNA, which is accessible for transcription into RNA. Ultrastructurally, heterochromatin appears as electron-dense granular masses while euchromatin is electron-lucent (Fig. 1-4). The proportion of heterochromatin to euchromatin varies between cells and is often an identifying feature.

Chromatin is packed by coiling at several levels of organization. The basic unit is the **nucleosome** that is formed from 200 base pairs of double-stranded DNA complexed with several histones. The exact number of base pairs involved is species variable. The nucleosomes are separated by shorter (about 50-base-pair) sequences of double-stranded DNA. Even during transcription, euchromatin is composed of nucleosomes and internucleosomal strands while transcriptionally inactive heterochromatin is further

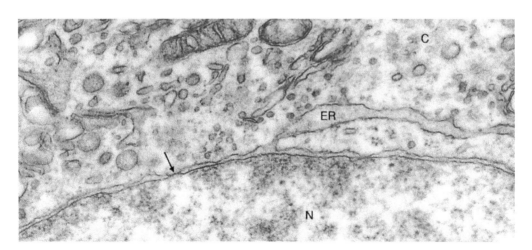

FIGURE 1-4   Part of the nucleus (N), with electron-dense heterochromatin and electron-lucent euchromatin, and the cytoplasm (C) of a neurohypophysial glial cell. The nuclear envelope is pierced by pores (arrow). The perinuclear space between the inner and outer nuclear membranes is continuous with a cisterna of the endoplasmic reticulum (ER) (×67,000).

coiled. Heterochromatin is characterized by 30-nm **chromatin fibers** consisting of spirals of coiled nucleosomes. Even more elaborate coiling and structuring of chromatin occurs in conjunction with mitosis or meiosis and results in recognizable chromosomes.

In all cells of female individuals, one of the two X chromosomes is permanently inactivated and does not participate in transcription. The inactive X chromosome is recognizable in epithelial cells from the oral cavity as a single granule called **sex chromatin-** (Barr body) that is attached to the nuclear lamina. In neutrophils, the sex chromatin takes the form of a drum stick-like appendage to the nucleus (Fig. 1-5). These structures have been used for gender testing in the past, but today, in situ hybridization techniques using labeled DNA probes that specifically bind to X chromosomes are preferred. The formula for genetic information encoded in the DNA is written using four letters representing the bases adenine (A), guanine (G), thymine (T), and cytosine (C). The sequence of these bases determines the information encoded in genes of the DNA, and this information is passed on (transcribed) to RNA. Hybridization refers to the unique sequence of bases of the applied probe that binds to the complementary sequence of nucleotides in the DNA being investigated (A binding to T and G to C). This technique affords a high degree of specificity and the probe can be labeled with a variety of substances that are detectable in either the light or electron microscope. Probes that are complementary to specific chromosome regions or genes can be used for prenatal diagnosis of hereditary diseases (Fig. 1-6).

The **nuclear matrix** refers to filamentous material remaining after enzymatic digestion and extraction of the nucleus. It is believed that the nuclear matrix is important for positioning chromosomes in the nucleus in a pattern resembling that observed during mitotic cell division.

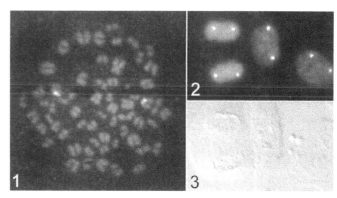

FIGURE 1-6 Bovine chromosome pair 7 identified by their intense (white) fluorescence using in situ hybridization on spread metaphase chromosomes (1), on cultured bovine endothelial cells, observed in fluorescence (2), and in interference contrast to bring out morphologic details (3). DNA has been gently counterstained by a more weakly fluorescent dye. Note in 2 and 3 the presence of a dividing cell (anaphase; left), in which the two pairs of chromosome 7 are being divided between the two daughter cells. Also note in 2 and 3 two interphase cells (right), which each contain two fluorescent dots corresponding to two copies of chromosome 7. By this approach, the number of chromosomes can easily be determined also in interphase cells, obviating lengthy preparation of metaphase chromosomes (×2000).

Nucleoli

The **nucleoli** are prominent, spherical structures involved in production of ribosomes (Fig. 1-7). At the light microscopic level, nucleoli range up to 1 μm in diameter and usually stain with basic dyes such as hematoxylin, depending on their RNA content. The number of nucleoli is determined by the number of active **nucleolar organizing regions** (NORs), which are chromosomal regions responsible for encoding **ribosomal RNA** (rRNA). Normally, there are fewer nucleoli than NORs because either some NORs are

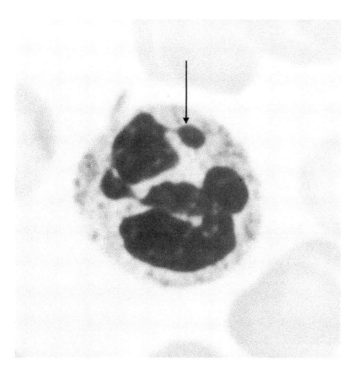

FIGURE 1-5 Sex chromatin (arrow) in the nucleus of a neutrophil (×3800).

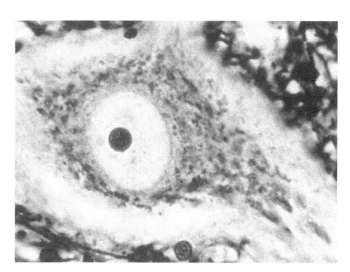

FIGURE 1-7 Motor neuron from the spinal cord. The euchromatic nucleus contains a distinct nucleolus. The ergastoplasm (chromatophilic or Nissl substance) is visible as dark, pleomorphic masses throughout the cytoplasm. Cresyl violet Luxol fast blue (×1100).

inactivated or several fuse to form one nucleolus. At the electron microscopic level, nucleoli have areas of varying electron density. A **granular component** representing maturing ribosomal subunits is often prominent. **Fibrillar components** representing NOR DNA and transcribed rRNA are also observed. Nucleoli, along with nuclear chromatin, are dispersed in a nuclear sap consisting of water, ions, free nucleotides, RNA, and protein.

CYTOSOL

The **cytosol** makes up about half of the cell volume and contains water, ions, sugars, amino acids, nucleotides, hundreds of soluble enzymes (e.g., of the glycolytic pathway), subunits for the cytoskeletal components, messenger RNA, transfer RNA, and myriad other molecules. Polymerization of actin is involved in regulating the viscosity of the cytosol. Transition of the cytosol from a gel state to a more soluble (gel-to-sol) state assists the formation of extensions (pseudopodia) involved in cell motility.

ORGANELLES

Rough and Smooth Endoplasmic Reticulum and Ribosomes

The endoplasmic reticulum (ER) forms an anastomosing (interconnected) network of membrane-delimited sacs (cisternae) and tubules. The **rough ER** (rER) is densely studded with ribosomes and is engaged in protein synthesis (Fig. 1-8), while the **smooth ER** (sER) lacks ribosomes and is engaged in lipid synthesis, calcium sequestration, steroid hormone synthesis, and detoxification of harmful agents. Both forms of ER are interconnected and the rER connects to the outer nuclear membrane. The ribosomes and membranes of the ER are below the resolution of the light microscope. However, the cytoplasm of cells that synthesize

large amounts of proteins is rich in ribosomes and mRNA and is therefore strongly basophilic. Accumulations of basophilic, well-developed rER are sometimes referred to as ergastoplasm in pancreatic cells or Nissl substance in neurons (Fig. 1-7).

The sER does not have attached ribosomes and is not engaged in protein synthesis. Instead, sER synthesizes lipids of cellular membranes and steroid hormones. Endocrine cells of the gonads and adrenal cortex have a well-developed system of tubular sER (Fig. 1-9). In addition, several drug-metabolizing enzymes that participate in detoxification of noxious and carcinogenic materials are present in sER. Finally, the sER performs calcium-sequestering functions in many cells. Release of calcium from the sER can be elicited by several external stimuli and may precipitate a variety of cellular actions. Skeletal and cardiac muscle cells contain an elaborate system of sER, referred to as the sarcoplasmic reticulum, which sequesters calcium ions that are released upon stimulation of muscle contraction.

Ribosomes are bound to membranes of rER or present in the cytosol as free ribosomes. Each individual ribosome is formed from two spherical subunits of different sizes. The subunits con-

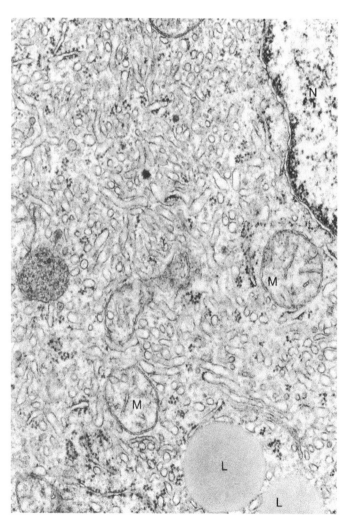

FIGURE 1-9 Adrenal cortical cell containing abundant smooth endoplasmic reticulum, mitochondria (M), and lipid droplets (L) in the vicinity of the nucleus (N) (×27,000).

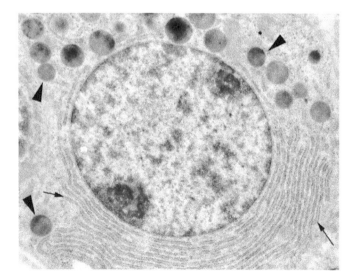

FIGURE 1-8 Electron micrograph of pancreatic zymogen cell, containing abundant cisternae of rough endoplasmic reticulum (rER) (arrows) and several secretory granules (arrowheads) (×6600).

tain several different proteins, all synthesized in the cytosol, and rRNA. A variety of cytosolic proteins enter the nucleus through the nuclear pores and are assembled with rRNA in the nucleolus. The immature ribosomal subunits then exit back to the cytoplasm through nuclear pores. Additional ribosomal proteins are added in the cytosol.

Proteins are formed through the transcription of genes in the nucleus, which results in the formation of **messenger ribonucleic acids** (mRNAs). The mRNAs are exported to the cytosol, where they combine with the ribosomal subunits. An mRNA may be simultaneously translated by multiple ribosomes, thus forming a **polyribosome** (polysome). Multiple polyribosomes are often scattered in the cytoplasm of cells.

The nucleotide sequence of the mRNA depends upon the sequence of the gene from which it was transcribed and will, in turn, encode different proteins. All mRNAs attach to ribosomes by their initiator codon (AUG representing adenine, uracil, and guanine), which encodes methionine. For every amino acid encoded in the mRNA sequence, there exists a corresponding **transfer RNA** (tRNA) that transports an amino acid to the mRNA–ribosome complex. The first tRNA carries methionine to the complex. Subsequently, the ribosome moves along the mRNA to the next codon and recruits the next corresponding tRNA. The amino acids released from the tRNAs join together by peptide bonds and form a growing peptide chain that emerges from the mRNA–ribosome complex.

If a protein is predestined for lysosome incorporation, membrane insertion, or export from the cell, it will start with a short hydrophobic **signal peptide** sequence. The signal peptide binds to a **signal recognition particle** (SRP) present in the cytosol. The ensuing complex then attaches to an **SRP receptor** on the cytosolic face of the rER, which results in threading of the protein into the cisternae of the ER. Once inside the rER, the protein undergoes several posttranslational modifications including the cleavage of the signal peptide as well as folding and glycosylation. Cytosolic proteins that are destined to remain in the cell lack signal peptides and are synthesized by free ribosomes (not attached to the rER) in the cytosol.

Golgi Complex and Vesicular Transport

The **Golgi complex** consists of a series (usually 3 to 10) of flattened cisternae with a convex or **cis** side that is usually oriented toward the nucleus and a concave or **trans** side that generally faces the cell periphery (Fig. 1-10). At the trans side, anastomosing tubules and cisternae form the **trans-Golgi network** (TGN) (Fig. 1-11). In addition, small vesicles are present at the periphery of the cisternae and larger vesicles or vacuoles are often detected at the trans side (Fig. 1-10). Although the Golgi complex can be visualized by silver impregnation in light microscopic preparations, electron microscopy is necessary to delineate its structure.

Transmembrane, secretory, and lysosomal proteins are transferred from the rER to the Golgi complex. Small transport vesicles filled with newly synthesized proteins bud off the cisternae of the rER and fuse with the cisternae on the cis side of the Golgi complex (Fig. 1-11). Subsequently, the protein from the vesicles

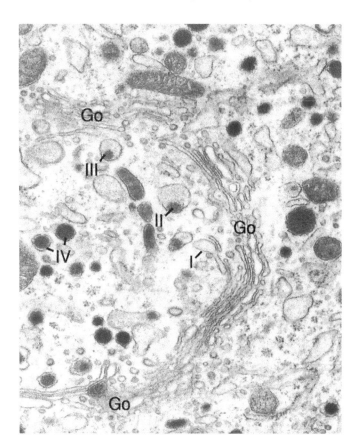

FIGURE 1-10 Electron micrograph of the Golgi complex (Go) and surrounding cytoplasm of an adenohypophysial cell. As the secretory granules mature, they move away from the concave (trans) side of the Golgi complex and their content becomes more electron-dense. In the sequence of maturation of the secretory vesicles, the newest vesicle is I while the most mature vesicle is IV (×23,700).

is transported through the Golgi complex in a cis-to-trans direction. During this transport, the protein becomes concentrated and undergoes posttranslational modifications, including glycosylation. At the trans side, appropriately modified proteins are sorted in the TGN and packaged in vesicles. Mannose-6-phosphate-containing lysosomal enzymes bind to specific mannose-6-phosphate receptors in the TGN and become packaged in vesicles that will become primary lysosomes. When budding off from the TGN, these vesicles are coated with a protein, **clathrin.**

In specialized digestive glands and hormone-producing cells, secretory products are packaged in condensing vacuoles that mature into **secretory granules** (Figs. 1-11 and 1-12). The granules remain in the cytoplasm until the cell receives a signal to secrete their contents. This type of secretion is referred to as **regulated secretion.** When a signal is received, the membranes of the secretory vesicles fuse with the cell membrane, resulting in the opening of an orifice through which the vesicle contents are expelled (secreted) through **exocytosis.** It is, of course, important that the vesicles fuse with the correct membrane in the cell, and to this end, vesicles and target membranes are equipped with complementary "address tags" referred to as **SNAREs** (Soluble *N*-ethylmaleimide-sensitive fusion protein *A*ttachment protein *RE*ceptors). The correct combination of vesicle SNAREs

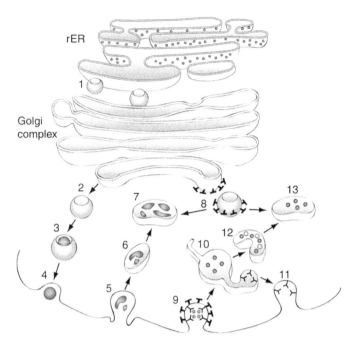

FIGURE 1-11   Schematic drawing illustrating transport of vesicles in the cell. Small transfer vesicles (1) bud off the (rER) and fuse with the cis-side of the Golgi complex. Secretory granules (2) form from vesicles budding from the trans-Golgi network (TGN). Mature secretory granules (3) release their contents through exocytosis (4). Particulate material is taken into the cell by phagocytosis (5), forming a phagosome (6). A Secondary lysosome (7) is formed as the phagosome fuses with primary lysosomes (8), derived from clathrin (T)-coated vesicles budding from the TGN. During receptor-mediated endocytosis (9), receptors (Y) and their bound ligands are transferred to early endosomes (10). Dissociated receptors recycle back to the cell membrane through exocytosis (11), while ligands are transported by multivesicular bodies (12) to late endosomes (13). Late endosomes also fuse with primary lysosomes and mature into secondary lysosomes. Secondary lysosomes that contain undigested material may remain in the cell as residual bodies (not shown).

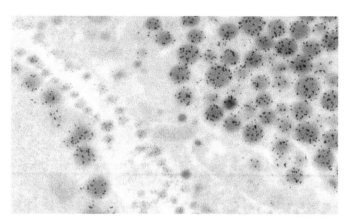

FIGURE 1-12   Electron micrograph of pituitary endocrine cells, immunohistochemically stained with antibodies to adrenocorticotropic hormone (ACTH), conjugated to small 5-nm gold particles and with antibodies to growth hormone (GH) conjugated to larger 12-nm gold particles. The gold particles appear as electron-dense black dots over secretory granules storing ACTH and GH, respectively. Cells involved in regulated secretion store numerous secretory granules in their cytoplasm, the different sizes and morphologies of which aid in cell identification (×42,000).

(vSNAREs) and target membrane SNAREs (tSNAREs) helps to ensure that the appropriate components will fuse.

While regulated secretion is the province of specialized secretory cells, all cells are capable of **constitutive secretion,** which is the continuous delivery of growth factors and components of membranes and the extracellular matrix to the cell surface. This delivery needs no specific stimulus and is exerted by small vesicles that continuously bud off from the trans region of the Golgi complex and fuse with the cell membrane to deliver their contents through exocytosis.

Both regulated and constitutive secretion result in the delivery of considerable amounts of membrane material to the plasmalemma. The accumulation of membranes is balanced by a reverse process referred to as **endocytosis** (Fig. 1-11). Via endocytosis, the plasmalemma invaginates and forms a small vesicle that buds off into the cytoplasm. Different types of endocytosis occur depending upon the material ingested, and endocytosis has many functions in addition to membrane exchange. Ingestion of solid

particulate material by endocytosis is referred to as **phagocytosis.** This process characteristically occurs in neutrophils and macrophages but can be executed by many different cell types. Phagocytosis is a defense mechanism against infectious organisms and also removes particles and cell debris. **Pinocytosis** refers to the uptake of fluid, while **receptor-mediated endocytosis** refers to the uptake of receptor-bound material. Cellular uptake of low-density lipoproteins (LDLs) exemplifies receptor-mediated endocytosis. LDL particles bind to cell surface receptors and accumulate in **coated pits,** which are clathrin-coated membrane invaginations (Fig. 1-11). The pits invaginate and form endocytotic vesicles with the receptor-bound LDL facing the inside. The vesicles transfer their contents to an **early endosome,** which is a system of membrane-delimited tubules and vesicles. The internal pH of the endosome is acidic, causing the LDL to dissociate from the receptors. Subsequently, free receptors become enriched in the tubular region of the endosome, which eventually pinches off to form a shuttle vesicle that returns the receptors to the cell surface. The free ligands are sorted to **multivesicular bodies** (MVBs) and are further transferred to **late endosomes.** Late endosomes fuse with primary lysosomes and transform into **secondary lysosomes.** Controversy exists as to whether the different components of the endosomal system (endocytotic vesicles, early and late endosomes, and lysosomes) represent a maturing system or are separate structures shuttling components between themselves.

Transcytosis is used for transporting material through cells. Endocytosed material on one surface of a cell is transported through the cytoplasm and exocytosed on the other surface (Fig. 1-13). An example of transcytosis is the transport of material from the blood to nearby tissue fluid.

Lysosomal enzymes eventually degrade most extracellular material taken up by phagocytosis, pinocytosis, or receptor-mediated endocytosis, but they do not break down material

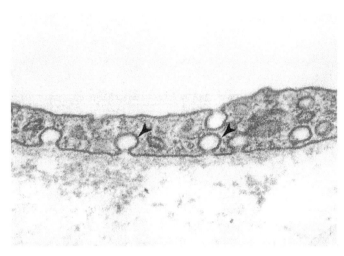

FIGURE 1-13 Transcytotic vesicles (arrowheads) form at the cell membrane and are present in the cytoplasm of a capillary endothelial cell (×76,000).

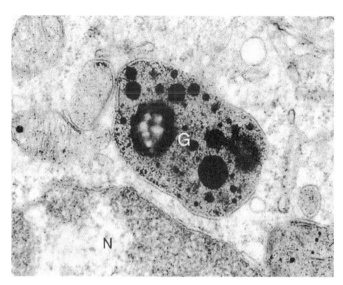

FIGURE 1-14 Lipofuscin granule (G) in an adenohypophysial cell. Nucleus (N) (×29,850).

undergoing transcytosis. The enzymes are sorted to primary lysosomes in the Golgi complex. **Primary lysosomes** are very small (down to 50 nm) and inconspicuous in most cells, but are larger (up to 500 nm) in specialized phagocytic cells like neutrophils and macrophages. Material undergoing receptor-mediated endocytosis or pinocytosis passes from early endosomes to late endosomes. The late endosomes receive enzymes from primary lysosomes and then mature into **secondary lysosomes** (Fig. 1-11). Phagocytosed material in phagosomes does not pass through the endosomal structure, but instead fuses directly with primary lysosomes. These fused structures are also referred to as **secondary lysosomes** or **phagolysosomes**. In addition, constituents of the cell itself can become engulfed into an **autophagosome**. This mechanism represents a way for the cell to digest aged or little-used organelles into useful metabolites. In secondary lysosomes, lysosomal hydrolytic enzymes digest the enclosed material. Such enzymes can digest most cellular material and include acid phosphatase, ribonuclease, deoxyribonuclease, proteases, lipases, sulfatases, and β-glucuronidase. All of these enzymes have an acidic pH, and a proton pump of the lysosomal membrane ensures that the lysosomal interior is optimally acidic. In spite of the multitude of enzymes, some indigestible material remains and is retained within the secondary lysosome, forming a **residual body**. In long-lived cells such as neurons, cardiac myocytes, and liver cells, gradual accumulation of residual bodies results in the formation of a yellowish-brown age pigment, **lipofuscin** (Fig. 1-14).

Mitochondria

Mitochondria are spherical to oblong membrane-delimited organelles that are 0.3 to 1 μm in diameter and up to 20 μm in length. They are visible in the light microscope if stained with cytochemical methods or vital dyes. Ultrastructurally, mitochondria are bounded by **outer** and **inner membranes** that are separated by an **intermembrane space** (Fig. 1-15). In the classical interpretation of mitochondrial ultrastructure, the inner membrane is folded into **cristae,** which limit a finely granular **matrix** in the intercristal space. Modern microscopic techniques have shown that the cristae also connect to the inner membrane with fine tubules. While most cells contain mitochondria having shelflike cristae (Fig. 1-15), steroid-producing cells are unique in that their mitochondrial cristae are tubular. While the outer mitochondrial membrane is permeable to many molecules,

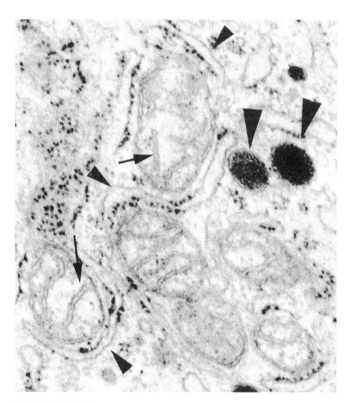

FIGURE 1-15 Mitochondria with cristae (arrows) in an intestinal endocrine cell, which also contains two secretory granules (large arrowheads) and several cisternae of rough endoplasmic reticulum (rER) (small arrowheads) (×52,000).

transport across the inner membrane requires specific channels or carriers. The mitochondrial matrix contains most of the enzymes of the citric acid cycle as well as enzymes involved in fatty acid oxidation. The inside of each crista is studded with 8.5 nm particles involved in the synthesis of **adenosine triphosphate** (ATP). The energy bound in ATP can easily be traded by the many energy-demanding reactions in the cell. The main function of mitochondria is to transform the inaccessible energy bound in fuels such as glucose and fatty acids into easily accessible energy bound within ATP. A process known as **oxidative phosphorylation,** which consumes about 80% of inhaled O_2 and produces CO_2, accomplishes this transformation. Metabolism of glucose (glycolysis) in the cytoplasm results in the formation of pyruvate, which is converted into acetyl-coenzyme A (acetyl-CoA) by the mitochondria. Additionally, mitochondrial fatty acid oxidation results in the formation of acetyl-CoA. Acetyl-CoA enters the **citric acid cycle,** which produces NADH and $FADH_2$. Electrons from these molecules move via carriers in the inner mitochondrial membrane to O_2, and this movement is coupled to the pumping of H^+ into the intermembrane space. This reaction generates an electrochemical gradient, resulting in flow of H^+ through a proton channel that is coupled to the 8.5-nm ATP synthase particles. The narrow tubular connections between the inner membrane and the cristae may serve to compartmentalize the proton gradient and minimize proton leakage through the outer mitochondrial membrane. The flow of protons drives ATP synthesis and large numbers of cristae increase the area that can harbor ATP synthase particles. Cells with high-energy demands, such as cardiac muscle cells and flight muscle cells, contain mitochondria with numerous cristae. A protein, **thermogenin,** creates a proton pore in the inner mitochondrial membrane and thus bypasses the transport of protons through the ATP synthase particles. This uncoupling of oxidative phosphorylation produces heat instead of ATP and is used by hibernating animals, animals adapted to cold climates, and newborns to maintain body temperature. Thermoregulation of this type mainly occurs in brown adipose tissue, which has mitochondria rich in thermogenin.

The mitochondrial matrix also contains electron-dense bodies that are rich in calcium in some cell types, but the function of these **dense bodies** is unknown. The matrix also contains the circular DNA of mitochondria, which is similar to bacterial DNA, as well as rRNA, mRNA, and tRNA. Some mitochondrial proteins are encoded by mitochondrial DNA and are synthesized inside the mitochondria themselves, while others are synthesized in the cytosol. The mitochondrial ribosomes are distinct from eukaryotic ribosomes and resemble bacterial ribosomes. Mitochondria are present only in eukaryotes, and it is believed that mitochondria are antecedents of aerobic bacteria that have entered a symbiotic relationship with primitive anaerobic eukaryotic cells. During cell division, mitochondria duplicate their own DNA and divide by a process similar to bacterial fission. Additionally, mitochondria divide when need arises, such as following exercise. Under special circumstances, changes in mitochondrial permeability lead to leakage of an electron carrier from the intermembrane space (cytochrome C), which activates programmed cell death (apoptosis).

Peroxisomes

Peroxisomes (microbodies) are 0.2- to 1.2-μm spherical, membrane-delimited organelles that contain a paracrystalloid inclusion in some species. Their name is derived from their ability to metabolize hydrogen peroxide. Peroxisomes contain catalase, which produces water and oxygen from hydrogen peroxide, as well as enzymes involved in oxidation of fatty acids. Like the fatty acid oxidation in mitochondria, peroxisomal fatty acid oxidation also produces acetyl-CoA. However, peroxisomal acetyl-CoA is not used for ATP synthesis but rather is transported to the cytosol where it participates in different synthetic pathways. Peroxisomes also contain enzymes that oxidize substrates like L- and D-amino acids while reducing oxygen and hydrogen peroxide. Peroxisomal proteins are synthesized in the cytosol and contain a short amino acid sequence that is recognized by a receptor in the peroxisomal membrane, leading to import of the protein into this organelle. Peroxisomes increase in number by division.

CYTOSKELETON

The term cytoskeleton is misleading in that it covers structures that function to maintain not only cell shape, but also the motility and intracellular transport functions of the cell. There are three main components of the cytoskeleton: microtubules, microfilaments, and intermediate filaments.

Microtubules

Microtubules (Fig. 1-16) are involved in the transport of vesicles and other organelles within the cytoplasm, chromosome separation during cell division, and the motility of cilia and flagella. Each microtubule is composed of 13 parallel rows of protofilaments that form hollow tubes that are 25 nm in diameter. Individual protofilaments consist of subunits formed from two proteins, **α-** and **β-tubulin** (Fig. 1-17). Microtubules grow outward from the **microtubule organizing center** (MTOC), or **centrosome,** located close to the nucleus (Fig. 1-16). Inside the centrosome, two **centrioles** are present. The centrioles are composed of microtubules arranged as nine peripheral triplets and are positioned with their long axes perpendicular to each other (Fig. 1-1). The centrioles are believed to attract centrosome proteins important for tubulin polymerization. Microtubules of the centrioles do not extend as cytoplasmic microtubules. Instead, microtubules in the cytoplasm polymerize on rings of γ-tubulin present in the vicinity of the centrioles. These microtubules are polarized and grow most rapidly at their plus (β-subunit) end. The minus end of the microtubule may either remain attached to the centrosome (e.g., during mitosis) or detach from it. Detached microtubules preserve their orientation with their minus end closest to the centrosome. Cytoplasmic microtubules are in equilibrium with free microtubular subunits in the cytosol, and they constantly grow and shrink by a process dependent upon the hydrolysis of guanosine triphosphate (GTP). In contrast, microtubules present in cilia and flagella are stable and do not change size.

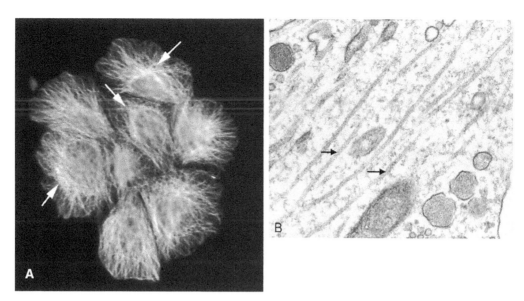

FIGURE 1-16   A. Immunohistochemical staining for tubulin in cultured mammary epithelial cells. Antitubulin antibodies labeled with a fluorescent dye have been used and microtubules appear in the fluorescence microscope as white structures on a dark background. Note that microtubules converge at microtubule organizing centers close to the nuclei (arrow). **B.** Microtubules (arrows) in axons of neurosecretory neurons (×63,000).

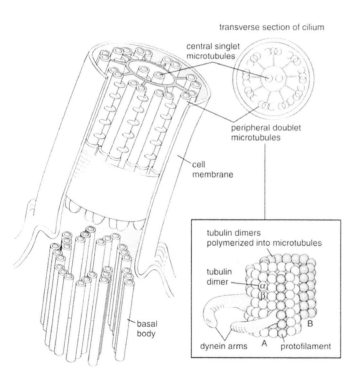

FIGURE 1-17   Diagram of the structure of a cilium. Nine doublet microtubules are found in the peripheral region of the cilium while two singlets occupy the center. α- and β-tubulin subunits are indicated in the paired microtubules (lower right drawing). Dynein arms extend from the A microtubule to contact the B microtubule of an adjacent doublet. A basal body with nine sets of triplet microtubules is shown at the base of the cilium.

Two **motor proteins**, kinesin and dynein, are important for microtubule function. Kinesin transports vesicles and other material from the minus end of the microtubules toward the cell periphery, while dynein transports vesicles and other material in the opposite direction. Both motor proteins bind their cargo and "walk" along the microtubule in either the plus (kinesin) or minus (dynein) direction, deriving energy from hydrolysis of ATP during the process. In developing cells, kinesins pull the ER outward toward the cell periphery while dyneins pull the Golgi complex in the opposite direction.

Microfilaments

Microfilaments (7 nm) are comprised of the protein **actin**. Together with thicker filaments (15 nm) composed of the protein **myosin**, actin constitutes the main protein involved in muscle contraction. In skeletal muscle, actin makes up 10% of all protein. However, actin is also an abundant protein (1 to 5%) in nonmuscle cells. Actin occurs as a monomer (G-actin), which can be polymerized to form 7-nm thick microfilaments (also referred to as actin filaments, or F-actin) (Fig. 1-18A). Like microtubules, actin filaments are polarized with a plus end and a minus end that makes directional movement of motor proteins (in this case, myosin) possible. Microfilaments are also numerous in the cell cortex underlying the plasmalemma. Here, actin filaments associate with transmembrane proteins and stabilize cell shape while simultaneously restricting protein mobility. Receptor-bound hormones and growth factors also interact with cortical actin filaments. At the end of mitosis, actin and myosin filaments form a band that eventually separates the daughter cells from each other. Exposure of cells to agents that stimulate cell migration results in reorganization of the actin cytoskeleton and overlying plasmalemma into finger- or leaflike projections known as

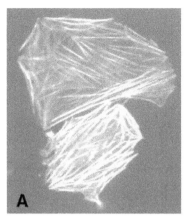
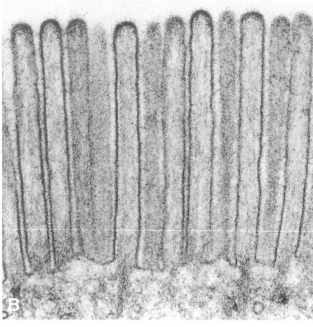

FIGURE 1-18 A. Osteosarcoma cells genetically engineered to express fluorescent actin. Note that actin filaments predominantly occur as straight stress fibers. **B.** The microvilli at the apical surface of a small intestinal absorptive cell contain numerous microfilaments that project into the terminal web (×51,000).

filopodia and lamellipodia, respectively. These projections probe the cell surroundings prior to the formation of specialized matrix receptors (integrins), which bind to ECM proteins and form focal adhesions. Integrins connect intracellularly to sturdy stress fibers consisting of multiple strands of actin filaments that anchor the cell to its site of attachment. Actin filaments also participate in cell-to-cell adhesion phenomena at zonulae adherens junctions and in the support of microvilli (Fig. 1-18B).

Intermediate Filaments

The diameter of **intermediate filaments** (10 nm) lies between that of thin microfilaments (actin, 7 nm) and thick microfilaments (myosin, 15 nm). Intermediate filaments are not polarized and therefore are not engaged in intracellular transport, but perform anchoring and structural functions instead. Several different families of intermediate filaments exist, including **keratins** (cytokeratins), **vimentin, desmin, glial fibrillar acidic protein,** and **neurofilaments**. In addition, filaments that associate with the nuclear lamina (**lamins**) belong to this group. Keratins are associated with most epithelial cells. Vimentin is expressed by most cells of mesenchymal origin, while desmin is typical in smooth, cardiac, and skeletal muscle cells. Glial fibrillar acidic protein is found in glial cells, while neurofilaments are present in neurons. Certain tumor cells can continue to express the original form of intermediate filaments, such that immunohistochemistry of the filaments can be used to determine the cell type of origin of the tumor.

INCLUSIONS

The cytosol contains a number of deposits of materials that do not perform any specific chemical reactions and, hence, are not classi-

fied as organelles. Such inclusions include: (a) **lipid droplets** (Fig. 1-9), which occur in, for example, adipocytes, adrenal cortical cells, and liver cells. In ordinary light microscopic preparations, lipid is dissolved leaving unstained areas in the cytoplasm. In frozen sections, lipid is retained and can be detected by special dyes. One of these is osmic acid, which imparts a dark coloration of lipids in light and electron micrographs; (b) **glycogen** deposits, which are frequent in liver and muscle cells. Glycogen is normally not discernible in the light microscope, but can be detected by special stains such as periodic acid-Schiff (PAS) or Best's carmine. In the electron microscope glycogen is seen as fine electron-dense granules and aggregates; and (c) pigments such as **lipofuscin** of aging cells, **melanin** of pigmented cells, and **hemosiderin,** which is derived from the breakdown of hemoglobin. Lipofuscin inclusions (residual bodies) appear light brown in the light microscope and are often seen close to the nucleus in aging cells. Their formation has been described in conjunction with lysosomes, which accumulate the pigment. Melanin inclusions are detectable as minute dark granules present in pigmented epidermal cells, melanocytes, and certain types of neurons, while hemosiderin is a golden-brown pigment detected in macrophages that have phagocytosed red blood cells.

CELL SURFACE MODIFICATIONS

Microvilli are fingerlike projections of the cell membrane that increase the surface area of absorptive cells. Microfilaments constitute the core structure of the microvilli (Fig. 1-18B). **Stereocilia** represent a long variant of microvilli. Both microvilli and stereocilia are nonmotile.

Ciliated cells have numerous, 2- to 10-µm long motile **cilia,** which are on the cell surface that beat in a synchronous manner to produce a unidirectional transport of material. Thus, in the respiratory tract, cilia transport mucus and particles in an oral direction. Flagellated cells, like spermatozoa, normally have a single flagellum. The structure of cilia and flagella is very similar (Fig. 1-17). Both cilia and flagella are delimited by the cell membrane and contain a central region (**axoneme**) characterized by nine peripheral pairs (doublets) of longitudinal microtubules plus one central pair. The central pair of microtubules is separated from the peripheral pairs by a central sheath. A peripheral doublet consists of one complete A microtubule (composed of 13 protofilaments) and one incomplete B microtubule that shares part of its wall with the A microtubule. The nine peripheral A plus B doublets are connected to each other by protein (nexin) bridges and to the central sheath by radial spokes. Arms of a special form of **dynein,** LR-dynein, extend from the A microtubules. During ciliary movement, the dynein arms attach to B microtubules of the adjacent doublet. Because nexin protein bridges connect the microtubules, they cannot slide past each other. Instead, the movement of dynein in the minus direction is translated into a bending motion, which forms the basis for the motility of flagella of spermatozoa and for the ciliary stroke of respiratory epithelium. At the base of each cilium or flagellum, a **basal body** is present. Like centrioles, basal bodies have nine peripheral triplets of microtubules and no central microtubules. The A and B microtubules of the cilium or flagellum continue directly into the corresponding microtubules of the basal bodies. The central microtubules of the axoneme terminate before the centriole, and the third microtubule of the basal body triplets does not extend into the axoneme. Certain plants contain colchicine, which prevents formation of microtubules. This substance inhibits cell division and vesicle transport and may cause death in cattle feeding on such plants.

CELL CYCLE, CELL DIVISION, AND APOPTOSIS

Somatic cells multiply by mitosis while gametes increase in number through a more complex process referred to as meiosis (see Chapter 12). Before a cell undergoes mitosis, it must duplicate its content of genetic information so that the resulting two daughter cells will contain the same amount of DNA as the parental cell. In addition, since the cytoplasm and organelles are divided between the daughter cells during cytoplasmic division, it is also necessary for the parental cell to increase its size through growth before division. The cell therefore goes through a series of definable steps referred to as the **cell cycle.** These steps are G1 (gap1), S (synthesis of DNA), G2 (gap2), and M (mitosis). During **G1,** the cell grows and receives signals (growth factors) from its surroundings that order it to commence preparations for mitosis. While in the **S** phase, the cell doubles its DNA. During **G2** the cell grows further, checks the quality of the DNA it replicated during the S phase, and synthesizes proteins (such as tubulin subunits) needed for the **M** phase. After mitosis, the daughter cells may enter either

a new cell cycle or a resting stage (G0). Ordered transition through each of these steps is required. At critical checkpoints, the cell will determine if it is of the correct size and if DNA has been correctly replicated. Before proceeding to the next step of the cell cycle, appropriate signals must be received from neighboring cells. Progression is controlled by special proteins called **cyclins.** Different cyclins are needed at different checkpoints and will activate enzymes (**cyclin-dependent kinases,** or CDKs) that make it possible for a cell to continue to the next step. Thus, the cell cycle is tightly controlled. Failure of the cell to produce the right cyclin at the right time will stop cell cycle progression and may even result in the demise of the cell through apoptosis. If the cell cycle progresses, the cell will enter mitosis.

Mitosis is characterized by the following morphologically distinguishable phases: prophase, prometaphase, metaphase, anaphase, telophase, and cytokinesis (Fig. 1-19). During **prophase** (Fig. 1-19), chromatin gradually becomes more condensed, resulting in the formation of individual, discernible chromosomes, which stain intensely with hematoxylin or other basic dyes. In addition, nucleoli disappear and the centrosome divides into two centrosomes that migrate to opposite poles of the cell and begin to organize microtubules into the mitotic spindle.

The next step, **prometaphase,** is characterized by the disappearance of the nuclear envelope (Fig. 1-19). This is brought about by phosphorylation of the nuclear lamins through an M-phase-promoting cyclin-dependent kinase, leading to electrostatic repulsion between lamin subunits and ensuing breakdown of the nuclear lamina. During **metaphase,** the chromosomes become oriented in the equatorial plane perpendicular to the centrosomes (Fig. 1-19). In metaphase spread-preparations (Fig. 1-20), the chromosomes are easily seen to be composed of two closely apposed, identical halves (**chromatids** or **sister-chromatids**). The sister-chromatids, formed earlier by DNA replication during the S phase, become visible due to increased coiling of the DNA. Chromatids are connected to each other at the **centromere,** which is a constricted, pale staining structure that contains a protein complex, the **kinetochore.** The kinetochore is an attachment point for microtubules emanating from opposite centrosomes. Colchicine prevents polymerization of microtubules and arrests mitosis in metaphase. Techniques using colchicine are sometimes employed to obtain metaphase chromosomes for cytogenetic investigation (Fig. 1-20).

During **anaphase,** the two sister-chromatids separate from each other and are drawn toward a centrosome by the kinetochore microtubules (Fig. 1-19). Anaphase ends when the sister-chromatids (now called daughter chromosomes) have separated toward opposite sides of the cell.

During **telophase,** the nuclear envelope reappears (assisted by dephosphorylation of lamins), chromosomes decondense, and nucleoli appear. **Cytokinesis** takes place concomitantly with telophase, resulting in a **cleavage furrow** around the equatorial plane of the cell (Fig. 1-19). This furrow is created by the contraction of actin and myosin filaments and will divide the cytoplasm into two halves surrounding each newly formed nucleus.

The frequency with which cells pass through the cell cycle and divide varies considerably. Certain cells in the adult animal

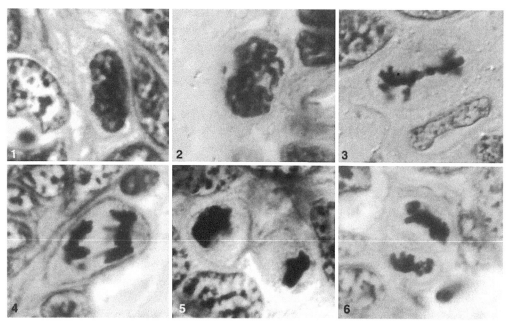

FIGURE 1-19 **1.** Prophase. **2.** Prometaphase. **3.** Metaphase. **4.** Anaphase. **5.** Telophase and cytokinesis. **6.** Late telophase in fetal oral epithelium, stained with iron-hematoxylin. Note the centrosome and part of the microtubules of the spindle apparatus in 3 and 4 and the cleavage furrow in 5.

are constantly renewed, such as intestinal absorptive cells, which are replaced every 3 to 5 days. Most cells are in either a permanent or a temporary resting (G0) phase. Some cells, such as neurons, lose their ability to divide in the adult animal and enter a permanent G0 state. Cells in a temporary G0 phase normally do not replicate but are able to do so if the need arises.

Induction of a cell to proliferate involves stimulation by growth factors that are important for activating the cell cycle in G1. In tumor cells, mutations may result in autonomous activa-

tion of growth factor–signaling mechanisms. This activation makes tumor cells oblivious to the controlled signaling mechanisms in the body, resulting in continuous proliferation of cells that take no heed of their surroundings. Since every round of cell division carries the risk of inducing mutations, it is likely that these uncontrolled cells will eventually acquire further mutations that result in invasive, malignant behavior.

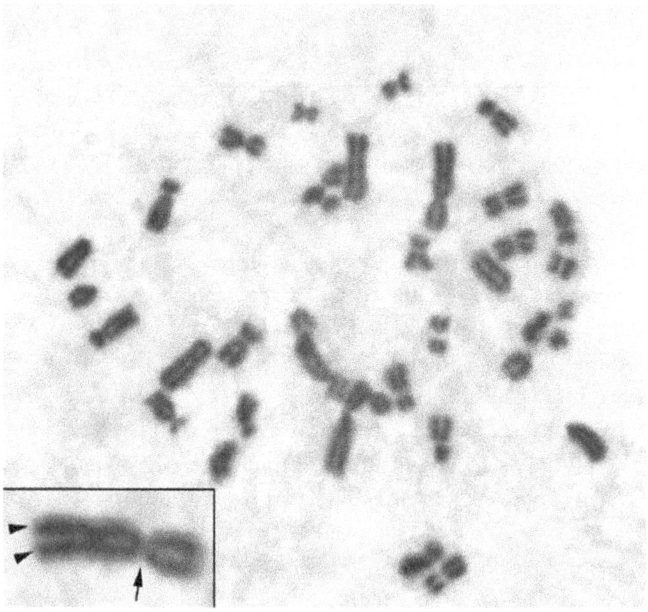

Safeguards to avoid mutation exist in the form of a cellular suicide mechanism termed **apoptosis**. Apoptosis is defined by a series of morphologic changes leading to the destruction of the cell. In tissue sections, apoptotic cells are recognized by the presence of condensed (**pyknotic**) nuclei that eventually break down into fragments (**karyorrhexis**). The nuclear fragments are encased by corresponding fragments of cytoplasm to form **apoptotic bodies** that are later phagocytosed by surrounding cells. If a cell contains mutated or damaged DNA, it will activate the apoptotic program, which, through a series of biochemical reactions, will ultimately destroy the cell's genetic material. Apoptosis also plays a major role for developmental sculpturing of the organism and for the replacement of aged or infected cells.

FROM CELLS TO TISSUES

In multicellular organisms, cells integrate themselves in a social context with other cells and assume specialized roles with functions that benefit the entire organism. The process of assuming specific functions is called cellular **differentiation**. Social interaction requires that cells make contact with other cells and with the ECM, resulting in the formation of tissues and organs. Moreover, the cells need to continue to communicate with each other by both local and global means.

FIGURE 1-20 Metaphase chromosomes from a boar. Note sister-chromatids and centromeres, which are identified by arrowheads and arrows, respectively, in the insert.

Intercellular Junctions

Several types of cell junctions (occluding, anchoring, and communicating) occur between cells (Fig. 1-21). Anchoring contacts are present between adjacent cells as well as between cells and the ECM. Occluding and communicating contacts only occur between cells. Intercellular contacts can be ring-shaped (zonulae) or spotlike (maculae).

The presence of occluding contacts between cells is characteristic of epithelial cells. In many epithelia, such as the lining of the gastrointestinal tract, the **zonula occludens** (tight junction) seals off the upper part of the epithelium. This mechanism prevents leakage of material from the lumen into the subepithelial

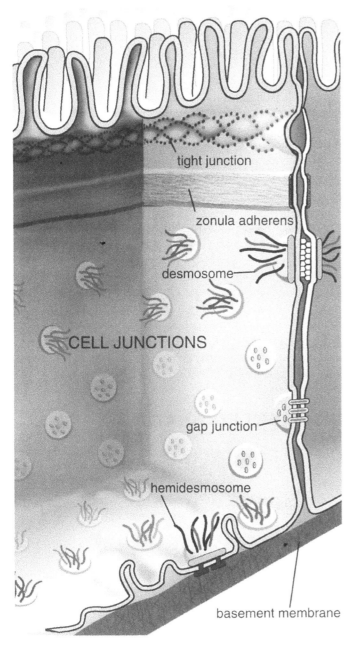

FIGURE 1-21 Diagrams of intercellular junctions: tight junction, zonula adherens, macula adherens (desmosome), hemidesmosome, and gap junction. *(From: Eurell J. Veterinary histology. Jackson, WY: Teton NewMedia, 2004.)*

space and vice versa. Additionally, the zonula occludens prevents free mobility of transmembrane proteins in the cell membrane. An individual zonula occludens joins two neighboring cells by a beltlike structure consisting of anastomosing ridges. The junction consists of transmembrane proteins, **occludin** and **claudin,** which join the two cell membranes together. Peripheral cytoplasmic proteins, ZO-1 and ZO-2, link claudin and occludin to spectrin, a structural protein within the cell.

Zonulae adherens and maculae adherens (desmosomes) form cell-to-cell anchoring contacts, while focal adhesions and hemidesmosomes form cell-to-ECM or cell-to-basement membrane contacts. **Zonulae adherens** are comprised of multiple, anchoring transmembrane proteins known as **cadherins.** The extracellular region of a cadherin molecule engages in homophilic binding with a cadherin molecule extending from an adjacent cell, thus forming a protein bridge between the cells. Cadherin binding requires Ca^{2+}. Therefore, cell dispersal can often be achieved by restricting Ca^{2+} from cells. On the inside of the cell membrane, cadherins attach to linker proteins, which, in turn, connect to microfilaments. In zonulae adherens junctions, cadherins join microfilaments of neighboring cells into a network. The microfilaments connect with the **terminal web** that represents a collection of actin, myosin, and keratin filaments (Fig. 1-18). This connection effectively anchors cells to each other. Moreover, by interacting with myosin, the actin filaments can contract and alter the shape of the epithelium. It is believed that the contraction of actin–myosin filaments connected to zonulae adherens plays a role in the folding of the neuroectodermal epithelium that results in formation of the neural tube. In tall columnar epithelium, zonulae adherens are present just below the zonulae occludens. Together, these structures form the **terminal bar,** which appears as a dense condensation of the cell membrane when viewed with light microscopy.

Maculae adherens, or desmosomes, are 200- to 400-nm disklike, cell-to-cell contacts that are particularly well developed in the epidermis of the skin. Like zonulae adherens junctions, maculae adherens have cadherins that function as junctional proteins. The cadherins attach to intracellular adaptor protein complexes that connect to intermediate filaments in neighboring cells, producing a very strong, pointlike cell adhesion (Figs. 1-21 and 1-22). Ultrastructurally, maculae adherens are characterized by two prominent, dark-staining plaques located on the inside of the two adjacent cell membranes. These plaques correspond to the adaptor protein complexes. Intermediate filaments extend from the plaques into the cytoplasm. The adjacent cell membranes in the macula adherens are separated by a gap of about 30 nm, which often contains an electron-dense line (Fig. 1-23).

Hemidesmosomes connect cells to the basement membrane complex by way of specific cell-surface matrix receptor proteins called **integrins.** Like maculae adherens, hemidesmosomes connect intracellularly via adaptor proteins to intermediate filaments. Ultrastructurally, hemidesmosomes look like half desmosomes with a plaque on the inside of the cell membrane from which **intermediate filaments** radiate into the cytoplasm. In the epidermis of the skin, maculae adherens anchor epidermal cells to each other along the lateral margins and hemidesmosomes anchor cells to the basement membrane above the dermis. Mutations in keratin genes, integrins, or ECM proteins can produce painful

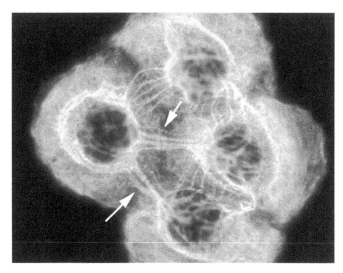

FIGURE 1-22 Immunohistochemical detection of keratins in mammary epithelial cells in culture using fluorescent antibodies. Arrows indicate maculae adherens (×1200).

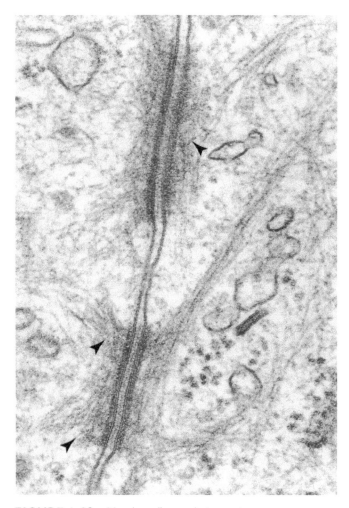

FIGURE 1-23 Maculae adherens between two neurohypophysial glial cells. Notice the distinct central electron-dense lines and the intermediate filaments (arrowheads) that insert into the dense plaques and then make a hairpin turn back into the cytoplasm (×87,500).

diseases (epidermolysis bullosa) characterized by blister formation due to defective anchoring of epidermal cells.

Focal adhesions also connect cells to the underlying matrix via integrins. The intracellular connection in focal adhesions is via microfilaments, similar to that of zonulae adherens junctions. Focal adhesions are not only involved in anchoring of cells, but also have been implicated in cell motility and signaling.

Gap junctions (nexus) are communicating junctions that allow the passage of electrical signals, ions, and small water-soluble molecules (up to 1000 daltons) between cells. At these junctions, neighboring cell membranes are separated by a 2- to 4-nm gap. Protein complexes known as **connexons** span the gap and form narrow channels through which small molecules may pass from one cell to another. Gap junctions occur in many cell types. For example, these communicating junctions are important for conducting electrical signals through intercalated disks of cardiac muscle cells, thereby contributing to a coordinated contraction wave throughout the heart muscle.

Cell Communication

Signals from other cells and from the ECM direct cellular functions and processes. Cell communication can be further described as endocrine, neurocrine, and paracrine. **Endocrine** signaling through hormones secreted into the blood and **neurocrine** signaling through neurotransmitters represent distant signaling pathways. **Paracrine** secretion is local transmission of signals to cells within diffusion distance. **Autocrine** signaling refers to a mechanism by which cells signal to themselves. This phenomenon is best known in cancer cells, which use autocrine secretion of growth factors to circumvent normal intercellular control, leading to increased tumor size. Signaling by endocrine, neurocrine, and paracrine mechanisms represents control mechanisms of the body that ensure that all differentiated cells function properly. Proliferation is only stimulated when need arises and is controlled by **growth factors** that have cell and tissue selectivity. Examples of growth factors include erythropoietin, epidermal growth factor, and platelet-derived growth factor.

SUGGESTED READINGS

Bornens M. Centrosome composition and microtubule anchoring mechanisms. Curr Opin Cell Biol 2002;14:25–34.

Frey TG, Manella, CA. The internal structure of mitochondria. TIBS 2000;25:319–324.

Gruenberg J. The endocytic pathway: a mosaic of domains. Nature Rev 2002;2:721–730.

Lodish H, Berk A, Zipursky LS, et al. Molecular Cell Biology. 4th Ed. New York: W. H. Freeman & Co., 2000.

Huang S. Building an efficient factory: where is pre-rRNA synthesized in the nucleolus? J Cell Biol 2002;157:739–741.

Marshall WF. Order and disorder in the nucleus. Curr Biol 2002;12: R185–192.

Perkins GA, Frey TG. Recent structural insight into mitochondria gained by microscopy. Micron 2002;31:97–111.

Purdue PE, Lazarow PB. Peroxisome biogenesis. Ann Rev Cell Dev Biol 2000;17:701–752.

2

Epithelium
BRIAN L. FRAPPIER

Introduction
  Cells, Tissues, and Organs
  Characteristics of Epithelium
Surface Epithelium
  Classification
  Microscopic Structure
    Simple squamous epithelium
    Simple cuboidal epithelium
    Simple columnar epithelium
    Pseudostratified epithelium
      Pseudostratified columnar epithelium
      Transitional epithelium
    Stratified squamous epithelium

    Stratified cuboidal epithelium
    Stratified columnar epithelium
    Sensory epithelium
Glandular Epithelium and Glands
  Classification of Glands
    Morphologic characteristics
      Simple glands
      Compound glands
        Parenchyma
        Stroma
      Nature of the secretory product
      Mode of release of the secretory product
  Myoepithelial Cells

INTRODUCTION

Cells, Tissues, and Organs

Epithelium is a tissue. A **tissue** is an aggregation of cells and intercellular substances specialized to perform particular functions. Despite its structural and functional complexity, the animal body is composed of only four basic types of tissue: **epithelium, connective tissue, muscle,** and **nervous tissue** (Table 2-1). **Organs** consist of various arrangements of the four basic tissues (Fig. 2-1).

Characteristics of Epithelium

Epithelium exists in two major forms: surface epithelium and glandular epithelium. **Surface epithelium** consists of sheets of aggregated cells of similar type that cover all of the external surfaces and line all of the internal surfaces of the body. **Glandular epithelium,** the secretory cells of endocrine and exocrine glands, results from the proliferation of surface epithelial cells into under-

lying connective tissue. Table 2-2 summarizes the main characteristics of epithelium as a tissue.

The characteristics of the cells of epithelium include specialization for a variety of different functions, including protection, absorption, secretion, excretion, and formation of barriers for selective permeability. The location of cellular organelles and variations in morphologic features of the luminal, basal, and lateral portions of the cell membrane indicate a definite polarization of epithelial cells. In mammals, essentially all epithelial cells contain cytoplasmic filaments composed of the protein **cytokeratin,** an exception being endothelial cells. Cells not of epithelial origin (e.g., mesenchymal cells) lack cytokeratin. This characteristic is used in diagnostic pathology to identify the cell of origin of malignant neoplasms (cancers), which consist of cells that are unrecognizable by routine histologic methods. In addition to functional diversity and specific structural characteristics, epithelial cells continuously proliferate via mitosis to replace cells lost through attrition.

At the basal surface of all epithelial cells that make contact with underlying connective tissue, a thin sheet of extracellular

TABLE 2-1   The Basic Tissues

Epithelium
Connective tissue
Muscle
Nervous tissue

TABLE 2-2   Characteristics of Epithelium

Covers body surfaces (surface epithelium)
Forms secretory cells of glands (glandular epithelium)
Cells are functionally diverse
Cells contain cytoplasmic cytokeratin filaments
Cells are capable of mitosis (regeneration)
Contacts a basement membrane
Devoid of blood vessels (avascular)
Derived from each of the three embryonic germ layers

matrix, the **basement membrane,** is present. The basement membrane usually is not visible in routine light-microscopic sections, but can be demonstrated with the periodic acid-Schiff (PAS) technique or silver stains. As seen with the electron microscope, the basement membrane invariably consists of two distinct layers: the **lamina lucida,** a low-density layer next to the epithelial cell membrane, and an underlying electron-dense **lamina densa** (**lamina basalis** or **basal lamina**) (Fig. 16-9). These two laminae are synthesized by the epithelial cells and are composed principally of proteoglycans (primarily heparan sulfate) as well as laminin, fibronectin, and type IV collagen. In most basement membranes, a third component, the **lamina fibroreticularis** (**subbasal lamina**), is present (Fig. 16-9). The lamina fibroreticularis is composed principally of reticular fibers (type III collagen) and connects the lamina densa to the subepithelial connective tissue. In addition to providing attachment for the epithelium, the lamina fibroreticularis permits stretching and recoil of the epithelium in distensible organs. The basement membrane is described in greater detail in Chapter 16.

In addition to underlying all epithelia that contact connective tissue, a basement membrane is found between two epithelial layers in both the renal corpuscle of the kidney and the pulmonary alveolus. In these locations, the lamina fibroreticularis is absent and the structure is referred to simply as the **basal lamina.** A basal lamina also surrounds many individual cells including smooth muscle cells, skeletal muscle cells, and cardiac muscle cells, as well as adipocytes and neurolemmocytes.

The basement membrane serves in a variety of capacities, for example, as an ultrafilter in capillaries, particularly those of the renal corpuscle; as a selective barrier to exchange of macromolecules; and as a guide to epithelial cell movements. Since blood and lymph vessels do not penetrate the basement membrane, overlying epithelial cells receive their nutritional support by diffusion through the basement membrane from capillaries located in the underlying connective tissue.

All three embryonic germ layers take part in the formation of epithelium. **Ectoderm** is the origin of the epithelium of the external body surfaces, such as the epidermis of the skin. Most of the lining epithelium (i.e., that lining the luminal surfaces of the digestive and respiratory systems) originates from **endoderm,** while **mesoderm** gives rise to the lining of the vascular system, the lining of the serous membrane body cavities, and parts of the urinary and reproductive systems.

SURFACE EPITHELIUM

Classification

The classification of the various surface epithelial types is based on the number of layers present and the shape of the epithelial cells. A surface epithelium consisting of a single layer of cells resting on the basement membrane is described as a **simple epithelium.** A **stratified epithelium** is composed of two or more layers of cells with only the basal layer resting on the basement membrane. The names given to the various types of stratified epithelia are based on the *shape of the surface cells* without regard to the shape of those within the deeper layers. A surface epithelium is considered **pseudostratified** if all of its cells contact the basement membrane but not all extend to the free surface. As a result, nuclei are located at different levels within a pseudostratified epithelium, giving the false impression of stratification. Figure 2-2 depicts the classification of epithelial tissue.

Microscopic Structure

Simple Squamous Epithelium

Simple squamous epithelium consists of a single layer of thin, flat, scalelike cells. On surface view (Figs. 2-3A and 2-4), the cells have an irregular shape with a slightly serrated border. They fit to-

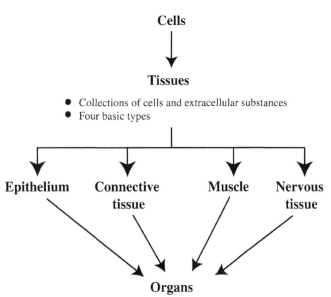

Cells

↓

Tissues

- Collections of cells and extracellular substances
- Four basic types

Epithelium   **Connective tissue**   **Muscle**   **Nervous tissue**

Organs

- Composed of various arrangements of the four basic tissues

FIGURE 2-1   Structural organization of the animal body.

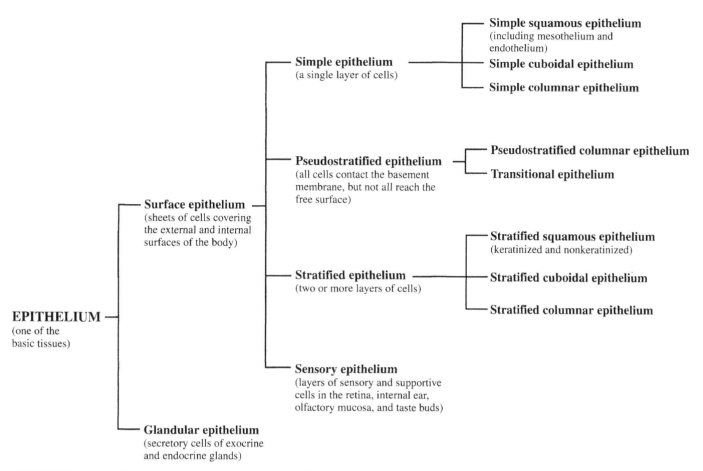

FIGURE 2-2   Classification of the various forms of epithelial tissue.

gether to form a continuous sheet. A spherical to oval nucleus is located near the center of the cell. On cross section, the cell appears thicker in the area of the nucleus and has thin attenuated strands of cytoplasm on either side (Fig. 2-4).

Simple squamous epithelium lines moist internal surfaces, such as the serous membrane body cavities, the internal surface of the heart, and the luminal surface of blood and lymph vessels. The simple squamous epithelium lining the serous membrane body cavities (pleural, pericardial, and peritoneal cavities) is referred to as **mesothelium**; that lining the heart, blood vessels, and lymph vessels is referred to as **endothelium**. Simple squamous epithelium is also found lining the pulmonary alveoli, the anterior chamber of the eye, the internal surface of the tympanic membrane, the membranous labyrinth of the internal ear, the glomerular capsule, and a portion of the loop of the nephron.

Simple Cuboidal Epithelium

Simple cuboidal epithelium is a single layer of cells whose width and height are approximately equal. These cells appear as squares in cross sections but are more hexagonal when seen from the surface (Figs. 2-3B and 2-5). When the height is slightly less than the width of a cell, it is known as low cuboidal epithelium, and when the height is slightly greater than the width, the epithelium is called tall cuboidal epithelium. The classification of epithelia is not always clear-cut, however, and many times

intermediate forms require some subjective judgment regarding classification.

Simple cuboidal epithelium can be found lining the ducts of many glands and the collecting ducts of the kidney, as a component of the choroid plexus in the brain and ciliary body of the eye, and lining the follicles of the thyroid gland. The epithelium of the lens of the eye and the retinal pigment epithelium are also examples of simple cuboidal epithelium.

Simple Columnar Epithelium

Simple columnar epithelium consists of tall, narrow cells with considerably greater height than width (Figs. 2-3C and 2-6). Usually, the nuclei are oval and are located near the base of the cell. Generally, simple columnar epithelium lines the luminal surface of organs that perform absorptive or secretory functions, for example, the glandular stomach, the small and large intestines, and the gallbladder in the digestive system; the bulbourethral gland in the male reproductive system; and the uterus and uterine tube in the female reproductive system.

Pseudostratified Epithelium

Pseudostratified epithelium exists in two forms: pseudostratified columnar epithelium and transitional epithelium. In both forms, *all of the cells contact the underlying basement membrane, but not all of them reach the free surface.*

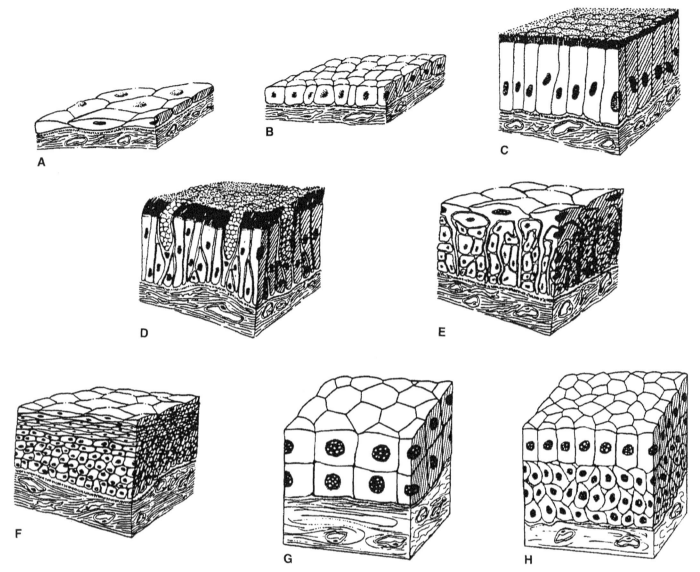

FIGURE 2-3   Schematic drawings illustrating the major types of surface epithelia. **A.** Simple squamous epithelium. **B.** Simple cuboidal epithelium. **C.** Simple columnar epithelium bearing microvilli. **D.** Pseudostratified columnar epithelium with cilia and goblet cells. **E.** Transitional epithelium. **F.** Stratified squamous epithelium, nonkeratinized. **G.** Stratified cuboidal epithelium. **H.** Stratified columnar epithelium.

Pseudostratified columnar epithelium

Pseudostratified columnar epithelium is composed of a single layer of cells, but because the cells are irregular in size and shape, their nuclei are located at various levels. Therefore, the epithelium appears to have several layers (Figs. 2-3D and 2-7). The cells that extend from the basement membrane to the surface of pseudostratified columnar epithelium are **ciliated** or **nonciliated epithelial cells** and **goblet cells** (unicellular mucous glands). **Basal cells** are attached to the basement membrane but do not reach the surface of the epithelium. By division and differentiation, basal cells replace the other epithelial cell types lost by attrition.

Ciliated, pseudostratified columnar epithelium with goblet cells lines the greater part of the nasal cavity, paranasal sinuses, and nasopharynx, as well as the auditory tubes, the trachea, and the larger bronchi. In the respiratory system, the goblet cells contribute to a thin mucous film over the epithelium. Dust particles in the inhaled air become trapped in this mucus, and the current created by the ciliated cells moves the dust-laden mucus to the body openings. A pseudostratified columnar epithelium with stereocilia but lacking goblet cells is found lining the duct of the epididymis and the ductus deferens.

Transitional epithelium

Transitional epithelium, a pseudostratified type with a wide variety of appearances, lines hollow organs capable of considerable distention, such as the renal pelvis and calices, ureter, urinary bladder, and urethra. Transitional epithelium may also be seen in the palpebral conjunctiva, larynx, and nasopharynx. *The cells increase in size from the basal "layers" to the superficial "layers" of transitional epithelium.* The shape of the epithelial cells depends on the degree of organ distention at the time of fixation. When the epithelium is under little tension, the surface cells are large and "pillow-shaped," whereas the deeper cells are smaller and irregularly shaped (Figs. 2-3E and 2-8). When the epithelium is

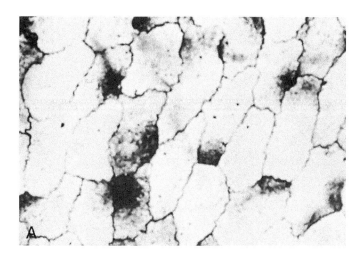

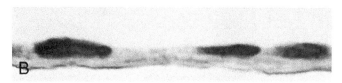

FIGURE 2-4 Simple squamous epithelium. **A.** Surface view of silver-impregnated mesothelium, mesentery. Silver stain (×500). **B.** Cross section of mesothelium, peritoneum on the surface of the urinary bladder. Hematoxylin and eosin (×1200). (**B:** *from Stinson AW, Brown EM. Veterinary Histology Slide Sets. East Lansing, MI: Michigan State University, Instructional Media Center, 1970.*)

stretched, the cells become flattened and elongated, and the total height of the epithelium decreases.

The luminal surface of transitional epithelial cells appears relatively smooth with the light microscope. In electron micrographs, however, areas of thickened plasmalemma (*plaques*) anchored by numerous cytoplasmic filaments are seen on the luminal

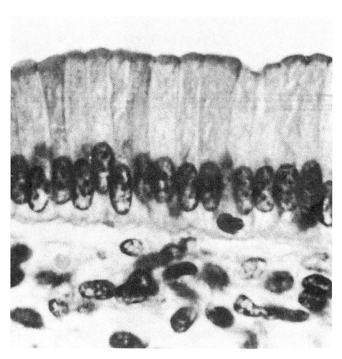

FIGURE 2-6 Simple columnar epithelium, lining of gallbladder (pig). Hematoxylin and eosin (×900).

surface of the cell. The region between the membrane plaques is a normal cell membrane, and when the bladder contracts, the plaques fold together much like a hinge, producing typical transitional epithelial surface ridges. Upon distention, the plaques unfold, allowing expansion of the luminal surface.

The surface epithelium of the urinary bladder is a barrier to the diffusion of water from the subepithelial tissue to the hypertonic urine stored in the lumen. Morphologic evidence of this

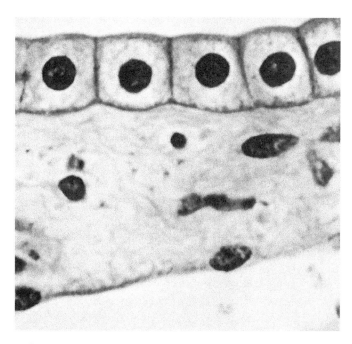

FIGURE 2-5 Simple cuboidal epithelium, collecting duct, kidney (horse). Hematoxylin and eosin (×900).

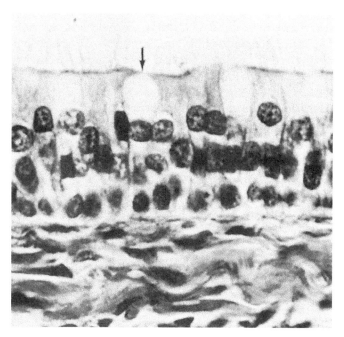

FIGURE 2-7 Pseudostratified columnar epithelium with cilia and goblet cells, trachea (dog). The arrow points to a goblet cell. Hematoxylin and eosin (×1200).

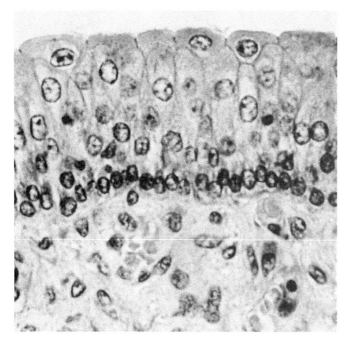

FIGURE 2-8 Transitional epithelium, urinary bladder (pig). Hematoxylin and eosin (×480). Note occasional pillow-shaped surface epithelial cells and that the cells increase in size as they approach the free surface.

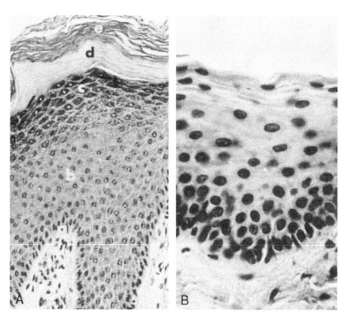

FIGURE 2-9 Stratified squamous epithelium. **A.** Keratinized stratified squamous epithelium, skin of teat (cow). Stratum basale (a), stratum spinosum (b), stratum granulosum (c), stratum lucidum (d), stratum corneum (e). Hematoxylin and eosin (×150). **B.** Nonkeratinized stratified squamous epithelium, lip (cat). Hematoxylin and eosin (×380).

diffusion barrier includes (a) the increased thickness of the outer lamina of the trilaminar cell membrane compared to the inner lamina; (b) a concentration of tonofilaments immediately beneath the luminal surface; and (c) junctional complexes located between the adjacent surface cells that prevent intercellular diffusion.

Detailed studies of transitional epithelium indicate that when the epithelium is relaxed, the cells elongate and overlap each other and the epithelium appears multilayered. All of the transitional epithelial cells remain attached to the basement membrane by slender cytoplasmic processes, much like the attachment in pseudostratified columnar epithelium (Fig. 2-3E). The attachment allows the cells to form a parallel alignment when the urinary bladder is distended; thus, fewer layers of cells are seen.

Stratified Squamous Epithelium

Stratified squamous epithelium consists of several layers of cells, but only the superficial cells have a squamous shape (Fig. 2-3F). Two types of stratified squamous epithelia are recognized (Fig. 2-9). **Keratinized stratified squamous epithelium** has cells in the surface layer that have lost their nuclei and are filled with keratin, a water-resistant protein that forms a protective barrier against the destructive forces of the environment. In **nonkeratinized stratified squamous epithelium,** contrary to the implication of the name, keratin is present in the epithelial cells. In contrast to the keratinized epithelium, the flattened superficial cells retain their nuclei.

Three to five distinct cell layers are present in stratified squamous epithelium (see also Chapter 16). The deepest layer of cells next to the basement membrane is the **stratum basale** (Figs. 2-3F and 2-9), which is a single layer of cuboidal to columnar cells. The

cells of the stratum basale are mitotically active and give rise to the cells that move into the upper layers of the epithelium.

The next layer is the **stratum spinosum** (Fig. 2-9), composed of a varying number of layers of polyhedral cells tightly adhered to each other by numerous **desmosomes (maculae adherens).** In ordinary histologic preparations, the cytoplasm between the desmosomal attachments shrinks, and wherever the cells remain attached, small spiny processes radiate from the surface of the cells. This appearance gives rise to the name of the layer, stratum spinosum, or "spiny layer." These spiny processes contain **cytokeratin filaments,** termed **tonofilaments,** which are condensed at the site of the desmosomes (Fig. 16-4).

As the cells of the stratum spinosum move toward the surface, they become more flattened and accumulate **keratohyalin granules** and **lamellar granules** in their cytoplasm. This layer of cells, known as the **stratum granulosum,** is absent from nonkeratinized stratified squamous epithelium as well as keratinized forms that produce hard keratin, such as those found in the wall of the hoof and in the horn of ruminants.

The **stratum lucidum** occurs only in nonhairy skin regions (Fig. 2-9). This layer of flattened keratinized cells between the stratum granulosum and the stratum corneum has a translucent appearance because it contains **eleidin,** a protein similar to keratin but with a different affinity for histologic stains.

The outermost layer of keratinized stratified squamous epithelium is the **stratum corneum,** which consists of dead, keratinized cells that are fairly resistant to environmental irritants. To reach the keratinized state, epithelial cells undergo a series of transformations as they move from the stratum basale to the stratum corneum. The process of **keratinization** involves the gradual disappearance of the nuclei, Golgi complexes, and mitochondria, along with decreased lysosomal activity and a concurrent accumulation of **tonofilaments.** Cells of the stratum basale are rich in polyribosomes that participate in the synthesis of cytokeratin. As these germinative cells move up into the stratum spinosum, the tonofilaments condense into bundles visible with the light microscope (**tonofibrils**) and become attached to desmosomes. The cells in the stratum granulosum are flat and contain numerous nonmembrane-bounded **keratohyalin granules,** which are readily visible with the light microscope. With the electron microscope, the tonofilaments are observed to extend into the periphery of the cell, intermingling with the granules. The cells of the stratum granulosum also contain unique, oval, membrane-bounded granules (100 to 500 nm) composed of alternating light and dark lamellae. These Golgi-derived **lamellar granules (membrane-coating granules)** are located at the cell periphery. By the time the cells reach the stratum lucidum, they are more elongated and flattened and all the organelles are gone. With the light microscope, only the cell outlines are visible, and the cytoplasm appears homogeneous. Ultrastructural examination reveals densely packed tonofilaments embedded in a dense matrix, probably derived from the keratohyalin granules. In the stratum corneum, the contents of lamellar granules are secreted by exocytosis, thereby giving rise to the intercellular substance between stratum corneum cells. This substance is a component of the barrier properties of the epithelium. Groups of cells in the outermost layer of the stratum corneum eventually become loose and separate. This process gives rise to the descriptive term **stratum disjunctum.**

A stratum corneum is not present in nonkeratinized stratified squamous epithelium found on moist surfaces. The layer of keratin-containing cells that fail to lose their nuclei as they migrate to the surface of the epithelium is termed the **stratum superficiale.**

Stratified Cuboidal Epithelium

Stratified cuboidal epithelium consists of two or more layers of cells with a surface layer of typical cuboidal cells. Frequently, it occurs as a distinct two-layered epithelium lining the excretory ducts of glands (Figs. 2-3G and 2-10).

Stratified Columnar Epithelium

Stratified columnar epithelium consists of several layers of cells. The superficial layer of tall, prismatic cells does not extend to the basement membrane (Figs. 2-3H and 2-11). The deeper layers are composed of smaller polyhedral cells that do not reach the surface. This type of epithelium may be found lining the distal portion of the urethra, as circumscribed areas in a transitional epithelium, in the parotid and mandibular ducts, and in the lacrimal sac and duct.

Sensory Epithelium

Epithelia containing supportive (sustentacular) cells and specialized receptor cells are found in the retina of the eye, the internal ear, the olfactory mucosa, and the taste buds. These highly specialized **sensory epithelia** mediate the senses of vision, hearing, equilibrium, smell, and taste. These epithelia are described in detail in Chapters 9, 10, 17, and 18.

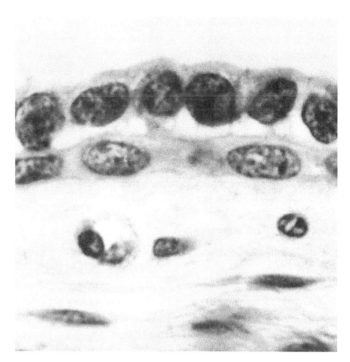

FIGURE 2-10 Stratified (two-layered) cuboidal epithelium, duct of carpal gland (pig). Hematoxylin and eosin (×1400).

GLANDULAR EPITHELIUM AND GLANDS

The secretory cells of endocrine and exocrine glands constitute **glandular epithelium.** These cells derive from the proliferation

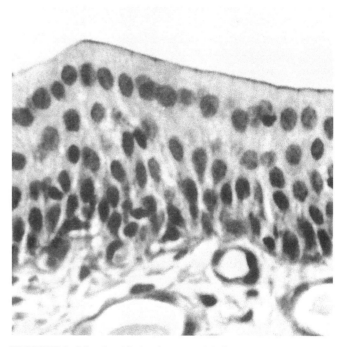

FIGURE 2-11 Stratified columnar epithelium, penile urethra (horse). Hematoxylin and eosin (×620). Note that the surface cells are columnar and the nuclei form a fairly regular row.

of surface epithelial cells into underlying connective tissue. A **gland** is a structure that may consist exclusively of glandular epithelium or may include a complex duct system, lined by surface epithelium, and a supportive framework of connective tissue, the **stroma.** Glands are found, in one form or another, in most organs of the body.

Classification of Glands

Glands are classified based on **morphologic characteristics,** the **nature of the secretory product,** and the **mode of release of the secretory product** (Table 2-3).

Morphologic Characteristics

Unicellular glands consist of a single secretory cell in a nonsecretory surface epithelium. An example of this type of gland is the **goblet cell,** a specialized epithelial cell that produces **mucinogen,** which is released onto the epithelial surface as **mucin,** a component of **mucus.** As this secretory material is synthesized, it fills and expands the apical portion of the cell and forces the nucleus into the slender basal portion, thus giving the cell a distinct goblet shape (Fig. 2-7). Unicellular endocrine glands are found scattered throughout the epithelial linings of the tubular organs of the gastrointestinal, respiratory, urinary, and reproductive systems, as well as in various other organs (adrenal gland, kidney, and thyroid gland). These cells are referred to as **APUD cells** because they are characterized by the uptake of amine precursors and their subsequent decarboxylation in the process of amine or peptide hormone synthesis (*a*mine *p*recursor *u*ptake and *d*ecarboxylation). APUD cells are described in detail in Chapter 15.

Multicellular glands are composed of more than one cell, and most glands belong in this classification. They may occur as a cluster of only a few secretory cells within a surface epithelium, forming **intraepithelial glands,** or as large accumulations of cells that have proliferated into the underlying connective tissue, forming **extraepithelial glands.**

Endocrine glands are multicellular glands that do not have a system of ducts to convey their secretory product to sites of utilization. Instead, the secretory products, often referred to as **hormones,** are released directly into the intercellular fluid, from which they are transported to a site of action by the blood and lymph.

Exocrine glands are multicellular glands with a system of ducts through which their secretory products are transported to the sites of utilization. Exocrine glands are either **simple glands,** consisting of one to several secretory units connected to the surface through an unbranched duct, or **compound glands,** with many secretory units emptying into a highly branched duct system.

Simple glands

Simple exocrine glands have secretory units of various shapes and dispositions. **Simple straight tubular glands,** such as those in the large intestine, pursue a straight, unbranched course in the surrounding tissue and open directly onto the surface (Figs. 2-12A and 2-13). **Simple coiled tubular glands** have a coiled or convoluted terminal portion. In histologic sections, the secretory unit appears as a cluster of cross-sectional profiles (Figs. 2-12B and 2-14). Sweat glands of the skin are good examples of this type. **Simple branched tubular glands** have a branched terminal portion (Figs. 2-12C and 2-15). The branches converge into a single duct near the opening onto the surface, and both portions are lined with secretory cells. The glands of the stomach are typical simple branched tubular glands.

Simple acinar and **simple alveolar glands** are similar because they have an enlarged, spherical secretory unit connected to the surface by a short duct (Figs. 2-12D, 2-12E, and 2-16). The lumen of the **acinus** is small and narrow, but that of the **alveolus** is large and distended (Fig. 2-17). Simple acinar and simple alveolar glands are rare; some sebaceous glands are of the simple acinar type, whereas simple alveolar glands are found in the respiratory system of the chicken. **Simple branched acinar** and **simple branched alveolar glands** are more common than unbranched glands. In these branched types, two or more acini

TABLE 2-3   Classifications of Glands

Based on Morphologic Characteristics	Based on the Nature of the Secretory Product
Unicellular Glands	Serous
Multicellular glands	Mucous
Intraepithelial	Seromucous (mixed)
Extraepithelial	
Endocrine	**Based on the Mode of Release of the Secretory Product**
Exocrine	Merocrine (eccrine)
Simple	Apocrine
Tubular—straight, coiled, branched	Holocrine
Acinar/Alveolar—single, branched	Cytocrine
Tubuloacinar/Tubuloalveolar	
Compound	
Tubular	
Acinar/Alveolar	
Tubuloacinar/Tubuloalveolar	

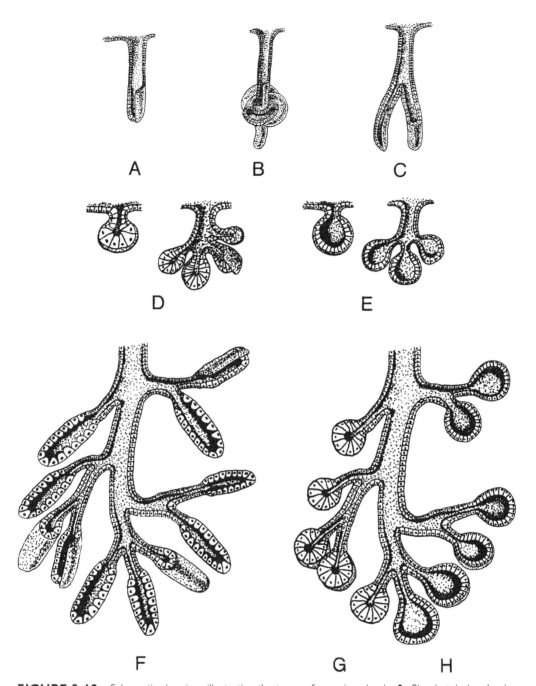

FIGURE 2-12 Schematic drawings illustrating the types of exocrine glands. **A.** Simple tubular gland. **B.** Simple coiled tubular gland. **C.** Simple branched tubular gland. **D.** Simple acinar gland and simple branched acinar gland. **E.** Simple alveolar gland and simple branched alveolar gland. **F.** Compound tubular gland. **G.** Compound acinar gland. **H.** Compound alveolar gland. Compound tubuloacinar/ tubuloalveolar glands consist of either a mixture of tubular and acinar/alveolar secretory units or tubular secretory units "capped" by acini or alveoli.

or alveoli occur together, and their secretory product empties through a common duct (Fig. 2-12D and E). Many of the larger sebaceous glands of the skin are of the simple branched acinar type. Simple branched alveolar glands are found in the respiratory system of the chicken.

Simple tubuloacinar and **simple tubuloalveolar glands** have secretory units composed of a tubular portion with a terminal acinus or alveolus and occur only in the branched form. The

minor salivary glands that empty into the oral cavity are classified as this type.

Compound glands

Compound glands contain the same types of secretory units as those of the simple glands but have *elaborate duct systems that branch repeatedly.* Compound glands are classified as tubular, acinar, alveolar, tubuloacinar, or tubuloalveolar types. For example,

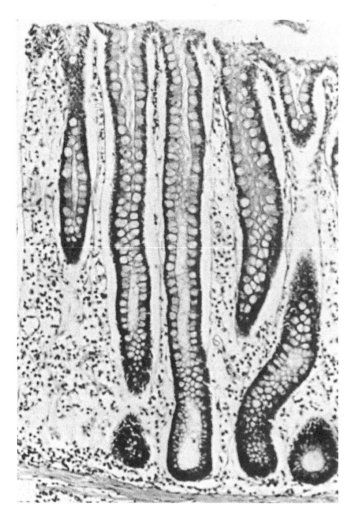

FIGURE 2-13 Simple tubular glands. Large intestine (dog). Hematoxylin and eosin (×120).

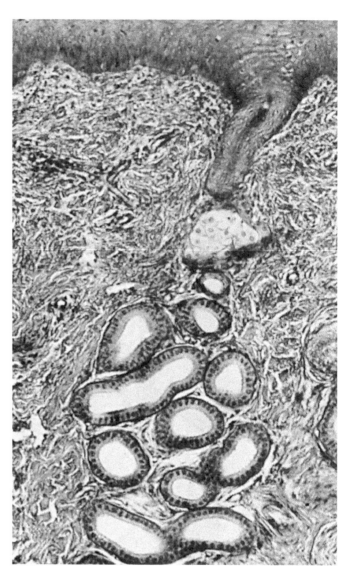

FIGURE 2-14 Simple coiled tubular gland. Ceruminous gland, ear canal (cow). Hematoxylin and eosin (×120).

a gland with a highly branched duct system whose secretory units consist of tubules of glandular epithelium would be classified as **compound tubular,** whereas a **compound tubuloacinar gland** contains either a mixture of acinar and tubular secretory units or tubular secretory units with terminal acini. Figure 2-12F, G, and H and Figure 2-18 illustrate the various types of secretory units and ducts found in compound glands.

Parenchyma. Compound glands are composed of secretory units and ducts, collectively termed **parenchyma;** the supportive or connective tissue elements comprise the **stroma.** Large glands are partly or completely divided into **lobes,** which are large, easily recognized structural units. The lobes are further subdivided by connective tissue into **lobules,** which in turn are composed of numerous **secretory units** (Fig. 2-18). Some of the smaller compound glands have only lobules and secretory units. The various segments of the duct system of compound glands are identified by their location within the gland.

Secretory product produced in tubules, acini, or alveoli of a compound gland flows first into an **intralobular duct,** usually located in the center of the lobule. Intralobular ducts continue as **interlobular ducts** as they emerge from the lobule to enter the

interlobular connective tissue. Interlobular ducts converge to form large **lobar ducts,** which drain individual lobes of the gland. The **main duct** is formed by the convergence of the lobar ducts (Fig. 2-18).

In some glands, such as the parotid salivary gland, portions of the intralobular ducts also contribute to the secretory product and thus are called **secretory ducts.** These ducts are also called **striated ducts,** because their cells contain many mitochondria oriented perpendicularly to the long axis of the cell and located between folds of the basal plasmalemma, thus giving the cells a striated appearance (Fig. 2-18G). **Intercalated ducts** are small, nonsecretory intralobular ducts that connect the secretory units with the secretory (striated) duct (Fig. 2-18C and E). Intercalated ducts are prominent in the parotid salivary gland and are also present in the mandibular and sublingual salivary glands as well as the pancreas.

The general term **excretory duct** describes any of the previously mentioned ducts that function only to transport the

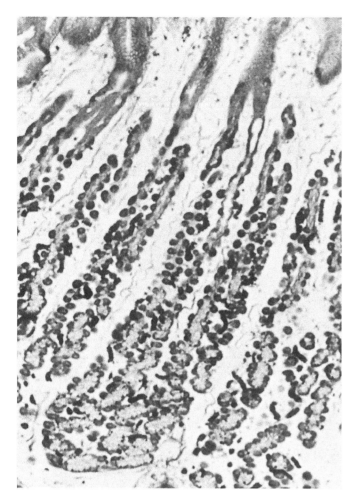

FIGURE 2-15 Simple branched tubular glands. Fundic stomach (dog). Hematoxylin and eosin (×120).

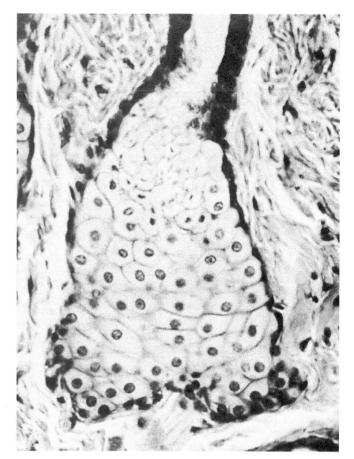

FIGURE 2-16 Simple acinar gland. Sebaceous gland, nostril (horse). Hematoxylin and eosin (×300).

secretory product to the site of utilization. They do not contribute to the secretory product as do the secretory ducts.

Stroma. The **stroma** of compound glands includes the capsule and the internal supportive framework. The **capsule,** composed of collagen, elastic, and reticular fibers, completely surrounds the gland and gives rise to connective-tissue sheets (**septa**) or strands (**trabeculae**) that extend well into the parenchyma. Septa clearly define the lobes and lobules and provide support for the various lobar and interlobular ducts. Fine **reticular fibers** encircle the individual secretory units.

Nature of the Secretory Product

Both simple and compound glands may be classified as mucous, serous, or seromucous (mixed), based on the nature of the secretory product. **Serous glands** produce a thin watery product. The cells of the secretory units usually have spherical nuclei near the center of the cells, and the apical cytoplasm is filled with small secretory granules (Fig. 2-18F). These granules are precursors of enzymes produced by many of the serous glands and are called **zymogen granules.** The parotid salivary gland and the exocrine part of the pancreas are typical serous glands.

Mucous glands produce a thick, viscous secretion, **mucin,** which contributes to a protective coating over the lining of hollow organs that communicate with the outside of the body (Fig. 2-18B). This protective coating is termed **mucus** and contains cast-off epithelial cells and leukocytes, in addition to mucin. The cells of the mucus-secreting units are filled with **mucinogen,** the precursor of **mucin,** which stains light with hematoxylin and eosin. The nuclei are displaced toward the basal part of the cell and are usually flattened against the cell membrane.

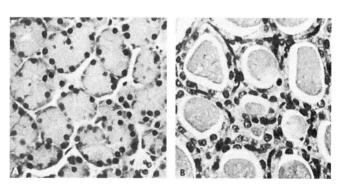

FIGURE 2-17 Types of secretory units. **A.** Acini, characterized by a small lumen, parotid salivary gland (horse). Hematoxylin and eosin (×480). **B.** Alveoli, mammary gland (sow). Note the large lumen. Hematoxylin and eosin (×480).

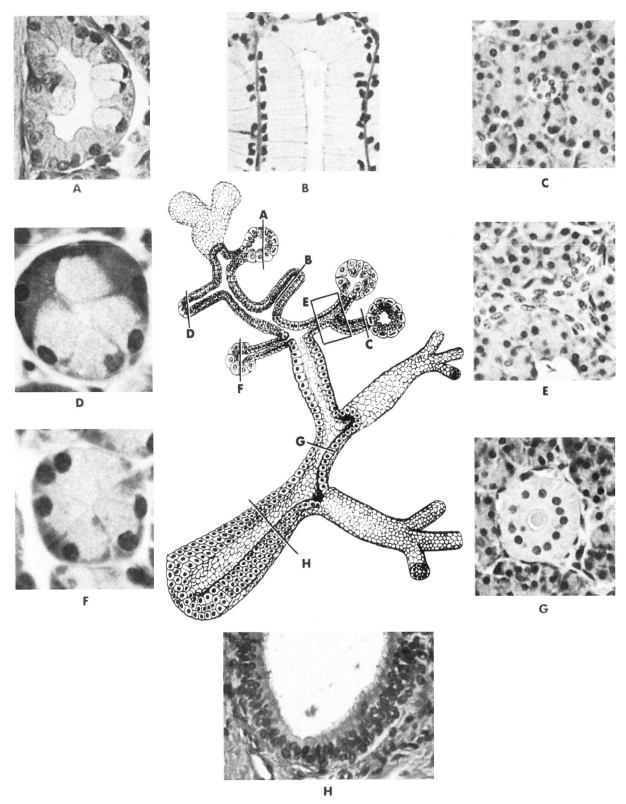

FIGURE 2-18   Schematic composite drawing and photomicrographs of the duct system and secretory units of a compound gland. The photomicrographs correspond to the areas labeled A through H. **A.** Seromucous alveolus, trachea (pig). Trichrome (×600). **B.** Mucous tubular secretory unit, bulbourethral gland (bull). Hematoxylin and eosin (×480). **C.** Cross section of intercalated duct, parotid salivary gland (horse). Hematoxylin and eosin (×480). **D.** Mucous acinus with serous demilunes, seromucous salivary gland (horse). Hematoxylin and eosin (×1000). **E.** Longitudinal section through intercalated duct, parotid salivary gland (horse). Hematoxylin and eosin (×480). **F.** Serous acinus, parotid salivary gland (horse). Hematoxylin and eosin (×1200). **G.** Striated intralobular duct, parotid salivary gland (horse). Hematoxylin and eosin (×480). **H.** Interlobular duct, mandibular salivary gland (dog). Hematoxylin and eosin (×300). *(Drawing from Stinson AW, Brown EM. Veterinary Histology Slide Sets. East Lansing, MI: Michigan State University, Instructional Media Center, 1970.)*

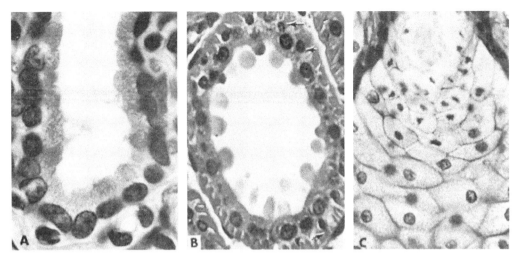

FIGURE 2-19 Secretory units illustrating the various modes of release of the secretory product. **A.** Merocrine (eccrine) gland, prostate (dog). Hematoxylin and eosin (×1200). **B.** Apocrine sudoriferous gland, skin (pig), with myoepithelial cells at arrows. Hematoxylin and eosin (×610). **C.** Holocrine gland, sebaceous gland (horse). Hematoxylin and eosin (×480).

Glands that contain both mucous and serous cells are described as **seromucous, mucoserous,** or simply "**mixed.**" The combinations of these two types of cells vary considerably from one gland to another. Some secretory units contain intermixed serous and mucous cells (Fig. 2-18A). Other seromucous glands are composed of a mixture of all-mucous acini and all-serous acini, rather than each acinus containing some serous and some mucous cells. Most commonly, the serous cells are located at the periphery of the mucous secretory unit and are half-moon- or crescent-shaped cells called **serous demilunes** (Fig. 2-18D). They empty their serous secretory product into the lumen of the secretory unit by way of small channels between the mucous cells called intercellular canaliculi. Some seromucous tubuloacinar glands have a mucous tubular unit with a terminal serous acinus.

Mode of Release of the Secretory Product

The mechanism by which the secretory product is released from the cell forms the basis for a third classification of glands. Four different modes of release are recognized: merocrine or eccrine, apocrine, holocrine, and cytocrine.

During the **merocrine** (sometimes called **eccrine**) mode of secretion, the contents of small secretory granules are released as the secretory product (Fig. 2-19A). The secretory granules are usually enclosed within a membrane. When the secretory granule reaches the cell surface, its membrane fuses with the plasmalemma, thereby discharging the secretory product via **exocytosis.**

In the **apocrine** mode of secretion, a large, single secretory granule migrates in the cytoplasm to the cell apex. The plasmalemma and a portion of the neighboring cytoplasm surround the granule. Eventually, the plasmalemma constricts beneath the granule, causing the projection containing the granule to bulge into the gland lumen (Fig. 2-19B). Constriction of the plasmalemma proceeds until the membrane-bounded granule and its

accompanying cytoplasm and plasmalemma are separated from the cell, leaving the rest of the cell plasmalemma intact.

Apocrine glands in the secretory state are easily recognized; however, when they are in a resting phase with no secretory "droplets," their differentiation from merocrine glands is difficult. Examples of apocrine glands include the mammary gland and the general body sweat glands.

In the **holocrine** mode of secretion, entire cells are released as the secretory product (Fig. 2-19C). The sebaceous glands of the skin are typical holocrine glands. The cells become filled with lipid granules and move toward the duct of the gland; the cells then disintegrate, and their contents are extruded into the duct.

In the **cytocrine** mode of secretion, secretory material is transferred from one cell to the cytoplasm of another cell. It is exemplified in the epidermis, where melanocytes transfer the brown pigment, melanin, into the cytoplasm of the keratinocytes.

Myoepithelial Cells

In some glands, **myoepithelial cells** are interposed between the base of the secretory cells and the basement membrane. As their name suggests, myoepithelial cells possess characteristics of both muscle cells (actin and myosin filaments) and epithelial cells (cytokeratin). When stimulated, these cells contract and force the secretory product of the epithelial cells into the duct system. Myoepithelial cells are especially well developed in sweat glands and mammary glands (Fig. 2-19B). In the mammary gland, myoepithelial cells are stimulated by oxytocin.

SUGGESTED READINGS

Bharadwaj MB, Calhoun ML. Histology of the urethral epithelium of domestic animals. Am J Vet Res 1959;20:841–851.

Franke WW, Jahn L, Knapp AC. Cytokeratins and desmosomal proteins in certain epithelioid and nonepithelial cells. In: Osborn M, Weber K, eds. Cytoskeletal Proteins in Tumor Diagnosis. Cold Spring Harbor, NY: Cold Spring Harbor Laboratory, 1989.

Griep EB, Robbins, ES. Epithelium. In: Weiss L, ed. Cell and Tissue Biology. 6th Ed. Baltimore: Urban & Schwarzenberg, Inc., 1988.

Hashimoto K. The eccrine and apocrine glands and their function. In: Jarret A, ed. The Physiology and Pathophysiology of the Skin. New York: Academic Press, 1978:5.

International Committee on Veterinary Gross Anatomical Nomenclature. Nomina anatomica veterinaria. 4th Ed. Ithaca, NY: International Committee on Veterinary Gross Anatomical Nomenclature, 1994.

International Committee on Veterinary Histological Nomenclature. Nomina histologica. 2nd Ed. (revised). Ithaca, NY: International Committee on Veterinary Histological Nomenclature, 1994.

Krstić RV. General Histology of the Mammal. New York: Springer-Verlag, 1985.

Krstić RV. Ultrastructure of the Mammalian Cell. New York: Springer-Verlag, 1979.

Martin BF, Wong YC. Development and maturation of the bladder epithelium of the guinea pig. Acta Anat 1981;110:359–375.

Petry G, Amon H. Licht- und elektronenmikroskopische studien über struktur und dynamik des übergangsepithels. Z Zellforsch 1966;69:587.

Phillips SJ, Griffin T. Scanning electron microscope evidence that human urothelium is a pseudostratified epithelium. Anat Rec 1985;211:153A.

Severs JJ, Hicks RM. Analysis of membrane structure in transitional epithelium of rat urinary bladder. 2. The discoidal vesicles and Golgi apparatus: their role in luminal membrane biogenesis. J Ultrastruct Res 1979;69:279–296.

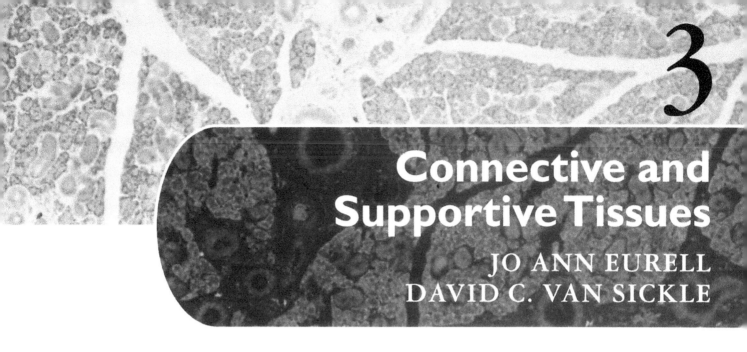

3

Connective and Supportive Tissues

JO ANN EURELL
DAVID C. VAN SICKLE

Connective Tissue Cells
  Mesenchymal Cells
  Fibrocytes and Fibroblasts
  Reticular Cells
  Adipocytes
  Pericytes
  Mast Cells
  Macrophages
  Plasma Cells
  Pigment Cells
  Other Cells of Loose Connective Tissue
Connective Tissue Fibers
  Collagen Fibers
  Reticular Fibers
  Elastic Fibers
  Fibrous Adhesive Proteins
Ground Substance
Embryonic Connective Tissues
  Mesenchyme
  Mucous Connective Tissue
Adult Connective Tissues
  Loose Connective Tissue
  Dense Connective Tissue
    Dense irregular connective tissue
    Dense regular connective tissue
      Collagenous tendons and ligaments
      Elastic ligaments
  Reticular Connective Tissue

Adipose Tissue
  White adipose tissue
  Brown adipose tissue
Adult Supportive Tissues
  Cartilage
    Cartilage cells
      Chondroblast
      Chondrocyte
    Cartilage matrix
    Classification of cartilage
      Hyaline cartilage
      Elastic cartilage
      Fibrocartilage
    Development of cartilage
    Nutrition of cartilage
  Bone
    Bone cells
      Osteoblast
      Osteocyte
      Osteoclast
    Bone matrix
    Structural and functional characteristics
      Macroscopic structure
      Histologic preparation
      Microscopic structure
    Osteogenesis
      Intramembranous ossification

Endochondral ossification
    Primary center of ossification
    Secondary centers of ossification
Growth in length
Growth in width and circumference
Bone modeling

Bone remodeling
    Fracture repair
Joints
    Fibrous Joints
    Cartilaginous Joints
    Synovial Joints

Connective and supportive tissues connect other tissues, provide a framework, and support the entire body by means of cartilage and bones. These tissues also play an important role in thermoregulation and in defense and repair mechanisms. Connective tissues are also a reservoir for various hormones and cytokines that play an important role in growth and development.

Most connective and supportive tissues are derived from mesoderm, which arises from the somites and lateral layers of the somatic and splanchnic mesoderm. In addition, neural crest cells from surface ectoderm form the head mesenchyme, which subsequently develops into the connective tissue of the rostral head. Connective and supportive tissues are composed of **cells, fibers,** and amorphous **ground substance** in varying proportions. Embryonic mesenchyme is a unique connective tissue because it lacks fibers during early development. Based on occurrence, connective and supportive tissues are classified as embryonic or adult with several subgroups.

CONNECTIVE TISSUE CELLS

The cells of connective tissue proper are diverse and have varied functions ranging from production of connective tissue components to phagocytosis and antibody formation. Many cells of connective tissue, such as fibrocytes, remain as resident cells in a fixed location within the tissue. Other connective tissue cells, such as macrophages, are capable of moving through the tissue as mobile or wandering cells.

Mesenchymal Cells

Mesenchymal cells are irregularly shaped with multiple processes (Fig. 3-1). They are smaller than fibroblasts and have fewer cytoplasmic organelles. The large, oval nucleus has a prominent nucleolus and fine chromatin. The mesenchymal cell population serves as a reservoir of pluripotent cells that can differentiate into other types of connective tissue cells as needed.

Fibrocytes and Fibroblasts

The most common cell of connective tissue is the **fibrocyte** (Fig. 3-2A). Fibrocytes are generally elongated and spindle-shaped, with processes that contact adjacent cells and fibers. Their heterochromatic nucleus is surrounded by a scant amount of pale

cytoplasm. Secretory vesicles in the cytoplasm discharge their contents (e.g., procollagen, proteoglycans, proelastin) into the surrounding microenvironment. At the transmission electron microscopic (TEM) level, the cytoplasm has sparse rough endoplasmic reticulum (rER) and a small Golgi complex. Free ribosomes, mitochondria, lysosomes, and vesicles are also present. Actin filaments occur as bundles in the cell processes. Fibrocytes maintain the connective tissue matrix by forming the fibers and constantly renewing the ground substance.

The **fibroblast** has a larger, more euchromatic nucleus and more abundant, basophilic cytoplasm than the fibrocyte (Fig. 3-2B). At the EM level, abundant rER and a prominent Golgi complex are present in the cytoplasm. These structural characteristics indicate more active connective tissue matrix production in comparison to the fibrocyte. Fibroblasts may arise directly from undifferentiated mesenchymal cells or are transformed from fibrocytes under the influence of microenvironmental factors (e.g., cytokines). In certain situations, fibroblasts may differentiate into adipose cells, chondroblasts, or osteoblasts.

Myofibroblasts are fibroblasts that contain actin filaments associated with dense bodies; hence, they resemble smooth mus-

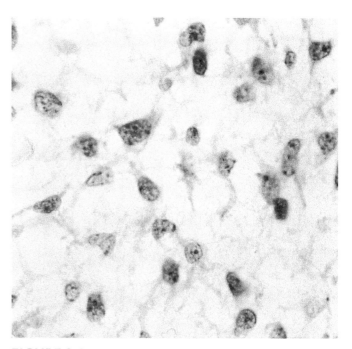

FIGURE 3-1 Mesenchyme (rat embryo). Note the stellate mesenchymal cells in an amorphous ground substance. Hematoxylin and eosin (×800).

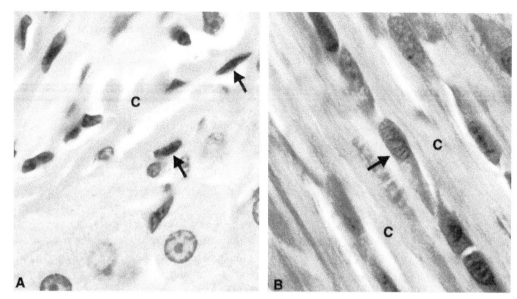

FIGURE 3-2 A. Fibrocytes (arrows), collagen fibers (C), connective tissue, liver (dog). **B.** Fibroblasts (arrow), tendon (young puppy). The cells are located between collagen fibers (C). Hematoxylin and eosin (×1520).

cle cells. It is believed that myofibroblasts play a role in contraction of the wound during healing.

Reticular Cells

Reticular cells are similar in appearance to the fibrocyte (Fig. 3-3). They are stellate-shaped cells with a spherical nucleus and basophilic cytoplasm. Reticular cells produce **reticular fibers,** which form the fine structural network of organs such as the lymph nodes, spleen, and bone marrow. These cells are fixed in the tissue and are capable of phagocytosis. Reticular cells should not be confused with the reticulocyte, an immature erythrocyte.

Adipocytes

Adipocytes are also referred to as fat cells or adipose cells (Fig. 3-4). Individual adipocytes or clusters containing multiple cells are normal components of loose connective tissue, but when the fat cells outnumber other cell types, the tissue is called **adipose tissue** (see more on adipose tissue later in this chapter). Mature **unilocular adipocytes** are spherical or polyhedral cells that measure up to 120 μm in diameter. Most of the cell is occupied by a single, large nonmembrane-bounded lipid droplet surrounded by a thin layer of cytoplasm. The cell nucleus is displaced to the periphery by the lipid droplet, which is surrounded by cytoplasm that contains a small Golgi complex, mitochondria, rER, and microfilaments.

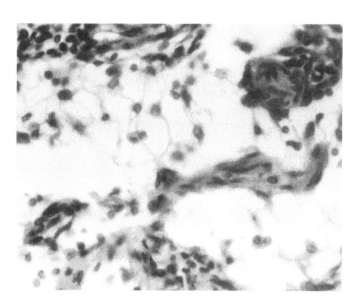

FIGURE 3-3 Reticular connective tissue, lymph node (sheep). Note the numerous interconnected reticular cells, which form a three-dimensional network. Hematoxylin and eosin (×600).

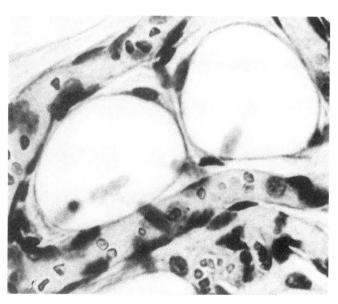

FIGURE 3-4 Two white adipocytes surrounded by capillaries. Hematoxylin and eosin (×630). *(Courtesy of A. Hansen.)*

In contrast, mature **multilocular adipocytes** contain a more centrally located nucleus with multiple lipid droplets in the cytoplasm (Fig. 3-5). Both the Golgi complex and rER are rather inconspicuous, but many mitochondria are present. The high concentration of cytochromes in the mitochondria is primarily responsible for the brown color of aggregates of multilocular adipocytes, which are referred to as brown fat (described below).

Unilocular adipocytes produce chemical energy, whereas multilocular adipocytes metabolize lipid to produce heat. Leptin, a protein produced by unilocular fat cells, regulates the amount of adipose tissue in the body. Thermogenin, a transmembrane protein in the mitochondria of brown fat, channels protons away from adenosine 5´-triphosphate (ATP) synthesis and into heat production instead.

Because fat is rapidly dissolved by most of the dehydration and/or clearing agents commonly used for the preparation of histologic sections, the lipid droplets appear as clear spaces surrounded by cytoplasm (Fig. 3-4). When rapidly processed, the lipid can be preserved and stained with certain agents, such as osmium tetroxide or Sudan III stain.

Pericytes

Pericytes, also known as Rouget cells or periendothelial cells, are elongated cells that are located adjacent to the endothelium lining capillaries and postcapillary venules. The cells are surrounded by the basal lamina of the blood vessel and make frequent contact with the underlying endothelial cells by extending processes through the lamina. Pericytes resemble fibrocytes in appearance but have contractile filaments similar to smooth muscle. Proposed functions of pericytes include regulating capillary blood flow; serving as multipotent mesenchymal cells with specific ability to form vascular smooth muscle cells; phagocytosing; and regulating

new capillary growth. Pericytes also have the ability to differentiate into adipocytes, osteoblasts, and phagocytes.

Mast Cells

Mast cells are common in loose connective tissue, especially around nerve endings and microcirculation. The cells are found in the dermis of the skin and connective tissue of the respiratory tract and gastrointestinal system.

Mast cells are large, polymorphic, spherical, or ovoid cells that contain a prominent, centrally located nucleus. Numerous secretory granules are present in the cytoplasm (Fig. 3-6). These cells can be identified with immunocytochemistry or a **metachromatic stain,** which has the capacity to stain elements of a cell or matrix a different color from that of the dye solution (e.g., toluidine blue, a blue dye that stains heparin-containing granules red). At the EM level, the mast cell granules are membrane-bounded and have crystalline, lamellar, or fine granular characteristics. The remaining cytoplasm is occupied by an extensive Golgi complex, cisternae of rER, free ribosomes, and mitochondria.

Mast cell granules contain histamine, heparin, and various proteases. **Histamine,** a biogenic amine, is a vasoconstrictor that causes increased permeability of small venules, thereby permitting leakage of plasma, resulting in tissue edema. This localized inflammatory reaction is designed to dispose of foreign antigens rapidly. Histamine also stimulates smooth muscle contraction in small airways. **Heparin,** a glycosaminoglycan, acts as an anticoagulant and is believed to stimulate angiogenesis. Mast cells can be activated to release their contents (degranulate) by physical stimuli such as trauma or sunlight; immunogenic stimuli including immunoglobulin (Ig) E, complement, or cytokines; and neurogenic stimuli such as neuropeptides.

Three populations of mast cells based on protease content have been identified. The **mucosal mast cell** (MC_T) contains tryptase only, while the **connective tissue mast cell** (MC_{TC}) contains tryptase, chymase, carboxypeptidase, and cathepsin. A

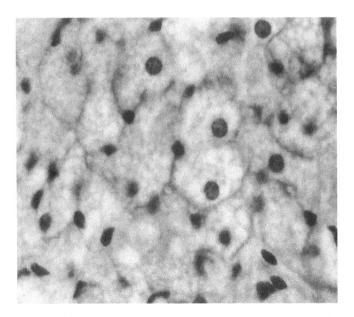

FIGURE 3-5   Brown adipose tissue. Note the numerous small lipid inclusions in the multilocular adipocytes. Hematoxylin and eosin (×600).

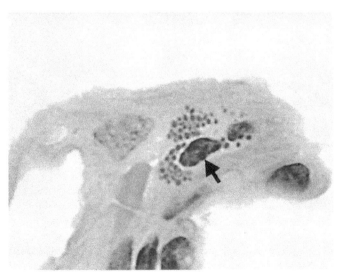

FIGURE 3-6   Mast cell (arrow), lung (rabbit). Note the characteristic granules. Hematoxylin and eosin, plastic section (×1200).

third mast cell type (MC_C) has chymase and carboxypeptidase. The dog and cat have about 70% MC_{TC} cells. Proteases can destroy nearby cells and tissue matrix and activate complement components. Arachidonic acid products (leukotrienes) and cytokines (e.g., various interleukins, stem cell factor, and tumor necrosis factor alpha [TNF-α]) are also produced by the mast cell and immediately released without storage in the cytoplasmic granules. In the past, the mast cell has been described as a "tissue basophil," but despite some similarities, the mast cell and basophil are different cells. Both cells develop from the same pluripotent stem cell (CD34+), and both have basophilic cytoplasmic granules that contain similar inflammatory products. However, basophils are terminally differentiated before they enter blood circulation, while mast cells leave the bone marrow, pass through the circulation, and differentiate in tissues outside the bone marrow. The mast cell can undergo mitotic division while the basophil cannot. Also, basophils have a short lifespan of days while most mast cells can survive for weeks to months.

Macrophages

Macrophages are phagocytic cells that are scattered throughout the body and form the **mononuclear phagocyte system.** They are derived from a bone marrow precursor cell (CFU-GM) that divides and produces monocytes that circulate in the blood. The monocytes then migrate across blood vessel walls into the connective tissue or organs and become macrophages. Mobile macrophages wander through the tissues performing their phagocytic function while fixed macrophages remain in one location. The fixed macrophage of connective tissues is also known as the **histiocyte.** Other macrophages located in specific tissues include the stellate macrophage of the liver (Kupffer cell), the microglial cell, the intraepidermal macrophage (Langerhans cell), and the osteoclast.

Macrophages are large, ovoid, or spherical cells that contain cytoplasmic vacuoles and are readily distinguishable with the light microscope (Fig. 3-7). At the EM level, they are characterized by numerous lysosomes, phagosomes, phagolysosomes, and pseudopodia (footlike extensions of the cell membrane) (Fig. 3-8). Abundant ribosomes, rER, smooth ER (sER), mitochondria, and a Golgi complex are also present. Histochemical stains for lysosomal enzymes, such as acid phosphatase, facilitate the identification of macrophages. Once activated, the macrophage changes morphology with increased microvilli and lamellipodia, which are sheetlike extensions of cytoplasm. The lamellipodia form transient adhesions with the surrounding substrate, enabling the cell to move.

A variety of chemotactic stimuli (e.g., infectious agents, cytokines) cause macrophages to migrate to locations in the body where foreign material must be removed. Macrophages engulf material such as cell debris, abnormal matrix components, neoplastic cells, bacteria, and inert substances by pinocytosis and phagocytosis. Phagocytosis may be indiscriminate (e.g., dust particles in the lung) or may involve specific interaction with receptors on the macrophage surface (e.g., Fc receptors, IgG, and IgM). Macrophages also act as antigen-presenting cells, which process and display foreign substances so that lymphocytes can recognize and respond more effectively to the challenge.

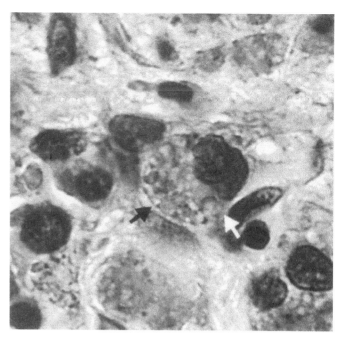

FIGURE 3-7 Macrophage (arrows), connective tissue. Note the numerous cytoplasmic vacuoles and phagolysosomes. Hematoxylin and eosin (×1200).

Inflammation can be characterized as acute or chronic based on the relative proportion of neutrophils to macrophages. Acute inflammation has more neutrophils than macrophages, whereas chronic inflammation has more macrophages than neutrophils. When stimulated, macrophages may form clusters of **epithelioid cells,** which resemble epithelial cells in morphology. **Multinucleated giant cells** or foreign-body cells (Fig. 3-9) arise during chronic inflammation and are a result of the fusion of several macrophages in response to the presence of foreign material.

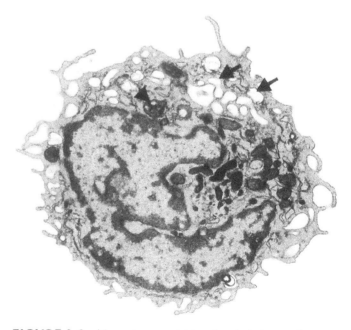

FIGURE 3-8 Macrophage containing abundant pinocytotic vacuoles (arrows) and phagolysosomes (arrowhead) (×8000). *(Courtesy of J. Turek.)*

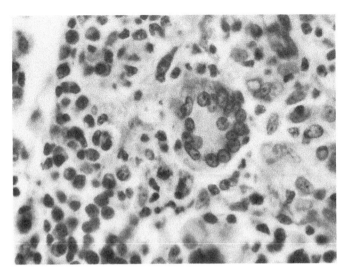

FIGURE 3-9   Multinucleated giant cell, lymph node (sheep). Crossman's trichrome (×435).

Macrophages synthesize and secrete many substances that are a reflection of their multiple functions. These substances include enzymes such as lysozyme, which lyses the wall of many bacteria; cytokines (interferons and interleukin); complement components (C2, C3, C4, and C5); coagulation factors; and reactive chemical species (hydrogen peroxide, hydroxyl radicals, nitric oxide), which are important components of the bactericidal and cytocidal (e.g., tumor cells) activities of macrophages.

Plasma Cells

Plasma cells are spherical, ovoid, or pear-shaped cells with a spherical, eccentric nucleus. The chromatin is often arranged in peripherally located clumps or in centrally converging strands that give the nucleus a "cartwheel" appearance (Fig. 3-10). The cytoplasm is intensely basophilic, and a negatively stained Golgi region is usually present. At the fine-structural level, in addition to an extensive Golgi complex, the cytoplasm has an abundant rER with

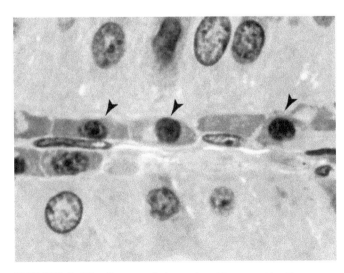

FIGURE 3-10   Plasma cells (arrowheads), connective tissue, duodenum. Hematoxylin and eosin (×900).

dilated cisternae containing slightly granular and moderately electron-dense material as well as spherical inclusions referred to as Russell bodies (Fig. 3-11). Russell bodies give a positive reaction for immunoglobulin. Free ribosomes and mitochondria are also present in the cytoplasm.

Plasma cells are most numerous in lymphatic tissue, especially in the center of medullary cords of lymph nodes. They are also particularly abundant in bone marrow, the loose connective tissue underlying the epithelium of the gastrointestinal tract, the respiratory system, and the female reproductive system.

Plasma cells do not originate in loose connective tissue but develop from B lymphocytes that immigrate into the connective tissue from the blood; they produce circulating or humoral antibodies (see Chapter 8).

Pigment Cells

Cells in connective tissue may contain pigments, including melanin in domestic animals or pteridines and purines in fish

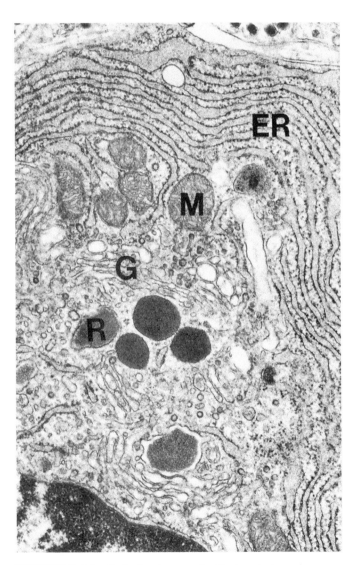

FIGURE 3-11   Part of a plasma cell with abundant rough endoplasmic reticulum (ER), mitochondria (M), extensive Golgi complex (G), and Russell bodies (R) (×19,500).

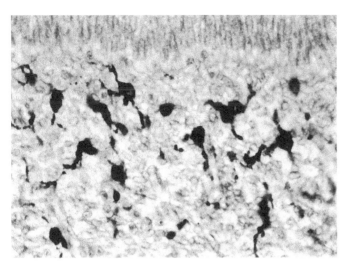

FIGURE 3-12 Pigment containing cells in the lamina propria of a uterine caruncle (sheep). Hematoxylin and eosin (×325).

and amphibians (Fig. 3-12). When present in large numbers, the cells impart color to the connective tissue. They occur in various locations such as the dermis, uterine caruncles of sheep, meninges, choroid, and iris. Their significance is described in connection with these organs.

Other Cells of Loose Connective Tissue

Depending on its location and various other factors (infestation by parasites, presence of bacteria, and the like), loose connective tissue may contain a varying number of lymphocytes, monocytes, and granulocytes (especially eosinophils and neutrophils). The structure and function of these immigrant cells are described in the section on blood (see Chapter 4).

Globule leukocytes are mononuclear cells with acidophilic and metachromatic cytoplasmic granules. These cells are found in epithelium and connective tissues of the respiratory, digestive, reproductive, and urinary systems. Globule leukocytes are believed to be mucosal mast cells, but their origin as a subpopulation of T lymphocytes has also been proposed.

CONNECTIVE TISSUE FIBERS

Structural connective tissue fibers include collagen, reticular, and elastic fibers. In addition, **fibrous adhesive proteins** such as fibronectin and laminin bind structural fibers together or help cells attach to the connective tissue matrix.

Collagen Fibers

Collagen is the principal fiber type in mature connective tissue. The turnover rate of collagen is tissue-specific and can vary within the same tissue. Most collagen digestion occurs through the action of metalloproteinases (e.g., collagenase) and serine proteases.

Collagen polypeptide chains are synthesized in the rER as pro-α chains that contain extension peptides (propeptides) at

both ends (Fig. 3-13). Multiple α chains have been recognized. Within the rER cisternae, these pro-α chains assemble into triple helices to form **procollagen** molecules. The molecules are then transferred to the Golgi complex, packaged into secretory vesicles, and released by exocytosis. At this point in synthesis, collagen can be classed as fibril-forming, FACIT (*fibril-associated collagens with interrupted triple helices*), sheet-forming, multiplexin, connecting and anchoring, or transmembrane collagen. Twenty-seven collagen types are currently recognized.

Fibril-forming collagen then undergoes extracellular enzymatic cleavage of the propeptides to yield collagen molecules. These molecules in turn assemble in the extracellular matrix (ECM) to form **collagen fibrils**. The fibrils are only visible with the electron microscope, are up to several micrometers in length, and vary in diameter (10 to 300 nm), with characteristic cross-striations repeated at 67-nm intervals (Figs. 3-13 and 3-14). Bundles of these fibrils form **collagen fibers** that are visible by light microscopy (Fig. 3-2B). Fibril-forming collagen includes types I, II, III, V, XI, XXIV, and XXVII. Fibers composed of type I collagen account for 90% of the body collagen. Type I collagen is found in skin, tendon, bone, and dentin, while type II collagen is specific for cartilage and vitreous humor. Frequently colocalized with type I collagen, type III collagen is essential for normal collagen I fibrillogenesis. Type V collagen is necessary for extracellular matrix assembly in connective tissues; it is present in fetal tissues and the placenta. Type XI collagen is found in hyaline cartilage and type XXIV is distributed in developing cornea and bone.

Fresh collagen fibers are white, and in histologic preparations, they stain with acid dyes. Thus, they are red to pink in hematoxylin and eosin (H&E)-stained sections, red with van Gieson's method, and blue in Mallory's and Masson's triple stains (green when light green stain is used). The fibers are flexible and can adapt to the movements and changes in size of the organs with which they are associated. Collagen fibers are characterized by a high tensile strength and a poor shear strength, and stretch is limited to approximately 5% of their initial length. Consequently, they are found wherever high tensile strength is required, such as in tendons, ligaments, and organ capsules.

Other collagens known as **FACIT collagens** (*fibril-associated collagens with interrupted triple helices*) include types IX, XII, XIV, XX, XXI, and XXII. These collagens serve as molecular bridges that are important in the organization and stability of extracellular matrices. Glycosaminoglycans are linked to type II collagen of hyaline cartilage by collagen IX. Type XX collagen is prevalent in corneal epithelium. The ECM of blood vessel walls contains type XXI collagen, while the ECM at tissue junctions contains type XXII collagens. Some FACIT collagens (types XVI and XIX) are unable to bind fibers and are referred to as FACIT-like collagens.

Sheet-forming collagen forms a flexible framework of sheets rather than fibrils. Collagen IV forms the basal lamina of epithelia. In the eye, the posterior limiting lamina (Descemet's membrane) of the cornea is formed from type VIII collagen. Type X collagen is found in the hypertrophic zone of the physis.

Multiplexins (*multiple triple-helix domains and interruptions*) are collagens that are associated with basement membranes. This subgroup includes types XV and XVIII.

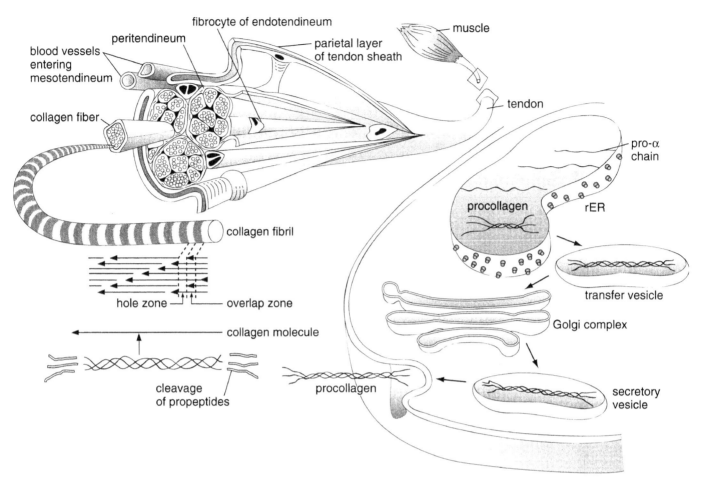

FIGURE 3-13 Collagen polypeptide chains are synthesized within the cell and released into the extracellular space as procollagen. In fibril-forming collagen, peptides are then cleaved from the procollagen, resulting in a collagen molecule. The collagen molecules are assembled in such a way that hole zones are created, which stain dark, in contrast to overlap zones, which exclude stain. Bundles of light- and dark-banded fibrils form collagen fibers. In a tendon, individual collagen fibers are surrounded by endotendineum and bundles of fibers are bound by peritendineum. In this drawing, the sheath surrounding the tendon is reflected to show the collagen fiber bundles (fascicles) inside. Blood vessels pass through the mesotendineum to supply the tendon.

Connecting and anchoring collagen binds to the surface of fibril-forming collagen and may mediate the interactions of fibrils with one another and with other matrix components. Collagen types VI and VII are believed to perform this function. Type VI collagen forms unique beaded filaments, while collagen VII forms anchoring fibrils that link collagen IV of the basal lamina of the epidermis to the collagen of underlying connective tissue.

Transmembrane collagens include XIII, XVII, XXIII, and XXV. Collagen XVII, a transmembrane collagen of the skin, is associated with hemidesmosomes and mutates in diseases that cause blisters (epidermolysis bullosa). Type XXIII collagen is associated with metastatic tumor cells while type XXV collagen is a neuronal collagen.

Collagen XXVI is unclassified and is found in the testes and ovary.

Reticular Fibers

In routine histologic preparations, reticular fibers cannot be distinguished from other small collagen fibers. These fibers can be

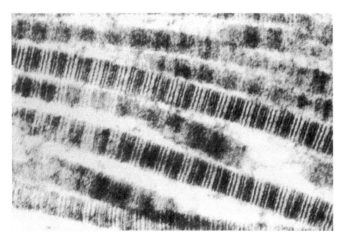

FIGURE 3-14 Electron micrograph of collagen fibrils with characteristic cross-striations (×88,000).

identified only with certain silver impregnations (thus the term **argyrophilic** or **argentaffin fibers**) or with the periodic acid-Schiff (PAS) reagent (Fig. 3-15). These fibers are actually individual collagen fibrils (type III collagen) coated by proteoglycans and glycoproteins. This coating increases the affinity of the fibers for silver salts. When individual reticular fibers are bundled to form collagen fibers, the coating is supposedly displaced and the argyrophilia decreases.

Reticular fibers form delicate, flexible networks around capillaries, muscle fibers, nerves, adipose cells, and hepatocytes and serve as a scaffolding to support cells or cell groups of endocrine, lymphatic, and blood-forming organs. They are an integral part of basement membranes.

Elastic Fibers

Elastic fibers and/or sheets (laminae) are present in organs in which normal function requires elasticity in addition to tensile strength. Elastic fibers can be stretched as much as two and one-half times their original length, to which they return when released. Found in the pinna of the ear, vocal cords, epiglottis, lungs, ligamentum nuchae, dermis, aorta, and muscular arteries, elastic fibers are one of the most resilient connective tissue fibers, withstanding chemical maceration and autoclaving.

Elastic fibers usually occur as individual, branching, and anastomosing fibers. Their diameters vary within a wide range, from 0.2 to 5.0 µm in loose connective tissue to as large as 12 µm in elastic ligaments, such as the ligamentum nuchae in the neck (Fig. 3-16). In H&E-stained histologic sections, the larger elastic fibers in elastic ligaments are readily distinguished as highly refractile, amorphous, light pink strands; they are stainable by certain selective dyes, such as orcein and resorcin-fuchsin.

The main component of elastic fibers is **elastin,** which contains a network of **fibrillin** microfibrils that form a supporting scaffold for the elastin. An amorphous protein rich in proline and glycine, elastin contains little hydroxyproline. One theory of elastin structure is that the molecules are randomly coiled and

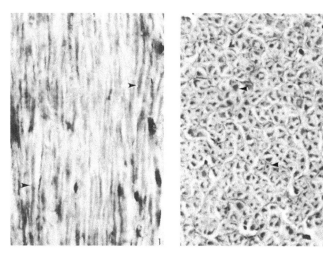

FIGURE 3-16   Ligamentum nuchae, large ruminant. **1.** Longitudinal section. **2.** Cross section. Note that the large elastic fibers (arrowheads) are surrounded by networks of collagen fibers. Crossman's trichrome (×600).

joined by stable, covalent cross-links containing **desmosine,** an identifying component of elastic fibers. The coils of elastin can stretch and then recoil as needed. Elastin is synthesized by fibroblasts and smooth muscle cells.

The secondary component of elastic fibers is 10-nm microfibrils that are embedded within and surround the elastic core (Fig. 3-17). The microfibrillar material is composed of a glycoprotein, **fibrillin,** which is necessary for elastic fiber integrity.

During development of the elastic fiber, fibrillin microfibrils are secreted before elastin and provide a scaffolding on which elastin is deposited. At this stage, the fiber is referred to as **oxytalan.** In the second stage of development, elastin is deposited between the microfibrils, forming **elaunin.** As more elastin accumulates within the developing fiber, mature **elastic fibers** are formed. Developmentally, the elastic fiber is the last fiber to appear in organs (e.g., lung) or connective tissue.

Fibrous Adhesive Proteins

The extracellular matrix contains noncollagenous fibrous proteins that play a role in organizing the matrix and help cells to adhere to it. **Fibronectin,** a major product of mesenchymal cells, is a fibril-forming protein that binds to various structures, including the cell membrane, collagen, elastin, and proteoglycans, and probably mediates the connection between the cytoskeleton and the ECM. Fibronectin plays a role in a variety of processes, such as cell adhesion, cell differentiation, cell growth, and phagocytosis.

Laminins are large glycoproteins. They are a major constituent of the basement membrane and are synthesized by the cells that are in contact with it (e.g., epithelial cells, smooth muscle cells, neurolemmocytes) (Fig. 16-6). Laminins are present in the lamina lucida (lamina rara) and lamina densa. They are connected to type IV collagen by the adhesive glycoprotein nidogen (entactin). Laminins form a structural network in the basement membrane to which other glycoproteins and proteoglycans attach. Also, they are signaling molecules that stabilize cell surface receptors.

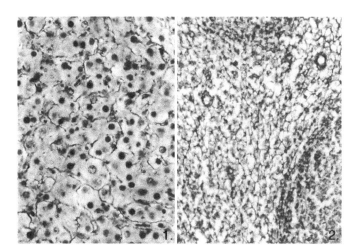

FIGURE 3-15   Reticular fibers. **1.** Liver (pig). Achucarro silver impregnation (×435). **2.** Lymph node (dog). Palmgren silver impregnation (×230).

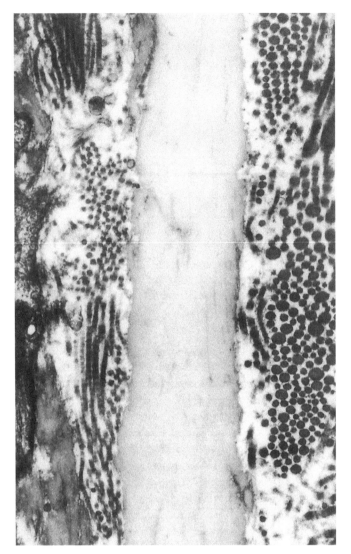

FIGURE 3-17 Electron micrograph of an elastic lamina between collagen fibrils (longitudinal and cross sections). The electron-dense thin lines in the elastic lamina are microfibrils (×21,000).

Other adhesive glycoproteins include fibrinogen (blood-clotting mechanism), link protein (linking of cartilage matrix components), mucins, tenascin (embryonic tissues, uncertain function), and thrombospondin (platelet aggregation).

GROUND SUBSTANCE

The cells and fibers of connective tissue are embedded in an amorphous ground substance composed of glycosaminoglycans (GAGs), proteoglycans, plasma constituents, metabolites, water, and ions. The ground substance forms a hydrated gel that, by virtue of its high water content, has unique properties of resiliency.

Glycosaminoglycans are comprised of unbranched polysaccharides of alternating uronic acid and hexosamine residues. Seven major types of GAGs can be distinguished. **Hyaluronan** (hyaluronic acid) is a nonsulfated GAG. It is a large, long molecule that forms networks with spaces that are filled with tissue

fluid. The resulting gel is particularly abundant in the vitreous humor of the eye and in synovial fluid; it is also found in the umbilical cord, loose connective tissue, skin, and cartilage. Hyaluronan binds proteoglycans into a larger molecule called an **aggrecan** (Fig. 3-18). **Chondroitin-4-sulfate** and **chondroitin-6-sulfate** are abundant in cartilage, arteries, skin, and cornea. A smaller amount is found in bone. **Dermatan sulfate** is found in skin, tendon, ligamentum nuchae, sclera, and lung. **Keratan sulfate** is present in cartilage, bone, and cornea. **Heparan sulfate** is found in arteries and the lung, whereas **heparin** is found in mast cells, the lung, the liver, and skin. The latter six GAGs are of the sulfated variety.

Proteoglycans are formed by covalently linking GAGs to a protein core and range in size from small molecules (decorin, m.w. 40,000) to large aggregates (aggrecan, m.w. 210,000) (Fig. 3-18). In addition to filling space in the connective tissue matrix and imparting its unique biomechanical properties, proteoglycans may regulate the passage of molecules and cells in the intercellular space. They are also believed to play a major role in chemical signaling between cells and may bind and regulate the activities of other secreted proteins.

Proteoglycans in low concentrations are not detected in H&E-stained sections, but when present in higher concentrations, as in hyaline cartilage, they stain with basophilic dyes.

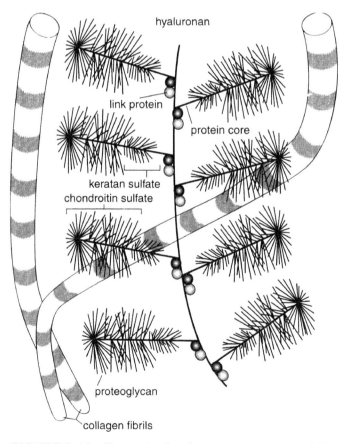

FIGURE 3-18 The matrix of cartilage contains aggrecans, which are composed of proteoglycans bound to a hyaluronic acid chain by link proteins. The proteoglycans are composed of glycosaminoglycans, such as chondroitin and keratan sulfate, bound to a protein core.

When stained with toluidine blue or crystal violet, a metachromatic change to pink or magenta occurs.

EMBRYONIC CONNECTIVE TISSUES

Mesenchyme

Mesenchyme, the connective tissue of the developing embryo, is composed of irregularly shaped mesenchymal cells and amorphous ground substance (Fig. 3-1). The cell processes contact adjacent cells and thus form a three-dimensional network. Mesenchymal cells undergo numerous mitotic cell divisions and continuously change their shape and location to adapt to the transformations that occur during embryonic growth. During early development, mesenchyme does not contain fibers, and the abundant amorphous ground substance fills the wide intercellular spaces. Mesenchyme gives rise to various types of adult connective tissues, as well as blood and blood vessels.

Mucous Connective Tissue

Mucous or gelatinous connective tissue is found primarily in the embryonic hypodermis and umbilical cord (Fig. 3-19). It is characterized by stellate fibroblasts that form a network. The large intercellular spaces are occupied by a viscous, gel-like amorphous ground substance that has a positive reaction for glycosaminogly-

cans or proteoglycans. Collagen fibers (types I and III) are also present. In the adult organism, gelatinous connective tissue occurs in the papillae of omasal laminae and reticular crests, the bovine glans penis, and the core of the rooster comb.

ADULT CONNECTIVE TISSUES

Adult connective tissues are classified based on the variation of quantity and arrangement of fibers within the matrix. The properties of cell structure and the biochemical composition of fibers and ground substance are similar across connective tissue types.

Loose Connective Tissue

Loose, or areolar, connective tissue is the most widely distributed type of connective tissue in the adult animal (Fig. 3-20A). The cells and fibers of loose connective tissue are widely separated by spaces filled with ground substance. Compared to other types of connective tissue, the cells in loose connective tissue are more abundant and include both fixed and mobile populations. All three fiber types (reticular, collagen, and elastic) are present. The relative abundance and orientation of fibers vary widely and depend primarily on the location and specific function of the tissue. In cases of injury, the stage of healing also causes variation in fiber arrangement. Early connective tissue is highly cellular with fine reticular fibers; later connective tissue has predominantly thick collagen fibers.

The amorphous ground substance of loose connective tissue is composed of proteoglycans that bind a significant quantity of tissue fluid. Substances dissolved in the tissue fluid can diffuse through the amorphous ground substance and thus have ready access to connective tissue cells. Circulating tissue fluid is formed at the arterial end of capillaries and absorbed by either venous or lymphatic capillaries.

Loose connective tissue is present beneath many epithelia, where it provides support and a vascular supply. This tissue forms the interstitial tissue in most organs, thereby allowing easy movements and shifting of organs. Loose connective tissue is present around nerve and skeletal muscle bundles as named tissue layers (e.g., epineurium) and is found between the layers of smooth musculature of hollow organs. The pia mater and arachnoid of the brain and spinal cord are also composed of loose connective tissue.

The functions of loose connective tissue range from the purely mechanical, such as support and dampening biomechanical effects in various locations (e.g., hypodermis), to more sophisticated functions, such as participation in tissue repair and defense activities (inflammation).

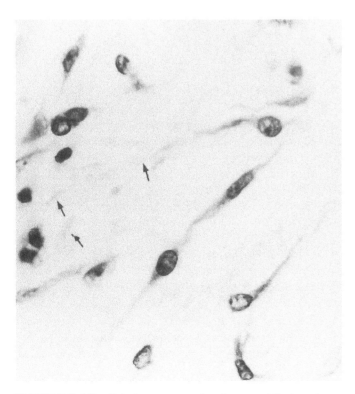

FIGURE 3-19 Gelatinous connective tissue, umbilical cord (pig). Fine collagen fibers (arrows) are present. Hematoxylin and eosin (×800).

Dense Connective Tissue

The fibers in dense connective tissue are more abundant than cells and amorphous ground substance. Dense connective tissue is commonly classified as either **dense irregular connective tissue,** with a random orientation of the fiber bundles, or **dense regular connective tissue,** in which fibers are oriented in a regular pattern.

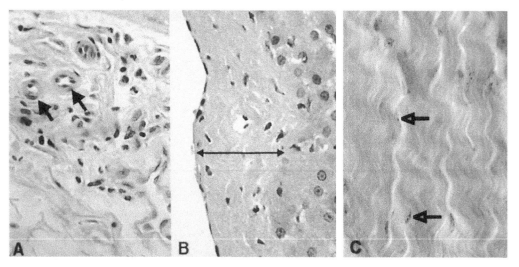

FIGURE 3-20 **A.** Loose connective tissue with blood vessels (arrows), liver (dog). **B.** Dense irregular connective tissue (arrow), liver (dog). **C.** Dense regular connective tissue with fibrocytes (arrows), tendon. Hematoxylin and eosin (×600).

Dense Irregular Connective Tissue

Fibrocytes are the predominant cell population in **dense irregular connective tissue** (Fig. 3-20B). Collagen fibers are generally arranged in bundles that cross each other at varying angles. In thin aponeuroses or muscle fasciae, these bundles are located in a single layer. In heavier aponeuroses, organ capsules, or dermis, the bundles are superimposed in several layers and interlace with one another in multiple planes. This irregular configuration allows adaptation to changes in the size of an organ or the diameter of a muscle, and stretching forces can be withstood in any direction. Continuation of surface connective tissue into the organ or muscle enhances strength. Elastic networks facilitate a rapid return to resting conditions.

Dense irregular connective tissue is found in a variety of locations, such as the lamina propria of the initial portions of the digestive system, the capsule of the lung (visceral pleura) and other organs (spleen, liver, kidney, testis), fasciae, aponeuroses, joint capsules, pericardium, and dermis. Special functional and morphologic features are described with the various organ systems.

Dense Regular Connective Tissue

Dense regular connective tissue occurs as collagenous tendons and ligaments or as elastic ligaments (Fig. 3-20C). In both types, all fibers are arranged in the same direction, according to specific functional requirements.

Collagenous tendons and ligaments

The great tensile strength of collagenous tendons is reflected in their structure. They consist of fascicles of parallel collagen fibers (Fig. 3-13). Individual collagen fibers are surrounded by fibrocytes, which form the **endotendineum.** These fascicles are bound together by sparse, loose connective tissue (the **peritendineum**) that forms a protective sheath around the blood vessels and nerves of the tendon. The peritendineum is continuous with the epi-

tendineum, the dense irregular connective tissue around the entire tendon. The fibrocytes between the collagen fibers of the tendon are long, flat cells of varying shape. Winglike cytoplasmic processes extend between adjacent collagen fibers and give the fibrocytes a stellate appearance in cross sections of tendon. Following injury, the fibroblasts of surrounding connective tissue sheaths proliferate and attempt to repair the damage.

The typical tendon structure may be altered at points of insertion into bone or cartilage or where the tendon courses around bones. Wherever tendons or ligaments insert on bone or cartilage, the dense regular collagenous tissue of the tendon gradually changes to fibrocartilage and then to mineralized fibrocartilage before the point of osseous penetration. Collagen fibers from the tendon or ligament are embedded in the bone matrix as **perforating fibers** (Sharpey's fibers). The function of this arrangement is to gradually transmit biomechanical forces from a flexible fibrous unit to a stiffer osseous unit. In areas where tendons course around bones, they are subject not only to tension but also to compression, which causes the cells to enlarge and to become encapsulated such that the tissue appears similar to fibrocartilage.

The mobility of the tendon is ensured either by the surrounding epitendineum or the **tendon sheath,** which consists of a visceral and a parietal portion (Fig. 3-13). The visceral portion is tightly anchored to the epitendineum of the tendon and is separated from the parietal portion by a fluid-filled synovial cavity. Both the parietal and the visceral portions of the tendon sheath comprise dense irregular connective tissue and a synovial layer, the structure of which is similar to that of synovial membranes (see synovial joints below). Blood vessels supplying the tendon pass through a gap between the opposing edges of the synovial sheath known as the **mesotendineum.**

Collagenous ligaments contain a lower percentage of ground substance than tendons and the collagen fibers are organized more randomly. Named connective tissue sheaths are not assigned to ligaments.

Elastic ligaments

Large elastic fibers that branch and interconnect predominate in **elastic ligaments.** The fibers are surrounded by loose connective tissue (Fig. 3-16). The ligamentum nuchae and some dorsal ligaments (ligamenta flava) of the vertebral column are examples of elastic ligaments.

Reticular Connective Tissue

The stroma of all lymphatic organs (spleen, lymph node, hemal node, tonsils), diffuse lymphatic tissue, solitary lymphatic nodules, and bone marrow is made of reticular connective tissue. This tissue is composed of stellate reticular cells and a complex three-dimensional network of reticular fibers (Fig. 3-15) (see Chapter 8).

Adipose Tissue

Adipose tissue, or fat, is a specialized type of connective tissue that, in addition to performing insulating and mechanical functions, plays an important role in the metabolism of the organism. One of the most important functions of adipose tissue is its participation in fat metabolism. The turnover of intracellular fat is rapid, with a continuous cycle of withdrawal and deposit, even if the organism has to draw on its fat reserves to supplement food intake.

Intracellular lipids are synthesized mainly from fatty acids but also from carbohydrates and proteins. The fatty acids necessary for lipid synthesis are derived from the enzymatic breakdown, by lipoprotein lipase, of the triglycerides contained in blood chylomicrons or lipoproteins; after their uptake by the adipocytes, the fatty acids are resynthesized to triglycerides.

Under hormonal (insulin) or nervous (norepinephrine) control, intracellular enzymatic hydrolysis of triglycerides takes place, and fatty acids and glycerol are released into the blood and catabolized in energy-yielding reactions. In brown adipocytes, mitochondrial respiration is uncoupled from ATP synthesis; thus, the oxidation of stored fat generates heat rather than ATP, causing a rise in body temperature in arousing hibernating mammals.

In mammalian subcutaneous connective tissue, the adipose-tissue component serves as a thermal and mechanical insulator. In the foot pads and digital cushions, adipose tissue is associated with bundles of collagen and elastic fibers. This combination of fibers and fat cells allows the adipose tissue to act as a dampening cushion, and at the same time, the cells are protected by the great tensile strength of the collagen fibers. After deformation, the elastic fibers allow the adipose cells to return to normal shape.

Two types of adipose tissue, white and brown, are distinguished in most mammals by differences in color, vascularity, structure, and function.

White Adipose Tissue

The cells of white fat are separated by septa of loose connective tissue into clusters of adipose cells referred to as lobules. Each adipose cell is surrounded by a delicate network of collagen and reticular fibers that supports a dense capillary plexus and nerve fibers (Fig. 3-4). In addition, the narrow intercellular spaces contain a few fibrocytes, mast cells, and sparse amorphous ground substance.

Brown Adipose Tissue

Brown adipose tissue (brown fat) is composed of aggregates of multilocular adipocytes (Fig. 3-5). The intercellular connective tissue consists of fibrocytes, collagen, and reticular fibers. Capillaries form a dense plexus, and the adipocytes are directly innervated by adrenergic axons.

Brown adipose tissue is particularly common and abundant in rodents and hibernating mammals. It is located primarily in the axillary and neck regions (interscapular fat body), along the thoracic aorta and in the mediastinum, in the mesenteries, and around the abdominal aorta and vena cava near the kidney. Brown fat may also be found in the same locations in other domestic mammals.

ADULT SUPPORTIVE TISSUES

Cartilage

Cartilage is specialized for a supportive role in the body. It possesses considerable tensile strength because the intercellular substance has a supportive framework of collagen and/or elastic fibers, and the firm but pliable ground substance enhances its weightbearing ability. In general, this tissue is avascular, alymphatic, and aneural. However, during development, blood vessels penetrate certain cartilage structures (e.g., cartilaginous epiphyses of developing bones).

Cartilage Cells

Two cell types are recognized in cartilage: the **chondroblast** and the **chondrocyte.**

Chondroblast

The **chondroblast** is found in growing cartilage (Fig. 3-21). The cell is oval-shaped with a spherical nucleus and a prominent Golgi apparatus. The cytoplasm is basophilic as a result of large quantities of rER. The chondroblast actively forms the matrix of cartilage that surrounds the perimeter of the cell.

Chondrocyte

After cartilage matrix formation is complete, the chondroblast becomes a less active cell, the **chondrocyte** (Fig. 3-22). The chondrocyte varies from elongate to spherical in shape, depending on the location within the cartilage. Each chondrocyte is located within a **lacuna,** a cavity within the semirigid cartilage matrix. In living cartilage or at the fine-structural level, the cell fills the lacuna. Short cytoplasmic processes extend into the intercellular substance. In most light microscopic preparations, the cell surface appears separated from the lacunar walls because of shrinkage. The chondrocyte has a spherical nucleus with one or more nucleoli and abundant rER and prominent Golgi complex. Glycogen and lipid accumulate in the cytoplasm of old chondrocytes, and

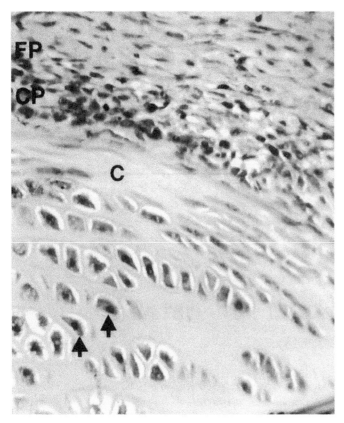

FIGURE 3-21 Immature hyaline cartilage (dog). The fibrous layer (FP) and cellular layer (CP) of the perichondrium border the cartilage (C) containing chondroblasts (arrows). Hematoxylin and eosin (×300).

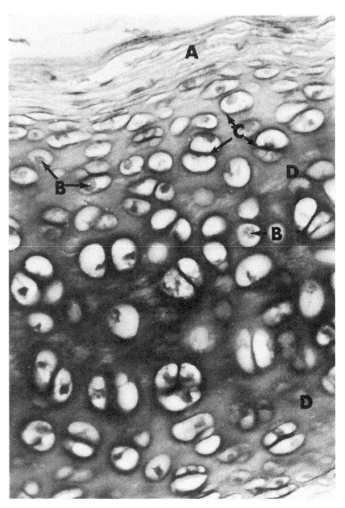

FIGURE 3-22 Mature hyaline cartilage (dog). The fibrous perichondrium (A) surrounds the cartilage mass. The chondrocytes (B) lie in lacunae. The territorial matrix (C) is darker than the interterritorial matrix (D). Hematoxylin and eosin (×425).

in routine preparations, the cells appear vacuolated. Although considered a less active cell than the chondroblast, the chondrocyte is responsible for continual ongoing maintenance of the surrounding matrix.

Cartilage Matrix

The matrix of cartilage is composed of fibers and ground substance as found in other connective tissues, but the **cartilage matrix** has unique biomechanical properties. Collagen forms the framework of the matrix. The major cartilage collagen is type II, but type I predominates in fibrocartilage and other collagen types are present in cartilage.

The ground substance contains the GAGs chondroitin sulfate, keratan sulfate, and hyaluronic acid, all of which play an important role in transporting water and electrolytes as well as in binding water to give hyaline cartilage its resiliency. GAGs complex with a protein backbone to form proteoglycans (Fig. 3-18). Numerous proteoglycans join to a hyaluronan core with the help of **link proteins,** thus forming a large **aggrecan.** The proteoglycans of the aggrecan are also bound to adjacent collagen fibrils, thereby forming a loose network that functions as a molecular sieve, limiting movement of larger molecules through the matrix.

Additional components of the cartilage matrix include the adhesive molecules, **chondronectin, anchorin CII,** and **fibronectin,** which are involved in the interaction between col-

lagen and chondrocytes. The matrix is mineralized by calcium phosphate, present in **hydroxyapatite** form, in the deep region of the articular cartilage and the zones of hypertrophy, resorption, and ossification of the physis.

Overall, the matrix is slightly basophilic when stained with H&E, reacts positively with PAS, and exhibits a marked metachromasia with metachromatic stains. Staining intensity varies across the matrix due to variations in biochemical composition of the matrix related to biomechanical stresses.

Classification of Cartilage

On the basis of different structural characteristics of the matrix, three types of cartilage are distinguishable: **hyaline cartilage, elastic cartilage,** and **fibrocartilage.**

Hyaline cartilage

Hyaline cartilage is found on the articulating surfaces of bones in synovial joints and provides support in the nose, larynx, trachea, and bronchi. It forms most of the entire appendicular and axial skeleton in the embryo.

The chondrocytes in mature hyaline cartilage vary in size (Fig. 3-22). Chondrocytes near the surface of cartilage are small, and their lacunae are elliptic, with their long axes parallel to the surface. Deep within the cartilage, the cells are larger and more polyhedral. Some lacunae contain only one cell; others contain two, four, or sometimes six cells. These multicellular lacunae are called **cell nests** or **isogenous cell groups.**

The amorphous ground substance of hyaline cartilage is a firm gel containing a network of type II collagen fibrils. Since the fibrils have the same refractive index as the amorphous ground substance, they cannot be seen in standard preparations. Surrounding each chondrocyte is a thin layer of **pericellular matrix** that has proteoglycans but lacks collagen. The **territorial matrix** surrounds the pericellular matrix and is composed of a network of fine collagen fibrils and ground substance. The **interterritorial matrix** lies outside the territorial matrix and fills the remaining matrix space. This matrix region contains large collagen fibrils and abundant proteoglycans. Differences in collagen and proteoglycan content account for the staining differences between regions as observed with the light microscope.

At the ultrastructural level, **matrix granules** are adjacent to the chondrocytes. These granules are proteoglycans secreted by the chondrocytes and represent early stages of matrix production. The proteoglycans later become components of aggrecans in the surrounding matrix.

Except on articular surfaces, hyaline cartilage is surrounded by vascular connective tissue called the **perichondrium,** which is composed of two distinct layers (Fig. 3-21). The layer immediately adjacent to the cartilage is composed of chondroblasts and a network of small blood vessels; it is called the **cellular** or **chondrogenic layer.** The outer **fibrous layer** of the perichondrium consists of irregularly arranged collagen fibers and fibroblasts.

Elastic cartilage

Elastic cartilage occurs where elasticity, as well as some rigidity, is needed, such as in the epiglottis and external auditory canal. It is also part of the corniculate and cuneiform processes of the larynx.

In addition to all of the structural components of hyaline cartilage, elastic cartilage possesses a dense network of elastic fibers that are visible in ordinary H&E preparations (Fig. 3-23). The elastic fibers are few in number near the perichondrium but form a dense network within the cartilaginous mass. Chondrocytes located away from the surface of elastic cartilage contain many fat vacuoles. Later in adults, these fat-containing cells often become adipose tissue.

Fibrocartilage

Of the three cartilage types, **fibrocartilage** occurs least frequently. It is often interposed between other tissues and hyaline cartilage, tendons, or ligaments. Fibrocartilage is found in the intervertebral disks and forms the menisci of the stifle joint. In dogs, fibrocartilage is found in the cardiac skeleton, which joins the atrial and ventricular heart muscles.

The most striking characteristic of fibrocartilage is the presence of prominent type I collagen fibers in the matrix (Fig. 3-24). The microscopic appearance of fibrocartilage may vary with location. Fibrocartilage that attaches ligaments and tendons to bone has large collagen fiber bundles dispersed in a plane parallel to the direction of the pulling forces, with rows of small lacunae containing chondrocytes between collagen bundles (Fig. 3-24A). In the fibrocartilaginous cardiac skeleton (fibrous trigone) of the dog, the chondrocytes and collagen fibers are distributed more randomly (Fig. 3-24B). The amorphous ground substance is most abundant in the vicinity of the cells, whereas the remainder of the matrix contains primarily collagen fiber bundles. Fibrocartilage lacks a distinct perichondrium; the cartilage is surrounded by collagen fibers in some locations, but a cellular layer is absent.

Development of Cartilage

The first indication of cartilage formation within the embryo is a clustering of mesenchymal cells. These cells enlarge, withdraw their processes, and synthesize and secrete amorphous ground substance and procollagen (type II). They are then referred to as chondroblasts, and the cell clusters are called **centers of chondrification.** As the intercellular matrix increases, the cells become spherical and isolated from each other in lacunae; at this point, they are called **chondrocytes.**

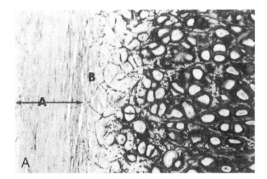
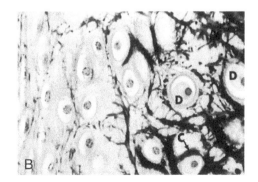

FIGURE 3-23 Elastic cartilage, external ear (dog). **A.** Perichondrium (A) with sparse elastic fibers (black) penetrating the cellular layer (B) (×80). **B.** High-power magnification illustrates elastic fibers (C) coursing through the matrix. The chondrocytes (D) nearly fill the lacunae. Verhoeff's stain (×425).

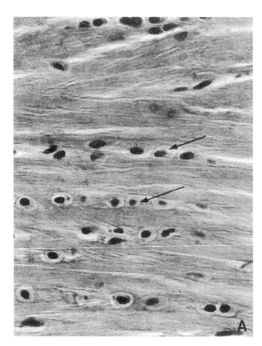 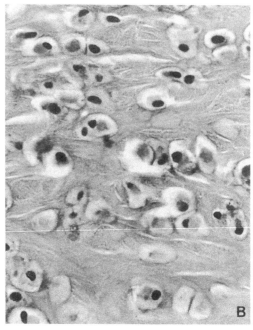

FIGURE 3-24 **A.** Fibrocartilage at ligament insertion on bone (dog). The lacunae (arrows) are oriented in the plane of pulling forces. Hematoxylin and eosin (×300). **B.** Cardiac skeleton (dog). The lacunae and collagenous fibers are randomly arranged. Hematoxylin and eosin (×570).

Chondroblasts undergo several mitotic divisions, and after each division, a new intercellular matrix separates the two resulting daughter cells. This process leads to substantial expansion of the cartilage from within and is referred to as **interstitial growth.** Concurrently, the mesenchyme surrounding the cartilage primordium differentiates into the perichondrium. Chondroblasts from the cellular layer of the perichondrium divide and secrete additional matrix on the surface of the cartilage. The process is called **appositional growth.** In the adult, the ability of the chondrogenic layer to produce cartilage persists, but it is dormant until a need arises for new cartilage.

During the development of elastic cartilage, fibroblasts initially produce undifferentiated fibrils. The fibroblasts later transform into chondroblasts and mature elastic fibers are identified in the matrix.

Nutrition of Cartilage

Unlike other connective tissues, most cartilage is avascular. Therefore, the chondrocytes must depend on diffusion of nutrients through the gelled matrix. These nutrients diffuse from nearby capillaries within the perichondrium or from synovial fluid bathing the cartilage surface. When the intercellular matrix becomes calcified, diffusion is no longer possible, and the chondrocytes die. This phenomenon occurs in aging and is natural in endochondral bone development.

If cartilage exceeds 3 mm³ in size, then vessels may penetrate the matrix. An example of vascularized cartilage is the hyaline cartilage of developing epiphyses of long bones, which contain blood vessels and nerves surrounded by connective tissue in structures called **cartilage canals.**

Bone

Bone is a connective tissue with cells and fibers embedded in a hard, mineralized substance that is well suited for supportive and protective functions. Functioning as an organ, bone provides internal support for the entire body as well as attachment sites for the muscles and tendons necessary for movement. It protects the brain and organs in the thoracic cavity and contains the bone marrow within its medullary space. Bone functions metabolically by providing a source of calcium to maintain proper blood calcium levels and various growth factors (e.g., transforming growth factor-beta [TGF-β]) that play a role in remodeling.

Bone is a dynamic tissue that is renewed and remodeled throughout the life of all mammals. Its construction is unique because it provides the greatest tensile strength with the least amount of weight of any tissue.

Bone Cells
Osteoblast

The **osteoblast** is the cell responsible for active formation and mineralization of bone matrix. The cells range from columnar to squamous in shape and are located on surfaces of bone where new bone is being deposited (Figs. 3-25 and 3-26). The nucleus is located in the basal region of the intensely basophilic cytoplasm. The Golgi apparatus and rER are prominent between the nucleus and the secretory surface of the osteoblast. The cell deposits **osteoid** (collagen I and proteoglycans), the unmineralized matrix of bone. In addition, the osteoblast produces various growth factors including fibroblast growth factor, insulin growth factor, platelet-derived growth factor, and TGF-β.

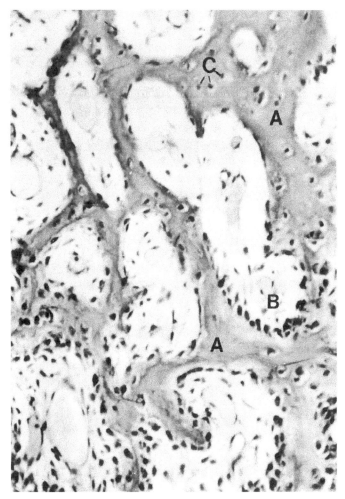

FIGURE 3-25 Trabecular bone (A) of intramembranous osteogenesis has osteoblasts (B) and osteocytes (C) within lacunae. Note the prominent blood vessels in the mesenchyme. Hematoxylin and eosin (×175).

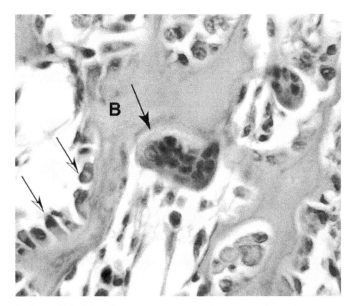

FIGURE 3-26 Osteoclast, in an erosion lacuna (arrow), resorbing bone. Osteoblasts (open arrows) are forming bone (B). Hematoxylin and eosin (×475).

Osteoblasts originate from pluripotent mesenchymal stem cells that also give rise to chondroblasts, fibroblasts, and other cell types. The **osteoprogenitor cell,** which ultimately develops into a differentiated osteoblast, does not have a typical morphologic appearance, but specific cell-surface molecules expressed during differentiation help identify the cell line. Bone morphogenetic protein (BMP), a protein from the bone matrix, plays an important role in the differentiation of stem cells into osteoblasts.

Flattened, resting osteoblasts are known as **bone lining cells.** These cells are found on the surfaces of adult trabeculae and compact bone. They are capable of becoming active osteoblasts when appropriately stimulated.

Osteoblasts have receptors for parathyroid hormone (PTH) on their surface. When PTH binds to the osteoblast, the cell releases factors that stimulate osteoclastic activity.

Osteocyte

As matrix secretion approaches completion, approximately 10% of the osteoblasts surround themselves with osteoid and modulate into osteocytes. The **osteocyte** is the principal cell in mature bone and resides in a **lacuna** surrounded by calcified interstitial matrix (Fig. 3-25). Numerous long, slender processes extend from the cell body into **canaliculi** within the matrix to contact adjacent osteocytes. Gap junctions are present at the contact points and provide communication between osteocytes. Further, the long cellular processes of the osteocyte are able to shorten and lengthen. This activity may serve as a "pump" to move fluid through lacunae and canaliculi to transfer metabolites from the surface of the bone. The organelles of young osteocytes resemble osteoblasts, but as they mature, the Golgi complex and rER are less prominent and lysosomes increase in number.

The exact way in which osteocytes preserve the integrity of bone matrix is not completely understood. Osteocytes are essential in preserving bone structure because, upon their death, osteoclasts immediately move to the area and resorb the bone. Therefore, signals from apoptotic osteocytes may be part of a signaling pathway to initiate bone remodeling.

Osteocytes may also play a role in calcium homeostasis, although the osteoclast is primarily responsible for calcium release through bone resorption. Osteocytes are believed to remove and replace perilacunar bone, a 1-μm layer immediately adjacent to the osteocyte. Perilacunar bone removal is called **osteocytic osteolysis.** The extent to which this process normally occurs is unclear.

The walls of the lacunae and canaliculi are covered with GAGs. The maintenance of this covering by osteocytes is important to maintain the integrity of this tissue.

Osteoclast

The **osteoclast** is a large, multinucleated cell located on the surface of bone (15 to 30 nuclei per cell, which is 40 to 100 μm in diameter) (Fig. 3-26). Occasional mononuclear osteoclasts are not easily recognized. The cytoplasm is acidophilic and contains a small amount of rER, ribosomes, numerous smooth vesicles, and mitochondria.

The activated osteoclast has a ruffled border created by extensive infoldings of the cell membrane that sweep across the bony surface. The cell secretes acid and lysosomal enzymes into this region. The cell membrane immediately adjacent to the ruffled border adheres tightly to the bony surface, thereby sealing the area of active bone resorption. As the osseous matrix is enzymatically digested, an **erosion lacuna** (Howship's lacuna) is formed. The lacuna remains after the osteoclast is no longer present, thus indicating prior areas of resorption. Osteoclasts may also be found in bone remodeling units as part of a cellular complex that remodels cortical bone in the adult (described later in this chapter). In addition to the release of mineral and protein components of bone, osteoclasts are also responsible for the release and activation of TGF-β from the matrix. Osteoclasts are stimulated by PTH, interleukins, and osteoprotegerin ligand (OPGL, RANKL); they are inhibited by calcitonin, osteoprotegerin (OPG), and gonadal steroids.

Osteoclasts are derived from pluripotent stem cells (CFU-GM) of the bone marrow that also give rise to monocytes and macrophages. Final differentiation to an osteoclast from a circulating monocyte occurs after the cells are recruited to bone resorption sites. At the end of their cell lifespan, osteoclasts undergo apoptosis.

Bone Matrix

The matrix of bone is composed of osteoid produced by the osteoblasts. Mineralization of the osteoid occurs as hydroxyapatite crystals are deposited in the osteoid framework.

The organic intercellular substance of bone contains sulfated glycosaminoglycans, glycoproteins, and collagen. Glycoproteins of bone include alkaline phosphatase, osteonectin, osteopontin, and sialoprotein. These glycoproteins are thought to play various roles in bone mineralization. Another noncollagenous protein, osteocalcin, regulates the activity of osteoclasts.

Type I collagen predominates in bone matrix with traces of types III, V, and X. The collagen fibrils in each osteonal lamella course in a spiral direction with respect to the long axis of the central canal. In addition to their spiral orientation, the collagen fibrils alternate at right angles to those in each adjacent lamella. This arrangement imparts considerable strength to each osteon.

The inorganic component of bone consists of submicroscopic hydroxyapatite crystals deposited as slender needles within the collagen fibril network. Such an efficient arrangement enhances the tensile strength that is characteristic of bone. The principal ions in bone salt are Ca, CO_3, PO_4, and OH, and the amounts of Na, Mg, and Fe are substantial. Bone, then, is a major storehouse for calcium and phosphorus, which are mobilized whenever they are needed.

Structural and Functional Characteristics

Adult bone is distinguished from cartilage by the presence of both a canalicular system and a direct vascular supply. The growth process of bone also differs from that of cartilage.

Adult cartilage depends entirely on diffusion for nourishment; bone, however, has a unique lacunar–canalicular system for supplying the bone cells with metabolites in a mineralized matrix in which diffusion is not an option (Figs. 3-27 and 3-28). Canaliculi extend from one lacuna to another and to the bone surface, where they open into the connective tissue surrounding the capillaries. The canalicular system provides a conduit system for nourishment of the mature osteocytes located deep in the bone, and the extensive capillary supply of bone further enhances the efficiency of the canalicular system.

Unlike cartilage, bone grows by apposition only. Because the intercellular substance mineralizes so rapidly, interstitial growth of bone is not possible. Therefore, bone changes shape and increases or decreases in size by adding layers to or removing layers from one or more of its existing surfaces.

Macroscopic structure

An adult long bone (e.g., humerus) consists of enlarged ends (**epiphyses**) connected by a hollow cylindrical shaft (**diaphysis**) (Fig. 3-29). The ends of the epiphyses are covered by a thin layer of hyaline cartilage known as the **articular cartilage,** whereas the remainder of the external surface of the bone is covered by a vascular fibrous membrane, the **periosteum** (Figs. 3-27 and 3-30). Each region of the bone is composed of lamellar bone, but it is arranged differently to best perform its biomechanical function. The epiphyses have a thin shell of dense bone (subchondral bone) under the articular cartilage. A network of **trabeculae** forms **spongy bone,** which extends from the subchondral bone to form the center of the bone. The wall of the diaphysis is composed of **compact bone,** which contains osteons. The inner (medullary) cavity of bone is lined by **endosteum** and contains adipose tissue or red (hemopoietic) or yellow (adipose) bone marrow, depending on the age of the animal or the region of the bone.

In the growing animal, the diaphysis and epiphysis are separated by the **physeal–metaphyseal** region (Fig. 3-31). This region consists of a specialized hyaline cartilage plate, the **physis** and the **metaphysis,** a region of trabecular bone underlying the physis. The physis, also referred to as the cartilaginous growth plate, is responsible for growth in length of the animal's bones. During the growth process, temporary trabeculae with cartilaginous cores are formed in the metaphysis and later modeled to permanent bony trabeculae (Figs. 3-29 and 3-31). Upon cessation of growth, the cartilage cells of the physis stop proliferating, but bone formation on the metaphyseal side of the physis continues. A transverse, perforated plate of bone (epiphyseal scar) takes the place of the physis in the skeletally mature animal. The epiphyseal scar may be visible on radiographs as the epiphyseal line.

Histologic preparation

Because of its dense mineral deposits, bone is difficult to section and process for histologic procedures. Decalcification before histologic processing removes the mineral from the bone, leaving behind the organic matrix and the bone cells for study (Fig. 3-32). If examination of osseous mineral content is required, undecalcified sections can be prepared using special techniques (Fig. 3-28).

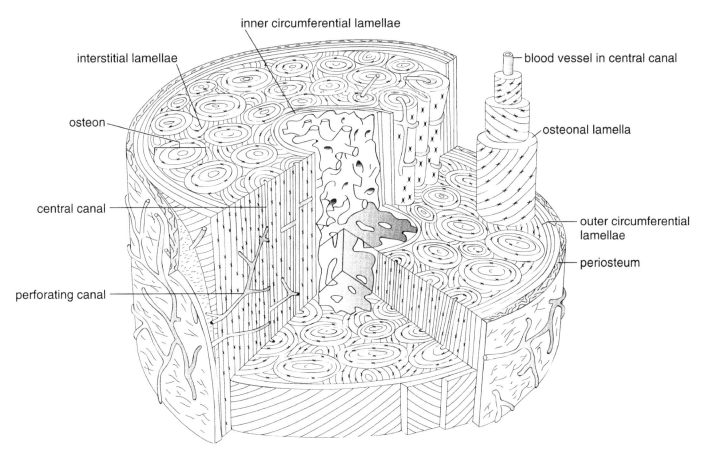

FIGURE 3-27 The structural unit of compact bone is the cylindrical osteon. In this drawing, an osteon is telescoped to show the concentric osteonal lamellae that surround the central canal. Blood vessels reach the central canal through perforating canals from either the periosteal or endosteal surface. The space between adjacent osteons is filled by interstitial lamellae, and inner and outer circumferential lamellae form the surfaces of compact bone.

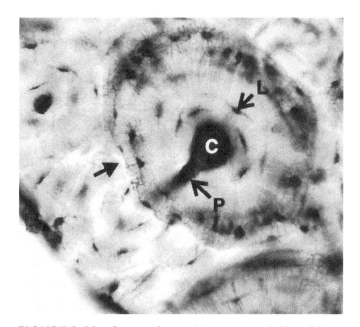

FIGURE 3-28 Osteon of ground bone surrounded by a light cement line (solid arrow). The central canal (C) carries blood vessels, lymphatics, and nerves, and branches into a transverse perforating canal (P). Lacunae (L) are located between lamellae of compact bone that surround the central canal. Fine canaliculi extend from each lacuna. Unstained (×230).

Microscopic structure

The outermost layers of the shaft of a long bone consist of compact bone arranged as **outer circumferential lamellae** (2 to 8 μm thick). Deep to the outer circumferential lamellae are **osteons** (Haversian systems) formed by concentric lamellae surrounding longitudinally oriented vascular channels (**central canals**) (Fig. 3-27). Internal surfaces of compact bone from adult animals are composed of **inner circumferential lamellae** encircling the medullary cavity.

Lacunae are located between each lamella of the compact bone (Fig. 3-28). Radiating from the lacunae are the branching **canaliculi** that penetrate and join canaliculi of adjacent lamellae. Thus, the lacunae and canaliculi form an extensive system of interconnecting passageways for the transport of nutrients.

The **central canal** (Haversian canal) of each osteon contains capillaries, lymphatic vessels, and nonmyelinated nerve fibers, all supported by reticular connective tissue. Central canals are connected with each other and with the free surface by transverse or horizontal channels called **perforating canals** (Volkmann's canals) (Figs. 3-27 and 3-28).

Most bones are invested with a tough connective tissue layer, the **periosteum** (Figs. 3-27 and 3-30). It has two layers: an inner **osteogenic layer** that provides cells necessary to form bone and an outer **fibrous layer** made of irregularly arranged

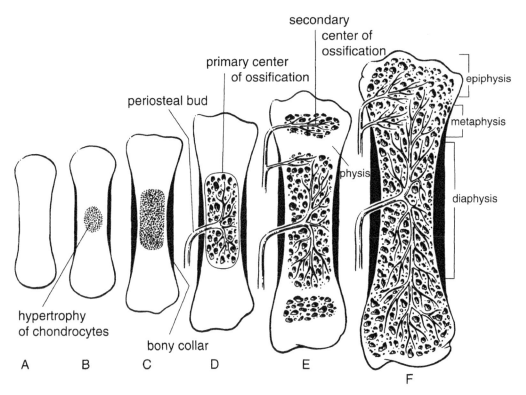

FIGURE 3-29 The stages of endochondral ossification of a long bone. **A.** A hyaline cartilage model forms initially. **B.** The chondrocytes in the center of the model hypertrophy. **C.** A bony collar begins to form around the cartilage model. **D.** Blood vessels from the periosteum (periosteal bud) invade the cartilage model, bringing bone-forming cells to initiate the primary center of ossification. **E.** The physis (growth plate) and secondary centers of ossification are established. **F.** The physis closes in the mature bone and a confluent marrow cavity from the epiphysis to the diaphysis is formed.

collagen fibers and blood vessels. The vessels branch and enter the perforating canals and ultimately reach the central canal of the osteons. The cellular layer is more evident in young animals than in adults. The periosteum is attached firmly to the bone by bundles of coarse collagen fibers that have been incorporated into the outer circumferential lamellae of the bone. These fibers are called **perforating (Sharpey's) fibers** (Fig. 3-30). A periosteum is absent over the surface of hyaline articular cartilage and at sites where tendons and ligaments insert on bones.

The marrow cavity and central and perforating canals are lined with a layer of squamous bone-lining cells, osteoblasts, and osteoclasts called the **endosteum.** Some cells of the endosteum send processes into canaliculi to join those of nearby osteocytes. Recently, the possibility has been suggested that these cells form an ion barrier so that the fluid flowing through the lacunae and canaliculi is separated from the interstitial fluid. In addition, endosteal cells may play a role in mineral homeostasis by regulating the flow of calcium and phosphate into and out of bone fluids, thus maintaining an optimum microenvironment for the growth of bone crystals.

Osteogenesis

Bone is formed by a two-step process. First, osteoid is deposited by osteoblasts, followed by mineralization of the osteoid several days later. Two theories exist for the initiation of bone mineral-

ization. The **nucleation theory** proposes that the hole regions of type I collagen fibrils serve as the major site of calcium phosphate crystal deposition. A second theory describes **matrix vesicles,** which are membrane-bounded structures that form along the osteoblast membrane. The vesicles contain lipid, accumulated calcium ions, and alkaline phosphatase, all of which are required to initiate and maintain the process of mineralization.

Bone is classified by the arrangement of collagen fibrils in the matrix (woven versus lamellar bone) or by the type of precursor connective tissue (intramembranous versus endochondral ossification).

Woven bone has collagen fibrils that are arranged in an irregular anastomosing fashion (Fig. 3-32), whereas **lamellar bone** has a more organized matrix, which is deposited in layers (Fig. 3-28). Woven bone is formed rapidly and is considered to be an immature form of bone; it is usually replaced by lamellar bone. Woven bone is found in developing bone, fracture repair sites, and certain bone tumors. Calcified cartilage and woven bone seem to mineralize in association with matrix vesicles, while the mineralization of lamellar bone appears to follow the nucleation theory.

Regardless of the site, bone develops by a process of transformation from an existing connective tissue. The two different types of bone development depend on specific cells differentiating within two different microenvironments. When bone forms directly from connective tissue, the process is termed **intramem-**

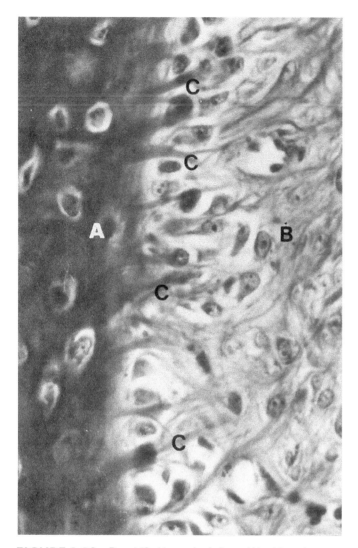

FIGURE 3-30 Decalcified bone (cat). Bone (A) with periosteum (B) attached by perforating fibers (C). Hematoxylin and eosin (×500). *(Courtesy of A. Hansen.)*

branous ossification (Fig. 3-32). This term arose because the soft tissue located where bone will form is arranged in a layer and, hence, is membranous. The process of bone formation in pre-existing cartilage models is termed **endochondral** or **intracartilaginous ossification** (Fig. 3-33). During this process, calcified cartilage is replaced by bone. The terms intramembranous and endochondral indicate the type of microenvironment in which the bone forms, rather than the type of adult bone. For example, both intramembranous and endochondral bone formation can give rise to spongy bone in the adult.

Intramembranous ossification

The process of intramembranous ossification takes place within well-vascularized connective tissue, such as that found in the diploë of the developing calvaria of the skull. Osteoprogenitor cells differentiate into osteoblasts. These cells begin to synthesize and secrete osteoid. The first secreted component of osteoid is collagen, and the remaining constituents of the ground substance are produced somewhat later. During early intramembra-

nous osteogenesis, osteoblasts become surrounded by a partially mineralized matrix containing visible collagen fibrils (Fig. 3-32). Gradually, more osteoid is produced, followed by complete mineralization. As a result, some osteoblasts become trapped within their lacunae and become osteocytes. These small, isolated pieces of developing bone within the connective tissue are called the **centers of ossification,** which ultimately radiate in several directions to form trabeculae (Fig. 3-25). Such bone is called **trabecular, spongy,** or **cancellous** bone.

The bony trabeculae increase in width and length by the addition of new lamellae, forming a primary spongiosa of trabecular bone. In areas of the spongiosa where compact bone forms, the mesenchymal space between trabeculae fills with osseous tissue except for a central canal containing the vasculature of the new osteon. In regions where spongy bone persists, the mesenchymal soft tissue located between trabeculae becomes bone marrow.

Endochondral ossification

Bones of the extremities, vertebral column, pelvis, and base of the skull are formed initially as hyaline cartilage models that are replaced by bone in the developing embryo.

Primary Center of Ossification. As the cartilage model grows both in width and in length, it reaches a stage when most of the remaining growth occurs at the ends of the model. The chondrocytes in the midsection mature and enlarge, so that the matrix between the hypertrophied cells becomes extremely thin (Fig. 3-33). At the same time, these chondrocytes release matrix vesicles, similar to those of osteoblasts, that promote calcification of the surrounding cartilage matrix. This calcification prevents the hypertrophied chondrocytes from receiving adequate nutrition and results in their degeneration and death.

In the meantime, the perichondrium is invaded by numerous capillaries. This event changes the microenvironment of the chondrogenic layer to one that favors osteogenesis on the surface of the cartilage model. The osteoprogenitor cells of this layer differentiate into osteoblasts and form a thin shell of bone around the midsection of the cartilage model. This **periosteal band** or **bony collar** forms by intramembranous ossification, and the perichondrium becomes the periosteum. Blood vessels are essential in activating the osteogenic potential of the inner layer of the perichondrium, the cells of which retain the ability to differentiate into either chondroblasts or osteoblasts throughout their life. This ability is especially significant in fracture healing, during which cartilage forms in areas that are relatively devoid of capillaries, but endochondral ossification occurs as soon as capillaries grow into the area.

After the bony collar forms around the midsection of the model, blood vessels from the periosteum invade the area of the degenerating hypertrophied chondrocytes, thereby raising the oxygen level (Fig. 3-29 and 3-34). Osteoprogenitor cells from the periosteum, pericytes, and undifferentiated mesenchymal cells all accompany the invading capillaries. These blood vessels and their associated cells constitute the **periosteal bud.** When the periosteal bud reaches the interior of the midsection of the cartilage model, the **primary center of ossification** is established.

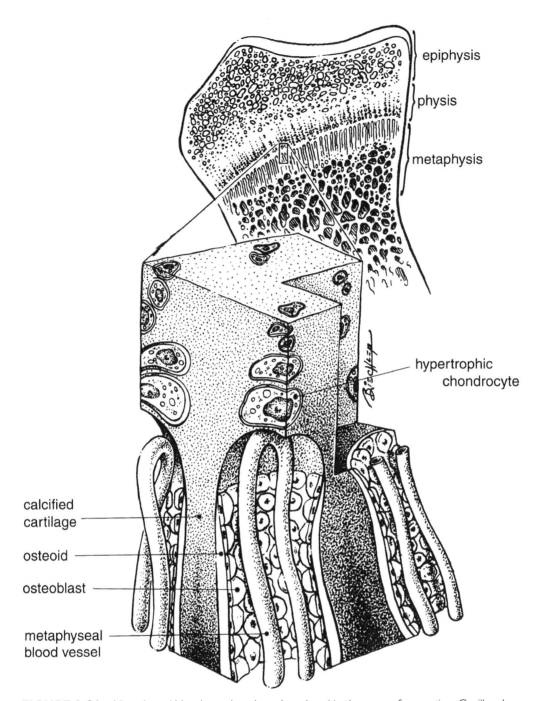

epiphysis

physis

metaphysis

hypertrophic
chondrocyte

calcified
cartilage

osteoid

osteoblast

metaphyseal
blood vessel

FIGURE 3-31 Metaphyseal blood vessels make a sharp bend in the zone of resorption. Capillary loops invade the lacunae of the degenerating hypertrophic chondrocytes. Osteoblasts form bone on the remnants of the calcified physeal cartilage.

Under the influence of inductive bone-forming factors in the blood plasma, the osteoprogenitor cells that accompany the capillaries differentiate into osteoblasts. These cells cluster around fragments of the calcified cartilage, begin to synthesize and secrete osteoid, and somewhat later contribute to the mineralization process. Such osteoblastic activity continues until bone trabeculae containing cores of calcified cartilage are formed.

While the primary center of ossification is forming, the cartilage at each end of the model continues to proliferate by interstitial growth, resulting in an increase in the length of the model. The bony collar surrounding the diaphysis continues to increase in thickness and length, hence the primitive bone in the primary center of ossification is no longer needed for support. Therefore, most of the bone in the primary center is resorbed by osteoclasts, thus forming the marrow cavity, which becomes filled with hemopoietic tissue developed from the undifferentiated mesenchymal cells brought in with the periosteal bud.

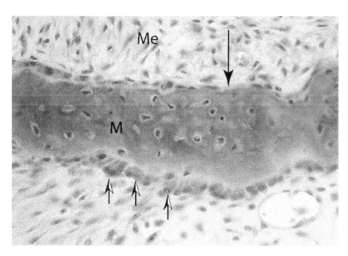

FIGURE 3-32 Intramembranous bone development. Bone is formed by osteoblasts (open arrows) surrounding the immature bone spicule (arrow). Irregularly arranged collagen fibrils are present in bony matrix (M); thus it is considered woven bone. Mesenchyme (Me) surrounds the forming bone. Hematoxylin and eosin (×600).

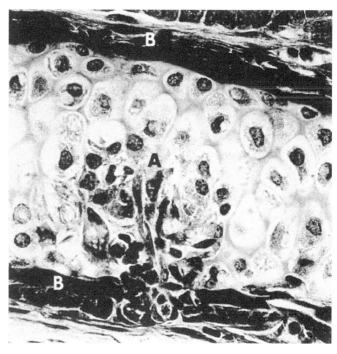

FIGURE 3-34 Primary center of ossification (cat). Periosteal bud (A) entering hypertrophied cartilage. Perichondrium (B). Crossman's trichrome (×570).

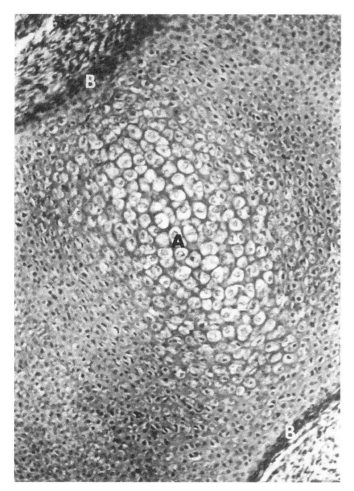

FIGURE 3-33 Endochondral ossification of a long bone (dog). Hypertrophied cartilage cells (A) are in the center of the model. Note the thin mineralized cartilage remnants between enlarged lacunae; perichondrium (B). Hematoxylin and eosin (×80).

Secondary Centers of Ossification. The cartilaginous epiphyses of the larger long bones develop additional centers of ossification referred to as **secondary centers** (Fig. 3-29). The epiphyseal cartilage of newborn animals is well supplied with **cartilage canals** containing arterioles, venules, and nonmyelinated nerve fibers, all surrounded by connective tissue (Fig. 3-35). These canals arise from the perichondrium and are evenly spaced throughout the epiphysis, providing nutrients to a given area. The blood vessels do not enter the physis or penetrate the future articular cartilage. The arterioles of these canals end in a capillary glomerulus, and the initial sites of ossification occur as multiple foci adjacent to the glomeruli. When ossification begins, the chondrocytes next to the glomerulus of the cartilage canal hypertrophy and degenerate, and the surrounding matrix calcifies. This process is followed by the appearance of circularly oriented layers of hypertrophic and dividing chondrocytes. Thus, this cellular arrangement resembles that of the growth zones in the physis. Because the connective tissue in the cartilage canals is continuous with the perichondrium, these cells have the same osteogenic potential for bone formation. Ultimately, these foci fuse into a single secondary center of ossification, forming spongy bone in the epiphysis.

Ossification does not replace all of the epiphyseal cartilage. Enough cartilage remains such that the epiphyseal portion serves as a template for enlarging the end of the bone, while the surface portion serves as the articular cartilage. A transverse plate of cartilage is left between the diaphysis and each epiphysis. In domestic animals, this physis persists until puberty, and then it too is replaced by bone.

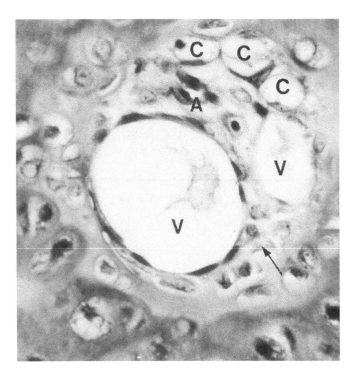

FIGURE 3-35 Cartilage canal in epiphysis of a 1-day-old puppy containing an arteriole (A), venules (V), and glomerular capillaries (C). Degenerating cartilage at arrow.

Growth in length

The physis and metaphysis function in bone growth in length and provide a scaffolding for constructing metaphyseal cancellous bone. Continued interstitial growth of the cartilage in the physis, involving chondrocytic hyperplasia, synthesis of proteoglycans, and chondrocyte hypertrophy, serves to lengthen the long bones.

Five distinct zones or regions are recognized in a longitudinal section through the physis (Fig. 3-36). From the epiphysis to the metaphysis, the following zones are present:

1. The **reserve zone** (resting zone) is adjacent to the bone and marrow cavity of the epiphysis (Fig. 3-37). Here, the small chondrocytes are dispersed in an irregular pattern and are nourished by epiphyseal blood vessels, which are arranged in glomeruli. Matrix vesicles, membrane-bounded structures similar to those produced by osteoblasts, are formed by chondrocytes in this zone, but matrix mineralization does not occur until deeper in the physis.

2. In the **zone of proliferation,** the chondrocytes are somewhat larger and form rows or columns parallel to the long axis of the developing bone (Fig. 3-37). New cells are produced through cell division at the top of the columns. The cells in the columns possess all the organelles necessary for synthesis of matrix, and each cell is separated from the cell in an adjacent lacuna by a layer of matrix.

3. As maturation progresses in the **zone of hypertrophy,** the cells increase in size and begin to accumulate calcium. The cellular calcium is released into the matrix of the deep hypertrophic zone and matrix vesicles begin calcium uptake. The action of alkaline phosphatase and neutral proteases re-

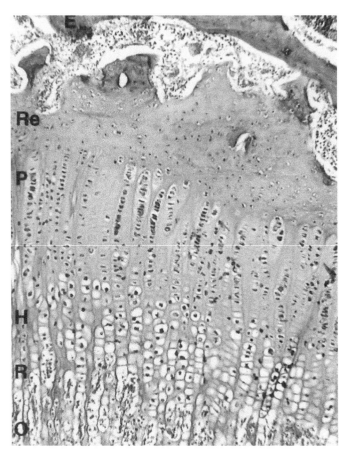

FIGURE 3-36 The physis is anchored to epiphyseal bone (E). Chondrocytes in the reserve zone (Re) are scattered in the matrix. In the zone of proliferation (P), chondrocytes are arranged in columns. The cells increase in size in the zone of hypertrophy (H). Metaphyseal capillaries enter the zone of resorption (R), and bone is formed on the cartilage remnants of the physis in the zone of ossification (O). Hematoxylin and eosin (×200).

leased from matrix vesicles causes a local increase of phosphate. Accumulation of calcium in the vesicles and the increase in phosphate leads to mineralization of the matrix, and the last two or three hypertrophied cells in the column are bordered by a wall of calcified matrix. Transverse septa between the cells do not calcify. Some of these hypertrophied cells become shrunken, and their pyknotic nucleus appears to attach to the transverse septum.

4. The metaphyseal capillaries make a sharp U-shaped bend in the **zone of resorption** and return to the medullary circulation (Figs. 3-31 and 3-38). Individual capillary loops and perivascular connective tissue invade the lacunae of the degenerating hypertrophic chondrocytes located at the base of the cell columns.

5. In the **zone of ossification,** osteoblasts differentiate from cells accompanying the invading capillaries. These cells deposit bone on the remains of the calcified walls of the chondrocytic lacunae. The resulting trabeculae of bone with calcified cartilage centers are known collectively as the **primary spongiosa** (Figs. 3-31 and 3-39).

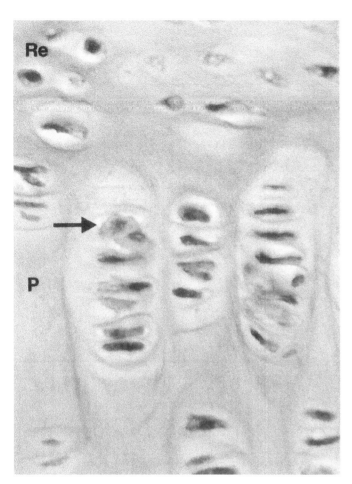

FIGURE 3-37 Chondrocytes of the reserve zone (Re) are scattered and spherical. New cells are produced at the top of the columns (arrow) in the zone of proliferation (P). Hematoxylin and eosin (×550).

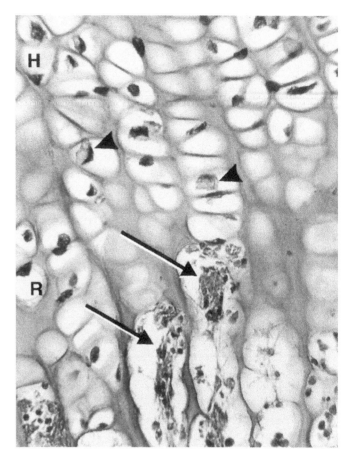

FIGURE 3-38 Hypertrophic chondrocytes (arrowheads) degenerate in the zone of hypertrophy (H) just above the zone of resorption (R). Metaphyseal blood vessels (arrows) invade the lacunae of the degenerating chondrocytes. Hematoxylin and eosin (×300).

The surface of many trabeculae of the primary spongiosa is covered with numerous osteoclasts for a short distance into the metaphysis. Precursors of these osteoclasts arrive with the invading metaphyseal vessels and differentiate into functional osteoclasts within the bone. The osteoclasts actively resorb bone from the surface of the trabeculae and reduce the number of trabeculae.

Because the cartilage cores of the trabeculae are continuous with the cartilaginous matrix of the physis, the new bony trabeculae are anchored firmly to the physis. In longitudinal sections through the growth plate, the bony trabeculae and their cartilage cores resemble separate stalks attached to the growth plate. In a cross section taken through the metaphyseal side of the physis, however, each trabecula is actually a wall between adjacent tubes filled with osteogenic cells and capillaries (Fig. 3-31).

Deeper in the metaphysis, trabeculae of the primary spongiosa decrease and trabeculae composed of lamellar bone predominate. Trabecular bone without cartilage cores is known as the **secondary spongiosa.**

Growth in width and circumference

The trabecular bone that formed in the original bony collar is converted to compact bone composed of primary osteons. Concurrent periosteal bone formation and endosteal bone resorption enlarge the marrow cavity and increase the width of the diaphysis. Because endosteal resorption lags behind periosteal production, the thickness of the shaft wall slowly enlarges as the circumference increases.

The outer surface of an actively growing bone is uneven, owing to numerous longitudinal ridges and grooves. Within these grooves, osteoblasts from the adherent periosteum deposit bone around the periosteal vessels. Eventually, the edges of the groove meet, forming a tube lined with osteogenic cells and enclosing the blood vessel derived from the periosteum. The osteogenic cells produce concentric layers of bone around the blood vessel within the new central canal. In this way, new **primary osteons** are added to the periphery of an actively growing young bone. Primary osteons comprising the cortical bone are gradually replaced with more orderly **secondary osteons.**

Primary osteons are smaller than secondary osteons, lack cement lines, and often have two or more blood vessels in their central canal. Secondary osteons are surrounded by basophilic **cement lines,** composed of mineralized matrix deficient in collagen (Fig. 3-28). Between the secondary osteons are many irregularly shaped groups of lamellae called **interstitial lamellae.**

Finally, the bone growth slows, and appositional growth in the subperiosteal and endosteal regions adds more layers, which

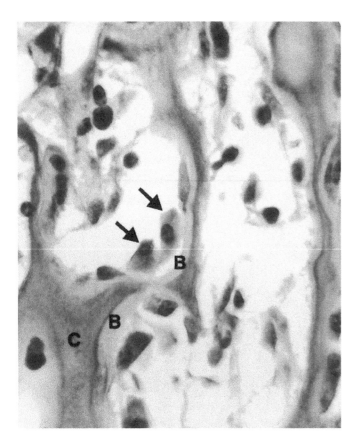

FIGURE 3-39   Osteoblasts (arrows) form bone (B) on darker staining calcified cartilage (C) in the zone of ossification. Hematoxylin and eosin (×475).

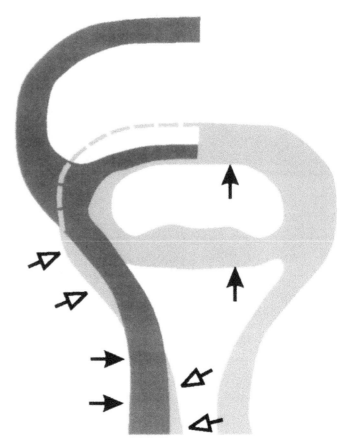

FIGURE 3-40   During growth, modeling occurs as new bone is added on the outer periosteal surface of the diaphysis and within the metaphysis and epiphysis (solid arrows). Bone is concurrently resorbed on both the endosteal and periosteal surfaces to shape the adult bone (open arrows).

smooth the surface. These layers are the inner and outer circumferential lamellae.

The important principle to note is that growth in length is the result of endochondral ossification, whereas growth in width is the result of intramembranous ossification. Each type of growth responds to different rules, and each can be affected separately without necessarily influencing the other.

Bone modeling

The changes in size and shape of bones during the growth process are called **modeling.** The concurrent action of bone resorption and formation on different surfaces of a bone alters the overall shape. The process of modeling continues over most of the skeleton until the adult shape of the bones is reached. Modeling is rapid and results in a net gain of bone in the body. Examples of modeling include the drifting of the diaphysis during growth, shaping of the metaphyseal funnel, and enlargement of the cranial vault.

In the diaphysis, bone formation occurs on the periosteal surface while bone is resorbed on the endosteal surface, resulting in a wider diaphysis and larger marrow cavity (Fig. 3-40). If the modeling process occurs in an eccentric fashion, the entire diaphysis may drift in a specific direction.

In contrast, the shaping of the metaphyseal region is accomplished by periosteal resorption on the external surface to narrow

the funnel shape in the direction of the diaphysis. Concurrent endosteal bone formation creates a thickened metaphyseal cortex.

Bone remodeling

Throughout life, bone is constantly being turned over. Early woven bone is of poorer quality than mature lamellar bone. In addition, as bone ages, the quality also diminishes. **Bone remodeling** is the process by which bone is constantly replaced.

In contrast to modeling, bone remodeling occurs in a cyclical fashion at a slower rate. The process generally does not alter the shape or size of the bone. Remodeling is coupled; it initiates and proceeds in only one way. First, activation of remodeling occurs, perhaps caused by a change in biomechanics. Osteoclastic bone resorption is then followed by osteoblastic bone formation. Balance between bone resorption and formation is important for healthy bone; however, bone resorption is often greater than bone formation, leading to net bone loss (e.g., osteoporosis related to aging).

Cortical bone is remodeled by **cortical remodeling units.** The unit, when viewed longitudinally, consists of a leading **cutting cone** composed of osteoclasts, which resorb compact bone without respect to osteonal barriers (Fig. 3-41). The cutting cone is followed by a **reversal zone,** in which resorption switches to

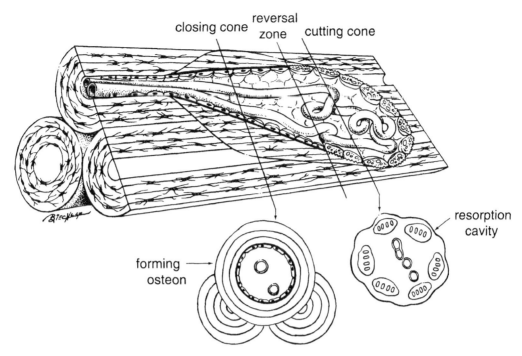

FIGURE 3-41   The remodeling unit of cortical bone is composed of a cutting cone of osteoclasts, which resorbs bone. Osteoclasts are followed by osteoblasts at the reversal zone and the osteoblasts of the closing cone fill in the resorption cavity to create a new osteon.

osteoblastic bone formation. The structure terminates as a **closing cone,** in which osteoblasts close the newly excavated osteon by adding centripetal layers of lamellar bone inward from the cement line boundary. The osteoclasts of the cutting cone are supported metabolically by a glomerulus, whereas the osteoblasts of the closing cone are within close diffusion distance from the blood vessel of the new central canal.

In spongy bone, remodeling is accomplished on the endosteal surface of the trabecula. Osteoclasts resorb bone from the surface of the trabecula. Osteoblasts then form new bone in either the same location where the resorption occurred or on the opposing surface of the trabecula. If bone is formed on the opposing surface, the alignment of the trabecula is changed in the direction of the bone formation.

Fracture repair

After a midshaft fracture of a bone, a certain sequence of events occurs during the healing process. Fracture repair involves changes in blood supply that affect cellular proliferation and differentiation as well as bone resorption.

The trauma that causes the bone to break also tears the adjacent soft tissues and blood vessels. The blood clot that forms at the fracture site stops circulation and results in necrosis or death of the surrounding tissue. Likewise, the interruption of the blood vessels within the osteons causes cessation of blood supply and death of the osteocytes on each side of the fracture site.

New tissue developing at the fracture site forms a bridge between the fragments. This formation is termed a **callus** and is composed of two parts. The **internal callus** develops between the opposing ends of the bone, and the **external callus** surrounds the outermost surface of the broken bone.

The cells involved in callus formation are osteogenic cells of the periosteum and endosteum. Early in the healing process, the cells of the periosteum proliferate to such an extent that the fibrous layer of the periosteum is lifted away from the bone. In addition, the endosteal cells proliferate, resulting in a thickened endosteum. The undifferentiated marrow cells increase in number in the same area. Differentiation of these cells takes place in one of two ways and depends on the vascular supply available. Those nearest to the bone fragments differentiate in the presence of blood vessels; consequently, they become osteoblasts and form bony trabeculae. Those farther away from the bone proliferate in an area relatively devoid of capillaries; consequently, they form chondroblasts, which produce cartilage in the external callus. The cartilage is a temporary splint that eventually is replaced by bone, following the same sequence of events that occurs in endochondral ossification. Gradually, the callus is remodeled by resorption of the trabeculae at the periphery, until the original outline of the bone is restored.

No external callus develops when a bone fracture has smooth, even, opposing surfaces that are perfectly aligned without any space between the fragments, and the fragments are held rigidly throughout the healing period. In this situation, dead bone extends for some distance on both sides of the fracture line. Osteogenic cells and capillaries in the living bone proliferate and grow into the adjacent dead bone. Simultaneously, osteoclasts invade the area and form cortical remodeling units that cross the fracture line. Resulting new osteons extend into the cortical bone on the other side of the fracture (primary osteosynthesis).

Fractures that are realigned in direct apposition but have a small space between the two fragments heal similarly, as long as rigid fixation is maintained. The only difference is that the two bone ends are joined initially by woven bone rather than by new osteons. Remodeling occurs as a secondary event.

JOINTS

Joints connect two or more bones. The various types of joints are classified according to the type of tissue that makes up the structure and the degree of movement permitted. As the result of aging, certain fibrous and cartilaginous joints may become **synostoses,** as the respective connective tissues are eventually replaced by bone.

Fibrous Joints

Bones held together by collagenous or elastic dense connective tissue are called **syndesmoses** or **sutures.** An example of a syndesmosis is the fibrous articulation between the radius and ulna. Sutures are typical of the skull.

Cartilaginous Joints

Joints in which the two bones are connected by cartilage are **synchondroses,** such as the physis. In the **symphysis** joint, the hyaline cartilage caps of adjacent bones are joined by thick fibrous bands. Between the hyaline cartilage and the collagen fibers is a transition zone of fibrocartilage. The pelvic symphysis is an example of this type of joint.

The intervertebral disk is a symphysis that consists of an outer lamellated **annulus fibrosus** and an inner dorsally eccentric cavity, which is filled with a gelatinous **nucleus pulposus** in young animals (Fig. 3-42). The nucleus becomes more rigid with age and may calcify in some breeds of dogs at approximately 5 years of age. The annulus is thicker ventrally than dorsally, and its fibers insert into a thin layer of hyaline cartilage covering the ends of adjacent vertebrae. The cells in the peripheral laminae of the annulus resemble fibrocytes, whereas the cells of the deeper lamellae are more representative of chondrocytes. The annulus is avascular and hence is sustained by diffusion from the vessels in the medullary cavity and periosteum of the vertebrae.

Synovial Joints

Synovial (diarthrodial) joints are characterized by the presence of articular cartilage on the opposing bony surfaces, a lubricating synovial fluid within the closed joint cavity, and a joint capsule enclosing the entire joint (Fig. 3-43).

The articulating surfaces of synovial joints are covered by a specialized complex, the **articular cartilage,** which consists of hyaline cartilage, tidemark, and calcified cartilage (Fig. 3-44). The hyaline cartilage segment is devoid of perichondrium and can be divided into three zones based on the morphology of the

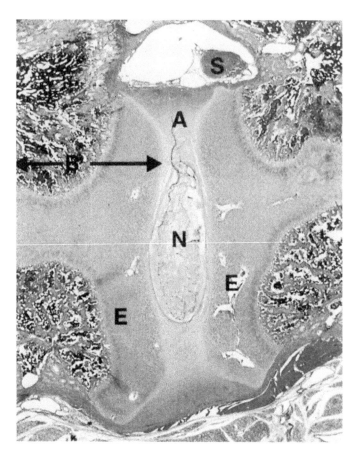

FIGURE 3-42 Vertebral column, longitudinal section (puppy). The central nucleus pulposus (N) of the intervertebral disk is surrounded by the annulus fibrosus (A). The disk attaches to the cartilaginous end plates (E) of the vertebral bodies (B). A spinal nerve (S) exits from the spinal cord through the intervertebral foramen above the disk. Hematoxylin and eosin (×8).

chondrocytes and the arrangement of the type II collagen fibrils in the matrix: (1) the **superficial zone** has flat cells that lie among layers of collagen fibrils oriented parallel to the surface; (2) the **middle zone** has larger, more spherical cells, displays a random arrangement of collagen fibrils, and stains the most intensely of all zones for GAGs; and (3) the **deep zone** has cells that are arranged perpendicular to the articular surface between columns of collagen fibrils. These fibrils are anchored into the calcified cartilage, which forms the deepest layer of articular cartilage. The calcified cartilage is joined to underlying subchondral bone by simple adherence without traversing collagen fibrils. Although uncalcified articular cartilage (superficial, middle, and upper deep zone) may vary in thickness during life, the thickness of the calcified cartilage layer remains constant.

The **tidemark** is a thin layer of clusters of mineral, glycoproteins, and lipids located between the calcified and uncalcified layers of the deep zone. In decalcified sections, the tidemark stains with hematoxylin. Multiple tidemarks may be present in older animals and indicate that mineralization of the cartilage was interrupted and then resumed several times. This contrasting interface between calcified and uncalcified tissues is prone to fracture.

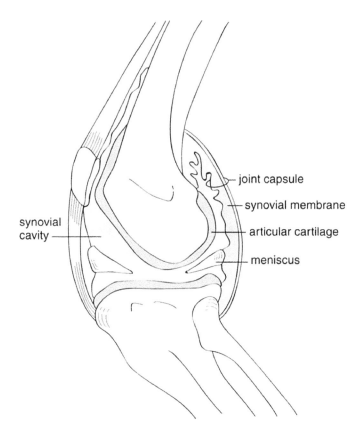

FIGURE 3-43 Articular cartilage covers the opposing bony surfaces of a synovial joint as shown in this diagram of a stifle. The joint space is filled with synovial fluid produced by the synovial membrane of the surrounding joint capsule. A meniscus composed of fibrocartilage extends into the joint cavity.

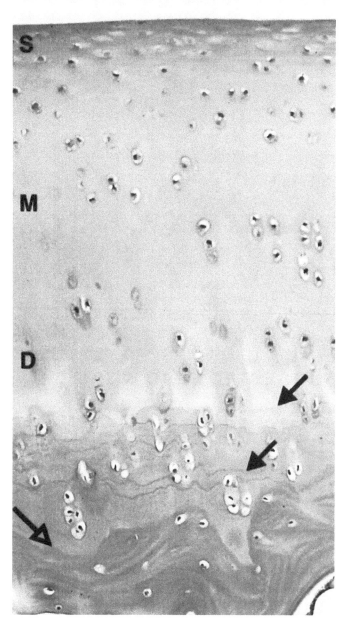

FIGURE 3-44 Articular cartilage zones: superficial (S), middle (M), and deep (D). Multiple tidemarks (closed arrows) are present in the calcified cartilage region. The junction of the articular cartilage with the subchondral bone is indicated by the open arrow. Hematoxylin and eosin (×290).

The highly anionic GAGs (e.g., chondroitin sulfate and keratan sulfate to a lesser degree) of articular cartilage normally bind water, which is released upon compression of the cartilage. Conversely, when the compression is released, the water is absorbed into the matrix and rebinds with the GAGs. This process provides a "weeping" lubrication of the articular surfaces, as well as a circulation of nutrients to and waste products from the articular chondrocytes. This fluid circulation is important since the articular cartilage is avascular and alymphatic.

The joint capsule encloses the entire joint and comprises an inner **synovial membrane** and outer **fibrous layer** (Fig. 3-45A). The synovial membrane, in turn, is composed of synovial cells and subcellular connective tissue, which may be loose (Fig. 3-45B), fibrous, or adipose. The predominating type of connective tissue in the synovial membrane varies with the location in the joint and classifies the type of synovial membrane. The outer fibrous layer is composed of dense irregular connective tissue and is continuous with the periosteum of adjacent bones.

The synovial cavity is filled with **synovial fluid**, which has a composition similar to plasma. This fluid is derived as an ultrafiltrate of the blood with the addition of a substantial amount of polymerized hyaluron from synovial cells. Synovial fluid provides the lubrication for the articulating surfaces of joints.

Some synovial joints (stifle) have intraarticular **menisci** composed of fibrocartilage (Fig. 3-43). Usually, menisci are anchored on one side to the fibrous layer of the joint capsule. If the cartilages are removed after traumatic injury, a new structure can develop from the fibrous layer of the capsule; however, it is composed of dense collagen rather than fibrocartilage. These structures are important to the biomechanics of the joint, and the ends (horns) are heavily innervated with proprioceptive nerves.

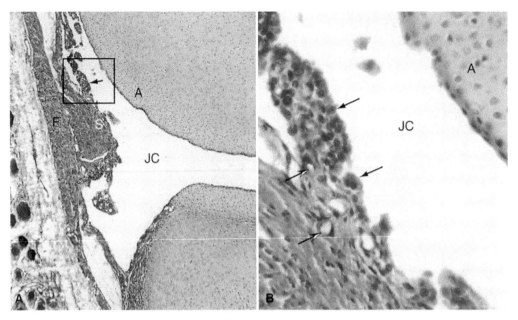

FIGURE 3-45 Phalangeal joint (dog). **A.** The articular cartilage (A) is developing adjacent to the joint cavity (JC). The synovial membrane (S) has synovial villi (arrow) and the fibrous layer (F) of the joint capsule is dense connective tissue (×100). **B.** Area outlined by rectangle in A. Synovial cells (closed arrows) rest on connective tissue containing numerous capillaries (open arrows). Hematoxylin and eosin (×800).

SUGGESTED READINGS

Alberts B, Bray D, Lewis J, et al. Molecular Biology of the Cell. 3rd Ed. New York: Garland Publishing, 1994.

Anderson C. Manual for the Examination of Bone. Boca Raton, FL: CRC Press, 1982.

Cheville NF. Cell Pathology. 2nd Ed. Ames, IA: Iowa State University Press, 1983.

Everts V, Van der Zee E, Creemers L, et al. Phagocytosis and intracellular digestion of collagen, its role in turnover and remodeling. Histochem J 1996;28(4):229–245.

Freeman MAR, ed. Adult Articular Cartilage. New York: Grune and Stratton, 1972.

Frost HM. Intermediary Organization of the Skeleton. Boca Raton, FL: CRC Press, 1986;I, II.

Ghosh P, ed. The Biology of the Intervertebral Disc. Boca Raton, FL: CRC Press, 1988;I, II.

Göthlin G, Ericsson JLE. The osteoclast. Clin Orthop 1976;120:201.

Hall BK, ed. Cartilage. San Diego: Academic Press, 1983;I, II.

Hirschi KK, D'Amore, PA. Pericytes in the microvasculature. Cardiovasc Res 1996:32:687–698.

Ibbotson KJ, D'Souza SM, Kanis JA, et al. Physiological and pharmacological regulation of bone resorption. Metab Bone Dis Rel Res 1981;2(3):177–189.

Jee WSS. The skeletal tissues. In: Weiss L, ed. Histology, Cell and Tissue Biology. 6th Ed. New York: Elsevier Biomedical, 1988:213.

Jee WSS, Parfitt AM, eds. Bone Histomorphometry. Paris: Societe Nouvelle de Publications Medicales et Dentaires, 1981.

Kimmel DB, Jee WSS. Bone cell kinetics during longitudinal bone growth in the rat. Calcif Tissue Int 1980;32:123–133.

Kincaid SA, Van Sickle DC. Bone morphology and postnatal osteogenesis—potential for disease. In: Alexander JW, Roberts RE, eds. Symposium on Orthopedic Diseases. Philadelphia: WB Saunders, 1983;13(1):3.

Kuettner KE, Schleyerbach R, Hascall VC, eds. Articular Cartilage Biochemistry. New York: Raven Press, 1986.

Malluche HH, Faugere M-C. Atlas of Mineralized Bone Histology. New York: S. Karger, 1986.

Piez KA, Reddi AH, eds. Extracellular Matrix Biochemistry. New York: Elsevier Biomedical, 1984.

Reddi AH, ed. Extracellular matrix: structure and function. In: UCLA Symposia on Molecular and Cellular Biology. New York: Alan R. Liss, 1985;25:1.

Ruggeri A, Motta PM, eds. Ultrastructure of the Connective Tissue Matrix. Boston: M. Nijhoff, 1984.

Scott MA, Stockham SL. Basophils and mast cells. In: Feldman BF, Zinkl JG, Jain NC, eds. Schalm's Veterinary Hematology. Philadelphia: Lippincott, Williams and Wilkins, 2000.

Simon SR, ed. Orthopaedic Basic Science. Chicago: American Academy of Orthopaedic Surgeons, 1994.

Stockwell RA. Biology of Cartilage Cells. Cambridge: Cambridge University Press, 1979.

Talmage RV. Morphological and physiological consideration in a new concept of calcium transport of bone. Am J Anat 1970;129:467–476.

Tizard IR. Veterinary Immunology. 5th Ed. Philadelphia: WB Saunders, 1996.

Urist MR, ed. Fundamental and Clinical Bone Physiology. Philadelphia: JB Lippincott, 1980.

Van Sickle DC, Kincaid SA. Comparative arthrology. In: Sokoloff L, ed. The Joints and Synovial Fluid. New York: Academic Press, 1979;I:1.

Weiss L, Sakai H. The hemopoietic stroma. Am J Anat 1984;170:447–463.

Wilsman NJ, Van Sickle DC. Cartilage canals, their morphology and distribution. Anat Rec 1972;173:79–93.

Woo SL-Y, Buckwalter JA, eds. Injury and Repair of the Musculoskeletal Soft Tissues. Park Ridge: AAOS, 1988.

4

Blood and Bone Marrow

JOANNE MESSICK

Blood
  Plasma
  Erythrocytes
  Leukocytes
    Neutrophil
    Eosinophil
    Basophil
    Monocyte
    Lymphocyte
  Platelets/Thrombocytes
Bone Marrow
  Structure and Function
  Hematopoiesis

  Hematopoietic stem cells
  Cytokines and regulation of hematopoiesis
Granulopoiesis
  Neutrophilic precursors
  Eosinophilic and basophilic granulocytes and mast cells
Monocytopoiesis
Erythropoiesis and Erythroid Precursors
Thrombopoiesis and Platelet Precursors
Lymphopoiesis and Lymphoid Precursors
Other Cells in Bone Marrow

BLOOD

The blood consists of specialized cells derived from the bone marrow that are suspended in a liquid called plasma. In an adult animal, the blood volume is about 8 to 10% of the body weight or approximately 40 mL of blood for each lb. of body weight. Thus, the total blood volume in a 1000-lb. horse is estimated at 40 L, whereas that of a 10-lb. dog or cat is only about 400 mL. Blood volume of some laboratory animals such as mice may be as low as 6% of body weight. The plasma component represents 55% of the blood volume, with the formed or cellular elements (red blood cells, leukocytes, and platelets) making up the remaining 45%.

The blood has several important functions. First, the hemoglobin contained within red blood cells carries oxygen to the tissues and collects carbon dioxide to facilitate its removal. Blood also conveys nutrients such as amino acids, sugars, and minerals to the tissues, and it is a conduit for byproducts and toxic substances that may be removed by the liver and kidney. Hormones, enzymes, and vitamins make their way to tissue targets by means of the blood. As a result of the phagocytic activity of leukocytes, the killing potential of their granules, and the humoral and cell-mediated immune responses mounted by lymphocytes, the blood provides a defense system for the animal. Finally, the platelets are tiny cellular elements that play a major role in hemostasis, preventing the entire blood volume from being lost during hemorrhage. When blood is freshly drawn into a test tube without anticoagulants, platelets and coagulation factors in the fluid portion are responsible for the formation of a clot.

Plasma

The addition of an anticoagulant such as ethylenediaminetetraacetic acid (EDTA) to a test tube of freshly drawn blood will prevent the formation of a clot. The **plasma,** or fluid portion of the blood, can be separated from its cellular components by centrifugation, resulting in plasma at the top of the centrifuged blood, the buffy coat in the middle, and the red cell mass at the bottom of the tube (Fig. 4-1). The plasma is colorless to lightly yellow depending on the animal species, and is a slightly alkaline fluid consisting of approximately 92% water and 8% solids

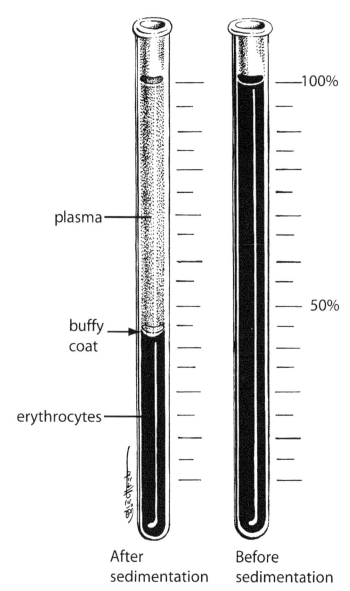

plasma

buffy coat

erythrocytes

—100%

— 50%

After sedimentation

Before sedimentation

FIGURE 4-1 Blood before and after sedimentation. The volume of packed erythrocytes is almost 45% of the total blood volume. The leukocytes and platelets form a buffy coat, accounting for approximately 1% of the blood volume. The remainder of the blood is the supernatant plasma.

or dry matter. About 90% of dry matter is organic substances such as glucose, lipids (cholesterol, triglycerides, phospholipids, lecithin, and fats), proteins (albumin, globulins, fibrinogen, and others), glycoproteins, hormones, amino acids, and vitamins. The inorganic or mineral portion of the dry matter of plasma is dissolved in ionic forms that can dissociate into positive and negative ions.

The cellular elements of blood form distinct layers following centrifugation. The lowest layer is red in color and represents about 45% of the blood volume. This layer consists of erythrocytes and represents the **packed cell volume** (PCV) or hematocrit. The PCV is a measure (%) of the volume of erythrocytes relative to the total volume of whole blood in a sample. The **buffy coat** is an off-white layer identified on top of the packed red cells. In the normal patient, the buffy coat accounts for about 1% of the

total blood volume and consists of platelets and leukocytes. The **platelet layer** is whiter and is located at the top of the buffy coat. This layer can be distinguished from the leukocyte layer, which is below and slightly pink due to an admixture with erythrocytes of low specific gravity, including reticulocytes. Although the numbers of leukocytes and platelets vary in domestic animals, 8000 to 12,000 leukocytes/µL of blood and 200,000 to 400,000 platelets/µL of blood are usual.

Erythrocytes

In general, the size of an **erythrocyte,** or red blood cell, in domestic animal species ranges from 3 to 7 µm. The red blood cells of the dog are largest at about 7 µm in size, whereas those of sheep and goats are only 4.5 µm and 3.2 µm, respectively. The shape of the erythrocyte and presence of a nucleus varies among animal species. Although mammalian red cells are reported to have a biconcave disk shape that results in a slight central pallor visible with light microscopy, this feature is only easily seen in the red blood cells of the dog (Fig. 4-2). The erythrocytes of family camellidae, including camels, llamas, and alpacas, have a characteristic oval shape. Red blood cells of amphibians, reptiles, and birds are also oval and, unlike mammalian cells, retain a nucleus in maturity. Fragments of the nucleus, or **Howell-Jolly bodies,** are normally seen in a few circulating red cells of the horse and cat. An increased number of circulating red cells with nuclei or Howell-Jolly bodies in other animal species may suggest that splenic function is abnormal or that the animal may have been splenectomized.

Red blood cells are rich in **hemoglobin,** a protein capable of binding oxygen and transporting it to the tissues. The lack of a nucleus allows more room for hemoglobin, and the biconcave shape of the red blood cell helps increase its oxygen-carrying capacity. The latter is likely related to increased surface area.

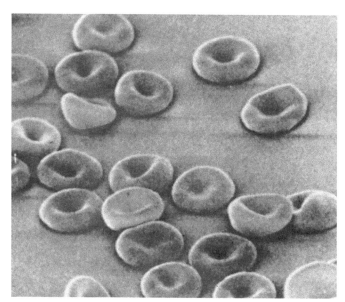

FIGURE 4-2 Scanning electron micrograph of erythrocytes from a clinically normal dog. The erythrocytes are biconcave disks. *(From Jain NC. Schalm's Veterinary Hematology. 4th Ed. Philadelphia: Lea & Febiger, 1983.)*

Erythrocytes are the most numerous of the formed elements in the blood. About 5 to 10 million red blood cells are typically present in every μL of blood in a healthy adult animal. In contrast, the number of red blood cells may be as high as 12 to 15 million/μL of blood in sheep and goats.

A few young **polychromatophilic red blood cells** (reticulocytes) are normally found in peripheral blood smears of dogs. In contrast, these cells are normally absent from the blood of horses and cows. The reticulocyte is slightly more bluish than the mature red blood cell in a Wright-Giemsa-stained blood smear, due to the presence of residual ribonucleic acid (RNA). The ribosomes, polyribosomes, and mitochondria retained in these cells are aggregated into a reticular mesh when stained with vital stains such as new methylene blue. The enumeration of reticulocyte numbers in the peripheral blood is used as an indication of bone marrow erythropoietic activity.

The lifespan of the red blood cells in circulation is variable in veterinary species. In mice, the lifespan of red blood cells is about 30 days, whereas the red blood cells of the cat and dog are reported to survive 68 days and 110 days, respectively. A longer lifespan has been reported in adult goats, cows, and horses, approaching 125 days, 145 days, and 160 days, respectively. The loss of these cells is continually balanced by the release of reticulocytes and mature red blood cells from the bone marrow.

A slight variation in the size of red blood cells, or **anisocytosis,** is a common finding in a peripheral blood smear. Although the presence of **poikilocytosis,** or variation in shape of red blood cells, is a normal finding in goats and sheep, it is uncommon in other animal species. **Crenated red blood cells,** which have numerous short, evenly spaced, blunt or sharp projections, are also a common finding. These changes are usually artifact, but may occur in animals with lymphoma and in patients that are uremic. **Rouleau formation,** or aggregates of red blood cells resembling "stacked coins," is a common finding in the blood smear of the horse. In the dog and cat, the presence of rouleau may suggest that certain total protein concentrations, such as immune globulins or fibrinogen, are increased. **Agglutination,** or irregular clumping of red blood cells rather than "coinlike" stacking, is abnormal and must be distinguished from rouleau formation.

Leukocytes

The blood leukocytes are divided into two categories: granulocytes and agranulocytes. The term **granulocyte** relates to the presence of specific granules in the cytoplasm of these cells, which can be used to differentiate the neutrophil, eosinophil, and basophil. The differing affinity of the granules for neutral, acidic, and basic stains gives them their characteristic color. **Agranulocytes** lack distinctive granules.

Neutrophil

Neutrophils are produced in the bone marrow and released into the blood once they mature. The mature neutrophil is approximately 12 to 15 μm in diameter and is distinguished by a segmented nucleus, often comprised of three to four lobes containing clumped or heterochromatic chromatin (Plate 4-1). Granules of

the neutrophil contain many hydrolytic enzymes and antibacterial substances needed to inactivate and digest phagocytosed microorganisms. The cell cytoplasm is rather transparent because the granules are small and neutral-staining in most mammalian neutrophils. In contrast, the cytoplasmic granules of the neutrophil in rabbits, guinea pigs, birds, amphibians, and reptiles are large and red, and the cell is called a **heterophil** (Plate 4-10).

Electron microscopic and cytochemical studies have revealed that neutrophils contain an active Golgi complex but few mitochondria. The cytoplasmic granules of the neutrophil vary in size and peroxidase activity. **Primary granules** (azurophilic granules) are larger and peroxidase-positive, whereas **secondary granules** (specific granules) are smaller and lack peroxidase activity (Fig. 4-3). The primary granules are membrane-bounded and contain enzymes such as acid hydrolases, neutral proteases, and elastase. Microbicidal elements, including myeloperoxidase, lysozyme, defensins, and bactericidal permeability–inducing protein, are also contained in primary granules. Interspecies variation in the cytochemical reactivity and content of the primary granules has been reported. The secondary (specific) granules of the neutrophil contain enzymes such as alkaline phosphatase, collagenase, and C5a splitting enzymes. Neutrophils also possess oxygen-dependent and oxygen-independent systems for destroying internalized microorganisms within their secondary granules. These antimicrobial elements include cationic proteins and enzymes such as hydrolases, proteases, lactoferrin, lysozyme, and defensins as well as enzymes that generate toxic metabolites of oxygen.

In most species, neutrophils are the most numerous of the circulating white cells, accounting for 40 to 80% of the total white cell numbers in most animal species. They function as the body's first line of defense against microbial infections.

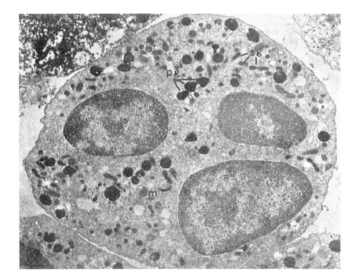

FIGURE 4-3 Electron micrograph of a mature neutrophil from canine bone marrow stained for peroxidase. The neutrophil contains large, spherical, peroxidase-positive primary granules (pg) and small, pleomorphic, peroxidase-negative secondary granules (sg). Some mitochondria (m) are present. The nuclear lobes show chromatin condensation. *(From Jain NC. Schalm's Veterinary Hematology. 4th Ed. Philadelphia: Lea & Febiger, 1983.)*

After spending a brief time of approximately 8 hours circulating in the blood, neutrophils enter the surrounding tissues and body cavities to carry out their specific functions. Thus, the entire circulating pool of neutrophils is turned over about three times daily. Physiologic stimuli, such as stress (corticosteroids), fear (epinephrine), infection, infarction, or trauma, can increase either the production or the release of neutrophils from the bone marrow.

The circulating neutrophilic cells in the normal, healthy animal include mature, segmented neutrophils with a few band neutrophils. The **band neutrophil** is approximately the same size or slightly smaller (12 to 15 μm) than the metamyelocyte. The nuclear chromatin pattern of the band is slightly less condensed and the nucleus is nonsegmented with a smooth contour and parallel-appearing sides. The **mature neutrophil (segmented neutrophil)** has features similar to the band neutrophil, but the nucleus has two to five distinct lobes connected by fine nuclear filaments. The cytoplasm of both band and segmented neutrophils is clear and contains pale- or neutral-staining granules. The numbers of band neutrophils and less mature cells of this series may increase in response to a disease process. If the numbers of bands are increased, but still less than the numbers of mature neutrophils, this type of blood count is called a "left-shift." Other morphologic indications of an inflammatory blood picture may include the presence of blue cytoplasmic inclusions known as **Dohle bodies** (aggregates of ribosomes and endoplasmic reticulum), cytoplasmic basophilia, and cytoplasmic vacuoles.

Eosinophil

Eosinophils are approximately the same size as the neutrophil, but are easily distinguished by the presence of bright reddish granules in their cytoplasm. The granules of the eosinophil have an affinity for eosin, a red acidophilic dye found in Wright stain. This staining characteristic is attributed to a high content of arginine-rich, highly basic proteins that attract the acidic dye. Another feature that is helpful in identifying the eosinophil is the presence of a nucleus that rarely has more than two lobes, whereas the neutrophil nucleus usually has three or four lobes.

The size, shape, number, and staining characteristics of the granules in eosinophils vary among the different animal species. In the dog, the granules rarely fill the cytoplasm of the cell and may vary from small, homogenous pinkish-orange to a vacuolated granule. The granules in the eosinophil of the cat are rod-shaped and numerous and stain reddish. Large, bright reddish granules are found in the horse, whereas smaller, less intensely stained granules that almost completely fill the cytoplasm are seen in the sheep, goat, cow, and pig (Plates 4-2 and 4-3).

Ultrastructural studies of the eosinophil have shown that the Golgi complex elaborates many **primary granules** (azurophilic granules). These granules are larger than primary granules in the neutrophil. The **secondary granules** (specific granules) of the canine eosinophil vary from dense homogenous granules surrounded by a narrow rim of lighter matrix to a clear vesicle with only a cap of dense material. A few mitochondria and remnants of rough endoplasmic reticulum are also found in the mature eosinophil (Fig. 4-4). Feline and guinea pig eosinophils have char-

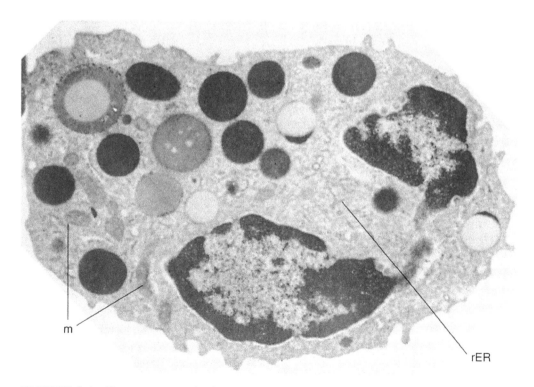

FIGURE 4-4 Electron micrograph of a canine eosinophil. The cell contains pleomorphic granules. Dense and light homogeneous granules and clear vesicles are present. A few mitochondria (m) and remnants of rough endoplasmic reticulum (rER) are scattered throughout the cell. *(From Jain NC. Schalm's Veterinary Hematology. 4th Ed. Philadelphia: Lea & Febiger, 1983.)*

acteristic crystalloid specific granules, whereas other species, including the cow and horse, have only homogenous granules.

Eosinophils usually account for only 0 to 8% of the total leukocyte count, giving absolute numbers of 0 to 500 eosinophils/µL of blood. The intravascular lifespan of the eosinophil is extremely short, estimated at less than 1 hour in the dog. The eosinophil plays an important role in acute inflammatory, allergic, and anaphylactic reactions, and in controlling infestations by helminthic parasites. In the process of regulating allergic and inflammatory responses, this cell phagocytizes immune complexes and inhibits the release and replenishment of histamine and other vasoactive amines. The phagocytic and bactericidal capabilities of eosinophils are limited when compared to those of neutrophils. It has been demonstrated that eosinophils may also induce damage in tissues and play a role in fibrosis when excessive numbers of eosinophils are present. Substances such as antigen–antibody complexes, fibrin, fibrinogen, and factors released from stimulated T lymphocytes, basophils, or mast cells may act as chemotactic factors for eosinophils. Histamine, released by both mast cells and basophils in response to tissue injury or allergic reactions, is the major chemotactic factor for eosinophils.

Basophil

The **basophil** measures 10 to 15 µm and has a segmented nucleus. Characteristic deep purple granules often fill the cytoplasm and obscure the nucleus. The purplish staining of the granules is ascribed to their content of sulfated glycosaminoglycans. Granules of the feline basophil are rod-shaped and usually stain dull purplish-gray due to lack of sulfated glycosaminoglycans, whereas granules of the canine basophil stain reddish violet (Plates 4-4 and 4-5). Basophil granules in the dog do not fill the cytoplasm of the cell, in contrast to the granules in basophils from cows, horses, and cats. In some species, the granules are water-soluble and may be partially dissolved or lost during the process of staining the blood smear.

The basophil is the least numerous granulocyte in the peripheral blood, rarely accounting for more than 0 to 1.5% of the total leukocyte count or 0 to 200 basophils/µL. Evidence supports the role of the basophil in allergic conditions, including urticaria, allergic rhinitis, allergic conjunctivitis, asthma, allergic gastroenteritis, and anaphylaxis caused by drug reactions or insect stings. Another function of the basophil is to promote lipolysis. Heparin released from the granules of the basophil promotes the release of lipoprotein lipase from endothelial cells of the blood vessel wall. This process causes clearing of chylomicra from the blood and facilitates the metabolism of triglycerides. Basophils also play a major role in mediating inflammatory responses. The anticoagulant actions of heparin and the procoagulant effects of protease-generated kallikreins that are secreted by basophils may antagonize and promote hemostasis, respectively.

Monocyte

Monocytes are the largest leukocytes in the blood and are closely related to the neutrophil, sharing the same precursor cell (CSF-GM). They are 12 to 18 µm in diameter and have a pleomorphic nucleus, which may appear elongated, folded, indented, horseshoe-shaped, and even lobed. The nuclear chromatin of the mono-

cyte is lacy or reticular with some areas of condensation, and nucleoli are inconspicuous. The cytoplasm is abundant and grayish blue in color, often containing a few discrete vacuoles and/or fine azurophilic granules (Plates 4-9 and 4-11).

Monocytes account for 3 to 8% of the total leukocyte count. Thus, the absolute number of monocytes is approximately 200 to 1000 cells/µL of blood. The circulating half-life of monocytes in the blood is variable among the species. They transiently circulate in the peripheral blood, exiting the vasculature either randomly or in response to an inflammatory stimulus.

Upon leaving the blood, monocytes differentiate into long-lived **macrophages** under the influence of specific tissue factors. The young macrophage is similar in morphology to that of the circulating monocytes, but with time, they become activated, increasing in size, phagocytic activity, and lysosomal enzyme content. Electron micrographic studies often show many short microvillus-like projections along the surface of the macrophage and the cytoplasm is frequently vacuolated (Fig. 4-5). Although tissue macrophages are capable of cell division, most of the macrophages at an inflammatory site have been recruited from the blood. The exact lifespan of macrophages in tissues is unknown. It appears that resident macrophages are long-lived; however, macrophages that accumulate in response to inflammatory stimuli are shorter lived.

Circulating monocytes and tissue macrophages comprise the **mononuclear phagocyte system** (MPS). These cells are widely distributed in tissues and serosal cavities throughout the body and include specific cells such as stellate macrophages (Kupffer cells) in the liver, alveolar and interstitial macrophages in the lung, sy-

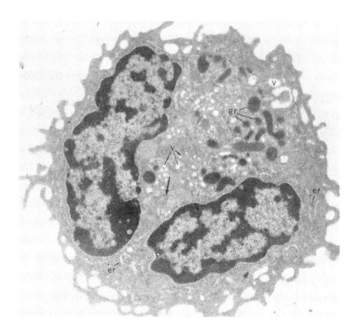

FIGURE 4-5 Electron micrograph of a canine monocyte. The cell contains many lysosomal granules (gr), several small to large vesicles (v), abundant ribosomes (arrow), and prominent rough endoplasmic reticulum (er), especially along the cell periphery. This cell also has many microvilluslike projections along the cellular outline. The nucleus appears bilobed and shows areas of chromatin condensation. *(From Jain NC. Schalm's Veterinary Hematology. 4th Ed. Philadelphia: Lea & Febiger, 1983.)*

novial cells in the joints, and microglia in the brain. Phagocytosis and digestion of cellular debris, microorganisms, and particulate matter are major functions of the macrophage. The MPS also plays an important role in the presentation of antigens to lymphocytes, which initiates an immune response, and in the regulation of granulopoiesis and erythropoiesis through the action of cytokines secreted by the macrophages.

Lymphocyte

Lymphocytes are variable in size. The smaller cells are 6 to 9 μm in diameter, which is only slightly larger than a red blood cell, while larger lymphocytes measure up to 15 μm in diameter (Plates 4-1, 4-6, 4-7, and 4-8). Small lymphocytes are the most numerous and may be found in the blood, lymphatic circulation, and lymphatic tissue. In the blood of dogs and cats, smaller lymphocytes are most common, whereas both small and large lymphocytes are present in the blood of cows, sheep, and goats. These large lymphocytes are mature and lack nucleoli.

The cell profile of the lymphocyte is normally round and smooth with light microscopy, but short microvilli may be observed on their surface with electron microscopy (Fig. 4-6). Lymphocytes have a round to slightly indented nucleus with clumped heterochromatin. Although lymphocytes are classified as agranular, some of them may have a few azurophilic granules in their cytoplasm. The nuclear-to-cytoplasmic ratio of small lymphocytes is high, with only a modest amount of pale blue cytoplasm.

The number of lymphocytes in the peripheral circulation varies among the species. These cells account for 20 to 40% of

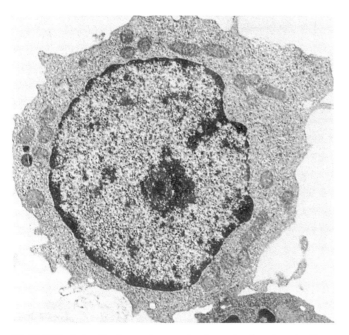

FIGURE 4-6 Electron micrograph of a canine lymphocyte. The cell has a moderate amount of cytoplasm surrounding a large nucleus with nucleolus. The cytoplasm is rich in free ribosomes, has some profiles of rough endoplasmic reticulum and scattered mitochondria, and contains dense granules (azurophilic granules). *(From Jain NC. Schalm's Veterinary Hematology. 4th Ed. Philadelphia: Lea & Febiger, 1983.)*

the total leukocyte count in dogs, cats, and horses, but may be 50 to 60% of the leukocyte differential in cows, mice, and pigs. Lymphocytes are key components of the adaptive immune response. They play an important role in cell-mediated (T lymphocytes) and antibody-mediated (B lymphocytes) immunity.

Platelets/Thrombocytes

Platelets vary in size from 5 to 7 μm in length and 1.3 to 4.7 μm in width among the animal species. A slight variation in platelet size is present in most species, but is greatly accentuated in the cat. Larger platelets, or **proplatelets,** up to 20 μm in length can be observed in the blood of the horse. In stained blood smears, platelets are discoid, oval, or elongated fragments of cytoplasm that lack a nucleus and have fine, reddish-purple granules. The term platelet and **thrombocyte** are often used interchangeably; however, when describing the nucleated platelet in fish, reptiles, and birds, the term thrombocyte is preferred (Plate 4-12).

When observed by electron microscopy, resting platelets have a smooth surface with random indentations that represent the membranous invaginations of the **open canalicular system** (OCS). This system opens to the platelet surface and is used for externalization of platelet secretory products and internalization of substances from plasma into the platelet. Bovine platelets are devoid of an OCS and secrete their contents directly to the exterior. Normal platelets are covered with amorphous material that forms a thin external glycocalyx. This glycoprotein-rich layer is responsible for the platelet's adhesive properties.

Beneath the surface membrane of the platelet, some microfilaments and a bundle of microtubules are observed. These cytoskeletal elements maintain normal platelet shape and make up the contractile system. Thus, they are responsible for the change in shape of platelets following activation and the subsequent secretion of platelet granules. Another series of channels, the **dense tubular system** (DTS), is found deep to the superficial cytoskeleton. The DTS provides a site for sequestration of calcium and localization of enzymes for prostaglandin synthesis. The internal structure of the platelet is composed of many α granules, electron-dense granules, and glycogen particles, with only a few mitochondria and lysosomes. The **α granules** are membrane-bounded and contain platelet factor 4, coagulation factors I (fibrinogen) and V (proaccelerin), platelet-derived growth factor, and many other components. **Electron-dense granules** are a storage pool for adenine nucleotides, histamine, serotonin, catecholamines, and calcium (Fig. 4-7).

The number of platelets in circulation ranges from about 200,000 to 400,000/μL of blood. In general, the lifespan of circulating platelets in domestic animal species is about 8 to 12 days. A key role of the platelet is maintenance of primary (platelet plug formation) and secondary (coagulation) hemostasis.

BONE MARROW

Structure and Function

The bone marrow is a mesenchymal-derived tissue that consists of hematopoietic cellular elements and a complex microenviron-

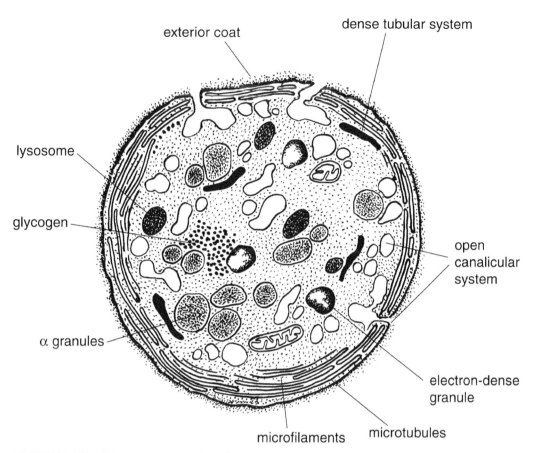

FIGURE 4-7   Schematic drawing of the fine structure of a platelet.

ment. In the adult animal, marrow is contained within the medullary cavity of flat and long bones and represents almost 5% of total body weight. It is a soft, gelatinous tissue that is divided into irregular, interconnected spaces by bony trabeculae. The rapidly dividing, hematopoietic precursor cells (erythroid, myeloid, and megakaryocytic lineages) are an extremely labile population that continuously undergoes a process of self-replication and/or differentiation. These precursor cells produce all of the peripheral blood cells, including erythrocytes, leukocytes, and platelets. Cells of the microenvironment, which include stromal cells (fibroblastlike reticular cells, endothelial cells, adipocytes, and macrophages), accessory cells (T lymphocytes, natural killer cells, and monocytes/macrophages), and their products (extracellular matrix and cytokines), are distributed throughout the bone marrow space. These components provide a scaffold as well as nutrient support for the developing hematopoietic cells. The supporting cells also play an active role in the regulation of hematopoiesis by direct cell-to-cell contact and/or by secreting regulatory molecules that influence the growth of hematopoietic precursor cells in a positive or negative manner. In addition, osteoblasts and osteoclasts of adjacent bone are present in the bone marrow.

Hematopoiesis is the process by which highly differentiated cells of the peripheral blood develop from specialized precursors in the bone marrow. Although the process occurs extravascularly in solid tissue that lies between the vascular spaces, the maturing cells are closely associated with thin-walled venous sinusoids.

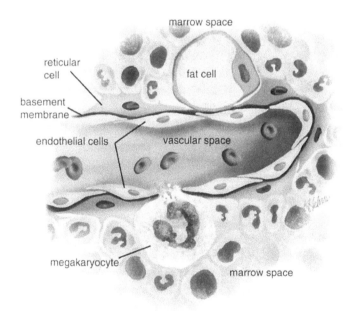

FIGURE 4-8   Schematic drawing of the bone marrow, showing vascular and cellular compartments. The hematopoietic cells are closely associated with thin-walled venous sinusoids. The walls of the sinusoids are trilaminar: endothelial cells on the inside, a basement membrane forming the middle layer and supporting the hematopoietic cells, and fibroblastlike stromal (adventitial reticular) cells on the outside. Cytoplasmic pseudopodia of the megakaryocyte extend through the sinus endothelium and release platelets directly into the vascular space.

The walls of the **sinusoids** in mature bone marrow are trilaminar (Fig. 4-8). Each sinusoid is lined by a single layer of endothelial cells on the inside (vascular space) with an overlying basement membrane and supporting reticular cells on the outside (bone marrow space). A selective barrier between the blood and bone marrow results from the loose intercellular junctions created by the overlap of adjacent endothelial cells. The basement membrane, which forms the middle layer of the sinusoid wall, is irregular and may be discontinuous or absent in some areas. As a result of the unique structure of the wall, the sinusoid may dilate readily to accommodate a highly active, hyperplastic bone marrow. The reticular cells covering the majority of the outer surface of the sinusoid wall appear to control access of cells from the marrow space into the circulation. When there is massive demand for peripheral blood cells, the amount of surface covered by these cells is markedly reduced. Reticular cells of the bone marrow are also phagocytic and can accumulate a substantial amount of fat, thereby reducing the marrow space available for hematopoiesis.

Excessive proliferation of stromal cells (myelofibrosis) in the sinusoid wall and/or within the marrow space may result in the failure of mature hematopoietic cells to gain access to the circulation. The peripheral blood of patients with myelofibrosis is often characterized by a severe pancytopenia (reduction in number of circulating blood cells). Myelofibrosis has been recognized in dogs and cats with underlying myeloproliferative diseases, as a terminal event in dogs with a red cell metabolic defect (pyruvate kinase deficiency), and in feline leukemia–infected cats; however, most cases in animals are idiopathic.

Fibroblastlike **reticular cells** branch from the sinusoid wall into the marrow space and may completely encircle developing precursor cells. The cells create a structural framework for adjacent hematopoietic cells and assist in hematopoiesis by binding essential growth factors. During development, a stratification of cells in the marrow space occurs, with immature cells in areas nearest the bone and mature cells at the vascular interface. Upon reaching maturity, hematopoietic cells migrate from the marrow space across the endothelium into the lumen of the sinusoid, thereby gaining access to the vascular or blood compartment. The migration occurs either through intercellular junctions between endothelial cells or through intracellular pores in the endothelial cells. In addition to the transmural migration of mature blood cells, the cytoplasmic processes of megakaryocytes penetrate the sinusoid wall. These projecting portions of the megakaryocyte dribble small cell fragments known as **platelets** into the circulation.

The vascular sinusoids of the bone marrow receive arterial blood from two major sources. One source of blood is the nutrient artery, which penetrates the bony shaft at the nutrient foramen. The artery traverses the cortical bone and then gives off several branches that extend throughout the marrow cavity. In the periphery of the bone marrow cavity, arterial capillaries feed a branching network of venules and sinusoids. The second source of blood supply to the bone marrow comes from the periosteal capillary network that sends small vessels into perforating canals in the cortical bone (Fig. 4-9). These transosteal vessels connect with sinusoids at the bone marrow junction. Blood drains from the sinusoids in the marrow into the longitudinal central vein,

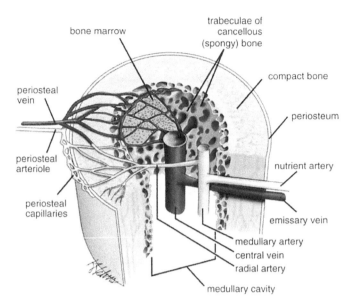

FIGURE 4-9 Schematic drawing of the microcirculation of the bone marrow. The sinusoids receive blood from two sources, the nutrient artery and a periosteal capillary network, which penetrate the cortical bone through numerous osteal canals.

which empties into venules in the perforating or nutrient canals, forming the major vascular outflow tracts from the marrow.

The concentration of small venules and sinusoids is higher near the bone than in central areas of the marrow space. This pattern parallels the distribution of hematopoiesis, which is highest in the subcortical areas and lowest in the area surrounding the central artery. Although the bone marrow is devoid of lymphatics, it has a rich nerve supply that accompanies the blood vessels. These nerve fibers respond to intramedullary pressure resulting from cellular proliferation, transmitting signals to the vessel walls. The signaling results in adjustments of blood flow and release of hematopoietic cells into the circulation.

Adipocytes are a major constituent of marrow tissue; however, the number of cells depends on the age of the individual animal and the location of the marrow. Marrow cellularity approaches 100% at birth and is hematopoietically active (red bone marrow) in the long bones of young animals. In contrast, the marrow cavity of long bones in adult animals is filled with fatty tissue (yellow bone marrow). Active bone marrow is found only in the sternum, ribs, vertebrae, scapulae, skull, pelvis, and proximal ends of the femur and humerus of adult animals. The proportion of fatty tissue increases with age, and cellularity declines such that hematopoietic cells may occupy as little as 25% of the marrow in older animals. The adipocyte in bone marrow acts as a passive storage site for energy; however, these cells also play a role in lipid metabolism and contribute to the promotion of hematopoiesis. Animals with certain diseases such as severe hemolytic anemia or chronic hypoxia may have a markedly reduced bone marrow fat content. In contrast, in other diseases such as aplastic anemia, excessive infiltration of yellow marrow has been reported.

Marrow stromal cells produce extracellular matrix (ECM) molecules such as collagen, fibronectin, laminin, thrombospondin, hemonectin, and proteoglycans. These substances facilitate cell–cell interactions and contribute to the up-regulation or down-regulation of hematopoiesis by binding and presenting growth factors to hematopoietic precursor cells.

Hematopoiesis

Hematopoietic stem cells move from blood islands in the yolk sac to developing organs in the embryo and fetus. Early in gestation, primitive nucleated red blood cells that produce embryonic hemoglobin are released into the circulation. The hematopoietic activity of the yolk sac is short lived and its declining production of blood cells is accompanied by a sharp increase in hematopoiesis by the liver. It is unclear whether hematopoiesis begins in the liver by differentiation of primitive mesenchymal cells into hematopoietic stem cells or by colonization with stem cells that migrate from the yolk sac. Definitive hematopoiesis, which develops in the liver, is characterized by hematopoietic stem cells that are capable of self-renewal and generation of progenitors that are committed to erythroid, myeloid, megakaryocytic, and lymphoid lineages. The spleen, lymph nodes, and thymus may contribute to hematopoiesis during this phase, but these organs generally are more active in lymphocyte production. The liver and spleen retain their potential for hematopoiesis throughout life. When hematopoiesis is present in these organs in the adult animal, the process is termed **extramedullary hematopoiesis** (EMH) and is considered an abnormal finding. EMH is a compensatory response to insufficient bone marrow production of blood cells. The most common conditions associated with marked splenic EMH in the dog are myelofibrosis, marrow failure or hypoplasia, and myeloproliferative disorders. Severe anemia in both the dog and cat may also play a role in the development of EMH in this organ. Rodents are notable exceptions, since their spleen normally serves as a hemopoietic organ.

It is likely that the concentration of growth factors and selective ECM components in organs supporting the production of blood cells changes with time. This alteration may explain the shifting of hematopoiesis from one organ to another during fetal life. The bone marrow begins to produce blood cells late in gestation and is the primary site of hematopoiesis at birth, continuing to increase cell production thereafter. The bone marrow in the adult animal is an extremely active tissue with a daily output of blood cells approaching 2.5 billion red cells, an equivalent number of platelets, and 1 billion granulocytes per kilogram of body weight.

Although not evident in histologic sections, the microenvironment of the bone marrow is a highly organized structure. The functional unit of erythropoiesis, the **erythroblastic island**, consists of a central macrophage (nurse cell) encircled by erythroid precursor cells. The macrophage provides erythropoietin and iron to the developing erythroid cells. Erythroblastic islands are usually located away from the bone trabeculae and close to vascular structures. Other components of the microenvironment, including the ECM, stromal cells, and a variety of regulatory cytokines, play an important role in supporting the proliferation and/or differentiation of hematopoietic progenitor cells. For example, in the ECM, certain proteoglycans (heparan sulfate, chondroitin sulfate, and hyaluronic acid) bind growth factors and present them to the progenitor cells. The modulation of erythropoiesis by fibronectin involves the attachment of this ECM component to early erythroid

progenitors, whereas hemonectin participates in the maturation and release of granulocytic cells from the bone marrow. These complex interactions also lead to certain topographic patterns in the bone marrow. For example, granulopoiesis takes place primarily in subcortical areas where the concentration of hemonectin is higher. Granulopoiesis also occurs in foci that are associated with alkaline phosphatase–producing stromal cells. In addition, stromal cells produce other growth factors that regulate granulopoiesis, including **granulocyte–macrophage colony stimulation factor** (GM-CSF), **granulocyte colony–stimulating factor** (G-CSF), and **macrophage colony–stimulating factor** (M-CSF).

Hematopoietic Stem Cells

All cells in the bone marrow, including erythroid, granulocytic-monocytic, lymphoid, and megakaryocytic lineages, originate from a population of **hematopoietic stem cells** (HSCs). Over the years, these cells have been given various names, including pluripotent stem cells and uncommitted stem cells. The HSCs are not morphologically distinct. However, these cells do have highly specific homing properties for the bone marrow and are able to undergo either self-renewal or differentiation into hematopoietic precursor cells. The HSCs may differentiate into two types of primitive, multipotent, committed precursor cells, which are the **colony-forming unit—lymphoid** (CFU-L) and the **colony-forming unit—granulocyte, erythrocyte, monocyte/macrophage, and megakaryocyte** (CFU-GEMM) (Fig. 4-10). The term **colony-forming unit** (CFU) has been adopted to describe an individual cell capable of giving rise to a colony of hematopoietic cells. With further differentiation, pluripotent CFUs give rise to committed progenitors that can only proliferate and mature along more restricted pathways. Thus, a bipotent progenitor cell for granulocytes and monocytes (**CFU-GM**) is derived from the multipotent precursor cell CFU-GEMM, which undergoes further proliferation and differentiation to result in an even more restricted progeny. Thereafter, some progeny are able to differentiate along the neutrophilic (**CFU-N**), eosinophilic (**CFU-Eo**), and basophilic (**CFU-Bas**) lineages while others differentiate along only the monocytic lineage (**CFU-M**). Megakaryocytes and erythrocytes are derived from a bipotent erythroid/megakaryocytic progenitor (**CFU-ME**). In addition, progenitors that are committed solely to the development of erythrocytes (**CFU-E**) and megakaryocytes (**CFU-Meg**) have been described. Similarly, further differentiation of CFU-L results in progeny that are committed to become T lymphocytes (**CFU-TL**) and B lymphocytes (**CFU-BL**).

The growth of unipotent progenitor cells (CFU-N, etc.) has been characterized both functionally and by membrane antigen expression. Ultimately, the commitment of progenitor cells to specific hematopoietic lineages is controlled through cell-specific transcription factors that initiate a pathway of distinct cellular signals.

Cytokines and Regulation of Hematopoiesis

A number of cytokines, including colony-stimulating factors, interleukins, and growth factors, are involved in the regulation of hematopoiesis (Fig. 4-10). The primary effects of these cytokines at different levels in the developmental pathways of blood cells and

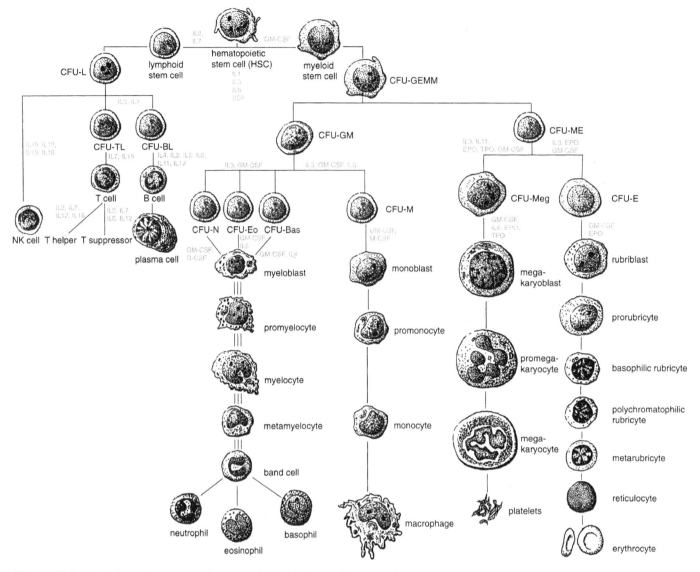

FIGURE 4-10 Schematic drawing of hematopoiesis including cytokines (gray).

their progenitors have been extensively studied. There is often a broad and overlapping spectrum of action for various hematopoietic target cells. Whether there is a stimulatory or inhibitory effect of the regulator on the target depends on the concentration and duration of exposure to the cytokine. The maturation stage of the target cell, existing cytokine milieu, and the physical relationship of the target cell to the marrow microenvironment may also influence this response.

For the most part, **colony-stimulating factor (CSF)** and **interleukins (ILs)** are growth-stimulatory cytokines. Synergy between stimulatory cytokines may result in important biologic responses. For example, stem cell factor (SCF), an essential growth factor in normal hematopoiesis, exerts potent effects when combined with granulocyte CSF (G-CSF). IL-3 also demonstrates synergistic effects with IL-1 and erythropoietin in the generation of erythroid progenitors, whereas IL-3 and IL-5 promote the development of eosinophils. In normal animals, the effect of **thrombopoietin (TPO)** in the peripheral blood is limited to marked increase in the number of platelets. However, the administration

of TPO to an animal with a suppressed bone marrow is associated with greatly accelerated recovery in all of the three cell lineages.

Cytokines that primarily act as negative regulators of hematopoiesis include **tumor necrosis factor-α (TNF-α)**, **interferon-γ (INF-γ)**, **transforming growth factor-β (TGF-β)**, and **lactoferrin**. There is strong evidence that TNF-α and INF-γ play a role in the development of anemia of chronic disease (ACD). However, the regulation of granulopoiesis by lactoferrin is controversial.

Granulopoiesis

Normal bone marrow has a heterogenous population of hematopoietic cells that are in various stages of differentiation; however, the most mature cells of a given lineage are present in the greatest numbers. The individual pathways and major cytokines involved in the production of each type of mature blood cell from a precursor or stem cell population are shown in Fig. 4-10 and described in detail hereafter. The characteristic heterogeneity of the marrow may be altered in various hematologic disorders, including myelodysplastic syndromes and hemato-poietic neoplasia.

The process of **granulopoiesis**, or white blood cell formation, begins with the proliferation and differentiation of the **myeloblast**, which is a progeny of the CFU-GM (Fig. 4-10). The transit time from the myeloblast stage to release of mature granulocytes into the circulation may be as short as 4 to 5 days or as long as 10 days. In general, as these cells mature, their size decreases progressively, nuclear chromatin condenses, and nucleoli disappear. Ultimately, the nucleus of the granulocyte becomes lobulated or segmented, the cytoplasm gradually loses basophilia, and specific or secondary granules accumulate.

The morphology and development of granulocytes in the bone marrow has been extensively studied. The first three cells of the myeloid lineage, the myeloblast, promyelocyte, and myelocyte, are capable of mitotic cell division. The **myeloblast** undergoes division and differentiates to produce two **promyelocytes**, each of which multiplies and differentiates into two **myelocytes** (Fig. 4-11). The myelocyte may undergo two or three successive mitotic cell divisions, without significant differentiation, to replicate additional myelocytes. One consequence of multiple, successive divisions is that the generation of granulocytes may be amplified at this step. On the other hand, successive divisions may be skipped to speed the production of mature granulocytes when there is great demand. Each myelocyte undergoes maturation without further cell division, generating the **metamyelocyte**, **band**, and **mature segmented granulocyte**.

Once released into the circulation, the mature granulocytes, which are mostly segmented neutrophils, are distributed between two peripheral blood pools. The **marginal granulocytic pool** (MGP) consists of granulocytes that line the walls of capil-laries and venules, whereas the **circulating granulocyte** pool (CGP) consists of cells that are more centrally located and free-floating in the vessels. The total and differential cell counts in the complete blood count (CBC) are a reflection of the CGP. The MGP and CGP are approximately equal in size but may freely exchange cells, thus altering the size of these pools. The granulocytes remain in the blood for a brief period of time, randomly leaving the circulation and moving into the tissues where they perform their specific functions. The neutrophils can also be specifically attracted (a process known as chemotaxis) to tissues that are infected by microorganisms. The function of the neutrophil is to phagocytize, digest, and kill the invading bacteria. Although the eosinophil is also phagocytic, this cell is primarily involved in limiting hypersensitivity reactions and defending against parasitic infections. The basophil is the source of mediators that promote immediate (allergic and anaphylactic) and delayed hypersensitivity reactions.

Neutrophilic Precursors

The earliest granulocytic precursor that can be morphologically identified is the **myeloblast**. The cell ranges in size from 15 to 20 µm and is characterized by a spherical nucleus, finely stippled chromatin, one or two nucleoli, and lightly to moderately basophilic cytoplasm. Cytoplasm of the myeloblast lacks or has few primary granules. The myeloblast also does not have a prominent light-staining perinuclear region, indicating a poorly developed Golgi complex.

Promyelocytes are slightly larger than myeloblasts and may range up to 25 µm in diameter. The nucleus is often eccentric and has slightly coarser chromatin and prominent nucleoli. A conspicuous light-staining Golgi zone is also characteristic of the promyelocyte. The cell cytoplasm is lightly basophilic, more abundant than the cytoplasm of the myeloblast, and contains numerous primary granules.

The nucleus of the **myelocyte** is spherical to ovoid, has coarse chromatin, and lacks distinct nucleoli. In most animal species, the synthesis of primary granules ceases at the myelocyte stage and the number of these granules decreases during subsequent cell divisions. The appearance of secondary granules in the myelocyte indicates a commitment to development along a specific cell lineage (neutrophilic, eosinophilic, and basophilic myelocytes).

The nucleus of the **metamyelocyte** may vary from a slightly indented sphere to a distinct "kidney-bean" shape with coarse chromatin and no obvious nucleoli. The cytoplasm of the cell is filled with secondary granules. Metamyelocytes are no longer capable of mitotic cell division.

Eosinophilic and Basophilic Granulocytes and Mast Cells

The stages of maturation of eosinophilic and basophilic granulocytes are similar to those of neutrophilic granulocytes. However, the size, shape, color, and number of specific granules vary greatly among the animal species. In general, the secondary granules of the **eosinophil** are considered to be lysosomes, containing enzymes such as peroxidase, acid phosphatase, and arylsulfatase. The granules also contain a variety of highly toxic proteins, such as major

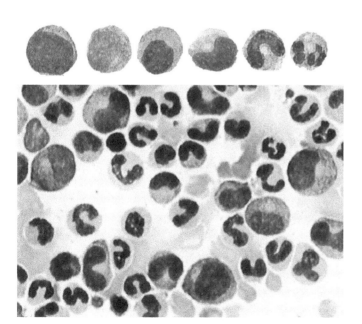

FIGURE 4-11 Granulocytic lineage (upper figure, left to right): myeloblast, promyelocyte, myelocyte, metamyelocyte, band, and neutrophil. Bone marrow smear (lower figure) showing the stages of granulocyte differentiation.

basic protein, eosinophil peroxidase, and eosinophilic cationic protein. Based on their affinity for anionic dyes such as eosin, the granules are reddish when stained with routine hematologic stains. The contents of the granules are released directly onto helminthic and protozoan targets to assist in killing the parasites. Eosinophils play a role in anaphylactic and allergic reactions and also have the ability to phagocytize particles such as immune complexes.

The primary substances stored in granules of the **basophil** include biogenic amines, heparin, hydrolytic enzymes, proteoglycans, and major basic protein. The granules are dark purple with routine hematologic stains and they obscure the nucleus in some species. The basophil is mainly involved in allergic and anaphylactic reactions. This process is mediated by cross-linking of surface immunoglobulin (Ig) E receptors on the basophil, which results in the release of the contents of the granules into the environment. Histamine, a major biogenic amine, contributes to local increases in vascular permeability, smooth muscle contraction, and bronchoconstriction. The basophil may also play a role in host defense against bacterial and viral infection, in some chronic and fibrotic disorders, and possibly in tumor cytotoxicity.

The **mast cell** originates from a pluripotent hemopoietic stem cell; however, the lineage is distinct from the monocyte and granulocyte precursors. The mast cell is larger than the basophil and has more abundant purplish granules and a spherical nucleus. Although mast cells are normal residents of the bone marrow, few are normally present. The committed mast cell precursors move from marrow to blood and then into the tissues, especially respiratory and mucosal tissues. In this location, the functions of mast cells include promoting hypersensitivity reactions, modulating immune responses, defending against tissue parasites, and promoting acute and chronic inflammatory responses. A subset of mast cells, often found adjacent to microvasculature and neural tissues, may also be involved in angiogenesis and tissue repair.

Monocytopoiesis

The stages of maturation of the monocyte progress through an undetermined number of mitotic cell divisions. The circulating monocyte may then migrate from the peripheral blood to become a macrophage in surrounding tissues. Therefore, both monocytes and macrophages are derived from a bipotent progenitor cell, the CFU-GM. The **monoblast** has a spherical to slightly indented nucleus with a fine chromatin pattern and nucleoli, but it is not easily distinguished from the **promonocyte**. The mature **monocyte** is characterized by an abundant amount of bluish-gray cytoplasm. Monocytes may also have small, indistinct primary granules and variable cytoplasmic vacuolation. The cytokines that are principally involved in monocyte development include IL-3, GM-CSF, and M-CSF. Canine and bovine GM-CSFs have been produced as recombinant proteins, and this growth factor produces a dose-dependent neutrophilia and monocytosis following administration.

Erythropoiesis and Erythroid Precursors

Erythropoiesis, the production of erythrocytes or red blood cells, is controlled by growth factors that permit cellular survival and proliferation and by nuclear regulators that activate lineage-specific genes. **Erythropoietin,** produced by the kidney and other tissues, is the primary physiologic regulator of red cell production. The apoptosis of newly formed erythroid progenitor cells is inhibited by erythropoietin, thereby allowing the cells to differentiate into mature erythrocytes. Erythropoietin also plays a role in the proliferation and differentiation of committed erythroid progenitor cells, and it enhances the release of more mature cells into the blood.

The **rubriblast,** which is derived from the CFU-E, is the earliest recognizable erythroid precursor (Fig. 4-12). The cell ranges in size from 15 to 25 μm and is characterized by a spherical nucleus, stippled chromatin, one or two nucleoli, and deeply basophilic cytoplasm with a perinuclear pale area and no granules. A single rubriblast undergoes division and differentiates to produce two **prorubricytes**. Although similar in appearance to the rubriblast, the nuclear chromatin of the prorubricyte may have minimal condensation and nucleoli are indistinct. The prorubricyte undergoes successive mitotic cell divisions and continues to mature, producing basophilic rubricytes and polychromatophilic rubricytes. The nuclear chromatin of the **basophilic rubricyte** is more condensed and separated by light streaks, and the cell is slightly smaller in size than the prorubricyte. In the **polychromatophilic rubricyte,** the change in color of the cytoplasm to a grayish-blue indicates that hemoglobin synthesis is well under way. Each polychromatophilic rubricyte undergoes maturation without further cell division, generating the **metarubricyte** and then a reticulocyte. A metarubricyte is the smallest nucleated erythrocyte, having condensed nuclear chromatin and gray to reddish cytoplasm. The **reticulocyte,** which contains a significant number of ribosomes and stains grayish-pink in Romanowsky stains, is released into the circulation. Within 1 to

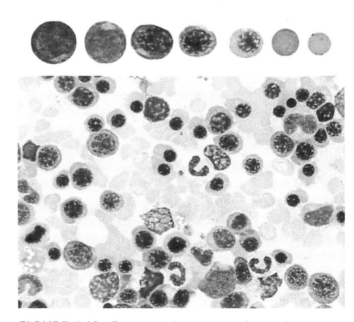

FIGURE 4-12 Erythrocytic lineage (upper figure, left to right): rubriblast, prorubricyte, basophilic rubricyte, polychromatophilic rubricyte, metarubricyte, reticulocyte, erythrocyte. Bone marrow smear (lower figure) showing the stages of erythroid differentiation.

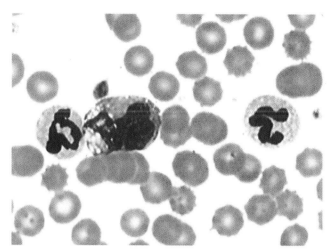

PLATE 4-1   Two canine neutrophils and one monocyte.

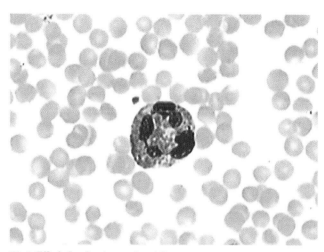

PLATE 4-2   Bovine eosinophil.

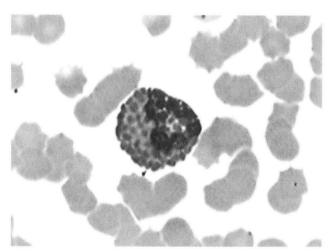

PLATE 4-3   Equine eosinophil. The granules of the equine eosinophil are the largest of all the domestic species.

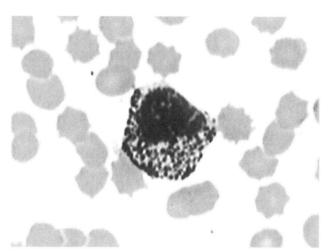

PLATE 4-4   Equine basophil.

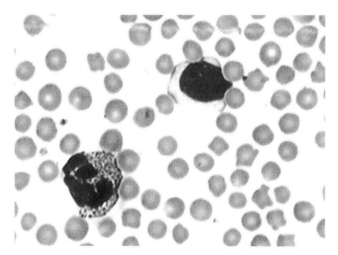

PLATE 4-5   Ovine basophil and lymphocyte.

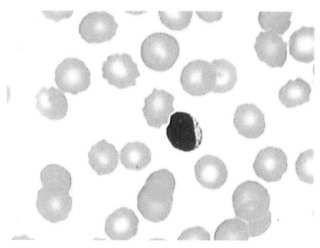

PLATE 4-6   Small canine lymphocyte.

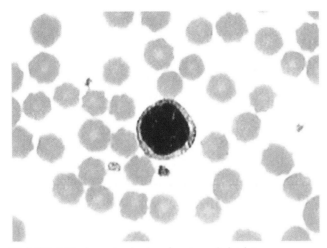

PLATE 4-7   Large bovine lymphocyte and platelets.

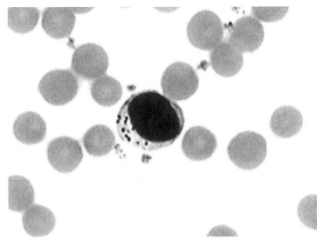

PLATE 4-8   Bovine lymphocyte with azurophilic granules and platelets.

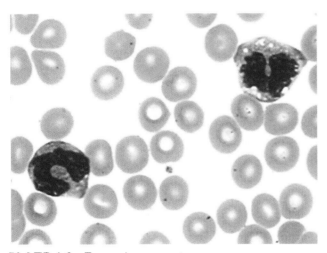

PLATE 4-9   Two canine monocytes.

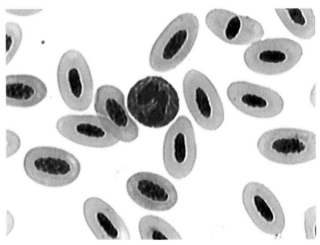

PLATE 4-10   Avian heterophil and nucleated erythrocytes.

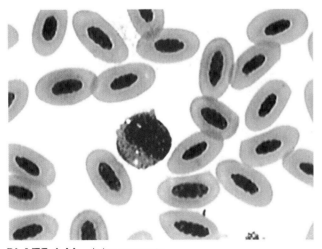

PLATE 4-11   Avian monocyte.

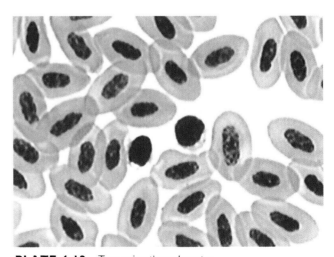

PLATE 4-12   Two avian thrombocytes.

2 days, the reticulocytes lose their ribosomes and become mature, circulating **erythrocytes** or red blood cells.

In general, erythroid cells become smaller with each successive mitotic division. Chromatin continues to condense until the nucleus becomes pyknotic and is eventually extruded from the cell. After 3 to 5 days, the rubriblast matures into the reticulocyte, and after 1 to 2 additional days, the reticulocyte is released into the circulation. When senescent, red blood cells are removed from the circulation by the MPS.

Thrombopoiesis and Platelet Precursors

Megakaryocytes arise from a multipotent progenitor cell, CFU-GEMM, in which lineage-specific genes have been activated (Fig. 4-10). **Thrombopoietin,** the primary physiologic regulator of the megakaryocytic lineage, stimulates the proliferation and differentiation of committed progenitor cells. This factor also enhances the release of platelets from mature megakaryocytes into the circulation. Stem cell factor (SCF), IL-3, GM-CSF, and other factors also regulate the proliferation of the **megakaryoblast,** the earliest recognizable progenitor cell of this lineage (Fig. 4-13). In response to these factors, the megakaryoblast undergoes **endomitosis,** a process of nuclear division and cytoplasmic maturation without cellular division. The process of megakaryocytic maturation occurs adjacent to vascular sinusoids in the marrow. During maturation, there is a progressive increase in cell size, nuclear ploidy (number of nuclei), and cytoplasmic volume. The cytoplasm becomes progressively less basophilic and acquires primary granules. The mature cell may contain as many as 16 to 32 nuclei that are discrete but connected.

Platelets are the end product of the megakaryocytic cell lineage. Although the exact mechanism by which platelets are formed is not well understood, cytoplasmic pseudopodia of the megakaryocyte have been observed extending through the sinusoid endothelium, dribbling platelets (fragments of their cytoplasm) into the vascular space. About two thirds of the total body platelet mass are found in the circulation and the remaining one third is present in the spleen.

Lymphopoiesis and Lymphoid Precursors

Lymphocytes, like other hematopoietic cells, originate from a population of pluripotent stem cells (Fig. 4-10). The earliest progenitor cell in this lineage, the **lymphoblast,** is present in low numbers in the marrow and is difficult to distinguish from rubriblasts and early myeloblasts. A spherical nucleus, fine chromatin, variable number of nucleoli, and a thin rim of deeply basophilic, agranular cytoplasm characterize this cell. The lymphoblast undergoes division and differentiates to produce **prolymphocytes** that subsequently divide and differentiate into **mature lymphocytes.** The number of mitotic cell divisions that occur between the progenitor and mature stage is not known. Most of the marrow lymphocytes are small with clumped nuclear chromatin and no apparent nucleoli. Up to 20% of the nucleated cells in feline bone marrow are mature lymphocytes, whereas less than 10% are mature lymphocytes in other species.

There are two populations of mature lymphocytes: **T lymphocytes** and **B lymphocytes** that function in cell-mediated and humoral immunity, respectively. B and T lymphocytes cannot be distinguished by their morphology alone; rather, special staining techniques, immunophenotyping, are required. In mammals, the bone marrow and ileal aggregated lymphatic nodules (Peyer's patches) are the site of B-lymphocyte maturation from stem cells to small lymphocytes that express cell surface immunoglobulin. B lymphocytes may undergo further differentiation in the marrow to become **plasma cells,** giving rise to low numbers of B cells in this location. Plasma cells are distinguished from resting lymphocytes by the presence of more abundant, deeply basophilic cytoplasm, a prominent light-staining perinuclear Golgi zone, and an eccentric nucleus. In birds, the process of B-lymphocyte maturation occurs in the cloacal bursa (bursa of Fabricius).

Some lymphoid precursors leave the marrow and seed the thymus, where they differentiate into thymic or **T lymphocytes.** In the bone marrow, a small population of lymphocytes with an abundant amount of lightly basophilic cytoplasm and azurophilic granules is often present. These cells are **large granular lymphocytes (LGLs)** and may be either natural killer cells or cytotoxic T lymphocytes, which play an important role in tumor resistance and host immunity to viral and other microbial infections.

Other Cells in Bone Marrow

Fibroblastlike cells support the walls of the bone marrow sinusoids and make up the "web" on which the hematopoietic cells grow within the marrow space. These supporting cells may be further named based on their location. Fibroblastlike cells occupying interstitial spaces are referred to as **reticular cells,** whereas those in the periphery of small vessels are called **adventitial cells.** Collectively, these supporting cells are also known as **adventitial**

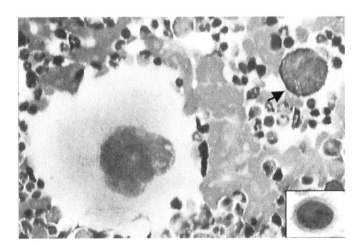

FIGURE 4-13 Megakaryocytic lineage: bone marrow smear showing a mature, granular megakaryocyte and a promegakaryocyte (arrow). A megakaryoblast is shown in the insert.

reticular cells. The morphology of these cells is somewhat variable. Because of their elongate processes, the cells may range up to 30 µm in overall diameter. A few primary granules and vacuoles are commonly found within the cytoplasm. The cell nucleus is typically spherical to ovoid in shape with a fine chromatin pattern and a variable number of nucleoli. Fibroblastlike cells are part of the marrow microenvironment and induce the proliferation of early myeloid and B-lymphoid progenitor cells.

Endothelial cells of the bone marrow sinusoids have been shown to support the proliferation and differentiation of myeloid and megakaryocytic progenitors. The primary function of sinusoid endothelial cells includes the regulation of the trafficking (outgoing) and homing (incoming) of hematopoietic cells into and out of the marrow. One consequence of this unique function is that only selected cells may gain access to a recipient's bone marrow after bone marrow transplant. Endothelial cells and fibroblastlike cells are often indistinguishable in a Wright's stained marrow smear.

The adipocyte is a prominent component of the marrow stroma. The nucleus of the adipocyte is often eccentric and compressed by fat-laden cytoplasmic vacuoles. Proliferating hematopoietic cells may rapidly replace this fatty tissue when there is increased demand for blood cell production. **Yellow marrow** increases in amount with age and is composed of adipocytes. In contrast, the **red marrow** of younger animals has few adipocytes. This age-related difference is important when interpreting marrow cellularity. Recent evidence suggests that adipocytes are secretory cells that produce cytokines such as IL-6 and TNF-α, which may be involved in control of adipose mass, inflammatory responses, and hematopoiesis.

In bone marrow biopsy specimens, osteoblasts and osteoclasts are found adjacent to bony trabeculae (Fig. 4-14). Osteoblasts, like stromal cells, are derived from a specific mesenchymal stem cell line that is distinct from the hematopoietic stem cell. The osteoblast has a large, eccentric nucleus with prominent nucleoli and abundant basophilic cytoplasm. These cells are involved in the deposition of osteoid and formation of new bone. Osteoblasts may be found in clusters in bone marrow biopsies of young animals but are rare in biopsies from adults. The osteoclast is involved in resorption and remodeling of bone. These cells are derived from the monocytic lineage and are multinucleated cells. The nuclei of the osteoclast are discrete and individual, which distinguishes them from the single nucleus of the megakaryocyte.

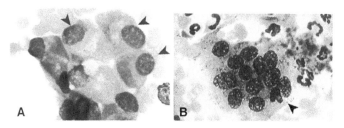

FIGURE 4-14 Bone marrow smears. **A.** Osteoblasts (arrowheads). **B.** A single multinucleated osteoclast (arrowhead).

SUGGESTED READINGS

Abboud CN. Human bone marrow microvascular endothelial cells: elusive cells with unique structural and functional properties. Exp Hematol 1995;23:1–3.

Bagby GJ Jr. Regulation of granulopoiesis: the lactoferrin controversy. Blood Cells 1989;15:386–399.

Bathija A, Ohanian M, Davis S, et al. The marrow fat cell: response to X-ray induced aplasia. Life Sci 1979;25:921–927.

Bertram TA. Neutrophil leukocyte structure and function in domestic animals. Adv Vet Sci Comp Med 1985;30:91–129.

Boosinger TR, Rebar AH, DeNicola DB, et al. Bone marrow alterations associated with canine parvoviral enteritis. Vet Pathol 1982;19:558–561.

Borish L, Joseph BZ. Inflammation and the allergic response. Med Clin North Am 1992;76:765–787.

Campbell AD. The role of hemonectin in the cell adhesion mechanisms of bone marrow. Hematol Pathol 1992;6:51–60.

Christian JA. Red cell survival and destruction. In: Feldman BF, Zinkl JG, Jain NC, et al., eds. Schalm's Veterinary Hematology. 5th Ed. Philadelphia: Lippincott Williams & Wilkins, 2000.

Colby CQ, Chang Y, Fuchimoto V, et al. Cytokine-mobilized peripheral blood progenitor cells for allogeneic reconstitution of miniature swine. Transplantation 2000;69:135–140.

Day MJ. Biology of lymphocytes and plasma cells. In: Feldman BF, Zinkl JG, Jain NC, et al., eds. Schalm's Veterinary Hematology. 5th Ed. Philadelphia: Lippincott Williams & Wilkins, 2000.

De Bruyn PP, Michelson PS, Thomas TB. The migration of blood cells of the bone marrow through the sinusoidal wall. J Morphol 1971;133:417–437.

Diebold J, Molina T, Camilleri-Broet S, et al. Bone marrow manifestations of infections and systemic diseases observed in bone marrow trephine biopsy review. Histopathology 2000;37:199–211.

Dines KC, Powell HC. Mast cell interactions with the nervous system: relationship to mechanisms of disease. J Neuropathol Exp Neurol 1997;56:627–640.

Draenert K, Draenert Y. The vascular system of bone marrow. Scan Electron Microsc 1980:113.

Duarte RF, Franf DA. The synergy between stem cell factor (SCF) and granulocyte colony-stimulating factor (G-CSF): molecular basis and clinical relevance. Leuk Lymphoma 2002;43:1179–1187.

Eckardt KU. The potential of erythropoietin and related strategies to stimulate erythropoiesis. Curr Opin Investig Drugs 2001;2:1081–1085.

Fernandez FR, Grindem CB. Reticulocyte response. In: Feldman BF, Zinkl JG, Jain NC, et al., eds. Schalm's Veterinary Hematology. 5th Ed. Philadelphia: Lippincott Williams & Wilkins, 2000.

Foucar K, Foucar E. The mononuclear phagocyte and immunoregulatory effector (M-PIRE) system: evolving concepts. Semin Diagn Pathol 1990;7:4–18.

Fridenshtein A. Stromal bone marrow cells and the hematopoietic microenvironment. Arkh Patol 1982;44:3–11.

Garland JM. Lymphocytes, lymphokines, and hematopoiesis. Immunol Ser 1990;49:297–328.

Gentry PA. Platelet biology. In: Feldman BF, Zinkl JG, Jain NC, et al., eds. Schalm's Veterinary Hematology. 5th ed. Philadelphia: Lippincott Williams & Wilkins, 2000.

Gevers EF, Loveridge N, Robinson IC. Bone marrow adipocytes: a neglected target tissue for growth hormone. Endocrinology 2002; 143:4065–4073.

Gimble JM, Robinson CE, Wu X, et al. The function of adipocytes in the bone marrow stroma: an update. Bone 1996;19:421–428.

Goldfarb AN, Flores JP, Lewandowska K. Involvement of the E2A basic helix-loop-helix protein in immunoglobulin heavy chain class switching. Mol Immunol 1996;33:947–956.

Gonzalez CL, Jaffe ES. The histiocytoses: clinical presentation and differential diagnosis. Oncology (Huntingt) 1990;4:47–60.

Gregoriadis AE, Heersche JN, Aurbin JE. Differentiation of muscle, fat, cartilage and bone from progenitor cells present in a bone derived clonal cell population: effect of dexamethasone. J Cell Biol 1988; 10:2139–2151.

Gulati GL, Ashton JK, Hyun BH. Structure and function of the bone marrow and hematopoiesis. Hematol Oncol Clin North Am 1988; 2:495–511.

Gullberg U, Bengtsson N, Bulow E, et al. Processing and targeting of granule proteins in human neutrophils. J Immunol Methods 1999;232:201–210.

Hofer M, Viklicka S, Tkadlecek L, et al. Haemopoiesis in murine bone marrow and spleen after fractionated irradiation and repeated bone marrow transplantation. II. Granulopoiesis. Folia Biol (Praha) 1989;35:418–428.

Jacobsen SE, Ruscetti FW, Ortiz M, et al. The growth response of Lin-Thy-1+ hematopoietic progenitors to cytokines is determined by the balance between synergy of multiple stimulators and negative cooperation of multiple inhibitors. Exp Hematol 1994;22: 985–989.

Kaushansky K. Small molecule mimics of hematopoietic growth factors: improving on mother nature? Leukemia 2001;15:673–674.

Kitamura Y, Jippo T. Biology of mast cells and basophils. Arerugi 1997;46:1003–1006.

Kurata M, Suzuki M, Agar NS. Antioxidant systems and erythrocyte life-span in mammals. Comp Biochem Physiol B 1993;106:477–487.

Laharrague P, Fontanilles AM, Tkaczuk J, et al. Inflammatory/haematopoietic cytokine production by human bone marrow adipocytes. Eur Cytokine Netw 2000;11:634–639.

Lotem J, Sachs L. Cytokine control of developmental programs in normal hematopoiesis and leukemia. Oncogene 2002;21:3284–3294.

MacKey MC. Cell kinetic status of haematopoietic stem cells. Cell Prolif 2001;34:71–83.

Marone G, Casolaro V, Patella V, et al. Molecular and cellular biology of mast cells and basophils. Int Arch Allergy Immunol 1997; 114:207–217.

McClugage SG Jr, McCuskey RS, Meineke HA. Microscopy of living bone marrow in situ. II. Influence of the microenvironment on hemopoiesis. Blood 1971;38:96–107.

McLeod DL, Shreeve MM, Axelrad AA. Chromosome marker evidence for the bipotentiality of BFU-E. Blood 1980;56:318–322.

Melchers F. B cell differentiation in bone marrow. Clin Immunol Immunopathol 1995;76:S188–191.

Messner HA. The role of CFU-GEMM in human hemopoiesis. Blut 1986;53:269–277.

Meuret G, Senn HJ, De Fliedner V, et al. Intravascular fate of granulocytes administered by granulocyte transfusions. Acta Haematol 1976;55:193–198.

Miyazaki H, Kato T. Thrombopoietin: biology and clinical potentials. Int J Hematol 1999;70:216–225.

Moreau I, Duvert V, Caux C, et al. Myofibroblastic stromal cells isolated from human bone marrow induce the proliferation of both early myeloid and B-lymphoid cells. Blood 1993;82:2396–2405.

Ogilvie GK. Clinical use of hemopoietic growth factors. In: Feldman BF, Zinkl JG, Jain NC, et al., eds. Schalm's Veterinary Hematology. 5th Ed. Philadelphia: Lippincott Williams & Wilkins, 2000.

Ohta M, Saito M. Regeneration of bone marrow tissue. Growth and differentiation of hematopoietic stem cells and the role of bone marrow microenvironment on hematopoiesis. Hum Cell 1991; 4:212–221.

Oni OO, Stafford H, Gregg PJ. An investigation of the routes of venous drainage from the bone marrow of the human tibial diaphysis. Clin Orthop 1988;230:237–244.

Palis J, Yoder MC. Yolk-sac hematopoiesis: the first blood cells of mouse and man. Exp Hematol 2001;29:927–936.

Prockop DJ. Marrow stromal cells as stem cells for nonhematopoietic tissues. Science 1997;276:71–74.

Reagan WJ. A review of myelofibrosis in dogs. Toxicol Pathol 1993; 21:164–169.

Riggs AD. DNA methylation and cell memory. Cell Biophys 1989; 15:1–13.

Roberts R, Gallagher J, Spooncer E, et al. Heparan sulphate bound growth factors: a mechanism for stromal cell mediated haemopoiesis. Nature 1988;332:376–378.

Saleque S, Cameron S, Orkin SH. The zinc-finger proto-oncogene Gfi-1b is essential for development of the erythroid and megakaryocytic lineages. Genes Dev 2002;16:301–306.

Scott MA, Stockham SL. Basophils and mast cells. In: Feldman BF, Zinkl JG, Jain NC, et al., eds. Schalm's Veterinary Hematology. 5th Ed. Philadelphia: Lippincott Williams & Wilkins, 2000.

Schultze AE. Interpretation of canine leukocyte response. In: Feldman BF, Zinkl JG, Jain NC, et al., eds. Schalm's Veterinary Hematology. 5th Ed. Philadelphia: Lippincott Williams & Wilkins, 2000.

Shivdasani RA. The role of transcription factor NF-E2 in megakaryocyte maturation and platelet production. Stem Cells 1996; 14S1:112–115.

Shmakova NL, Yarmonenko SP, Shapiro IM. Cytological analysis of radiation damage and recovery of bone marrow in mammals. Nature 1967;214:719–720.

Slavin BG, Yoffey JM, Yaffe P. Response of marrow adipocytes to hypoxia and rebound. Prog Clin Biol Res 1981;59B:231–241.

Smith GS. Neutrophils. In: Feldman BF, Zinkl JG, Jain NC, et al., eds. Schalm's Veterinary Hematology. 5th Ed. Philadelphia: Lippincott Williams & Wilkins, 2000.

Tablin F, Castro M, Leven RM. Blood platelet formation in vitro. The role of the cytoskeleton in megakaryocyte fragmentation. J Cell Sci 1990;97:59–70.

Takamoto M, Sugane K. Synergism of IL-3, IL-5, and GM-CSF on eosinophil differentiation and its application for an assay of murine IL-5 as an eosinophil differentiation factor. Immunol Lett 1995; 45:43–46.

Tanlin F. Platelet structure and function. In: Feldman, BF, Zinkl JG, Jain NC, et al., eds. Schalm's Veterinary Hematology. 5th Ed. Philadelphia: Lippincott Williams & Wilkins, 2000.

Tavassoli M, Aoki M. Localization of megakaryocytes in the bone marrow. Blood Cells 1989;15:3–14.

Thiele J, Galle R, Sander C, et al. Interactions between megakaryocytes and sinus wall. An ultrastructural study on bone marrow tissue in primary (essential) thrombocythemia. J Submicrosc Cytol Pathol 1991;23:595–603.

Thiele J, Timmer J, Jansen B, et al. Ultrastructure of neutrophilic granulopoiesis in the bone marrow of patients with chronic myeloid leukemia (CML). A morphometric study with special emphasis on azurophil (primary) and specific (secondary) granules. Virchows Arch B Cell Pathol Incl Mol Pathol 1990;59:125–131.

Vaananen HK, Zhao H, Mulari M, et al. The cell biology of osteoclast function. J Cell Sci 2000;113:377–381.

Valledor AF, Borras FE, Cullell-Young M, et al. Transcription factors that regulate monocyte/macrophage differentiation. J Leukoc Biol 1998;63:405–417.

Verfaillie C, Hurley R, Bhatia R, et al. Role of bone marrow matrix in normal and abnormal hematopoiesis. Crit Rev Oncol Hematol 1996;16:201–224.

Voermans C, van Hennik PB, van der Schoot CE. Homing of human hematopoietic stem and progenitor cells: new insights, new challenges? J Hematother Stem Cell Res 2001;10:725–738.

Vogt C, Noe G, Rich IN. The role of the blood island during normal and 5-fluorouracil-perturbed hemopoiesis. Blood Cells 1991; 17:105–121.

Vuillet-Gaugler MH, Breton-Gorius J, Vainchenker W, et al. Loss of attachment to fibronectin with terminal human erythroid differentiation. Blood 1990;75:865–873.

Weiss L. The structure of bone marrow. Functional interrelationships of vascular and hematopoietic compartments in experimental hemolytic anemia: an electron microscopic study. J Morphol 1965;117:467–537.

Weiss L. The histophysiology of bone marrow. Clin Orthop 1967; 52:13–23.

Weiss L, Geduldig U. Barrier cells: stromal regulation of hematopoiesis and blood cell release in normal and stressed murine bone marrow. Blood 1991;78:975–990.

Wellman ML. Lymphoproliferative disorders of large granular lymphocytes. In: Feldman, BF, Zinkl JG, Jain NC, et al., eds. Schalm's Veterinary Hematology. 5th Ed. Philadelphia: Lippincott Williams & Wilkins, 2000.

Wineman J, Moore K, Lemischka I, et al. Functional heterogeneity of the hematopoietic microenvironment: rare stromal elements maintain long-term repopulating stem cells. Blood, 1996;87: 4082–4090.

Wolber FM, Leonard E, Michael S, et al. Roles of spleen and liver in development of the murine hematopoietic system. Exp Hematol 2002;30:1010–1119.

Young KM. Eosinophils. In: Feldman BF, Zinkl JG, Jain NC, et al., eds. Schalm's Veterinary Hematology. 5th Ed. Philadelphia: Lippincott Williams & Wilkins, 2000.

Zhu Y, Ye D, Huang Z. The correlation of cytokines TNF alpha, IFN-gamma, Epo with anemia in rheumatoid arthritis. Zhonghua Xue Ye Xue Za Zhi 2000;21:587–590.

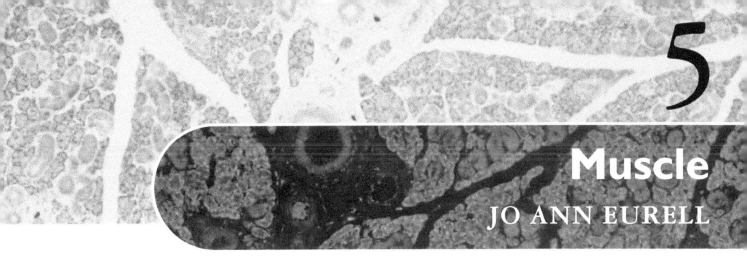

5

Muscle

JO ANN EURELL

Smooth Muscle
    Light Microscopic Structure
    Fine Structure
    Contraction
    Myogenesis, Hypertrophy, and Regeneration
Skeletal Muscle
    Light Microscopic Structure
    Fine Structure
    Contraction

Classification of Skeletal Muscle Fibers
Myogenesis, Hypertrophy, Atrophy, and Regeneration
Cardiac Muscle
    Light Microscopic Structure
    Fine Structure
    Cardiac Nodes and Impulse Conduction Fibers
    Contraction
    Myogenesis, Hypertrophy, and Regeneration

Many cells in the body are capable of contraction and limited movement, but only specialized collections of cells known as muscle are capable of strong, concerted contraction to produce integrated movement. Muscular tissues are present in three principal areas of the vertebrate body: the walls of hollow organs (e.g., viscera of the gastrointestinal tract, urogenital tract, blood vessels), the skeletal muscles, and the heart.

The specialized cells of muscular tissues have distinct morphologic characteristics directly related to their contractile activity. Muscle cells, also known as **myocytes** or **myofibers**, are elongated cells with spindle-shaped or fiberlike profiles. The term **fiber** in association with muscle refers to cells, in contrast to connective tissue fibers, which are condensed extracellular substances dispersed between cells.

The myocytes are arranged in bundles with their long axes aligned parallel to the direction of their contractions. The shape of the profiles of myocytes is dependent on the angle of sectioning. Myocytes sectioned parallel to their long axes appear as long rods or spindles, whereas those sectioned at right angles are polygonal. Oblique sectioning results in various elliptic profiles.

Within the cytoplasm of all myocytes are abundant fibrous proteins that stain intensely eosinophilic. The arrangement of these fibrous proteins is highly ordered in skeletal and cardiac muscular tissue, resulting in characteristic cross-striations of longitudinally sectioned fibers. Other muscular tissue in the walls of hollow organs is composed of myocytes without cross-striations and hence has a smooth appearance. Therefore, three basic types of muscle fibers are recognized: (1) nonstriated **smooth muscle,** which forms the contractile portion of the walls of most viscera; (2) striated **skeletal muscle,** which comprises the skeletal muscles that originate and insert on the bones of the skeleton; and (3) striated **cardiac muscle,** which is the major tissue of the walls of the heart. Skeletal muscle is considered to be voluntary in control, whereas cardiac muscle and smooth muscle are involuntary.

SMOOTH MUSCLE

Light Microscopic Structure

Smooth muscle cells are elongated, spindle-shaped cells (Fig. 5-1). Each cell contains a single, centrally located nucleus. The cells range from 5 to 20 μm in diameter and from 20 μm to 1 mm or more in length. The cytoplasm of smooth myocytes is acidophilic.

Within a tissue section, the cross-sectional size of cells is highly variable due to the tapered shape of the cells. Many cross sections of the cell lack nuclear profiles because of the extent of the cell beyond the central nuclear region (Fig. 5-1A).

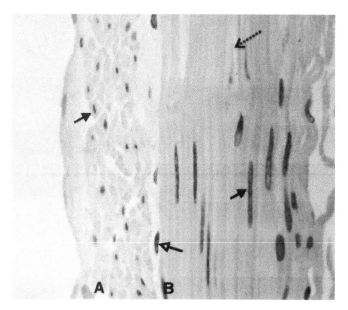

FIGURE 5-1 Smooth muscle. **A.** Cross section. **B.** Longitudinal section. The central myocyte nuclei (solid arrows) are absent in several cross sections due to sectional geometry. The tip of a spindle-shaped cell is visible at the dotted arrow. Fibroblast nuclei (open arrow) are dark and smaller than smooth muscle nuclei. Hematoxylin and eosin (×490).

Individual myocytes are surrounded by a fine network of reticular fibers, blood vessels, and nerves. In smooth muscle, reticular fibers are produced by myocytes rather than fibroblasts. Although the connective tissue is analogous to the endomysium of skeletal muscle described below, it is not termed as such.

Fine Structure

The cytoplasm of the smooth muscle myocyte contains numerous myofilaments in various orientations (Figs. 5-2 and 5-3). **Thin myofilaments** of smooth muscle contain **actin** and **tropomyosin** but lack **troponin,** which is present in skeletal and cardiac muscle. **Thick myofilaments,** composed of **myosin-II,** are sparse. The thick and thin myofilaments are not arranged in a highly ordered pattern as in striated muscle. **Dense bodies** in the cytoplasm and the cell membrane serve as anchor sites for the myofilaments. **Intermediate filaments** (desmin and vimentin) further link the dense bodies into a meshwork array. The myofilament attachment sites on the cell membrane also form junctions that connect adjacent cells.

Numerous pear-shaped invaginations (caveolae) and vesicles are present along the cell membrane and are believed to play a role in calcium transport (Figs. 5-2 and 5-3). Transverse T tubules found in striated muscle are lacking and smooth endoplasmic reticulum is sparse. Gap junctions, which allow for cell coupling, occur at frequent periodic sites in the cell membrane. Other cellular organelles, including mitochondria, Golgi complex, rough endoplasmic reticulum (rER), and free ribosomes, are located near the nucleus. Each myocyte is surrounded by a basal lamina, except at intercellular junctions (Fig. 5-3).

Contraction

The contractile apparatus of smooth muscle is capable of greater shortening in length and more sustained contractions than that of striated muscle. Contraction is governed by the phosphorylation of the myosin-II molecule in contrast to striated muscle, which is regulated by a troponin–tropomyosin complex described below.

The contraction sequence begins with an increase of calcium in the smooth muscle cell cytoplasm. Calcium increases by entering the cell through voltage-dependent calcium channels in the cell membrane or by inositol 1,4,5-triphosphate (IP_3)-induced release of calcium from the smooth endoplasmic reticulum. The rise in cytosolic calcium leads to subsequent binding of the calcium to **calmodulin.** The calcium–calmodulin complex then interacts with myosin light-chain kinase, which initiates phosphorylation of myosin-II and interaction between the actin and myosin-II myofilaments. The overall process leading to actin–myosin interaction is longer when compared with other muscle types, which results in the relatively slow contraction of smooth muscle.

Hormones that act via cyclic adenosine monophosphate (cAMP) can affect smooth muscle contraction. cAMP activates myosin light-chain kinase, leading to phosphorylation of myosin and cell contraction. Estrogen increases cAMP and subsequently smooth muscle contraction, while progesterone decreases cAMP, resulting in decreased smooth muscle contraction.

Contraction of smooth muscle is involuntary. Innervation is both parasympathetic and sympathetic, and the effects of neural input on smooth muscle are variable. **Unitary smooth muscle,** found in the wall of visceral organs, behaves as a syncytium that contracts in a networked fashion. Cells of this arrangement of smooth muscle are extensively connected by gap junctions but sparsely innervated. In contrast, **multiunit smooth muscle,** found in the iris of the eye, is capable of precise contractions due to individual innervation of each myocyte. The multiunit myocytes lack gap junctions, resulting in reduced coordinated communication between cells.

Myogenesis, Hypertrophy, and Regeneration

Smooth muscle tissue increases in size by both hypertrophy (increase in size) and hyperplasia (increase in number) of myocytes. New smooth muscle cells can form through mitosis or by derivation from pericytes. Formation of new myocytes is limited, so healing of smooth muscle is mainly through connective tissue scar formation.

SKELETAL MUSCLE

Light Microscopic Structure

Skeletal muscle myocytes are elongated cells that range from 10 to 110 μm in diameter and can reach up to 50 cm in length. These fibers are derived from the prenatal fusion of many individual mononuclear myoblasts. As a result of the fusion, a single myocyte

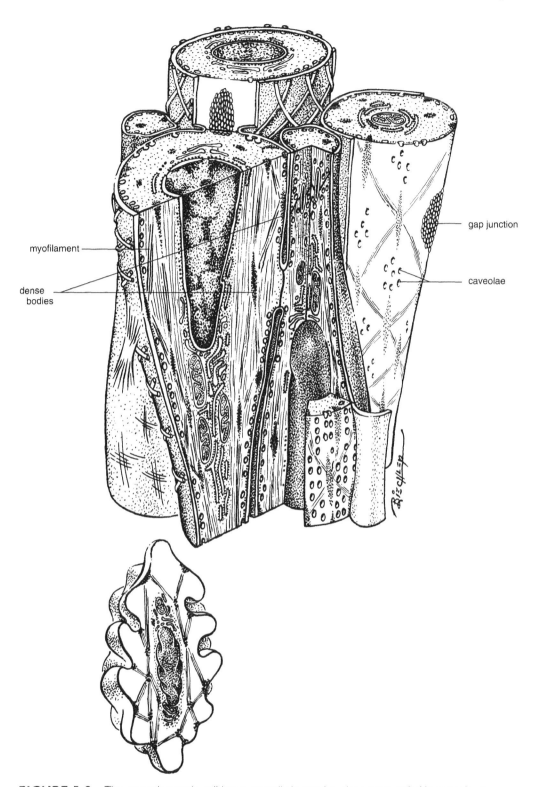

FIGURE 5-2 The smooth muscle cell has a centrally located nucleus surrounded by cytoplasm containing myofilaments in various orientations. The contractile myofilaments anchor into dense bodies on the cell membrane and within the cytoplasm of the smooth muscle cell. When the myofilaments contract, the cell shortens (lower diagram). Numerous caveolae, vesicles, and gap junctions are present along the cell membrane.

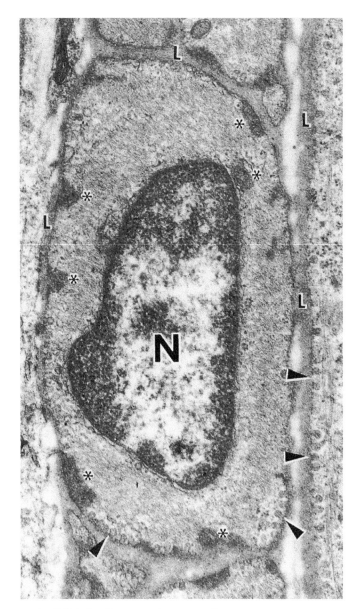

FIGURE 5-3 Electron micrograph of a cross-sectioned smooth muscle cell. The nucleus (N) is centrally located, and the cytoplasm contains numerous myofilaments. Electron-dense bodies (*) serve as attachment sites for the myofilaments. Numerous caveolae (arrowheads) are present along the plasma membrane of an adjacent cell. The basal laminae (L) are visible between the two cells and appear fused at points (×23,900). *(Courtesy of W. S. Tyler.)*

contains multiple oval nuclei, which are peripherally located within the cell (Fig. 5-4). When viewed in longitudinal section, transverse striations are present as alternating light and dark bands. In transverse section, the myocyte has an angular outline and a stippled cytoplasm (Fig. 5-5). Peripheral nuclei may be absent in some planes of the cross section of the myocyte. The surrounding cell membrane is visible at higher magnification.

Each muscle cell contains **myofibrils,** which form the dots in cross sections of the fiber at the light microscopic level (Fig. 5-6). The myofibrils are cylindrical and 1 to 2 μm in diameter. Individual myofibrils are composed of thick and thin **myofilaments,** which

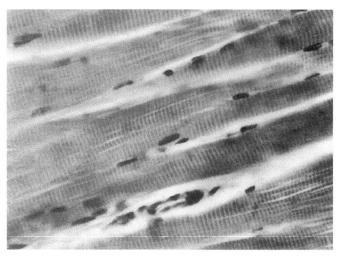

FIGURE 5-4 Skeletal muscle, longitudinal section. Notice the cross-striations and the nuclei located in the periphery of the myocytes. Hematoxylin and eosin (×435).

are responsible for contraction. The myofibrils align in a longitudinal direction to create the light and dark banding pattern of the myocyte. Thick and thin myofilaments overlap in the darker **A band** (anisotropic), whereas only thin myofilaments are present in the lighter **I band** (isotropic). The myofibrils are connected by intermediate filaments of desmin and vimentin, such that the light and dark bands of all myofibrils within a fiber are in register.

Satellite cells are spindle-shaped cells located adjacent to the cell membrane of the myocyte and within its basement membrane. Their nuclei are heterochromatic in contrast to the lighter-staining nuclei of the myocyte. Satellite cells are best recognized with electron microscopy. They are thought to represent a population of inactive myoblasts, which can be activated upon injury to initiate regeneration of muscle fibers.

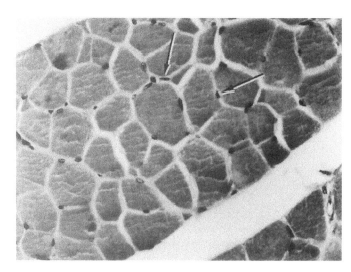

FIGURE 5-5 Skeletal muscle, cross section. The nuclei in the sparse endomysium (arrows) belong to either fibroblasts or satellite cells. Hematoxylin and eosin (×435).

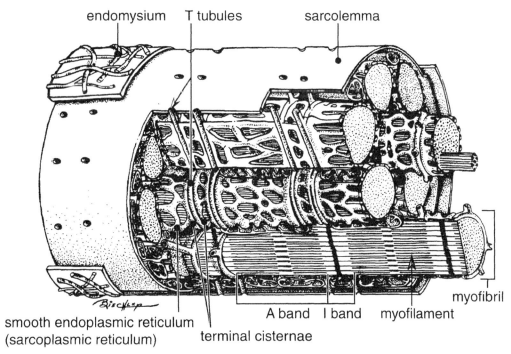

endomysium T tubules sarcolemma

smooth endoplasmic reticulum
(sarcoplasmic reticulum) terminal cisternae

A band I band myofilament myofibril

FIGURE 5-6 The myofibrils of skeletal muscle are comprised of myofilaments. Smooth endoplasmic reticulum surrounds each myofibril and forms terminal cisternae near the T tubule. T tubules extend into the cytoplasm from the cell membrane and surround the myofibrils at the A–I junction. A T tubule plus two terminal cisternae form a triad structure. Peripheral nuclei of the skeletal muscle myofiber are not shown in this illustration.

Individual myocytes are bound together into primary bundles or fascicles (Fig. 5-7). Within a fascicle, an individual myocyte is surrounded by reticular fibers, which form the **endomysium.** Nerve fibers and an extensive network of continuous capillaries are also present in the endomysium. Each fascicle is surrounded by dense irregular connective tissue, termed the **perimysium.** Supplying blood vessels and nerves plus muscle stretch receptors (muscle spindles) are located in the perimysium. Most muscles are surrounded on the outer surface by a dense irregular connective tissue layer, the **epimysium.** The connective tissues of skeletal muscle are interconnected and provide a means by which contractile forces are transmitted to other tissues.

Fine Structure

Contractile myofilaments of skeletal muscle cells are primarily actin or myosin-II. In addition, the myofilaments contain other proteins involved in either binding the primary filaments together (e.g., actinins, M-line proteins) or regulating the actin and myosin-II interaction (e.g., tropomyosin, troponin).

Thin myofilaments of skeletal muscle are composed of actin, troponin, and tropomyosin (Fig. 5-8). Globular molecules (G-actin) within the myoblast polymerize to form filamentous strands (F-actin). Each globular molecule has a binding site for myosin-II. Two filamentous strands twist together to form a double helix. Filamentous **tropomyosin** molecules lie in the groove between the two twisted strands of F-actin. The tropomyosin covers the

myosin-II binding sites on the actin. In addition, triple globular units of **troponin** are spaced at regular intervals along the tropomyosin. The globular subunits include TnT, which binds troponin to tropomyosin; TnC, which binds calcium; and TnI, which binds to actin and prevents interaction with myosin. When calcium increases and binds to TnC, tropomyosin moves off the actin-binding site and allows myosin-II to interact with actin.

Thick myofilaments are composed of myosin-II, formed by two heavy chains and four light chains of amino acids. The two heavy chains twist together to form a rodlike tail with two protruding globular heads. Two light chains are associated with each head. The heads have binding sites for actin and for adenosine triphosphate (ATP). In addition, they have adenosine triphosphatase (ATPase) activity. Individual thick filaments are bound by bands of **C protein,** which stabilize the filament.

The myofilaments are arranged to form the light and dark banding pattern visible in a longitudinal section of the myofibril (Fig. 5-9). Adjacent thick myofilaments and overlapping thin myofilaments form the A band. Thin myofilaments do not extend to the center of the A band, leaving a more lucent region known as the **H band.** The thick myofilaments are interconnected down the center of the H band by an **M line.** The M line contains **myomesin,** which links the M line to desmin, and **creatine phosphokinase,** which helps maintain levels of ATP for contraction. The **pseudo-H zone** is present on either side of the M line. In this region, thick myofilaments lack protruding cross-bridges and the area appears more electron-lucent.

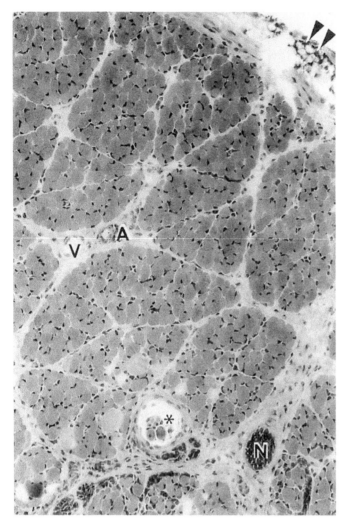

FIGURE 5-7 The myofibers are organized into fascicles (bundles) and separated from other fascicles by perimysium. Within the larger divisions of the perimysium, notice the arteriole (A), venule (V), intramuscular nerve branch (N), and muscle spindle (*). At the margin of the section is a portion of the epimysium (arrowheads) (×125).

In a cross section of the myofibril within the A band, groups of six thin myofilaments surround one thick myofilament to form a hexagonal lattice. The thick myofilaments are linked to each other by myosin-II cross-bridges (side arms that protrude from the filaments) in the A band, except in the pseudo-H zone, where cross-bridges are absent.

The I band is composed of the portion of the thin filaments that do not extend into the A band. These thin myofilaments are interconnected in the center of the I band by a **Z line** composed of **α-actinin**. A **sarcomere** extends from one Z line to the next and represents the repeating unit of myofilament arrangement within the myofibril.

Several structural proteins that link the contractile myofilaments are found within skeletal muscle. Springlike **titin** anchors the Z line to myosin-II filaments and the M line and helps maintain the A band width when muscle is stretched. **Nebulin**

is associated with actin and may regulate the assembly and length of actin filaments. **Desmin** filaments, located at the Z line, link adjacent myofibrils together side by side, and also attach the myofibrils to the cell membrane at specializations called costameres. **Dystrophin**, a transmembrane complex of proteins, stabilizes the cell membrane of the myocyte and links the cell to the surrounding basement membrane. On the cytoplasmic side of the cell membrane, the dystrophin complex is linked to actin myofilaments.

The cell membrane (previously termed sarcolemma) invaginates at several sites to form a tubular network, the **T tubules** (Figs. 5-6 and 5-10). Within the cytoplasm of the myocyte, individual myofibrils are surrounded by highly specialized smooth endoplasmic reticulum (sER) (sarcoplasmic reticulum), which stores calcium. The sER forms an anastomosing network of tubules around the myofibrils and dilates to create **terminal cisternae** at the A–I band junction. The membranes of the terminal cisternae have voltage-gated channels to release the stored calcium when needed. Each T tubule courses adjacent to two terminal cisternae and the three structures collectively form a **triad**. Mitochondria and glycogen granules are located in the cytoplasm between the myofibrils and provide energy during muscle contraction.

Contraction

A **motor unit** is composed of a nerve fiber (axon) and the muscle cells it innervates. One nerve fiber may innervate multiple myocytes. The axon contacts the skeletal muscle fiber and branches to form a **motor end plate** on the surface of the myocyte. When stimulated, an action potential travels down the axon and causes release of **acetylcholine** from the motor end plate into the synaptic cleft adjacent to the muscle fiber. Acetylcholine binds to receptors on the cell membrane and opens receptor-gated sodium channels into the myocyte. Sodium influxes into the muscle fiber and initiates a wave of depolarization that spreads across the cell membrane.

In the resting state before depolarization of the cell membrane, the tropomyosin–troponin complex covers the myosin-II binding sites on the actin filament (Fig. 5-8). Myosin-II heads are bound to ATP. As depolarization begins, an action potential spreads across the cell membrane and extends into the T tubules. The depolarization causes the adjacent terminal cisternae to release stored calcium into the cytoplasm around the myofibrils. The calcium binds to troponin (TnC) on the thin myofilaments, causing the troponin to undergo a conformation change. The change in troponin results in the movement of tropomyosin to expose the myosin-II binding sites. Actin and myosin-II interact, allowing the increased hydrolysis of ATP. Energy from the ATP hydrolysis is used to bend the head of the myosin-II complex. The movement of the head pulls the attached actin toward the center of the sarcomere, thus shortening the sarcomere and contracting the myocyte overall. The myosin-II head binds to a new ATP and then detaches from the actin filament and the cycle repeats. If ATP is depleted, the filaments cannot detach and rigor mortis sets in. After depolarization ends, calcium is actively transported back into the terminal cisternae and contraction ceases.

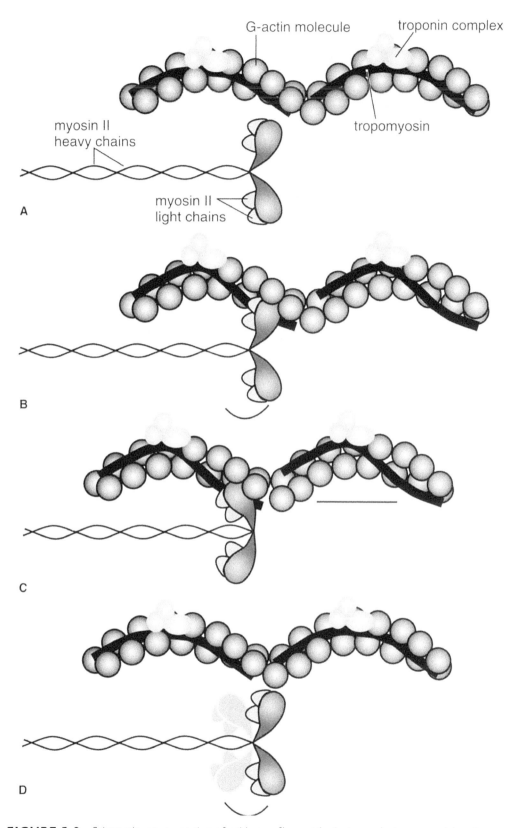

FIGURE 5-8 Schematic representation of a thin myofilament (actin, troponin, tropomyosin) and a myosin-II molecule. Several myosin-II molecules aggregate to form a thick myofilament. **A.** The muscle is relaxed; actin and myosin-II are not linked. **B.** As contraction begins, the troponin–tropomyosin complex moves off the actin-binding site and allows myosin-II to bind. The myosin-II head then bends. **C.** The thin myofilament is pulled toward the center of the sarcomere (to the left in this drawing). **D.** The actin–myosin complex then dissociates, troponin–tropomyosin covers the actin-binding site, and the myosin head swings forward to repeat the cycle.

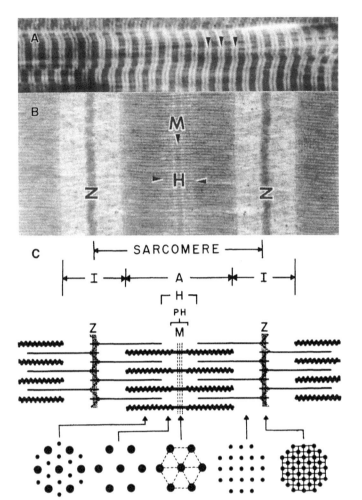

FIGURE 5-9 Light micrograph (**A**) and electron micrograph (**B**) of longitudinally oriented skeletal muscle and schematic representation (**C**) of a sarcomere. In **A,** transverse striations consisting of alternating light bands (I bands) and dark bands (A bands) are present. Each I band is bisected by a Z line (arrowheads) (×1150). In **B,** the transverse striations can be further resolved into Z lines (Z) that define a sarcomere and bisect the light I band (not labeled). The A band is electron-dense and is bisected by the M line (M, arrowhead), which connects adjacent thick myofilaments. On either side of the M line, an electron-lucent area represents the H band (H), where there is no overlap of thick and thin myofilaments (×22,500). In **C,** the arrangement of myofilaments is shown in relation to the electron micrograph. PH is the pseudo-H zone, a more electron-lucent region in which thick myofilaments lack cross-bridges. The bottom diagram represents a cross section of the region indicated by the arrows. Large dots represent thick myofilaments and small dots represent thin myofilaments.

During contraction, the I and H bands narrow and the Z lines move closer together. When muscle is stretched, opposite changes occur. In contrast, the width of the A band remains constant during either contraction or stretching.

Classification of Skeletal Muscle Fibers

Skeletal muscle fibers can be classified based on speed of contraction, gross anatomic appearance, and fatigue resistance. Within in-

dividual muscles, variable distribution of fiber types occurs. The fiber types are identified by using antibodies against either fast- or slow-twitch myosin isotypes. **Fast** muscle fibers contract quickly while **slow** muscle fibers contract more slowly. **Red** skeletal muscle fibers contain large amounts of **myoglobin**, which contributes to their red color. Myoglobin is an oxygen-carrying protein similar to hemoglobin. The red fibers have extensive mitochondria, which are densely packed under the sarcolemma and between myofibrils. This type of skeletal muscle fiber depends on the oxidative pathway for energy production. Most red muscle fibers contract and fatigue slowly and are termed slow-twitch fibers; however, some fast-twitch red fibers do exist. In contrast to red muscle fibers, **white** muscle fibers have less myoglobin and are lighter in color. Fewer mitochondria are present, often clustering as pairs between myofibrils near the I bands. The sER is more extensive, allowing for rapid release of calcium to initiate contraction. The energy for white muscle fiber contraction is primarily from anaerobic glycolysis. White muscle fibers contract and fatigue more rapidly compared with red muscle fibers and are known as fast-twitch fibers. Intermediate muscle fibers have characteristics of both red and white fibers.

Myogenesis, Hypertrophy, Atrophy, and Regeneration

During development, mesenchymal cells differentiate into skeletal muscle **myoblasts.** Myoblasts may migrate to remote locations from their original site of development. As development progresses, multiple myoblasts fuse and form elongated **myotubes.** Within the myotube, contractile myofibrils are formed. As additional myoblasts fuse to the developing myocyte and myofibrils increase in number, the nuclei peripheralize within the cell. Satellite cells remain as potential myogenic cells within the basal lamina next to the mature myocyte.

Hypertrophy of mature muscle cells occurs through the activity of satellite cells. One satellite cell divides into two daughter cells. One daughter cell remains as a satellite cell, whereas the other fuses with the muscle cell and adds additional nuclei. The new nuclei direct the synthesis of additional myofibrils and other cytoplasmic elements. Neither the myocyte nor its nuclei divide during the process of hypertrophy. In contrast, during atrophy of skeletal muscle, myofibrils and nuclei are lost.

Regeneration of muscle is dependent on the extent of injury. Small areas of muscle can be regenerated through fusion of satellite cells with each other to form new muscle cells or fusion with existing muscle cells. If damage is extensive, muscle is replaced by connective tissue instead.

CARDIAC MUSCLE

Light Microscopic Structure

The striated myocytes of cardiac muscle branch and anastomose (Fig. 5-11). At the end-to-end junction of adjacent cells, dense

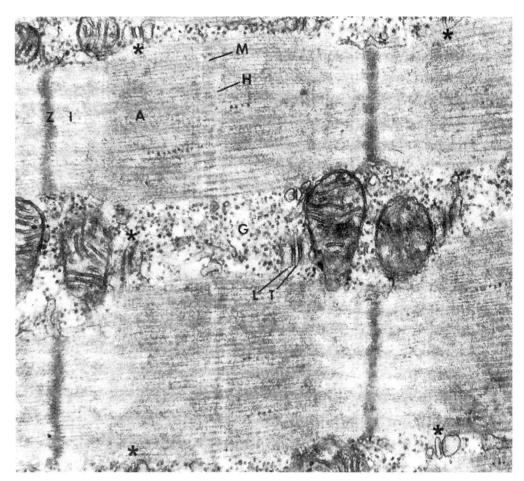

FIGURE 5-10   Electron micrograph of a longitudinal section through a skeletal muscle cell. Structures identified include: A band (A); I band (I); Z line (Z); M line (M); pseudo-H band (H); glycogen (G) within the cytoplasm adjacent to mitochondria; terminal cisternae (L); T tubule (T); and other triads (*) located at the A–I junction (×34,000).

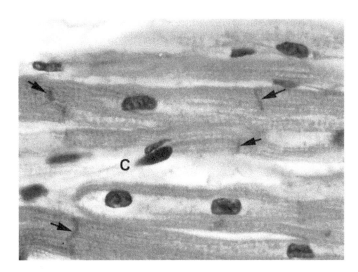

FIGURE 5-11   Cardiac myocytes in longitudinal section. Note the transverse striations and branching of the myocytes, the central location of their nuclei, and the dark-stained intercalated disks (arrows). This muscle type has many capillaries (C) (×700).

intercalated disks are present. Cardiac myocytes are approximately 15 μm in diameter and 85 to 100 μm in length. The single nuclei of cardiac muscle cells are located in the center of the cell and the cytoplasm is acidophilic (Fig. 5-12).

A network of fine reticular and collagenous fibers surrounds each cardiac muscle fiber. The network corresponds to endomysium of skeletal muscle but is more irregular. In the heart, cardiac myocytes are subdivided into groups by dense connective tissue analogous to the perimysium of skeletal muscle. No tissue that corresponds to skeletal muscle epimysium is present. Individual cardiac myocytes are surrounded by a well-developed capillary network (Figs. 5-11 and 5-12).

Fine Structure

Cardiac myocytes have myofibrils similar to skeletal muscle (Fig. 5-13). The same banding pattern of myofilaments is present. T tubules, located at the Z line, are larger than in skeletal muscle (Fig. 5-14). The sarcoplasmic reticulum is usually present on one side of the T tubule, forming a **diad** instead of a triad as found in skeletal muscle.

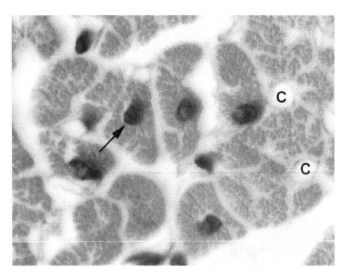

FIGURE 5-12 Cardiac muscle, cross section. Note the centrally located nuclei (arrow) and numerous capillaries (C). Hematoxylin and eosin (×800).

The mitochondria of cardiac myocytes are larger and more numerous than in skeletal muscle, indicating the degree of aerobic metabolism that occurs in this tissue (Fig. 5-14). The cytoplasm also contains lipid droplets and glycogen.

The intercalated disk is the means by which cardiac muscle cells are linked (Figs 5-13 and 5-15). The disk is formed by a complex interdigitation of the adjacent cell membranes. The longitudinal region of the disk contains gap junctions, which allow transfer of chemical signals between adjacent cells. Desmosomes and fasciae adherens are present in the transverse region of the disk. The desmosomes have intermediate filaments that extend into the cytoplasm and result in strong attachment between cells. Actin filaments of the myofibrils anchor into a specialized region of the myocyte membrane, the **fascia adherens,** located between the desmosomes (Fig. 5-15).

Atrial myocytes are smaller and have fewer T tubules than myocytes of the ventricle. In addition, atrial cardiac muscle has membrane-bounded dense granules in the cytoplasm that contain **atrial natriuretic peptides** (ANPs). ANPs stimulate the inner medullary collecting ducts of the kidney to excrete sodium

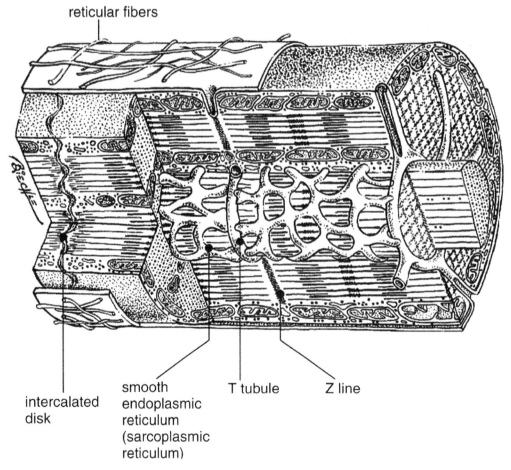

reticular fibers

intercalated disk

smooth endoplasmic reticulum (sarcoplasmic reticulum)

T tubule

Z line

FIGURE 5-13 The T tubules of cardiac muscle are located at the Z line. Smooth endoplasmic reticulum surrounds the myofibrils and contacts the T tubules, forming a diad structure. The ends of the adjacent muscle fibers are joined by an intercalated disk. A nucleus, which is centrally located in the cardiac muscle fiber, is not shown in this drawing.

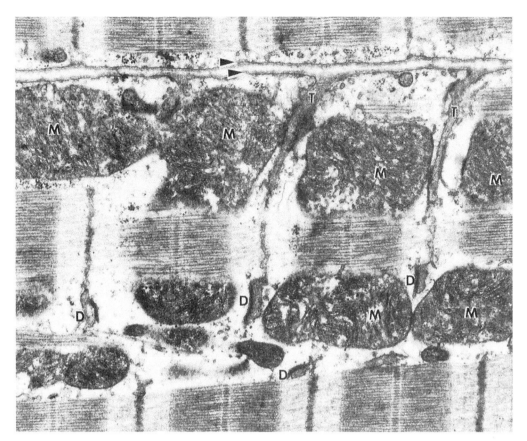

FIGURE 5-14   Electron micrograph of a longitudinal section of cardiac muscle. The cell membrane and basement membrane of each myocyte are indicated with arrowheads. Large mitochondria (M) with densely packed cristae are located just below the cell membrane. Note the two large T tubules (T) entering the lower myocyte at the Z lines. Diads (D) composed of a T tubule and smooth endoplasmic reticulum are present deeper in the cell between the myofibrils (×22,500). *(Courtesy of W. S. Tyler.)*

(natriuresis) and water (diuresis). The peptides also cause vascular smooth muscle to relax.

Cardiac Nodes and Impulse Conduction Fibers

Modified cardiac muscle cells form the **cardiac nodes** and **impulse conduction fibers** (Purkinje fibers) (Fig. 5-16 and Chapter 7). The cells of the sinoatrial and atrioventricular nodes are clustered together and have more cytoplasm and fewer myofibrils than cardiac myocytes, accounting for their light-staining cytoplasm. A large, pale area near the nucleus represents the storage site of glycogen, which is removed during tissue processing. The cells stain positively for acetylcholinesterase, which relates to their conductive function. At the ultrastructural level, the cells have mitochondria and sarcoplasmic reticulum but lack T tubules. The atrioventricular bundle, composed of impulse conduction fibers similar to nodal cells, originates from the atrioventricular node and supplies both ventricles. As the fibers course toward the apex of the heart, they become larger than adjacent cardiac myocytes and are a prominent feature of the subendocardium.

Contraction

Cardiac muscle is stimulated to contract by a mechanism similar to skeletal muscle. As there is less sER in cardiac muscle, an action potential triggers the release of calcium from both the sER and T tubules. Contraction is activated through the interaction of actin and myosin myofilaments. Sequential contraction of heart chambers is stimulated by the orderly spread of the action potentials via gap junctions in the intercalated disks. The number, size, and distribution of the gap junctions plus the type of connexin (the structural protein of the gap junctions) influence the rate of impulse conduction.

Myogenesis, Hypertrophy, and Regeneration

Cardiac muscle develops from splanchnic mesoderm surrounding the endocardial heart tube. The fibers arise by differentiation and growth of single cells. As the cells grow, new myofilaments form. The ability of cardiac muscle cells to divide is lost soon after birth. Enlargement of the heart wall during exercise or cardiac

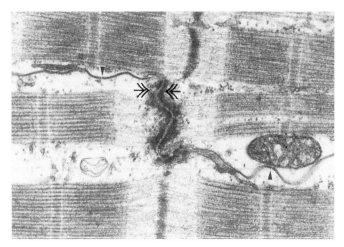

FIGURE 5-15   Electron micrograph of an intercalated disk from cardiac muscle. The fascia adherens junction (*) is oriented transversely to the long axis of the myofibril. Desmosomes are indicated by the double arrow. Gap junctions (arrowheads) are oriented parallel to the long axis (×42,100). *(Courtesy of W. S. Tyler.)*

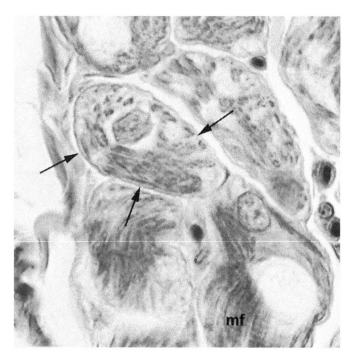

FIGURE 5-16   Cardiac impulse conduction fibers (one is outlined by arrows) are larger than myocytes. They have a centrally located nucleus and sparse myofibrils (mf) in their cytoplasm. PTAH stain (×1200).

insufficiencies is primarily through hypertrophy rather than hyperplasia. Damage to a section of the heart wall, with the resulting death of that section, is repaired primarily by proliferation of connective tissue rather than by regeneration of any significant number of new cardiac myocytes. Stem cells are under investigation as a possible source of replacement cells for damaged cardiac muscle cells.

SUGGESTED READINGS

Alberts B, Bray D, Lewis J, et al. Molecular Biology of the Cell. 3rd Ed. New York: Garland Publishing, 1994.

Allt G, Lawrenson JG. Pericytes: cell biology and pathology. Cell Tiss Org 2001;169:1–11.

Cardinet GH III, Leong DL, Means PS. Myocyte differentiation in normal and hypotrophied canine pectineal muscles. Muscle Nerve 1982;5:665.

Cardinet GH III, Orvis JA. Skeletal muscle function. In: Kaneko J, ed. Clinical Biochemistry of Domestic Animals. New York: Academic Press, 1980.

Dellmann HD, Carithers JR. Cytology and Microscopic Anatomy. Baltimore: Williams & Wilkins, 1996.

Ebashi S. Excitation-contraction coupling. Ann Rev Physiol 1976;36: 293–313.

Guyton AC, Hall JE. Textbook of Medical Physiology. Philadelphia: WB Saunders, 1996.

Hill M, Wernig A, Goldspink, G. Muscle satellite (stem) cell activation during local tissue injury and repair. J Anat 2003:203:89–99.

Horowitz A, Menice CB, Laporte R, et al. Mechanisms of smooth muscle contraction. Physiol Rev 1996;76:967–1003.

Huxley HE. Electron microscopy studies of the structure of natural and synthetic protein filaments from striated muscle. J Mol Biol 1963; 7:281–308.

Huxley HE. The structural basis of contraction and regulation in skeletal muscle. In: Heilmeyer LMG, Rüegg JC, Wieland T, eds. Molecular Basis of Motility. New York: Springer-Verlag, 1976.

Jones DA, Round JM. Skeletal Muscle in Health and Disease. New York: Manchester University Press, 1990.

Pardo JV, Siliciano JD, Craig SW. A vinculin-containing cortical lattice in skeletal muscle: transverse lattice elements ("costameres") mark sites of attachment between myofibrils and sarcolemma. Proc Natl Acad Sci U S A 1983;80:1008–1012.

Peachey LD, ed. Handbook of Physiology. Section 10: Skeletal Muscle. Bethesda, MD: American Physiological Society, 1983.

Pollard TD, Earnshaw WC. Cell Biology. Philadelphia: Saunders, 2002.

Severs NJ. Cardiac muscle cell interaction: from microanatomy to the molecular make-up of the gap junction. Histol Histopathol 1995; 10:481–501.

Tokuyasu KT, Dutton AH, Singer SJ. Immunoelectron microscopic studies of desmin (skeleton) localization and intermediate filament organization in chicken cardiac muscle. J Cell Biol 1983;96: 1736–1742.

Wang K, Ramirez-Mitchell R. A network of transverse and longitudinal intermediate filaments is associated with sarcomeres of adult vertebrate skeletal muscle. J Cell Biol 1983;96:562–570.

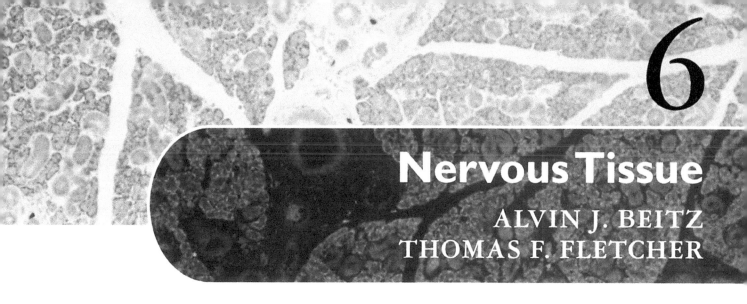

6

Nervous Tissue

ALVIN J. BEITZ
THOMAS F. FLETCHER

Neurons
  Neuronal Structure
    Cell body
      Nucleus
      Cell body cytoplasm
    Neuron processes
      Dendrites
      Axon
      Terminal branches (telodendrites)
  Classification
  Regions of a Neuron
  Neuronal Communication
    Interneuronal chemical synapses
    Synaptic ultrastructure and function
Neuroglia
  Central Nervous System Gliocytes
    Astrocytes
    Oligodendrocytes
    Microglia
    Ependymal cells

Peripheral Nervous System Gliocytes
    Ganglionic gliocytes
    Neurolemmocytes
  Myelin Sheath
Peripheral Nervous Tissue
  Nerves
  Ganglia
  Efferent Neurons
  Receptors
    Nonencapsulated receptors
    Encapsulated receptors
Central Nervous Tissue
  Cerebral Cortex
  Cerebellum
  Spinal Cord
Meninges, Blood Vessels, and Cerebrospinal Fluid
  Meninges
  Blood Vessels
  Cerebrospinal Fluid

Nervous tissue parenchyma consists of **neurons** and supportive cells called **neuroglia.** Nervous tissue forms the nervous system, which may be divided into the central nervous system and the peripheral nervous system. The **central nervous system** (CNS) includes the brain and spinal cord. The **peripheral nervous system** (PNS) consists of cranial and spinal nerves, including associated nerve roots and ganglia. Nerves and ganglia that innervate viscera are designated the **autonomic nervous system.**

NEURONS

Neurons are the structural and functional units of the nervous system. They are also trophic units because often they transform and sustain what they innervate. Generally, neurons must last a lifetime because, with some exceptions (e.g., olfactory neurons and neuronal stem cells), mature neurons are incapable of mitosis. However, recent evidence of new neuron formation in several regions of the brain has been discovered.

Morphologically, neurons feature elongated processes, termed axons and dendrites, that extend variable distances from the cell body (perikaryon) (Fig. 6-1). Metabolically, neurons are actively involved in maintaining their structural integrity and in synthesizing, packaging, transporting, and releasing secretory products.

Neurons specialize in excitability and they communicate by releasing chemical agents (neurotransmitters, neuromodulators, or neurohormones). Excitation involves ions passing through protein channels embedded in neuronal plasma membrane that otherwise acts as a hydrophobic barrier to ion flow. Via chemical secretion, neurons transmit excitation to other neurons or to muscle or glands.

Neuronal Structure

Neurons assume a variety of shapes and sizes, related to their functional roles. Neuronal processes are configured according to the connections that must be made. Neurons with processes that extend long distances must necessarily be larger than less extensive neurons. Also, because larger processes conduct more rapidly than smaller ones, neurons that convey urgent information are large.

Cell Body

The **cell body** (perikaryon; soma) of a neuron consists of the nucleus plus the surrounding cytoplasm and plasma membrane (Fig. 6-1). In routinely stained histologic sections, the cell body is the most identifiable feature of a neuron. Cellular constituents are synthesized within the cell body and then flow distally into neuronal processes (axon and dendrites).

Cell bodies range from less than 10 μm to more than 100 μm in diameter. Cell body size is proportional to neuronal total volume, although the cell body itself represents a minor portion of the total volume (and an even smaller fraction of total surface area). In multipolar neurons, where the cell body plasma membrane integrates synaptic input, smaller cell bodies are more

easily excited to threshold than larger ones; that is, less synaptic activity is required to trigger action potentials in small neurons (which have high input impedance, by virtue of their size).

Nucleus

Typically, the nucleus of a neuron is centrally positioned, spherical or ovoid, and relatively euchromatic, reflecting its high synthetic activity. Small neurons have rather heterochromatic nuclei. Neurons in autonomic ganglia have eccentric nuclei. Nuclear size is proportional to neuron size. The nucleus appears relatively large in a neuron because the cell body cytoplasm surrounding it represents only a minor fraction of total cell volume.

A prominent nucleolus is evident within the nucleus. In females of some species, **sex chromatin** (Barr body) may be evident in the vicinity of the nucleolus (cats, rodents) or nuclear membrane (primates).

Cell body cytoplasm

Many proteins are synthesized in the cell body cytoplasm of the neuron, including cytoskeletal proteins (e.g., for neurofilaments and microtubules), membrane proteins (e.g., for ion channels and active transport), enzymatic proteins (e.g., for glucose metabolism and neurotransmitter synthesis), and secretory peptides (e.g., neuromodulators and neurohormones).

The cell body cytoplasm of large neurons stained with aniline dyes and examined by light microscopy features clumps of **chromatophilic substance** (Nissl substance), which represent aggregations of rough endoplasmic reticulum (rER), free ribosomes, and polyribosomes. Chromatophilic substance extends into the trunks of dendrites, but it is absent from the axon and **axon hillock**, a pale-staining region of the cell body where the axon originates. Instead, the hillock contains neurofilaments and grouped microtubules. In small neurons, cytoplasmic chromatophilia appears relatively pale and diffuse.

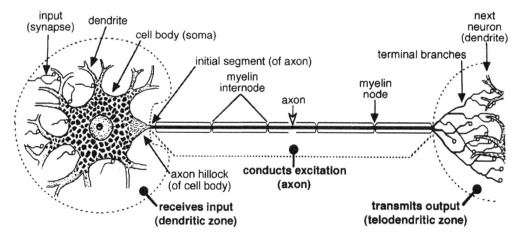

FIGURE 6-1 Schematic illustration of a typical (multipolar) neuron, showing multiple dendrites and one axon emanating from the cell body. Functional regions include a dendritic zone (cell body and dendrites), which receives synaptic input; telodendritic zone (axon terminals), which makes synaptic contact with other neurons; and the axon, which conducts excitation between the two zones. This axon is drawn myelinated. The myelin insulation is interrupted by nodes (gaps). The myelin of each internode is formed by individual glial cells (not shown).

When a neuron is injured (e.g., by transection of its axon), the cell body swells, the nucleus shifts to an eccentric position, and ribosomes disperse so that chromatophilic substance disappears from the center of the cell body (**chromatolysis**). This response to injury, called the **axonal reaction** (Fig. 6-2), begins within days of the injury and may persist several weeks. The reaction is considered pathologic evidence of nervous tissue damage in the CNS.

Organelles in the cell body cytoplasm of the neuron include plentiful mitochondria, which support the aerobic energy needs of the cell, and a prominent Golgi complex. **Secretory vesicles** originate from the complex and are transported through the axon to synaptic boutons (expansions of the axon terminal). Secretory vesicles commonly contain neuroactive peptides that influence the excitability or growth of target cells. In the case of certain hypothalamic neurons, secretory vesicles contain neurohormones that are released in proximity to blood vessels and ultimately enter the bloodstream.

Synaptic vesicles containing neurotransmitters are concentrated in axon terminals, where they fuse with plasma membrane and release neurotransmitter into a synaptic cleft. Long-lived neurons may accumulate **lipofuscin granules** in the cytoplasm as a residue of lysosomal activity.

Microtubules (25 nm in diameter) and **neurofilaments** (10 nm in diameter) are numerous in the cell body. Microtubules are involved in the rapid transport of membrane-bounded organelles within the neuron. Groups of neurofilaments, referred to as neurofibrils, can be visualized with light microscopy.

Neuron Processes

A typical neuron has a single axon and multiple dendrites originating as processes from its cell body (Fig. 6-1). The axon ends in terminal branches that synapse with dendrites and cell bodies of other neurons or innervate muscle or glandular epithelium. Each type of neuronal process has a distinct functional role within the neuron. Thus, the processes have different populations of plasma membrane proteins (channels, receptors, transporters, pumps).

Dendrites

Dendrites are highly branched processes designed to receive numerous synaptic contacts from other neurons. Treelike, each dendrite emerges as a main trunk that branches repeatedly into smaller and smaller twigs. The trunk has an organelle content similar to that of the cell body. Small dendritic branches feature predominantly microtubules, augmented by neurofilaments, mitochondria, and smooth endoplasmic reticulum (sER).

Synaptic sites on dendrites are distinguished by a band of electron-dense cytoplasm of variable thickness that lines a region of **postsynaptic membrane** that faces a **presynaptic element** across a **synaptic cleft** (Fig. 6-3). The dense material represents proteins (receptors, channels, enzymes, etc.) responsible for postsynaptic activity.

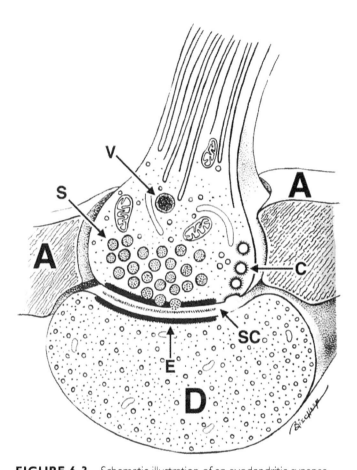

FIGURE 6-3 Schematic illustration of an axodendritic synapse. The terminal bulb of an axon is separated from a dendrite (D) by a synaptic cleft (SC) containing glycoprotein material. Astrocyte processes (A) border the synaptic cleft bilaterally. Within the terminal bulb, synaptic vesicles (S) are clustered around an active zone in which an electron-dense band lines the plasma membrane. As a consequence of Ca++ influx, synaptic vesicles are able to dock with the plasma membrane and release neurotransmitter molecules by exocytosis. Vesicle membrane is recovered from the plasma membrane and conveyed, as coated vesicles (C), to smooth endoplasmic reticulum (sER) for recycling. A solitary, large, dense-core secretory vesicle (possibly containing a peptide or monoamine neuroactive substance) is also shown (V), along with mitochondria, microtubules, and neurofilaments. The transverse section of the dendrite features an electron-dense band (E) along the postsynaptic membrane. Numerous microtubules and neurofilaments and a few sER profiles are evident in the dendrite.

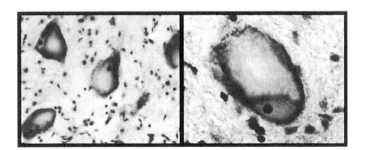

FIGURE 6-2 Two light micrographs at different magnifications of chromatolytic cell bodies from the spinal cord of a dog that had spinal nerves transected. The cell bodies are swollen, nuclei are shifted to an eccentric position, and chromatophilic substance is lost except for small amounts accumulated marginally. Nissl's stain (left, ×200; right, ×400).

Many neurons display numerous **dendritic spines** (gemmules), the postsynaptic partner in many excitatory synapses. A spine is a short expanded process attached to the dendritic branch by a narrow stalk, like a bud on a twig (Fig. 6-4). **A spine apparatus,** consisting of alternating membrane sacs and dense material, may be found within the spine. Spines increase dendritic surface area and act to restrict the spread of postsynaptic excitation. For a century or more, dendritic spines were considered very static structures, but within the last 5 years, research has shown that the structure of the spine is very dynamic. Time-lapse imaging shows that adult spines can change shape by as much as 30% of their length or width within a few seconds to minutes. Furthermore, high-frequency stimulation induces protrusion of new dendritic processes as well as spine bifurcation, also within minutes. These data suggest that changes in spine number or shape may contribute to synaptic plasticity, perhaps by providing a lasting structural substrate for newly encoded memories.

Axon

The **axon** is a relatively long, cylindrical process that originates from the axon hillock of the cell body and ends in terminal branches and synaptic boutons, which are described below. While the axon typically emerges from the cell body, in some neurons

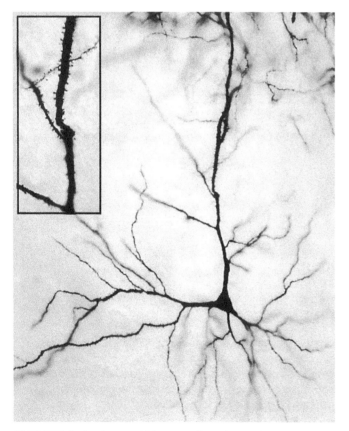

FIGURE 6-4 A pyramidal neuron from the cerebral cortex is shown (Golgi silver impregnation). This multipolar neuron has a pyramidal cell body from which apical and basal dendrites arise. A single axon (not visible) leaves the lower surface of the cell body. The insert, an enlargement of the middle of the apical dendrite, shows dendritic spines.

found in parasympathetic ganglia or in the brain, the axon originates as a branch of a dendrite. Except at its termination, axonal branches are sparse. When branches are present along the course of the axon, they emerge at right angles (from nodes in the case of myelinated axons) and are called **collateral branches. Axoplasm,** the cytoplasm of the axon, contains microtubules, neurofilaments, mitochondria, and sER. Devoid of rER, axoplasm is not well stained by hematoxylin and eosin and other routine histologic stains.

The **initial segment** of the axon is a site just distal to the axon hillock, where action potentials normally originate. It is narrower than the rest of the axon. Ultrastructurally, bundled microtubules are present and electron-dense material is evident along the inner surface of the plasma membrane of the initial segment. The density represents protein accumulation associated with ion channels and pumps. Similar electron-dense protein accumulations are also found at nodes of myelinated axons.

A slow flow of cytoplasm (1 mm/day) and a slow transport of cytoskeletal elements (10 mm/day) progress along the axon, from axon hillock to terminal branches (anterograde transport). In addition, axons have a fast transport capability (up to 400 mm/day) involving microtubule-linked movement of mitochondria and constituents packaged in vesicles. There is also a retrograde transport mechanism that rapidly conveys remnants of organelles from terminal branches back to lysosomes within the cell body. Viruses (e.g., rabies) and neurotoxins (e.g., tetanus toxin) can also be carried to the cell body by this route.

Axons are capable of regenerative conduction; that is, they convey an excitation signal to the end of the axon with the same magnitude as it had when it began at the initial segment. Large axons conduct more rapidly than small ones, but to further increase conduction velocity, large axons are myelinated (coated with a myelin sheath formed by glial cells). Small nonmyelinated axons are ensheathed by glial cells in peripheral nerves, but they are not ensheathed at all in the CNS.

Axon degeneration may be causally linked to the documented physiologic and behavioral deficits observed in aged animals. Traditionally, the decline in memory function and behavioral dysfunction that accompany normal aging in animals have been attributed to loss of neurons in certain areas of the brain. Recent data, however, show that aging does not induce prominent cell loss in the brain, but rather leads to degeneration of axons that innervate certain forebrain structures.

Terminal branches (telodendrites)

Axons terminate by successively branching (Fig. 6-1). The collective terminal branches constitute the axon terminal (telodendritic) zone of a neuron. Each terminal branch ends in an expansion called a **terminal synaptic bulb** (synaptic bouton). Along the nonmyelinated terminal branches, synapses occur at multiple focal swellings called axonal varicosities (preterminal boutons). The number of axonal varicosities is not insignificant; a single hippocampal cell axon makes 50,000 synapses over a distance of only 200 mm. Both axonal varicosities and terminal synaptic boutons are sites where neurotransmitter molecules are packaged and stored within synaptic vesicles.

The most common **synaptic vesicle** is spherical (40 to 50 nm in diameter) with an electron-lucent (agranular) core (Figs. 6-3 and 6-5). Such vesicles may contain any one of a number of neurotransmitters. Electron-lucent synaptic vesicles that appear flattened when exposed to solutions of high osmolarity are associated with inhibitory synapses. Some neurons have spherical vesicles (40 to 60 nm in diameter) with an electron-dense (granular) core. The electron-dense synaptic vesicles usually contain dopamine or norepinephrine molecules.

Synaptic vesicle proteins are synthesized in the cell body and transported rapidly to axon terminal sER, where they supplement local production of synaptic vesicles from recycled vesicular membrane. Transporter proteins in vesicle membrane load newly formed synaptic vesicles with neurotransmitter molecules that were also recycled. Linked by cytoskeletal actin filaments, synaptic vesicles are clustered together, in ready reserve for plasma membrane docking and exocytosis during synaptic activity (Fig. 6-3). In addition to synaptic vesicles, terminal branches may contain **secretory vesicles** that store neuroactive peptides (several dozen have been identified). Peptides are found in spherical, electron-dense vesicles that are relatively large (100 to 200 nm in diameter). The secretory vesicles are synthesized in the cell body and transported to preterminal and terminal synaptic boutons for storage and release. The peptides generally act as neuromodulators (agents that augment neurotransmitter effects). Secretory vesicles of certain hypothalamic neurons contain peptide hormones (e.g., vasopressin and oxytocin are stored and released in the neurohypophysis).

Sprouting of new terminal branches and degenerations of existing branches in response to environmental change is a major mechanism of neural plasticity, enabling neural development and subsequently behavioral modification and learning.

Classification

Neurons are anatomically classified as unipolar, bipolar, or multipolar according to the number of processes that emanate from the cell body (Fig. 6-6).

In a **unipolar** neuron, the cell body gives off a single axon that soon bifurcates into central and peripheral branches. The peripheral branch terminates in receptors that are sensitive to environmental energy. The central branch conveys the environmentally induced excitation into the CNS. Unipolar cell bodies are found in sensory ganglia located in roots of cranial and spinal nerves. Mammalian unipolar neurons are often referred to as pseudounipolar, because they originate as bipolar cells and only become unipolar during development. The unique geometry of unipolar sensory neurons can lead to the generation of spontaneous discharge in the cell bodies, potentially disrupting the fidelity of afferent signaling in normal animals. More importantly, following nerve injury, discharge originating ectopically within spinal ganglion cells is greatly augmented and can be a major contributor to neuropathic dysesthesias and chronic pain.

In a **bipolar** neuron, two processes emanate from the cell body, which is situated either within the axon (vestibulocochlear afferent neurons; bipolar cells of the retina) or at the juncture of the axon and a solitary dendrite (olfactory afferent neurons). Like unipolar neurons, bipolar neurons are afferent neurons that convey sensory information to the CNS.

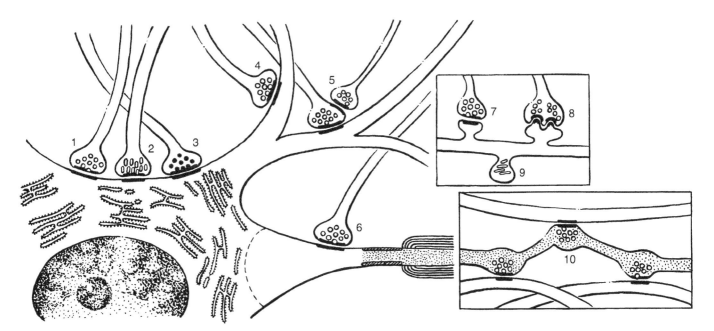

FIGURE 6-5 Schematic illustrations of types of central nervous system synapses. **1.** Axosomatic synapse with electron-lucent, spherical, synaptic vesicles. **2.** Axosomatic synapse with synaptic vesicles that are flattened (an artifact associated with inhibitory synapses). **3.** Axosomatic synapse with electron-dense synaptic vesicles. **4.** Axodendritic synapse. **5.** Axoaxonic synapse in which one terminal bulb synapses on another (associated with presynaptic inhibition). **6.** Synapse on an axon hillock, close to the initial segment of the axon. **7.** Axodendritic synapse on a dendritic spine. **8.** Relatively elaborate synapse on a dendritic spine. **9.** Dendritic spine exhibiting a spine apparatus (smooth endoplasmic reticulum plus electron-dense material). **10.** Three axonal varicosities making synapses in passing (en passant).

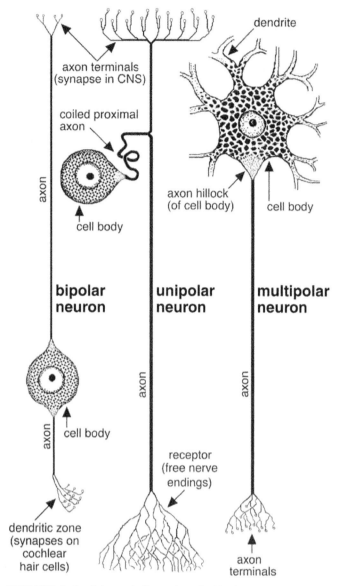

FIGURE 6-6 Schematic illustration of a bipolar neuron (left), a unipolar neuron (center), and a multipolar neuron (right). Neurons are anatomically classified according to the number of processes emanating from the cell body. Unipolar and bipolar neurons are sensory. Most neurons are multipolar; however, their shapes vary considerably. The cytoplasm of the cell bodies features clumps of chromatophilic substance (Nissl substance).

In a **multipolar** neuron, the cell body gives rise to multiple branches, several dendrites, and an axon. Nearly all of the billions of neurons comprising the CNS are multipolar, as are the neurons contained in autonomic ganglia of the PNS.

Regions of a Neuron

A typical neuron becomes excited at its input region, conducts excitation to its output region, and transmits excitation via chemical secretion at synapses (Fig. 6-1). Reception, conduction, and transmission of excitation require functionally different ion channels and cellular features. Thus, an individual neuron has distinct regions: (a) an input region or **dendritic zone**, where excitation is initially received; (b) an output region or **telodendritic (axon terminal) zone**, where excitation is transmitted to other cells; (c) an **axon**, which conducts excitation between the dendritic and axon terminal zones; and (d) a **cell body**, which nurtures the cell.

In a typical multipolar neuron (Fig. 6-1), the receptive dendritic zone features a large surface area encompassing the cell body and highly branched dendrites. An elongated, cylindrical axon originates from the cell body. The axon terminal zone is a highly branched region located at the distal end of the axon. The terminal branches feature localized expansions (boutons or bulbs) where neurotransmitter molecules are stored and released at synapses.

In the case of a unipolar afferent neuron, the cell body is situated along the axon and the dendritic zone consists of receptors that change environmental energy into neural excitation. Dendritic zones of bipolar afferent neurons may involve receptors (olfaction) or synaptic contact with receptor cells (in the retina and inner ear). From dendritic zones, excitation is conveyed along the axon to terminal branches within the CNS.

The protein composition of the plasma membrane is necessarily different at each functional region of a neuron. For example, dendritic zone membrane has ligand-reactive protein receptors that open ion channels, either directly or through second messengers. Here the term "receptor" refers to membrane proteins interacting with extracellular physiologic signals and converting them into intracellular effects. Axon membrane has voltage-gated Na^+ channels that enable membrane polarity reversal and regenerative conduction. The membrane of terminal branches and synaptic boutons has voltage-gated Ca^{++} channels (Ca^{++} is involved in the release of neurotransmitter molecules) and membrane-associated receptors for reuptake of released neurotransmitter.

Neuronal Communication

Neurons communicate with one another, with glial cells, and with the muscles and glands that neurons innervate. Alterations in excitation communicated from neuron to neuron (neural circuits) constitute the basis of nervous system function.

Among the billions of neurons that comprise the nervous system, the primary means of communication is localized release of neurotransmitter molecules at interneuronal chemical synapses. Chemical synaptic arrangements are also encountered between efferent neurons and the muscles and glands they innervate (see Peripheral Nervous Tissue section). A few neurons communicate through gap junctions (electrotonic synapses), especially in invertebrates and fish. In mammals, gap junction communication is common between neuroblasts during embryonic development, but it is relatively rare between mature neurons. Other neurons communicate by producing a gas that passes freely through neuronal membranes (e.g., the gases nitric oxide and carbon monoxide are increasingly appreciated as major neurotransmitters; NO and CO transmit signals between neurons by binding to a heme moiety at the active site of soluble guanylyl cyclase, leading to an increase in the intracellular second messenger molecule cyclic guanosine 5′-monophosphate [cGMP]).

Interneuronal Chemical Synapses

An **interneuronal chemical synapse** is a site of morphologic specialization where one neuron influences the excitability of another by releasing neurotransmitter molecules from synaptic vesicles. A majority of **neurotransmitters** are biogenic amines (e.g., glutamate, glycine, dopamine, norepinephrine, serotonin, acetylcholine, etc.). Generally, each neurotransmitter can interact with a variety of membrane receptors.

A **receptor** is a site on a membrane protein to which a neurotransmitter binds briefly. The receptor protein may be a channel that undergoes reconfiguration to allow passage of selective ions, or the receptor may be coupled to a G-protein cascade that opens ion channels either directly or indirectly by activating second messengers (such as cyclic adenosine monophosphate [cAMP]). Second messengers provide a means of amplifying the scope and impact of a neurotransmitter signal as well as prolonging its time course. Autoreceptors (receptors in presynaptic plasma membrane that influence neurotransmitter synthesis and release) and neuromodulators (peptides released from secretory vesicles) typically act via second messengers.

Ionotropic membrane receptors represent one large class of neurotransmitter receptors in which the receptor protein is part of an ion channel–receptor protein complex. When activated, the complex opens or closes the ion channel, resulting in a change in membrane permeability. **Metabotropic receptors** represent the other large class of neurotransmitter receptors in which the receptor protein acts via another protein such as a G protein to activate or inhibit enzymes and possibly open, close, or modify ion channels, ultimately leading to a change in cell function.

Based on the ion channel or the G protein to which a receptor is coupled, the receptor may be excitatory or inhibitory. Thus, it is the nature of the receptor type, rather than the neurotransmitter itself, that determines the function of a synapse (e.g., excitatory or inhibitory, short or long acting, etc.). Nonetheless, some neurotransmitters (e.g., glutamate) are associated with excitatory synapses, and others (e.g., glycine) are associated with inhibitory synapses. It is worth noting that glutamate receptors are the most prevalent excitatory neurotransmitter receptors in the brain, and they mediate almost all excitatory communications between CNS neurons. Thus, it is perhaps not surprising that epileptic seizures are a problem of overactivation of brain neurons that are driven mainly by glutamate synapses.

Most synapses between neurons involve terminal synaptic boutons of one neuron contacting the input region of another neuron, forming axodendritic or axosomatic synapses (Fig. 6-5). However, among the trillions of synapses in the nervous system, every synaptic combination has been observed, including axoaxonic, dendrodendritic, dendrosomatic, somatodendritic, and somatosomatic synapses.

The input region of a typical multipolar neuron receives thousands of synaptic contacts. Excitatory and inhibitory synaptic effects are collectively summated and integrated at the cell body of the target neuron, so that the cell body membrane potential continually registers the net effect of total synaptic input to the neuron. In turn, the cell body affects the membrane potential at the nearby initial segment of the axon. At any moment, the collective synaptic input to a neuron will be sufficient to trigger an action potential at the initial segment of the axon or be insufficient to do so.

The influence that one neuron has on another depends on the number of synaptic contacts it makes with the target neuron and where the synapses are positioned. Synapses close to the initial segment will have much greater influence triggering an action potential than will synapses on distal dendrites.

Synaptic Ultrastructure and Function

Ultrastructurally, an interneuronal chemical synapse may be identified by the juxtaposition of a presynaptic element, a synaptic cleft, and a postsynaptic membrane (Fig. 6-3). The **presynaptic element** contains multiple synaptic vesicles clustered around an active zone indicated by electron density (protein accumulation) just inside the plasma membrane. The **synaptic cleft** (in the CNS, approximately the same width as the general intercellular space, 20 to 30 nm wide) contains a protein that holds presynaptic and postsynaptic membranes together. The **postsynaptic somatodendritic membrane** contains many types of protein receptors that accumulate to form functional microdomains opposite presynaptic terminal boutons that release neurotransmitters. These domains are associated with postsynaptic densities that, under the electron microscope, appear as electron-dense material facing the presynaptic active zone. The **postsynaptic density,** which consists of adhesive proteins, such as cadherin–catenin complexes, receptor proteins, subsynaptic scaffolding proteins, and associated components of the cell's cytoskeleton, is involved in the stabilization and trafficking of receptors and in signal transduction.

When an action potential arrives at the end of an axon, it passively depolarizes the presynaptic element (e.g., terminal synaptic bouton). Voltage-sensitive channels in the presynaptic membrane open to allow Ca^{++} influx. Elevated cytoplasmic Ca^{++} activates enzymes that phosphorylate synaptic vesicle proteins responsible for reversibly linking vesicles to cytoskeletal actin filaments and merging vesicles with plasma membrane. This mobilizes synaptic vesicles, enabling them to dock with the plasma membrane and release several thousand neurotransmitter molecules by exocytosis. The molecules diffuse into the synaptic cleft and bind with various receptors and transporters.

Synapses are very dynamic structures and there is constant movement of receptors into and out of synaptic membranes. Recent data have shown that rapid gain and loss of neurotransmitter receptors from synaptic sites are accounted for by endocytosis and exocytosis, as well as by lateral diffusion in the plane of the membrane. These events are interdependent and are regulated by neuronal activity and interactions with scaffolding proteins. Thus, it is known that activity-dependent elevation in postsynaptic intracellular calcium concentration triggers rapid receptor immobilization and local accumulation on the neuronal surface. Neurotransmitter receptor movement into and out of the synaptic membrane is one of the core mechanisms for rapidly changing the number of functional receptors during synaptic plasticity.

Synaptic activity ceases when neurotransmitter molecules are removed from the synaptic cleft (or degraded in the case of acetylcholine). Molecules are actively transported intracellularly by transporters (protein pumps) located in the presynaptic membrane or in membranes of adjacent glial cells. Thus, neurotransmitter molecules are recycled to minimize the need for synthesis within presynaptic cytoplasm. As well, synaptic vesicle membrane is recycled. Vesicle membrane is extracted from the presynaptic plasma membrane and transported as coated vesicles to sER within the presynaptic cytoplasm (Fig. 6-3).

NEUROGLIA

Neuroglia (gliocytes) comprise over 90% of the cells that make up the nervous system. Recent studies have shown that glia are not simply the support structure in which neurons are embedded. While the biology of glial cells is poorly understood, it is clear that glial–neuronal and glial–glial interactions are essential for many of the critical functions that occur in the nervous system. Neurons communicate with glial cells by releasing ATP at synapses and from axons during conduction. Glial cells have vital roles in neuronal development, activity, plasticity, and recovery from injury.

Neuroglia are endowed with a rich assortment of ionic channels, neurotransmitter receptors, and transport mechanisms that enable the gliocytes to respond to many of the same signals acting on neurons and also to modulate the neuronal response. In parallel to the serial flow of information along chains of neurons, glia communicate with other glial cells through intracellular waves of calcium and via intercellular diffusion of chemical messengers. By releasing neurotransmitters and other extracellular signaling molecules, glia can affect neuronal excitability and synaptic transmission and perhaps coordinate activity across networks of neurons. Moreover, glia secrete cytokines, growth factors, and other trophic factors that dictate long- and short-term survival of neurons as well as the elaboration and retraction of synaptic connections.

From a histologic perspective, neuroglial cells are relatively small. With routine histologic stains, only their nuclei and cell bodies are evident, and thus in tissue sections they are distinguished primarily by the size and shape of their cell bodies and the size and chromatin pattern of their nuclei. However, the use of modern immunocytochemical staining for specific cell surface or internal markers allows definitive identification of glial cells in brain sections. It should be noted that unlike mature neurons, glial cells remain capable of mitosis, and thus they can give rise to tumors of the nervous system.

Except for microglial cells, which migrate into the CNS from mesoderm, CNS gliocytes are derived from the ectodermal cells that form the embryonic neural tube. Neurolemmocytes of the PNS are derived from the embryonic neural crest (as are neurons that have cell bodies in ganglia).

Central Nervous System Gliocytes

The gliocytes of the CNS include astrocytes, oligodendrocytes, microglia, and ependymal cells.

Astrocytes

With routine stains, **astrocytes** are identified by their pale, ovoid nuclei, which are largest among glial nuclei. With silver stains, astrocytes exhibit numerous processes that contain glial fibrils. In white matter, the processes are long, slender, and moderately branched; in gray matter, the processes appear shorter and highly branched. Thus, white matter is said to contain **fibrous astrocytes,** whereas gray matter contains **protoplasmic astrocytes** (Fig. 6-7).

Under the electron microscope, astrocytes feature packed bundles of intermediate filaments (8 nm in diameter) and pale cytoplasm. The **glial filaments,** which are composed of glial fibrillar acidic protein (GFAP), are unique to astrocytes and form the **glial fibrils** seen with light microscopy. The filaments are denser in fibrous astrocytes than in protoplasmic ones.

Adjacent astrocytes are joined by gap junctions. In response to local stimulation, a widening excitatory wave of elevated cytoplasmic Ca^{++} can spread outward from cell to cell via the gap junctions. The adjacent astrocytes are also linked by small, button-like adhering junctions (spot desmosomes).

Astrocyte processes terminate in expansions called **end feet.** Collections of end feet form a **glial-limiting membrane** to which pia mater is attached at the CNS surface. End feet are prominent in the subependymal glial layer, and they form septa in the spinal cord. End feet cover vessels within the brain and spinal cord, and they are believed to be responsible for inducing formation of tight junctions between capillary endothelial cells (a basis for the blood-brain barrier further described on page 115).

Astrocytes provide structural support through their glial fibrils, but in addition, these cells play a critical role in several aspects of brain function. By storing glycogen and releasing glucose, they represent a source of reserve energy. Astrocyte plasma membranes have ionic pumps that regulate K^+ throughout the narrow extracellular space of the CNS. Astrocyte processes insulate synapses and release substances that modulate synaptic sensitivity. Astrocytes can also take up neurotransmitter molecules from the synaptic cleft to stop ongoing synaptic activity.

Recent data have revealed that astrocyte activity is probably determined by neuronal activity and that astrocytes have the capacity to signal not only to each other, but also back to the neurons. Furthermore, since astrocytes can sense synaptic activity, it is thought that they are pivotal intermediaries between neurons and the brain microcirculation. In this regard, increased synaptic activity triggers calcium waves in astrocytes, causing their end feet to release substances that cause local vasodilation. Thus, astrocytes can act to couple brain activity not only to energy demands but also to blood flow requirements.

Finally, astrocytes seem to have an immune function; they can present antigens to T lymphocytes and can secrete a wide array of chemokines and cytokines, allowing them to influence T helper cell response and monocyte/microglia effector functions. It should be noted that the reaction of astrocytes following brain trauma or in certain pathologic states is characterized by astrocyte proliferation and hypertrophy, elongation of astrocyte processes, up-regulation of various intermediate filaments, and, in cases of severe trauma or pathology, the formation of a

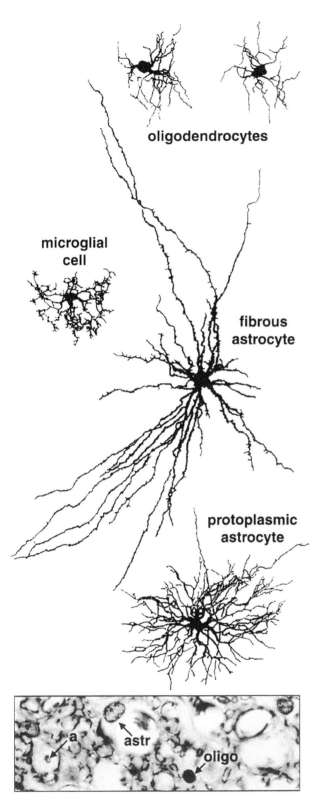

oligodendrocytes

microglial
cell

fibrous
astrocyte

protoplasmic
astrocyte

FIGURE 6-7 Central nervous system gliocytes are drawn as they appeared following Golgi silver impregnation of monkey cerebral cortex (×700). The insert at the bottom shows an astrocyte nucleus (astr) and an oligodendrocyte nucleus (oligo) as they appear in white matter stained with Luxol blue and hematoxylin. An axon (a) surrounded by a myelin vacuole and neurokeratin can be seen. *(Adapted from Weiss L. Cell and Tissue Biology. A Textbook of Histology. 6th Ed. Baltimore: Urban & Schwarzenberg, Inc., 1988.)*

dense glial scar. This process is referred to as astrogliosis and the glial scar is formed by the hypertrophied processes of reactive astrocytes filling in the space that results from loss of myelin and neurons.

Oligodendrocytes

Oligodendrocytes have relatively few branches (Fig. 6-7). In routine stains, they are recognized by their small, spherical, densely stained nuclei. Ultrastructurally, oligodendrocyte cytoplasm is electron-dense and rich in microtubules and organelles, especially rER and mitochondria. Oligodendrocytes lack gap junctions.

In gray matter, oligodendrocytes serve as perineuronal satellites. New data indicate that oligodendrocytes act as growth factor providers. Oligodendrocytes synthesize defined growth factors and provide trophic signals to nearby neurons. They also appear to be quite sensitive to neurotrauma.

In white matter, oligodendrocytes form **myelin sheaths** around axons, speeding action potential propagation in the CNS. Intracellular trafficking of membrane constituents plays an essential role in the biogenesis and maintenance of myelin. The requisite proteins and lipids are transported from their sites of synthesis to myelin via intracellular carrier vesicles transported along elements of the cytoskeleton.

Microglia

Microglia are cells of mesodermal origin that invade the CNS when it is vascularized embryologically. They are sparse and difficult to find in normal tissue. In routine stains, microglia are identified by their small, elongated, chromophilic nuclei. With silver impregnation, they are seen as small, elongated cells with polar processes (Fig. 6-7). Under physiologic conditions, microglia synthesize and release trophic factors; however, in response to CNS injury, microglia react, proliferate, and express protective or, in some situations, cytotoxic properties. Microglia activation often precedes reactions of any other cell type in the brain and once activated, they transform into macrophages with antigen-presenting and phagocytic capabilities. Reactive microglia secrete cytokines, including tumor necrosis factor and IL-1β, which can affect synaptic transmission and have trophic effects on neurons. Microglia have been recognized to play crucial roles in important diseases such as viral infections, autoimmunity, and neurodegenerative disorders.

In addition to microglia, other cell types also respond to CNS damage. Hematogenous macrophages can invade the CNS. Pericytes, cells associated with CNS capillaries and believed to have contractile capability, are also thought to be phagocytic. Although the functional role of glial scarring is not completely understood, it has been suggested to be an attempt by the CNS to restore homeostasis through isolation of the damaged region.

Ependymal Cells

Ependymal cells form an epithelium that lines ventricular cavities within the brain and the central canal of the spinal cord. The cells are typically cuboidal or columnar with numerous motile cilia on their apical surfaces (Fig. 6-8). Ependymal cells are linked by zonulae adherens and gap junctions near their luminal borders. In the adult brain, mature ependyma is not merely an inert lining but may instead regulate the transport of ions, small molecules, and water between the cerebrospinal fluid and neuropil. Ependyma serves an important barrier function that protects neural tissue from potentially harmful substances by mechanisms that are still incompletely understood. Ependymal cells have only limited regenerative capacity and thus typically do not undergo mitotic proliferation. Tearing of the epithelium leaves discontinuities that become filled with processes of subventricular astrocytes.

Specific modified ependymal cells, called **choroid plexus epithelium,** cover the surfaces of choroid plexus villi and produce cerebrospinal fluid by a mechanism that involves active secretion of Na^+. Modified ependymal cells are also present at certain sites (circumventricular organs) within brain ventricles. In both cases, the modified ependymal cells are cuboidal and have microvilli instead of cilia extending into cerebrospinal fluid. Adjacent cells are linked by relatively impermeable junctions (zonulae occludens), establishing a localized ependymal barrier in association with a locally reduced blood-brain barrier due to the presence of fenestrated capillaries.

Tanycytes are modified ependymal cells found in the hypothalamic wall of the third ventricle. The luminal border of a tanycyte has microvilli; the basal border features an elongated process that makes contact with capillaries and neurons. Tanycytes are thought to guide hypothalamic axons and to be involved in transport mechanisms between the ventricle and blood vessels of the hypothalamic–hypophysial portal system. Thus, tanycytes can influence the release of hypothalamic hormones.

At certain sites, neuronal processes extend between ependymal cells to contact cerebrospinal fluid. The processes, which end

in bulbs with stereocilia, are presumed to serve a receptive function. Also, neurons containing secretory vesicles can be found among ependymal cells; they are believed to release catecholamines.

Peripheral Nervous System Gliocytes

The gliocytes of the PNS include ganglionic gliocytes and neurolemmocytes (Schwann cells).

Ganglionic Gliocytes

Ganglionic gliocytes (satellite cells) encapsulate neuron cell bodies in the PNS. In cranial nerve and spinal (sensory) ganglia, a tight capsule is formed around each neuron cell body (Fig. 6-9). In autonomic ganglia (Fig. 6-10), capsules formed by ganglionic gliocytes are incomplete and may enclose more than one postganglionic cell body. Away from the cell body, ganglionic gliocytes are replaced by neurolemmocytes that sheathe or myelinate axons.

Neurolemmocytes

Neurolemmocytes (Schwann cells) are gliocytes of the PNS that sheathe and myelinate axons. Neurolemmocytes provide a protected immediate environment for PNS neurons and are vital for axonal function and survival. Each neurolemmocyte is enclosed

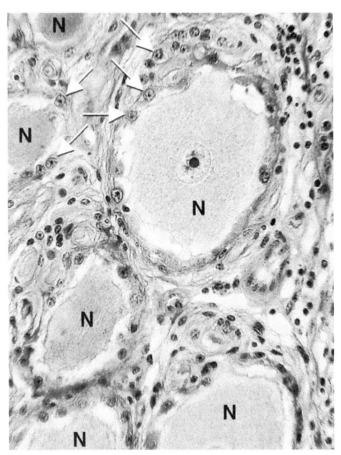

FIGURE 6-9 Canine spinal ganglion. Unipolar neuron cell bodies (N) are surrounded by ganglionic gliocytes (satellite cells) (arrows) within the ganglion. Triple stain.

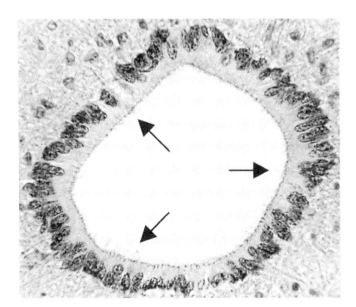

FIGURE 6-8 Ependymal cells (simple columnar epithelium) line the central canal of a canine spinal cord. Motile cilia projecting into the lumen of the central canal are evident (arrows). Hematoxylin and eosin stain.

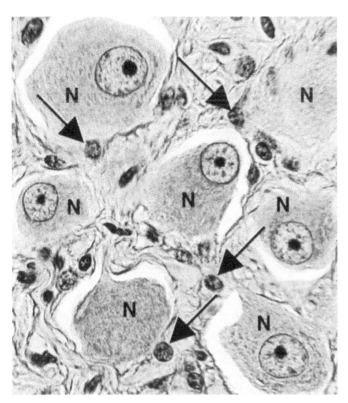

FIGURE 6-10 Canine autonomic ganglion. Cell bodies (N) of postganglionic neurons are multipolar and have their nuclei positioned eccentrically. Ganglionic gliocytes (satellite cells) (arrows) form an incomplete capsule around individual neuron cell bodies. Triple stain.

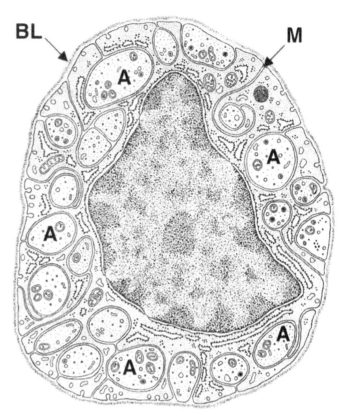

FIGURE 6-11 Drawing of the ultrastructure of a peripheral nerve neurolemmocyte sheathing 22 nonmyelinated axons (A). Each axon is enveloped by neurolemmocyte processes. Mesoaxons (M) are formed where the processes meet. A basal lamina (BL) surrounds the entire cell. *(From Lentz TL. Cell Fine Structure. Philadelphia: WB Saunders, 1971.)*

within a basal lamina. Neurolemmocytes can proliferate and become phagocytic in the event of nerve damage.

Every axon in the PNS is sheathed or myelinated along its entire length by neurolemmocytes (except for the most terminal branches in some cases). Because an individual neurolemmocyte is less than 1 mm in length, a tandem series of many neurolemmocytes is required to enclose the entire length of a long axon.

In the case of small axons, an individual neurolemmocyte sheathes a number of axons simultaneously and the axons (nerve fibers) are considered **nonmyelinated** (Fig. 6-11). Each axon resides in a furrow, protected by a pair of neurolemmocyte processes so that the space surrounding the axon communicates with the general interstitial space only by means of a narrow gap known as the **mesaxon.** For PNS axons larger than 1 μm in diameter, each neurolemmocyte encloses a single axon and glial processes wrap around the axon to form a **myelin sheath** (Fig. 6-12).

Myelin Sheath

The term **myelin sheath** (myelin) refers to wrappings of gliocyte plasma membrane that surround an axon and insulate it to speed conduction. Myelin is formed by oligodendrocytes in the CNS and neurolemmocytes in the PNS.

In the PNS, a transverse section of a myelinated fiber viewed by light microscopy reveals an axon enclosed in a myelin sheath surrounded by neurolemmocyte cytoplasm (Fig. 6-13). With

electron microscopy, one can see that the myelin sheath is composed of multiple layers of neurolemmocyte plasma membrane and the neurolemmocyte is within a basal lamina (Fig. 6-12).

Myelin formation in the PNS begins with a neurolemmocyte draped around a solitary axon, establishing a simple mesaxon (Fig. 6-14). Induced by the axon itself, neurolemmocyte processes elongate, slide past one another, and proceed to produce multilayered neurolemmocyte wrappings around the axon. Cytoplasm is extruded from the wrappings, thereby leaving the concentric lamellae of plasma membrane that constitute the myelin sheath.

At high magnification, the myelin sheath exhibits a periodicity of concentric **major dense lines** separated by intraperiod lines. Each major dense line is formed by fusion of inner surfaces of plasma membrane as cytoplasm is extruded during myelin sheath formation. An **intraperiod line** is formed where the outer surfaces of adjacent plasma membranes are separated by a small gap. The gap is continuous with the **inner mesaxon** and the **outer mesaxon,** all of which are derived from the original simple mesaxon of early myelin sheath development. Occasionally, a major dense line appears to split and contain a pocket of cytoplasm. Adjacent pockets of cytoplasm may extend throughout the thickness of the myelin sheath, thereby establishing a **myelin incisure** in the sheath.

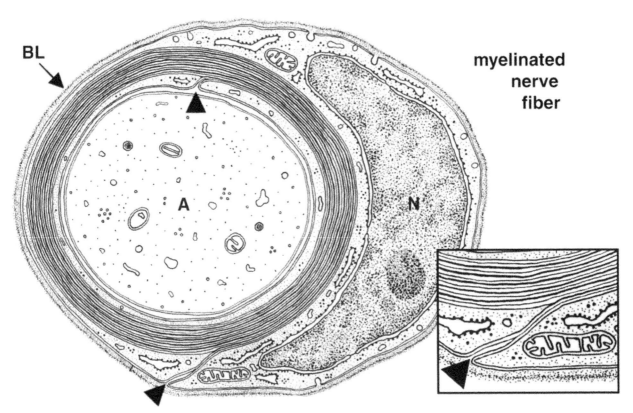

FIGURE 6-12   Ultrastructural drawing of a transected myelinated nerve fiber from the peripheral nervous system. A neurolemmocyte has produced a myelin sheath around a single axon (A). The myelin sheath consists of multiple wrappings of neurolemmocyte plasma membrane produced by paired neurolemmocyte processes that ultimately form outer and inner mesaxons (arrowheads at 12 and 6 o'clock, respectively). The nucleus of the neurolemmocyte is labeled (N). A basal lamina (BL) surrounds the neurolemmocyte. The insert (lower right) shows the outer mesaxon and myelin sheath enlarged. Notice that stained myelin exhibits major dense lines (formed by merger along the inner surface of neurolemmocyte plasma membrane), separated by intraperiod lines (formed by apposition of outer surfaces of neurolemmocyte plasma membrane). *(From Lentz TL. Cell Fine Structure. Philadelphia: WB Saunders, 1971.)*

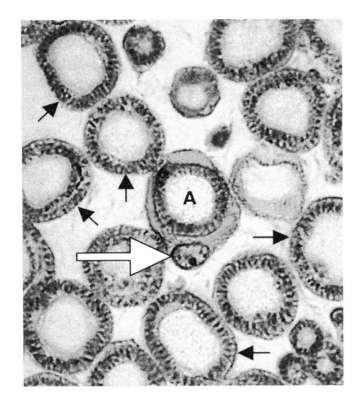

FIGURE 6-13   Transverse section through myelinated fibers of a canine peripheral nerve. Myelin sheath neurokeratin presents a radial pattern in this nerve (black arrows). The white arrow points to the nucleus of a neurolemmocyte. Its cytoplasm can be seen surrounding a myelinated axon (A). Hematoxylin and eosin stain.

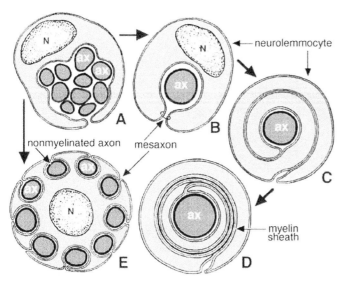

FIGURE 6-14 Schematic illustration of myelinated and nonmyelinated developmental relationships between axons (ax) and neurolemmocytes in cross-sectional perspective. **A.** Early in development, several axons are sheathed in common by a neurolemmocyte. **B.** After neurolemmocyte proliferation, a solitary large axon that is destined to be myelinated is sheathed by a neurolemmocyte; a mesaxon is formed where neurolemmocyte processes meet. **C.** Neurolemmocyte processes elongate and encircle the axon, thereby lengthening the original mesaxon. **D.** A myelin sheath is formed when cytoplasm is extruded from encircling neurolemmocyte processes, thereby leaving layers of plasmalemma. Cytoplasm is generally retained internal and external to the myelin sheath, where an inner mesaxon and an outer mesaxon are evident. **E.** In the case of nonmyelinated axons, neurolemmocyte invaginations provide a separate compartment and mesaxon for each sheathed axon. Neurolemmocyte nucleus (N). *(Adapted from Copenhaver WM, Bunge RP, Bunge MB. Bailey's Textbook of Histology. 16th Ed. Baltimore: Williams & Wilkins, 1971.)*

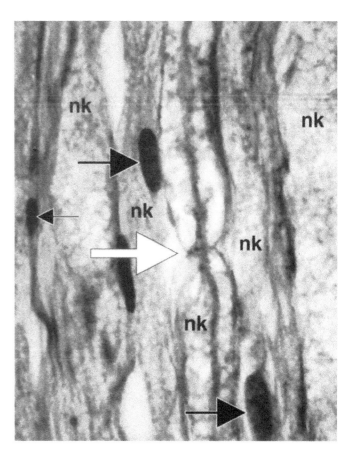

FIGURE 6-15 Light micrograph of a longitudinal section of a canine peripheral nerve. An axon passing through a myelin node (white arrow) is evident at the center. Lipid extraction during tissue preparation disintegrates myelin, leaving a protein residue (neurokeratin) that presents a foamy appearance (nk). Nuclei in the section belong to fibrocytes (small black arrow) or neurolemmocytes (large black arrows). Triple stain.

A longitudinal view of a myelinated nerve fiber shows myelin sheath gaps at the juncture of adjacent gliocytes (Fig. 6-15). Each gap is referred to as a **node** (of Ranvier), and the myelin sheath between nodes is called an **internode.** The internodal transition region immediately adjacent to a node is referred to as a **paranode** (Fig. 6-16). At the paranode, major dense lines split and cytoplasm is retained in processes that overlap one another as each contacts the axon plasma membrane. Outermost cytoplasmic processes of adjacent neurolemmocytes make contact, thus enclosing the node in the PNS. A continuous basal lamina is present external to the neurolemmocytes. At the node, the axon bulges slightly and exhibits subplasmalemmal electron-dense material. In normal axons, sodium channels are present at high density within the nodal gap, and voltage-dependent potassium channels are sequestered on the internodal side of the paranode—a region known as the juxtaparanode. The juxtaparanode and its associated potassium channels appear to stabilize nerve conduction and help maintain the internodal resting potential.

In the CNS, where myelin sheaths are formed by oligodendrocytes, nodes are not covered by cytoplasmic processes and they are exposed to the extracellular space (Figs. 6-16 and 6-17). Internodes are shorter and nodes are wider in the CNS compared to the PNS. A single oligodendrocyte is known to contribute internodes to as many as 50 myelinated fibers and the outer cytoplasm of the internode is restricted to a single ridge that is connected to the oligodendrocyte perikaryon by a thin process.

It is well established that myelin sheaths provide electrical insulation so that action potentials jump from node to node instead of progressing continually, as in nonmyelinated axons. The jumping process, called **saltatory conduction,** is much faster than nonmyelinated conduction, and the longer the internode is, the faster is the conduction. Internode length is proportional to myelin sheath thickness, and both are proportional to axon diameter. However, because neurolemmocytes develop an association with axons early in development, axons that subsequently grow farther (e.g., in the limbs) have longer internodes than axons (e.g., in the head) that do not grow as far.

The recent discovery of tight junctions and adhering junctions between myelin lamellae may help elucidate other roles played by this compact multilamellar structure. Whereas in epithelial cells these junctions are formed between different cells, in

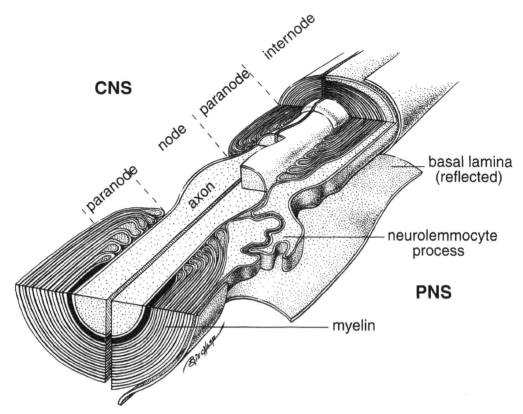

FIGURE 6-16 Schematic illustration of nodal and paranodal regions of myelinated fibers from the central nervous system (CNS) (left) and the peripheral nervous system (PNS) (right). In the CNS, myelin is formed by oligodendrocytes and nodes are broadly exposed to the extracellular space. In the PNS, outer cytoplasmic processes of adjacent neurolemmocytes (Schwann cells) overlap to restrict node exposure to the extracellular space. Also, neurolemmocytes are surrounded by a continuous basal lamina. Myelin consists of compressed membranes of glial cells, distinguished by a series of major dense lines separated by intraperiod lines. At each paranode, major dense lines split to contain terminal cytoplasmic "loops" that contact the axon plasma membrane and impede ionic flow beyond the node.

myelinating glia these so-called autotypic junctions are found between membrane lamellae of the same cell. Such junctions were initially proposed to link adjacent membranes for increased mechanical strength. However, tight junctions in other cell types play critical roles in paracellular nonbarrier function, including signal transduction, and fluid movement between cells via aqueous pores and channels. This knowledge, taken together with evidence from studies of normal and pathologic myelin, supports the possibility that in addition to mechanical strength, a primary function of junctional plaques in myelin is to regulate perfusion of the periaxonal space.

PERIPHERAL NERVOUS TISSUE

Tissue of the PNS consists of cranial and spinal nerves, including their roots, distal branches, and ganglia. **Cranial nerves** originate from the brain and exit from the cranial cavity. **Spinal nerves** originate from the spinal cord and exit from the vertebral canal. A **nerve root** is the proximal region of a cranial or spinal nerve that is enveloped by meninges within the cranial cavity or verte-

bral canal. The term **nerve fiber** refers to one axon within a nerve. In the case of a myelinated axon, the term **nerve fiber** (myelinated nerve fiber) includes the axon plus the myelin sheath and surrounding neurolemmocyte.

Individual nerve fibers may be classified as either afferent or efferent. **Afferent fibers** are sensory because they conduct excitation to the CNS. Typical afferent neurons have unipolar cell bodies located in cranial nerve and spinal (sensory) ganglia. The dendritic zone of an afferent neuron consists of receptors or postsynaptic endings on sensory epithelial cells in the case of sense organs. **Efferent axons** arise from multipolar cell bodies located in the brain or spinal cord or in autonomic ganglia. They activate muscle or gland or neurons in autonomic ganglia.

Individual nerve fibers are classified also as somatic or visceral. The **somatic fibers** innervate skin, skeletal muscles, and joints, whereas **visceral fibers** innervate cardiac and smooth muscles and glands. Visceral efferent fibers, in particular, (and often visceral fibers in general) are designated the **autonomic nervous system**. The visceral efferent pathway involves two neurons. The first (preganglionic) neuron has its cell body in the CNS. The cell body of the second (postganglionic) neuron is located in an autonomic ganglion.

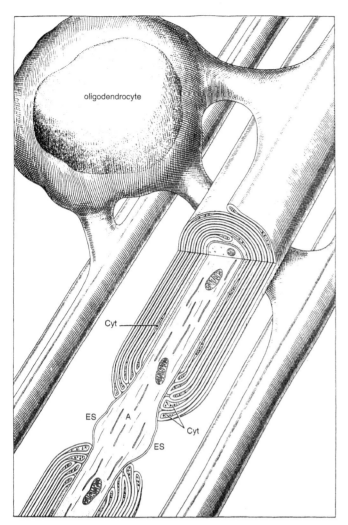

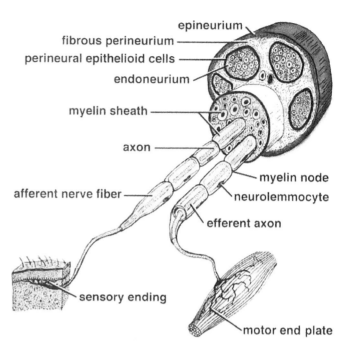

FIGURE 6-18 Diagram of peripheral nerve constituents: five fascicles constitute this peripheral nerve. The fascicles are united by a surrounding epineurium (connective tissue). Each fascicle is encircled by perineurium, which consists of layers of perineural epithelioid cells surrounded by fibrous perineurium. Within a fascicle, endoneurium surrounds individual myelinated fibers. A myelinated fiber consists of an axon surrounded by a myelin sheath that is formed by a series of neurolemmocytes and interrupted by nodes. Somatic afferent and efferent myelinated fibers are illustrated. *(Modified from Jenkins TW. Functional Mammalian Neuroanatomy. 2nd Ed. Philadelphia: Lea & Febiger, 1978.)*

FIGURE 6-17 Illustration of an oligodendrocyte providing myelin internodes to three axons. A bisected view of a node, adjacent paranode regions, and part of an internode is shown in the foreground. The axon (A) bulges at the node and is exposed to extracellular space (ES). Loop profiles containing cytoplasm (Cyt) contact the axon at the paranodal regions. Cytoplasm is retained along the ridges associated with inner and outer mesaxons, and small cytoplasmic pockets may be seen interrupting major dense lines. *(Adapted from Bunge MB, Bunge RP, Ris H. Ultrastructural study of remyelination in an experimental lesion in adult cat spinal cord. J Biophys Biochem Cytol 1961;10:67–94.)*

Nerves

A **nerve** typically consists of thousands of axons, each sheathed or myelinated by neurolemmocytes and all organized into fascicles enveloped by connective tissue (Fig. 6-18). A **nerve fascicle** is delimited by **perineurium,** which consists of fibrous tissue surrounding epithelioid cells. The multiple fascicles of a nerve are bound together by connective tissue called **epineurium.** Within a nerve fascicle, the fibrocytes and collagen fibers surrounding individual neurolemmocytes constitute **endoneurium.** Blood vessels supplying a nerve are designated **vasa nervorum.**

Individual perineural epithelioid cells are joined by zonulae occludens and enveloped by basal laminae. Multiple concentric sheets of the squamous cells, along with interposed collagen fibrils, form a continuous tube enclosing nerve fibers and endoneurium within a fascicle. A perineural epithelioid tube may have a dozen concentric layers at its origin, at the juncture of the nerve with its meningeal-covered root. The number of layers gradually decreases as a nerve branches. A single layer surrounds terminal branches, but epithelioid cells proliferate to encapsulate certain receptors. A **blood-nerve barrier** exists, constituted by the epithelioid cells and the endothelium of endoneurial microvessels. This barrier serves to protect axons and the internal nerve environment from fluctuations in blood plasma levels of hormones and ions and from toxic substances. While the perineural epithelioid tube affords nerve fibers a protected environment, the enclosed intrafascicular space may also serve as a channel for infectious or toxic agents once they invade the epithelioid cell barrier.

The **perineural epithelioid cells** are squamous and arranged in concentric sheets. The **fibrous perineurium** is collagenous connective tissue. The morphologic distinction between fibrous perineurium, which surrounds individual fascicles, and epineurium, which binds fascicles together, varies with the species. In the dog, for example, nerves are composed of a few relatively large fascicles and fibrous perineurium is dense compared to epineurium, which is a flimsy, fatty connective tissue. In contrast, fibrous perineurium and epineurium tend to blend indistinguishably in bovine nerves, which feature multiple small fascicles.

Ganglia

A **ganglion** is a localized enlargement of a nerve produced by the accumulation of neuron cell bodies. Spinal ganglia located in dorsal spinal roots and ganglia in cranial nerve roots are referred to as **sensory ganglia,** because they contain cell bodies of primary afferent neurons (Fig. 6-9). Afferent neurons are unipolar, except in the case of sense organs (vestibular apparatus, cochlea, retina, and olfactory epithelium), in which afferent neurons are bipolar.

Within a sensory ganglion, unipolar cell bodies are distributed superficially and nerve fibers course through the center of the ganglion. These unipolar cell bodies range in size from large (30 to 50 μm in diameter) to small (15 to 25 μm in diameter), and each cell body gives rise to a single axon that may coil initially before bifurcating into central and peripheral branches; the peripheral branch is usually thicker than the central branch. Large cell bodies give rise to myelinated axons that bifurcate at a node. Each cell body is tightly encapsulated by ganglionic gliocytes.

Autonomic ganglia are accumulations of multipolar cell bodies within autonomic nerves (Fig. 6-10). The neuron cell bodies, which have eccentric nuclei and marginally distributed chromatophilic substance as normal features, are loosely encapsulated by ganglionic gliocytes. Synapses occur in autonomic ganglia, where terminals of cholinergic preganglionic neurons synapse on dendritic zones of postganglionic neurons. Microscopic accumulations of postganglionic cell bodies within nerve plexuses of visceral organs (especially the gut) constitute terminal autonomic ganglia.

Postganglionic neurons are classified either as **cholinergic** if they synthesize and release acetylcholine or as **adrenergic** if their associated neurotransmitter is noradrenaline (norepinephrine). Adrenergic neurons feature dense-core synaptic vesicles. Some autonomic ganglia contain a few **small intensely fluorescent (SIF) cells.** These SIF cells feature numerous large, dense-core vesicles containing dopamine, which is released under neural control. The significance of SIF cells is unknown, but they form somatodendritic synapses and thus appear to function as interneurons.

Efferent Neurons

Somatic efferent neurons (α motor neurons) innervate skeletal muscle. One such neuron, together with all the muscle fibers it innervates, is regarded as a **motor unit,** because the muscle fibers contract as a unit when the neuron is excited. A motor unit may have few or several hundred muscle fibers, depending on muscle size. Typical muscles have a range of large and small motor units. **Small motor units** have fatigue-resistant muscle fibers innervated by small neurons that are the first to begin firing and the last to cease firing during muscular contraction. **Large motor units** have hundreds of muscle fibers innervated by large neu-

rons. The muscle fibers are readily fatigued and, because large neurons require additional synaptic input to reach threshold, they fire only when strong muscle contractions are needed.

A **neuromuscular synapse** consists of a presynaptic neuronal end plate overlaying a postsynaptic muscle sole plate at the midregion of a muscle fiber (Fig. 6-19). A **motor end plate** is formed by very short branches within a circumscribed zone (plate) at the end of one terminal branch of an efferent neuron. Each branch of the end plate lies in a corresponding trough of the **sole plate.** The width of the neuromuscular gap is 40 to 50 nm; however, the gap is increased by junctional folds, where sarcolemma of the trough undergoes transverse enfolding. Neurolemmocytes cover the end plate, and associated basal lamina extends into the neuromuscular gap and junctional folds (Fig. 6-20).

End-plate cytoplasm contains many mitochondria and numerous agranular synaptic vesicles (40 nm in diameter). The vesicles contain acetylcholine, which is released at active sites opposite the junctional folds. Acetylcholine molecules diffuse across the neuromuscular gap and bind to postsynaptic receptor sites that open cation channels, leading to muscle fiber depolarization. Some binding sites are cholinesterase enzymes that degrade acetylcholine and thereby stop synaptic activity. Transporter protein molecules are present in the presynaptic membrane to recapture choline and recycle it.

The **fusimotor** or **γ motor neuron** is another type of somatic efferent neuron. It innervates intrafusal muscle fibers within muscle spindles. These relatively small neurons have myelinated axons that terminate as end plates or trail endings (multiple synaptic contacts along the muscle fiber surface).

Preganglionic autonomic neurons originate in the CNS and synapse on postganglionic neurons in autonomic ganglia, making typical interneuronal synapses. **Postganglionic autonomic neurons** have nonmyelinated axons that innervate cardiac muscle, smooth muscle, or glands. The postganglionic axons terminate in branches that individually wander long distances without evidence of specialized contact with muscle or gland cells.

Ultrastructurally, terminal autonomic nerves consist of isolated neurolemmocytes sheathing one or more terminal branches. The terminal branches have numerous preterminal synaptic varicosities along their course. Each preterminal varicosity bulges beyond the confines of the sheathing neurolemmocyte and contains a concentration of synaptic vesicles. Thus, neurotransmitter is released from multiple sites and diffuses variable distances to bind with receptors on target cells. Postsynaptic specializations are not evident.

There are several lines of evidence indicating that postganglionic sympathetic axons innervating immune organs, such as the spleen and lymph nodes (see Chapter 8), can regulate cytokine production by immune cells in these organs. This occurs via the release of noradrenaline from nonsynaptic axonal varicosities, resulting in the suppression of immune responses. Conversely, immune cells can release neurotrophic factors, such as nerve growth factor and brain-derived neurotrophic factor, that act on appropriate receptors present on neurons and astrocytes and that have

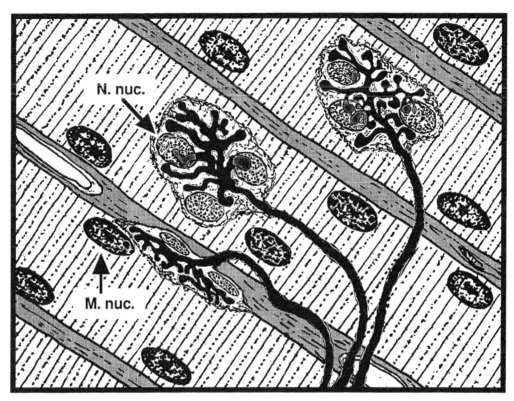

FIGURE 6-19 Drawing of three motor end plates synapsing on skeletal muscle fibers. Each of three terminal branches of an axon ends in a perfusion of short branches collectively designated an end plate. The bottom end plate is viewed from its edge. Neurolemmocytes that ensheathe axon terminal branches proceed to overlay the end plate branches. Neurolemmocyte nucleus (N. nuc.); muscle fiber nucleus (M. nuc.). *(Adapted from Krstić RV. General Histology of the Mammal. New York: Springer-Verlag, 1985.)*

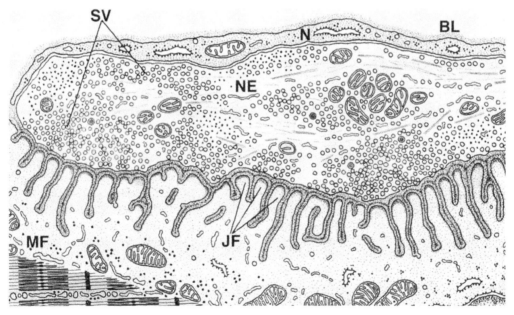

FIGURE 6-20 Ultrastructural drawing of one nerve ending (NE) of a branched motor end plate synapsing on a muscle fiber (MF). The nerve ending contains numerous synaptic vesicles (SV). The muscle fiber plasma membrane features junctional folds (JF) that greatly expand the synaptic cleft. The cleft contains basal lamina (BL) continuous with that covering the muscle fiber and the neurolemmocyte (N) overlaying the nerve ending. *(From Lentz TL. Cell Fine Structure. Philadelphia: WB Saunders, 1971.)*

neuroprotective effects. This highlights the fact that the nervous and immune systems are closely interlinked such that physiologic or pathologic effects on one system may affect the other.

Receptors

Afferent axons convey information to the CNS from receptors or from sense organs. Sense organs are organized collections of sensory epithelial cells, neurons, and supporting cells that detect visual, auditory, olfactory, or taste stimuli. In contrast, **receptors** are individual, isolated stimulus detectors that are widely distributed in the body (Fig. 6-21). Generally, the peripheral branch of an afferent axon branches repeatedly, and a receptor is located at the termination of each branch. All receptors of a single neuron have the same structure and function.

Receptors are classified in several ways. By location, **exteroceptors, proprioceptors,** and **enteroceptors** are found at the body surfaces, in musculoskeletal structures, and in viscera, respectively. Receptors are classified according to the type of stimulus they are sensitive to as **mechanoreceptors, chemoreceptors,** and **thermoreceptors.** Morphologically, receptors may be classified as **encapsulated** and **nonencapsulated.** The following is a list of common receptors.

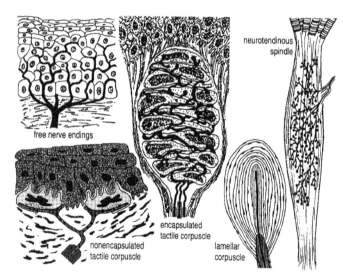

FIGURE 6-21 Schematic drawings of five receptors at various magnifications. Free nerve endings branch among cells of the epidermis. Two nonencapsulated tactile corpuscles are shown at the base of the epidermis; each corpuscle consists of a terminal branch making contact with a specialized tactile cell (Merkel's cell). An encapsulated tactile corpuscle (Meissner's corpuscle) is located in the dermis; dendritic branches from multiple myelinated axons weave among flattened neurolemmocytes within a capsule of perineural epithelioid cells. A lamellar corpuscle (Pacini's corpuscle) features the dendritic branch of a myelinated axon encased in a core of flattened neurolemmocytes within a laminated capsule composed of perineural epithelioid cells. A neurotendinous spindle splays among the collagen bundles of a small tendon; the receptor has a thin capsule and is associated with a myelinated axon (not shown). *(Encapsulated tactile corpuscle and neurotendinous spindle from Krstić RV. General Histology of the Mammal. New York: Springer-Verlag, 1985.)*

Nonencapsulated Receptors

Free nerve endings are found throughout the body. They detect stimulation described as pain (noxious), warmth, cold, or touch. Simultaneously, the same stimulus information is used for subconscious reflex activity. The receptors are associated with nonmyelinated or thinly myelinated axons that branch extensively to innervate a wide area (receptive field). The actual receptors are simply unsheathed terminal branches enveloped by basal lamina (Fig. 6-21).

Hair follicle terminals, which detect body hairs being displaced, are derived from myelinated axons that branch extensively to innervate hundreds of follicles. Each follicle is encircled by a nonmyelinated plexus that disperses free nerve endings among follicle epithelial cells. (A different situation prevails for tactile hair follicles [vibrissae], each of which receives several myelinated axons, giving rise to several kinds of receptors.)

Nonencapsulated tactile corpuscles are often collected at the base of a slight skin elevation called a tactile pad (Fig. 6-21). Each tactile corpuscle consists of an expanded axonal terminal branch that is embraced by processes of an epithelioid tactile cell (Merkel cell). The epithelioid cell, which develops under the trophic influence of the nerve ending, contains large dense core vesicles. Individual tactile corpuscles are innervated by a myelinated axon that distributes to a restricted receptive field. The tactile corpuscles are capable of persistent firing (tonic receptors).

Encapsulated Receptors

Encapsulated tactile corpuscles (Meissner's corpuscles) are oval, encapsulated phasic mechanoreceptors for touch and superficial pressure, found in the dermal papillae of mammalian skin (Fig. 6-21). Several myelinated axons give rise to nonmyelinated branches that permeate a stack of flattened neurolemmocytes encapsulated by perineural epithelioid cells. Tactile corpuscles and their associated afferent nerve fibers adapt rapidly and provide great sensitivity to minute skin deformation.

Lamellar corpuscles (Vater's corpuscles, Pacini's corpuscles) are widely distributed throughout the body and are large enough to be seen without magnification (0.5 × 1.0 mm). A terminal branch of a myelinated axon is encased in several layers of flattened neurolemmocytes that are surrounded by a fluid space and multiple concentric layers derived from perineural epithelioid cells (Fig. 6-21). The layered lamellae of these corpuscles function as an extremely selective high-pass filter, which serves to dampen the large, dynamic stresses and strains applied to the skin, allowing these receptors to be extremely sensitive to transient pressure, such as vibratory stimuli. Thus, these lamellar corpuscles are able to provide a neural image of vibrations transmitted to the skin.

Bulbous corpuscles (Krause's corpuscles, Golgi–Mazzoni corpuscles, genital corpuscles) vary in location, size, and shape. They are mechanoreceptors derived from myelinated axons that have highly coiled terminal branches enclosed in a relatively thin capsule derived from perineural epithelioid cells.

Neurotendinous spindles (Golgi tendon organs) are located at muscle–tendon junctions and are activated by tension. Derived from a large myelinated axon, the receptor consists of terminal branches traveling on bundles of collagen fibers within a fluid-filled, thin capsule derived from perineural epithelioid cells (Fig. 6-21). Ruffini's corpuscle, a tonic mechanoreceptor found in dermis, fascia, and ligaments, is structurally similar to the neurotendinous spindle.

Neuromuscular spindles (muscle spindles) are so elaborate that they could qualify as sense organs. Located in most skeletal muscles, the spindle has an elongated (1.5 mm) capsule derived from perineural epithelioid cells. The capsule encloses afferent and efferent innervation as well as two kinds of intrafusal muscle fibers, designated nuclear bag and nuclear chain fibers (Fig. 6-22). A typical spindle has one or two **nuclear bag** fibers, each with a dilated middle zone filled with nuclei and striated polar ends that project beyond the spindle capsule. Several **nuclear chain** fibers are also present within the spindle. These fibers are smaller than nuclear bag fibers, contained entirely within the spindle capsule, and characterized by a chain of nuclei at the middle of the fiber. The middle nuclear region of both types of intrafusal muscle fibers lacks myofilaments and is stretched when the striated polar regions contract. The striated regions are innervated by fusimotor (γ) motor neurons that establish either endplate or trail-type neuromuscular synapses. Trail endings form multiple synaptic contacts as terminal branches ramify on the surface of a muscle fiber.

Two types of receptors are found on intrafusal muscle fibers (Fig. 6-22). **A primary ending**, also called an **annulospiral ending**, is derived from a single, large myelinated axon that has terminal branches that spiral around the nuclear regions of intrafusal muscle fibers. **A secondary ending** is derived from a myelinated axon with dendritic branches arranged in a flower-spray configuration and situated on nuclear chain fibers adjacent to the annulospiral endings. Collectively, the receptors are activated by the rate and degree of stretch that occurs when either the polar ends of intrafusal muscle fibers contract or the whole muscle is stretched. Information from spindle receptors is primarily subconscious and important for regulating muscle tone, adjusting posture, and coordinating movements.

CENTRAL NERVOUS TISSUE

The CNS consists of the brain and spinal cord (plus the optic nerve and retina, which originate embryologically as an extension of the brain). The brain may be divided into brainstem, cerebellum, and cerebrum. When the CNS is sliced and observed grossly, one can identify white-matter regions, gray-matter regions, and regions where white and gray matter are mixed.

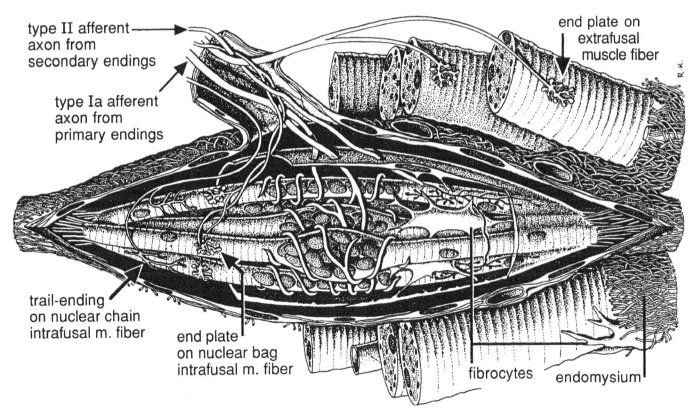

FIGURE 6-22   Schematic drawing of a muscle spindle and several extrafusal muscle fibers linked by collagen fibrils of the endomysium. Perineural epithelioid cells that surround nerve fibers continue to form the spindle capsule (cut open). The contents of the spindle include nuclear bag and nuclear chain intrafusal muscle fibers, primary and secondary receptors, two types of neuromuscular synapses, and fibrocytes and collagen fibrils. Primary or annulospiral endings, which spiral around nuclear bag and chain regions of intrafusal muscle fibers, arise from a large (myelinated) axon. Secondary or flower-spray endings, which contact nuclear chain fibers adjacent to the primary ending, arise from a medium-sized (myelinated) axon. Small (myelinated) axons of fusimotor (γ) neurons synapse on the polar regions of intrafusal muscle fibers. They form small end plates and trail endings. The trail endings are on nuclear chain fibers. Terminal branches of an α motor neuron form end plates on extrafusal muscle fibers. *(From Krstić RV. General Histology of the Mammal. New York: Springer-Verlag, 1985.)*

White matter is formed by dense accumulations of myelinated axons (myelin is rich in lipid and has a white appearance). Individual myelin sheaths are relatively thin in the CNS compared to the PNS. Nonmyelinated axons of the CNS are not sheathed; they are totally exposed to the CNS extracellular space. White matter is composed of collections of tracts (called fasciculi or lemnisci in particular cases). A tract consists of functionally related nerve fibers with a similar origin and destination.

An absence or scarcity of myelin results in CNS tissue having a gray appearance. **Gray matter** is rich in neuronal cell bodies, glial cells, and neuropil. **Neuropil** refers to the axons, terminal branches, dendrites, and glial processes that collectively form a background matrix for the cell bodies seen with light microscopy. Most synapses occur in the neuropil. Neuropil appears dense because the CNS extracellular space is uniformly narrow (approximately 20 nm wide).

Gray matter on the surface of the cerebellum and cerebrum is called **cortex**. Distinctive gray matter masses within the CNS are usually designated **nuclei**. Generally, a nucleus receives input from one or more tracts and projects output to other tracts, which, in turn, are input to a different nucleus or to cortex. For a given nucleus, incoming terminals typically synapse on small neurons with short axons, called **interneurons** because they are interposed between the input and output of the nucleus. Ultimately, the interneurons in a nucleus determine the appropriate output for a particular input.

Nervous tissue exhibits a variety of configurations among the different regions of the CNS. Gray and white matter features of three major CNS regions will be presented: cerebral cortex, cerebellum, and spinal cord.

Cerebral Cortex

The cerebrum of the brain is composed of paired cerebral hemispheres (Fig. 6-23). The surface of each hemisphere has **gyri** (ridges) demarcated by **sulci** (grooves). The surface is coated by gray matter called cerebral cortex. The characteristic neuron of the cerebral cortex has a pyramid-shaped cell body, oriented with its apex directed toward the surface (Fig. 6-4). Dendrites emerge from the apex and basal edges of the pyramidal cell; the axon leaves the center of the base and enters the white matter.

In mammals, all but the ventral cerebral cortex is designated neocortex, because it is phylogenetically recent. Cerebral **neocortex** is divisible into six layers, although the layering is evident only in thick sections and the prominence of individual layers varies from region to region. From superficial to deep, the six layers are as follows (Fig. 6-24):

1. **Molecular layer**—predominantly neuropil-oriented tangentially; composed of apical dendrites from pyramidal cells and terminal branches of superficial cortical afferent fibers.
2. **External granular layer**—predominantly small neurons that serve as interneurons.
3. **External pyramidal layer**—small and medium pyramidal neurons that send axons to adjacent cerebral cortex.
4. **Internal granular layer**—small stellate neurons that receive specific sensory input, a thick layer in sensory areas of cortex (e.g., primary visual area).

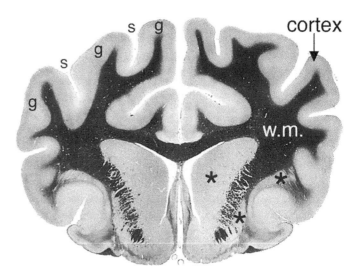

FIGURE 6-23 Transverse section through the cerebrum of a canine brain; white matter is stained dark. The cerebrum is composed of two cerebral hemispheres joined across the midline by white matter (corpus callosum). The cerebral surface features elevations, called gyri (g), separated by grooves, called sulci (s). Gray matter at the surface of the cerebrum is cerebral cortex. Cerebral white matter (w.m.) is deep to the cortex. Internal masses of gray matter at the base of the cerebrum constitute basal nuclei (*).

5. **Internal pyramidal layer**—medium to large pyramidal neurons that send axons into the white matter; a thick layer in the motor area of the cortex.
6. **Fusiform (multiform) layer**—many spindle-shaped neurons that send axons into the white matter; deep to this layer, cerebral white matter is composed of nerve fibers going to and coming from the cortex.

The basic functional unit of the neocortex is the 40- to 50-µm **minicolumn,** separated from adjacent minicolumns by vertical, cell-sparse zones that vary in size in different cortical areas. Minicolumns extend vertically from the white matter to the cortical surface and are linked into larger units called **cortical columns** (approximately 0.3 mm in diameter). Cortical columns are formed by the binding together of approximately 50 to 80 minicolumns by common input and short-range horizontal connections. Individual cortical columns are not histologically distinct. Physiologically, all neurons within a column become active in response to a certain feature of a stimulus and are inactive in the absence of that feature. The pyramidal neuron is the anatomic basis for vertical column organization. Pyramidal neurons have basal dendrites for making radial connections within a column, and they establish vertical contact by means of superficially directed apical dendrites and deeply directed axons.

Two types of afferent fibers enter a cortical column from the white matter. Nonspecific afferents, which lack specific information content, ramify in all cortical layers, but especially in superficial layers. These fibers produce background excitation as a means of alerting cortical columns. Specific afferents, the other fiber type, convey the modality-specific information with which the column is functionally concerned. The fibers synapse on the

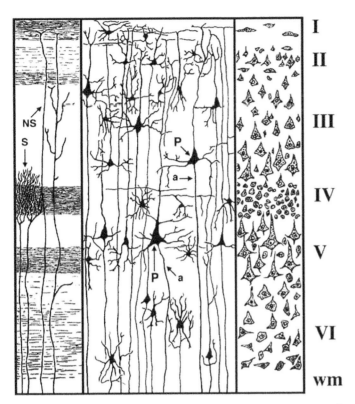

FIGURE 6-24 Schematic illustration of the six layers (I to VI) of cerebral cortex (neocortex), shown in three perspectives. The left panel illustrates nerve fibers (axons, telodendria, and dendrites) in the cortex. From the white matter (wm), modality-specific input fibers (S) terminate in layer IV; nonspecific input fibers (NS) terminate especially in the superficial layers. The middle panel displays individual neurons as they are seen with silver impregnation (Golgi stain). The characteristic neuron of the cerebral cortex has a pyramidal shape. Notice that pyramidal neurons (P) have an apical dendrite that ascends to the surface, radially oriented basal dendrites, and a single axon (a) that courses into the white matter. The right panel shows neuron cell bodies in the different layers of cerebral cortex (I to VI) as they appear in a Nissl stain. *(Modified from Crosby EC, Humphrey T, Lauer EW. Correlative Anatomy of the Nervous System. New York: The Macmillan Co., 1962.)*

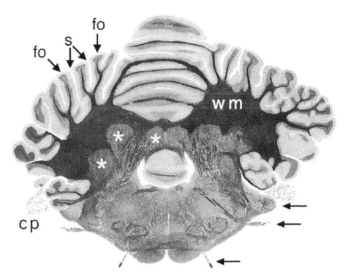

FIGURE 6-25 Transverse section through a canine hindbrain. The cerebellum (above) is joined to the brainstem (below). The cerebellar surface features elevations called folia (fo) separated by grooves called sulci (s). Cerebellar cortex, the surface gray matter, appears two-toned because of a cell-sparse molecular layer covering a cell-dense granule layer. Three cerebellar nuclei (*) are located bilaterally deep to the white matter (wm). The brainstem exhibits white matter tracts, gray matter nuclei, regions in which white and gray matter are mixed, and emerging cranial nerve roots (arrows). On each side, the tip of a choroid plexus (cp) is seen within the surrounding subarachnoid space.

small neurons of the internal granular layer, which serve as interneurons to distribute excitation throughout the column.

Output from the cortical column is predominantly from pyramidal neurons, which send their axons into the white matter. Superficial neurons send axons to neighboring regions of cortex (short association fibers). Neurons in the deepest two layers of the cortex send long axons to the brainstem (projection fibers), to the contralateral cerebral hemisphere (commissural fibers), or to distant regions of the same hemisphere (long association fibers).

Cerebellum

The cerebellar surface features **folia** (narrow ridges) separated by **sulci** (grooves). The surface is coated by gray matter, called **cerebellar cortex.** White matter is located deep to the cortex, and three bilateral pairs of cerebellar nuclei are embedded within the white matter (Fig. 6-25).

The cerebellar cortex is divisible into three layers (Fig. 6-26). The **molecular layer,** composed predominantly of neuropil, is most superficial. The **granule cell layer,** situated adjacent to white matter, features densely packed granule cells (small neurons with heterochromatic nuclei). Because of the extremely dense packing of the granule cells, the cerebellum contains about five times more neurons than the cerebral cortex. Finally, a single layer of large cell bodies is located at the interface of the molecular and granule cell layers. This is called the **piriform cell layer** (Purkinje cell layer).

The **piriform neurons (Purkinje cells)** send axons into the white matter to synapse on neurons of cerebellar nuclei. Each piriform neuron has an elaborate dendritic tree that projects into the molecular layer (Fig. 6-27) and makes more than 200,000 synaptic contacts with granule cell axons. Axons of **granule cells** enter the molecular layer, bifurcate, travel longitudinally within a folium, and synapse on numerous dendritic trees of the piriform neurons. Another neuron of the cerebellar cortex is called a **basket cell** because its terminal branches form "baskets" surrounding cell bodies of adjacent piriform neurons. The cell bodies of basket cells are found in the deep molecular layer; their axons course transversely in the folium and inhibit laterally positioned piriform neurons.

Two major types of input fibers enter the cerebellar cortex. One type (climbing fibers) has terminal branches that climb like vines on piriform dendritic trees, each fiber making numerous synapses-in-passing on one dendritic tree. The other type of input fiber has terminal expansions (mossy endings) within the granule cell layer. Neighboring granule cells send dendrites to synapse

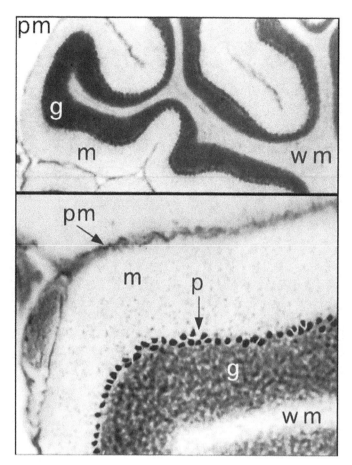

FIGURE 6-26 Two light micrographs at different magnification of cerebellar cortex (pig). Nissl stain. **Top:** white matter (wm) extends into the center of a cerebellar folium. Cortex covering the white matter exhibits a dense cell layer (g) and a relatively acellular layer (m). Pia mater (pm) covers the cerebellar surface and extends into sulci separating folia (×15). **Bottom:** cerebellar cortex, situated between white matter (wm) and pia mater (pm), is composed of three layers. From deep to superficial: the granule cell layer (g); the piriform cell layer (p); and the molecular layer (m) (×55).

with each terminal expansion, thereby creating a synaptic complex known as a **glomerulus**.

The cerebellum regulates muscle tone, posture, and movement so that these are expressed in an appropriate, coordinated pattern. It operates in the following manner: neurons of cerebellar nuclei are spontaneously active; they send their axons out of the cerebellum to excite brain neurons responsible for initiating posture and movement. Input to the cerebellum comes from these brain neurons and from muscle and joint proprioceptors. Input fibers excite cerebellar nuclei and specific regions of cerebellar cortex. Excitatory granule cells and inhibitory basket cells interact to produce a localized pattern of active piriform neurons in the cerebellar cortex. Piriform neuron axons, the only output from the cortex, inhibit neurons of cerebellar nuclei. Thus, the cerebellar cortex continuously compares movement initiation with movement performance and regulates movement execution by selectively inhibiting the generalized excitatory influence of cerebellar nuclei.

Spinal Cord

The cylindrical spinal cord is divisible into segments that are demarcated by the bilateral emergence of dorsal and ventral roots of spinal nerves. A transverse section of the spinal cord has a **central canal** surrounded by an H-shaped profile of gray matter, which is in turn surrounded by white matter (Fig. 6-28). The spinal cord is divided in the median plane by a **ventral median fissure** and a **dorsal median septum** (the septum is replaced by a fissure in the caudal half of the cord). Spinal cord and particularly spinal gray matter are enlarged at segments supplying limbs because limb innervation requires additional nervous tissue.

Spinal gray matter contains three categories of neurons: interneurons (contained within the gray matter, connecting afferent and efferent neurons), projection neurons (which project axons through white matter tracts to the brain), and efferent neurons (which send axons into ventral roots). A group of related neuron cell bodies is designated a **nucleus** (e.g., the intermediolateral nucleus is composed of sympathetic preganglionic neuron cell bodies). Spinal gray matter is sometimes subdivided into 10 defined laminae (boundaries of laminae are indistinct in ordinary tissue sections).

Bilaterally, spinal gray matter consists of dorsal and ventral gray columns connected by intermediate gray matter. In transverse sections, gray column profiles are usually called **horns**. The **ventral gray column** (horn) contains somatic efferent neurons that innervate skeletal muscle. The **dorsal gray column** (horn) contains interneurons and projection neurons on which primary afferent neurons synapse to convey sensory information related to pain, temperature, pressure, touch, etc. Intermediate gray matter features visceral neurons. In thoracolumbar segments, a **lateral gray column** (horn) containing sympathetic preganglionic neurons (intermediolateral nucleus) is present.

Spinal white matter is composed of fibers that form ascending and descending tracts plus fibers entering from dorsal roots or exiting to ventral roots. Ascending tracts terminate in the brain. Axons of descending tracts originate in the brain and mainly synapse on interneurons within the gray matter. Afferent axons of dorsal roots enter white matter at a dorsolateral sulcus and terminate principally in the dorsal gray column. Axons of efferent neurons exit ventrolaterally as ventral root fibers.

Bilaterally, spinal white matter is divided into three anatomic regions. The **dorsal funiculus** is located between the midline and dorsal root attachments. The **ventral funiculus** is situated between the midline and ventral root attachments. The **lateral funiculus** is positioned between dorsal and ventral root attachments.

MENINGES, BLOOD VESSELS, AND CEREBROSPINAL FLUID

Meninges

The brain and spinal cord and the roots of peripheral nerves are enveloped by a series of connective tissue sheaths termed **meninges**. Meninges also surround the entire optic nerve (which is CNS tissue). Meninges contain cerebrospinal fluid and constitute a protective barrier. Inflammation of the meninges results in a condition termed meningitis.

cerebellar cortex

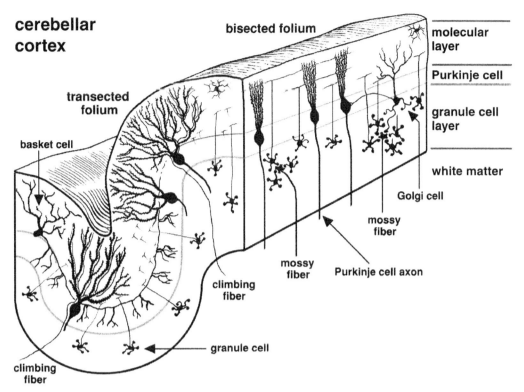

FIGURE 6-27 Schematic diagram of cerebellar cortex. The three layers of cortex (labeled on the right) are shown in bisected (right side) and transected (left side) views of a folium. The molecular layer of cerebellar cortex is composed of neuronal processes plus a few small stellate neurons (upper right, unlabeled). The piriform (Purkinje) cell layer features cell bodies of piriform cell neurons, which send their axons into the white matter. The piriform cell dendritic tree is flattened and oriented perpendicular to the long axis of the folium. The granule cell layer is packed with small granule cell neurons that send axons into the molecular layer to synapse on piriform cell dendrites. Two additional neurons include the Golgi cell (right edge) and the basket cell (left edge). The Golgi cell (great stellate cell) is an inhibitory interneuron located in the upper part of the granule cell layer. The basket cell, an inhibitory neuron located in the depths of the molecular layer, has axonal branches that form "baskets" around piriform cell bodies. Cerebellar white matter is composed of piriform cell axons leaving the cortex and two types of cortical afferents: mossy and climbing fibers. A mossy fiber makes synaptic contact with granule cell dendrites; the mossy ending forms the center of a synaptic glomerulus. Climbing fibers make many synaptic contacts on one Purkinje dendritic tree. *(Modified from Jenkins TW. Functional Mammalian Neuroanatomy. 2nd Ed. Philadelphia: Lea & Febiger, 1978.)*

Traditionally, three meningeal layers are described, from superficial to deep: dura mater, arachnoid, and pia mater (Fig. 6-29). **Dura mater** is sometimes called **pachymeninx** because it is thick and strong. The **arachnoid** and **pia mater** are collectively termed **leptomeninges,** because they are delicate and connected both embryologically and physically. A **subarachnoid space** containing cerebrospinal fluid separates arachnoid from pia mater.

Dura mater contains thick collagen bundles and elastic fibers, oriented longitudinally in spinal dura, but more irregularly in cranial dura. The dura mater also contains fibrocytes, nerves, and lymph and blood vessels. The inner surface of dura mater is lined by multiple layers of flattened fibrocytes to which outer cells of the arachnoid membrane adhere. Although there is no subdural space, hemorrhage can result in the accumulation of blood between fibrocyte layers (subdural hematoma), giving the false impression of a subdural space.

Spinal dura mater is surrounded by an epidural space that separates the dura mater from periosteum lining the vertebral canal. Collagen and elastic fibers in the spinal dura are oriented parallel to the long axis of the spine, providing the dura with longitudinal tensile strength, stiffness, and the property of relaxation.

Cranial dura mater is composed of two laminae. The internal lamina is comparable to spinal dura mater; the external lamina serves as periosteum for the cranial cavity. The two laminae are distinct only where the inner lamina separates from the outer one to form partitions between parts of the brain (Fig. 6-29). Endothelium-lined spaces, called **dural venous sinuses,** are present where the internal and external laminae separate. Venous blood drains into the sinuses, which resist collapse because of their rigid walls.

Arachnoid (arachnoid membrane) consists of outer layers of flattened fibrocytes and inner, loosely arranged, flattened fibrocytes associated with small bundles of collagen fibers. **Arachnoid**

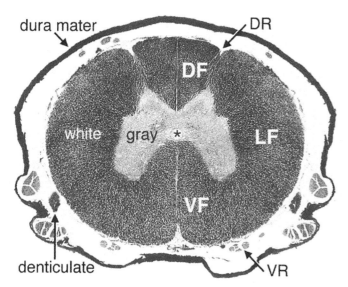

FIGURE 6-28 Transverse section through a canine spinal cord at the midthoracic region (stained with Luxol blue and hematoxylin). The central canal (*) is surrounded by butterfly-shaped gray matter (gray), which is surrounded by darkly stained white matter (white). In this thoracic segment, gray matter features a small dorsal horn, a subtle lateral horn, and a large ventral horn, bilaterally. Meninges and transected nerve roots are external to the white matter. Bilaterally, a process of denticulate ligament (denticulate) is evident between pia mater and dura mater. The spinal cord is divided into bilateral halves by a ventral median fissure and a dorsal median sulcus and septum. In each half, white matter is divided into three regions: dorsal funiculus (DF), lateral funiculus (LF), and ventral funiculus (VF). A prominent dorsolateral sulcus, where dorsal roots (DR) would enter, separates dorsal and lateral funiculi. The boundary between lateral and ventral funiculi is demarcated by the emergence of ventral roots (VR).

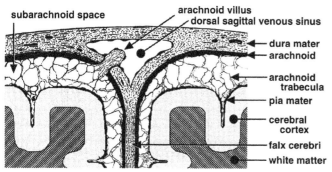

FIGURE 6-29 Schematic illustration of meningeal relationships at the dorsal midline of the cranial cavity. The internal lamina of dura mater separates from the external (periosteal) lamina and forms a partition, the falx cerebri, between cerebral hemispheres. The separation also encloses a venous sinus lined by endothelial cells (into which veins drain). Arachnoid merges with flattened fibrocytes lining the internal surface of dura mater. Arachnoid trabeculae connect to pia mater by traversing the subarachnoid space, which is filled with cerebrospinal fluid. The fluid drains into venous blood through an arachnoid villus that expands or collapses according to the pressure differential across it. (*Adapted from Weed LH. The absorption of cerebrospinal fluid into the venous system. Am J Anat 1923;31:191–221.*)

trabeculae are thin strands of inner arachnoid that traverse the subarachnoid space and establish continuity with pia mater. **Arachnoid villi** are microscopic projections of arachnoid that penetrate walls of dural venous sinuses and act as one-way valves for drainage of cerebrospinal fluid (Fig. 6-29). When cerebrospinal fluid pressure exceeds sinus blood pressure, arachnoid villi expand to facilitate fluid transfer into the bloodstream. The villi collapse to preclude blood reflux when venous pressure exceeds cerebrospinal fluid pressure. Cerebrospinal fluid can also drain into lymphatics of peripheral nerves.

The pia mater is a highly vascular layer that covers the spinal cord and brain, lining every sulcus and fissure. It is characterized by wide intercellular spaces containing variable amounts of interlacing collagen fibers and fine elastic networks with a few fibrocytes, lymphocytes, and mast cells. A basal lamina separates pia mater collagen from the underlying glial limiting membrane (astrocyte processes). The pia is covered on its outer surface by a layer of flat fibrocytes.

Together with arachnoid, pia mater bounds the subarachnoid space, which contains cerebrospinal fluid. The entire subarachnoid space, including the surfaces of nerves and vessels that traverse the space, is lined by flattened fibrocytes joined by zonulae adherens. The fibrocytes are capable of phagocytosis, and macrophages are sporadically found on the lining of the subarachnoid space. Since the fibrocytic layer lining the subarachnoid space lacks a basal lamina, a limited exchange of fluid, small molecules, and immunocompetent cells between the cerebrospinal fluid and the arachnoid and pia compartments is possible.

Along each midlateral surface of the spinal cord, an increase in the amount of pia mater collagen creates an elongated ligament called the **denticulate ligament.** A periodic series of projections extends laterally from the ligament and attaches to spinal dura mater (Fig. 6-28). Thus, bilateral denticulate ligaments act to suspend the spinal cord within the dura mater so the spinal cord is completely surrounded by the cerebrospinal fluid within the subarachnoid space.

As nerve roots converge to form cranial and spinal nerves at cranial and intervertebral foramina, there is a transition from meninges surrounding the nerve root to neural connective tissue around the nerves. Flattened fibrocytes of the leptomeninges are continued by the epithelioid cells of the perineurium. Dura mater is continued by fibrous perineurium and epineurium. Pia mater collagen is continued by endoneurium.

Blood Vessels

Blood vessels in the subarachnoid space are covered by leptomeningeal tissue derived from arachnoid trabeculae or pia mater (Fig. 6-30). When a vessel penetrates the CNS, it is surrounded by a **perivascular space** (i.e., a space situated between the vessel wall and the glial limiting membrane). The space persists to the level of small vessels, where the basal lamina associated with the glial limiting membrane merges with vascular basal lamina. Leptomeninges, particularly pia mater collagen fibers, fill the perivascular space so that a space is not obvious, except when it fills with inflammatory cells under

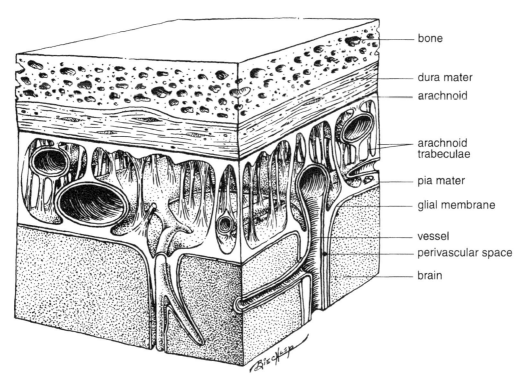

— bone

— dura mater
— arachnoid

— arachnoid trabeculae

— pia mater

— glial membrane

— vessel
— perivascular space

— brain

FIGURE 6-30 Schematic illustration showing cranial meninges and perivascular space around vessels. The entire subarachnoid space, including surfaces of vessels, is coated by leptomeninges (arachnoid and pia mater). The perivascular space that is present between the glial limiting membrane and the vessel wall is filled with pia mater collagen fibers.

pathologic conditions. Communication between perivascular spaces and the subarachnoid space is blocked by a continuous barrier of leptomeningeal cells, formed by cells on surfaces of vessels uniting with those on the pia mater surface.

In contrast to most endothelial cells in the body, endothelial cells of CNS capillaries are generally nonfenestrated and joined by tight junctions. These endothelial features are responsible for the **blood-brain barrier,** which impedes diffusion of hydrophilic molecules from the bloodstream to the CNS (polar molecules must be specifically transported into the CNS). The trophic influence of astrocyte end feet in contact with the basal lamina surrounding CNS capillaries induces CNS endothelial cells to become nonfenestrated and joined by tight junctions. A blood-brain barrier is not present either neonatally or at the few sites in the adult brain where modified ependymal cells are found (choroid plexuses and circumventricular organs).

A blood-brain barrier is also present in peripheral nerves. Capillaries within the endoneurium of peripheral nerves (but not ganglia) exhibit zonulae occludens. Perineural epithelioid cells surrounding nerve fascicles also have zonulae occludens. These tight junctions establish a blood-nerve barrier for hydrophilic molecules.

Cerebrospinal Fluid

Cerebrospinal fluid is produced by choroid plexuses in brain ventricles. A region of each ventricular wall is formed by **tela choroidea,** a term that refers to ependyma in contact with pia mater without intervening nervous tissue. A **choroid plexus** arises from tela choroidea as a mass of villi that collectively forms a fuzzy tufted growth extending into the ventricle. Each villus consists of pial vasculature in loose connective tissue covered by modified ependymal cells, called **chorioid plexus epithelium.** Although choroid plexus capillaries have fenestrated endothelial cells, choroid plexus epithelial cells are joined by zonulae occludens near their luminal surfaces. These tight junctions contribute to the formation of a **blood-cerebrospinal fluid barrier** regulating the extent to which proteins and drugs enter the cerebrospinal fluid.

Cerebrospinal fluid is produced by choroid plexus epithelium through a process that involves active Na^+ secretion. Choroid plexus epithelial cells exhibit pinocytotic vesicles, which originate at the base of each cell and migrate toward the luminal surface. In accordance with its location between two circulating fluid compartments (the blood and the cerebrospinal fluid), the choroid plexus epithelium is involved in numerous exchange processes that either supply the brain with nutrients and hormones or clear deleterious compounds and metabolites from the brain. Choroid plexuses also participate in neurohumoral brain modulation and neuroimmune interactions, thereby contributing greatly to the maintenance of brain homeostasis.

Cerebrospinal fluid flows through brain ventricles. The fluid leaves the ventricles by exiting through lateral apertures of the fourth ventricle and entering the subarachnoid space, where it surrounds the brain and spinal cord. Besides offering the physical protection of a fluid buffer, cerebrospinal fluid compensates for the absence of lymphatics in the CNS because large molecules from the CNS extracellular space are able to pass between ependymal cells and into the cerebrospinal fluid.

Dendritic cells are a subclass of antigen-presenting cells critical in the initiation and regulation of adaptive immunity against pathogens and tumors (see Chapter 8). Recent studies have indicated that dendritic cells are present in normal meninges, choroid plexuses, and cerebrospinal fluid, but absent from normal brain parenchyma. CNS inflammation is accompanied by recruitment of dendritic cells from the blood into the affected brain tissue. Dendritic cells present in different CNS compartments are likely to play an important role in the defense against CNS infections, but also may contribute to relapses or chronicity of CNS inflammation and to breakdown of tolerance to CNS autoantigens. Manipulation of dendritic cell recruitment and function within the CNS may represent a new strategy for treating neuroinflammatory diseases.

SUGGESTED READINGS

Bergman RA, Afifi AK, Heidger PM Jr. Atlas of Microscopic Anatomy. 2nd Ed. Philadelphia: WB Saunders, 1989.

Bruni JE. Ependymal development, proliferation, and functions: a review. Microsc Res Tech. 1998;41:2–13.

Calakos N, Scheller RH. Synaptic vesicle biogenesis, docking, and fusion: a molecular description. Physiol Rev 1996;76:1–29.

Choquet D, Triller A. The role of receptor diffusion in the organization of the postsynaptic membrane. Nat Rev Neurosci 2003;4: 251–265.

Cooper JR, Bloom FE, Roth RH. The Biochemical Basis of Neuropharmacology. 7th Ed. New York: Oxford University Press, 1996.

Dong Y, Benveniste EN. Immune function of astrocytes. Glia 2001; 36:180–190.

Dyer CA. The structure and function of myelin: from inert membrane to perfusion pump. Neurochem Res 2002;27:1279–1292.

Fawcett DW. A Textbook of Histology. 12th Ed. Philadelphia: WB Saunders, 1994.

Fields RD, Stevens-Graham B. New insights into neuron-glia communication. Science 2002;298:556–562.

Friedman EM, Irwin MR. Modulation of immune cell function by the autonomic nervous system. Pharmacol Ther 1997;74:27–38.

Hansson E, Ronnback L. Glial neuronal signaling in the central nervous system. FASEB J 2003;17:341–348.

Kazarinova-Noyes K, Shrager P. Molecular constituents of the node of Ranvier. Mol Neurobiol. 2002;26:167–182.

Kerschensteiner M, Stadelmann C, Dechant G, et al. Neurotrophic cross-talk between the nervous and immune systems: implications for neurological diseases. Ann Neurol 2003;53:292–304.

Kurosinski P, Gotz J. Glial cells under physiologic and pathologic conditions. Arch Neurol 2002;59:1524–1528.

Jones EG. The nervous tissue. In: Weiss L, ed. Cell and Tissue Biology. 6th Ed. Baltimore: Urban & Schwarzenberg, 1988.

Junqueira LC, Carneiro J, Kelly RO. Basic Histology. 8th Ed. Norwalk, CT: Appleton & Lange, 1995.

Krstić RV. General Histology of the Mammal. New York: Springer-Verlag, 1985.

Larocca JN, Rodriguez-Gabin AG. Myelin biogenesis: vesicle transport in oligodendrocytes. Neurochem Res 2002;27:1313–1329.

Messlinger K. Functional morphology of nociceptive and other fine sensory endings (free nerve endings) in different tissues. Prog Brain Res 1996;113:273–298.

Morgan CW. Axons of sacral preganglionic neurons in the cat: I. Origin, initial segment, and myelination. J Neurocytol 2001; 30:523–544.

Mountcastle VB. Introduction. Computation in cortical columns. Cereb Cortex 2003;13:2–4.

Nimchinsky EA, Sabatini BL, Svoboda K. Structure and function of dendritic spines. Annu Rev Physiol 2002;64:313–353.

Orlin JR, Osen KK, Hovig T. Subdural compartment in pig. A morphologic study with blood and horseradish peroxidase infused subdurally. Anat Rec 1991;230:22–37.

Pannese E. Neurocytology. Fine Structure of Neurons, Nerves Processes, and Neuroglial Cells. New York: Thieme Medical Publishers, 1994.

Parri R, Crunelli V. An astrocyte bridge from synapse to blood flow. Nat Neurosci 2003;6:43–50.

Pashenkov M, Teleshova N, Link H. Inflammation in the central nervous system: the role for dendritic cells. Brain Pathol 2003;13: 23–33.

Peters A, Palay SL, Webster HD. The Fine Structure of the Nervous System: Neurons and Supporting Cells. 3rd Ed. New York: Oxford University Press, 1991.

Segal M. Changing views of Cajal's neuron: the case of the dendritic spine. Prog Brain Res 2002;136:101–107.

Shepherd GM, Raastad M, Andersen P. General and variable features of varicosity spacing along unmyelinated axons in the hippocampus and cerebellum. Proc Natl Acad Sci U S A 2002;99: 6340–6345.

Sternberg SS. Histology for Pathologists. New York: Raven Press, 1992.

Sternini C. Organization of the peripheral nervous system: autonomic and sensory ganglia. J Investig Dermatol Symp Proc 1997;2:1–7.

Stevens, B, Porta, S, Haak LL, et al. Adenosine: a neuron-glial transmitter promoting myelination in the CNS in response of action potentials. Neuron 2002;36:855–868.

Strazielle N, Ghersi-Egea JF. Choroid plexus in the central nervous system: biology and physiopathology. J Neuropathol Exp Neurol 2000;59:561–574.

von Bohlen und Halbach O, Unsicker K. Morphological alterations in the amygdala and hippocampus of mice during ageing. Eur J Neurosci 2002;16:2434–2440.

7

Cardiovascular System

JOHANNA PLENDL

Blood Vessels
   Structure–Function Relationships of Blood Vessels
   General Structural Organization of Blood Vessels
   Vascular Endothelium
   Arteries
      Elastic arteries
      Muscular arteries
   Microvasculature
      Arterioles
      Capillaries
      Venules
      Arteriovenous anastomoses
   Veins
      Small veins
      Medium veins
      Large veins

Specialized Blood Vessels
Sensory Receptors
   Carotid body
   Carotid sinus
Heart
   Endocardium
   Myocardium
   Epicardium and Pericardium
   Cardiac Conduction System
   Cardiac Blood Vessels, Lymph Vessels, and Nerves
Lymph Vessels
   Lymph Capillaries
   Small and Medium Lymph Vessels
   Large Lymph Vessels and Collecting Ducts

Most tissues and organs of domestic animals are permeated by a network of tubular passages that conduct the more fluid components of the body. Highly cellular and viscous blood flows through the **blood vascular system** while the relatively acellular and watery lymph passes through the **lymph vascular system**. In domestic mammals, the blood vascular system forms circulatory arcs emanating from and returning to the heart. The lymphatic vascular system forms drainage channels, which join the major veins at the thoracic inlet and through which accumulating tissue fluid returns to the circulating blood.

Blood and lymph flow because of the pressure gradients within the lumina of their respective vascular networks. These pressure gradients arise from several forces including gravity, the pumping action of the heart, and the movements of musculoskeletal body parts. The pressure inside the vascular tubes differs from the pressure outside, and the resulting pressure gradients, coupled with the shearing forces of fluid flow, probably determine the structure of the various tubular portions comprising the vascular system.

BLOOD VESSELS

Structure–Function Relationships of Blood Vessels

The blood vessels of the **macrovasculature** are visible with the naked eye and include elastic and muscular arteries and accompanying veins. Arteries of the macrovasculature carry the blood from the heart to the **microvasculature**, which includes arterioles, metarterioles, capillaries, venules, and arteriovenous anastomoses. Functioning as return vessels of the macrovasculature, veins then carry the blood from the microvasculature back to the heart.

Blood vessels are commonly defined by their position in the vascular circuit. They are further characterized histologically by their individual structure, which reflects the particular forces withstood during blood flow and the mechanisms of control over vascular function. Arteries control flow to the microvasculature where blood flows slowly and can stop intermittently because blood pressure is only slightly above or below the counteracting pressure of surrounding tissues. In veins, the velocity of the blood flow returns to at least half that of the corresponding arteries, but the blood pressure is reduced.

Contractions of the heart ventricles are the greatest impelling force to blood circulation. The thick conducting **elastic arteries,** such as the aorta, receive the first surge of blood from each contraction, during which both velocity of flow and pressure reach their peaks. The high pressure of the cardiac blood pumped out during contraction of the cardiac ventricles (systole) is largely absorbed by the stretch of the highly elastic arterial walls. At the time of ventricular dilation (diastole), arterial wall tension lowers while maintaining blood pressure, and the volume of blood is distributed into more numerous **muscular arteries.** These vessels lead to specific organs or body parts and eventually into the smallest branches of the arterial tree, the **arterioles.** The velocity of flow is gradually reduced as additional distributive branches greatly expand the total blood vessel volume, but pressure in the muscular arteries remains high. Peripheral outflow is regulated by the sympathetic division of the autonomic nervous system, which determines contraction or relaxation of the smooth muscle cells in the walls of these arteries.

Frequently, the elastic, muscular, and arteriolar arteries are referred to as **large, medium,** or **small arteries,** respectively. On a comparative anatomic basis, the latter nomenclature is confusing because an elastic artery of a cat may be of smaller caliber than a muscular artery of a large ruminant. But within one species, the assumption of a relationship between structure and relative size is valid.

From the arterial tree, the vessels open into voluminous networks of small, uniformly thin-walled tubules called **capillaries.** In the liver, bone marrow, and certain endocrine glands, the capillaries are called **sinusoids.** The total blood volume in capillaries and sinusoids is much greater than in arterioles, such that the velocity of blood flow decreases from meters per second in the arterial tree to less than 1 mm per second in capillaries. The shearing forces generated by viscous blood flowing within the narrow arterioles decrease the pressure of the blood until it exceeds the pressure of the surrounding tissue fluid by 10 mm Hg or less. Thus, capillaries only oppose small-scale forces and therefore can have thin walls structured from single cells. Blood-tissue exchanges take place within the capillary network, as well as across the wall of postcapillary venules, which have a comparable structure.

Blood from the capillaries and sinusoids returns to the heart via the **veins.** Veins of increasing size, usually classified simply as **small, medium,** or **large veins,** form inverse vascular trees that are analogous to, and in most instances parallel with, the arterial trees. Consequently, arteries and their accompanying veins are seen adjacent to each other in most tissue sections. Usually, a nerve and sometimes a lymphatic vessel are seen along with the paired blood vessels. There are, however, specific exceptions, such as in the lung where arteries and veins group independently.

Because veins receive blood from low pressure capillaries, they oppose little residual pressure from the pumping action of the heart. They do, however, withstand pressures caused by gravity and surrounding tissues such as muscle. Flow of blood through the veins is caused by the minimal pressure of blood flowing from the capillaries into the veins and by pressure differences with surrounding tissues. This flow is augmented by a series of **valves** in the long veins of the extremities that facilitate movement of blood toward the heart.

The small pressure gradients within the veins provide relatively low velocities of flow as compared to flow velocity in arteries. However, the venous channels are large in comparison to those of companion arteries; consequently, the rate of flow through the two different vessel types is equal.

Because veins are larger than arteries, they hold nearly half of the total blood volume in the body, and the contractile state of the walls of the larger veins is an important determinant of total vascular volume.

General Structural Organization of Blood Vessels

The walls of all blood vessels larger than capillaries are composed of three concentric layers or tunics that include an inner **tunica interna** (intima), a middle **tunica media,** and an external **tunica externa** (adventitia) (Fig. 7-1). Arteries and veins are distinguished from each other on the basis of the composition of the various tunics, particularly the tunica media (Fig. 7-2).

The **tunica interna** (tunica intima) is lined with a simple squamous epithelium known as **endothelium** and its underlying basal lamina. A **subendothelial layer** includes collagen and elastic fibers, fibrocytes, and in some vessels, smooth muscle cells. The outermost layer of the tunica interna is the **internal elastic membrane.** This membrane is a sheet of elastin that has gaps that permit diffusion of nutrients into the tunica media; it is usually absent in the smaller veins and thin or inconspicuous in the larger ones. The internal elastic membrane is often indistinct under the light microscope but can be identified readily by electron microscopy (Fig. 7-3). The tunica interna is avascular and is nourished through transendothelial transport of substances from the circulating blood.

The **tunica media** consists of several layers of smooth muscle in helical arrangement, interspersed with varying numbers of elastic laminae, elastic fibers, and collagen fibers. Most of the inner half of the tunica media receives nutrients from the tunica interna; the remainder is supplied by **vasa vasorum** (small blood vessels that supply the vessel wall). An **external elastic membrane,** similar in structure to the internal elastic membrane, is clearly distinguishable in only the largest muscular arteries (Fig. 7-1).

In the outermost **tunica externa** (adventitia), collagen and elastic fibers predominate, and smooth muscle cells may be present. This tunic also contains vasa vasorum that extend into the outer layers of the tunica media (Fig. 7-4). Vasomotor nerves (**nervi vasorum**) form plexuses in the externa of most large blood vessels. A few axons penetrate the tunica media and terminate near smooth muscle cells (Fig. 7-5).

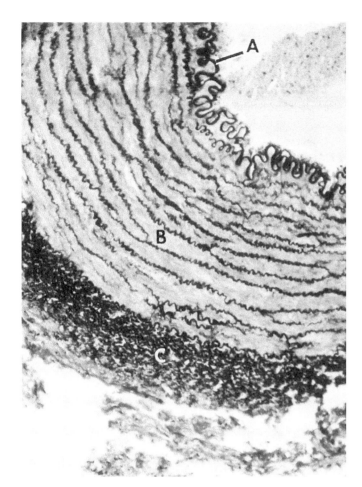

FIGURE 7-1 Cross section through part of the wall of a canine muscular artery. The most prominent layer of the tunica interna is the internal elastic membrane (A); the tunica media consists of several alternating layers of smooth muscle cells and elastic lamellae or fibers (B). In the tunica externa, elastic fibers predominate (C). Verhoeff's elastic stain (×130).

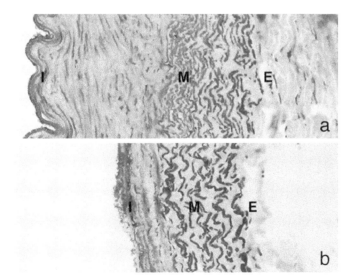

FIGURE 7-2 Cross section through part of the canine femoral artery (a) and vein (b). Arteries and veins are distinguished from each other on the basis of the thickness of the vascular wall and differences in the composition of the various tunics, particularly the tunica media (M). Tunica interna (I); tunica externa (E). Resorcin-fuchsin (×400).

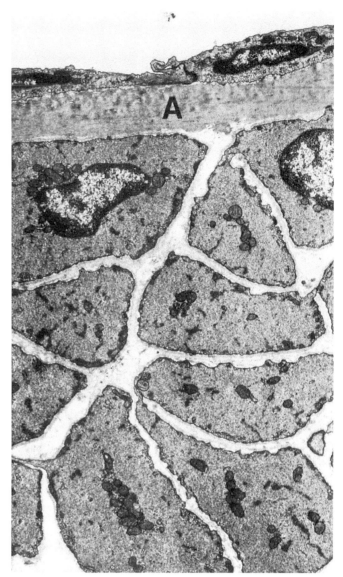

FIGURE 7-3 Electron micrograph of part of the wall of a muscular artery (rat). The endothelium rests on a thick internal elastic membrane (A). The smooth muscle cells of the tunica media are surrounded by a basal lamina and collagen fibrils are present in the intercellular spaces (×7800).

Vascular Endothelium

The vascular endothelium is interposed between the blood in circulation and the surrounding tissues or organs. Endothelial cells have been shown to be functionally interactive with other cells in many complex ways. The endothelial cytoskeleton, a complex network of actin microfilaments, microtubules, and intermediate filaments, combines to change and transduce signals between cells and regulate cell shape (Fig. 7-6).

Endothelial cells manifest extensive heterogeneity. Morphologic heterogeneity of these cells is found in arteries versus veins and can be demonstrated by corrosion casts that exhibit details of the endothelium. In arteries, endothelial cells are usually very elongated and lie parallel to the long axis of the vessel (Fig. 7-7). In contrast, endothelial cells of veins and capillaries are more rounded and less highly oriented.

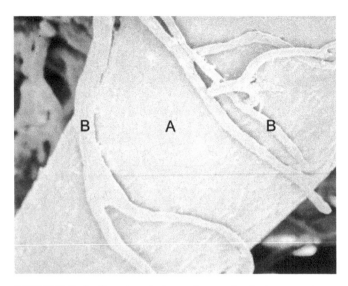

FIGURE 7-4 Scanning electron micrograph of microcorrosion cast showing bovine pododermal vein (A) with accompanying vasa vasorum (B) (×220). *(Courtesy of Dr. R. Hirschberg, Berlin.)*

Immuno- and glycohistochemical studies have led to the recognition of species-, organ-, and age-specific endothelial cell surface receptors. Selectivity in the seeding of metastatic cells from tumors and site-specificity of lymphocyte homing are examples of preferential adhesion to the endothelial cell surface. Structural heterogeneity such as the presence or absence of certain cellular organelles like Weibel-Palade bodies (rod-shaped bundles of microtubules in Fig. 7-8), differences in the synthesis of specific enzymes or cytokines, and variability in the production of vascular regulatory products such as prostaglandins are testimony to the complexity of the endothelium.

Arteries

Elastic Arteries

The tunica interna of elastic arteries is often thicker than the interna of other types of arteries (Fig. 7-9). The endothelial cells often appear to have a bricklike shape. The subendothelial layer contains smooth muscle cells, fibroblasts, primarily longitudinally oriented collagen fibers, and numerous fine elastic fibers. In the large domestic mammals, this layer is particularly thick.

The internal elastic membrane is often split into lamellae that may merge with the elastic laminae of the tunica media.

The tunica media is the thickest of the three tunics of the vessel wall and consists primarily of concentrically arranged, fenestrated elastic laminae (Fig. 7-10). Smooth muscle cells lie between adjacent laminae to which they are attached by collagen fibrils. The amorphous ground substance is basophilic due to the high quantity of sulfated glycosaminoglycans. All intercellular fibers and ground substance of the media are synthesized by the smooth muscle cells. With increasing distance from the heart, the number of smooth muscle cells in the tunica media of elastic arteries increases and the amount of elastic tissue decreases. The external elastic membrane is either absent or indistinct.

In the tunica externa, longitudinally arranged bundles of collagen fibers predominate and are intermixed with a few elastic fibers and fibroblasts. The interlacing of the collagen fibers limits the elastic expansion of the vessel.

Transition from elastic to muscular arteries may be either gradual or abrupt. In the dog, typical muscular renal arteries arise immediately at right angles from the elastic abdominal aorta. Carotid, femoral, vertebral, and brachial arteries commonly begin as elastic arteries and gradually transform into the muscular type in peripheral regions. The site of the transitional zone for each vessel varies among species and individual animals.

Muscular Arteries

The tunica interna of muscular arteries consists of the endothelium with an underlying thin subendothelial layer composed of collagen and elastic fibers. In large muscular arteries, a few fibroblasts and smooth muscle cells are present. With decreasing vessel size, the subendothelial layer gradually becomes thinner. The prominent, thick internal elastic membrane (Figs. 7-1 and 7-3) has fenestrations through which cytoplasmic processes of endothelial cells contact the smooth muscle of the tunica media. Blood vessel tone is determined by both smooth muscle and endothelial function. The two cell types interact in a dynamic manner to regulate blood vessel diameter.

Muscular arteries are characterized by a thick tunica media, composed mainly of smooth muscle cells in the form of circular or helical wrappings from three to more than 40 cell layers in thickness. Interspersed between these smooth muscle cells are elastic

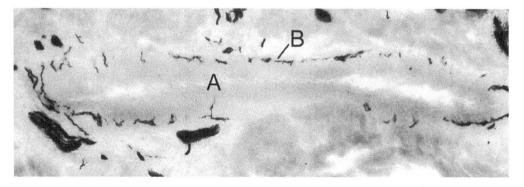

FIGURE 7-5 Longitudinal section through a bovine pododermal arteriole (A). Nervi vasorum (B) form a plexus around the vessel and few axons penetrate the tunica media. Acetylcholinesterase counterstained with nuclear fast red (×100). *(Courtesy of Dr. S. Buda, Berlin.)*

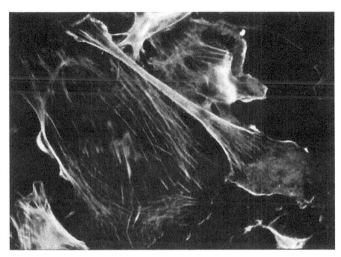

FIGURE 7-6 Cytoskeleton of endothelial cells, cultured in vitro and labeled by immunocytochemistry (i.e., a fluorescein-coupled monoclonal antibody to actin) (×600).

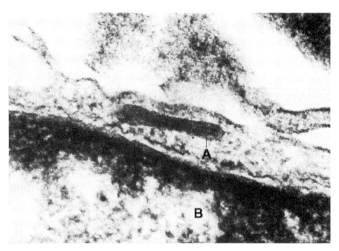

FIGURE 7-8 Electron micrograph of a porcine endothelial cell of the chorioid containing a so-called Weibel-Palade body (A), longitudinally cut. These endothelial-specific bundles of microtubules are located in the cytoplasm. Cell nucleus (B) (×150,000).

fibers or lamellae, as well as collagen fibers (Figs. 7-1, 7-3, and 7-10). The external elastic membrane is often discontinuous and not always clearly defined. It consists of a dense feltwork of elastic fibers adjacent to the tunica externa (Fig. 7-1).

The tunica externa is composed of collagen fibers, fibroblasts, and elastic fibers that decrease in number with decreasing size of the vessel.

When living tissues are prepared for fixation or when an animal dies, the muscular arteries contract considerably and blood is forced out of the lumina into the more expandable venous circulation. The tunica interna, including the underlying internal elastic membrane, and the external elastic membrane are thrown into longitudinal folds. Consequently, the cross-sectional profiles of muscular arteries in most histologic preparations have relatively small lumina containing little blood, the elastic membranes appear scalloped, and endothelial cells have a bricklike shape (Fig. 7-1).

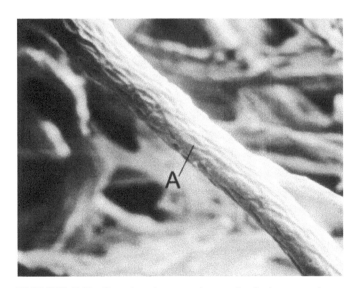

FIGURE 7-7 Scanning electron micrograph of microcorrosion cast showing bovine pododermal artery with elongated endothelial cell imprints (A) lying parallel with the long axis of the vessel (×320). *(Courtesy of Dr. R. Hirschberg, Berlin.)*

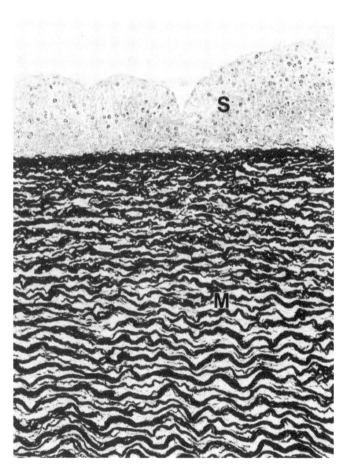

FIGURE 7-9 Cross section through part of the wall of the equine thoracic aorta. A particularly thick subendothelial layer (S) contains many longitudinally oriented elastic fibers. In the tunica media (M), elastic laminae predominate. Resorcin–fuchsin–van Gieson's stain (×50). *(Courtesy of A. Hansen.)*

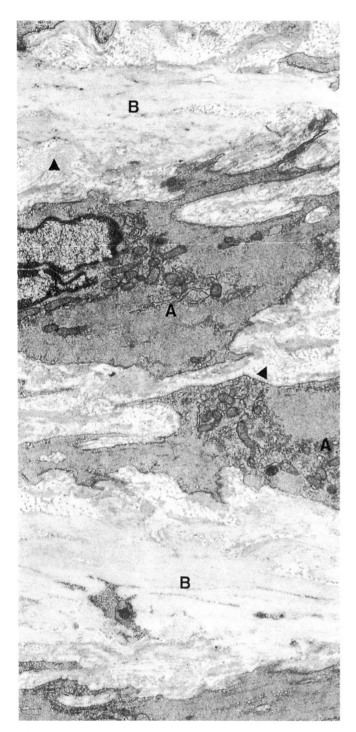

FIGURE 7-10 Electron micrograph of part of the tunica media of the aorta (rat). Smooth muscle cells (A) surrounded by collagen fibrils (arrowheads) alternate with elastic laminae (B) (×9000).

Microvasculature

In its simplest form, the microvasculature comprises afferent arterioles that lead to capillary networks drained by efferent venules. Shunts may exist between arterioles and venules in the form of either arteriovenous anastomoses or central channels that create preferential flow through capillary beds. In many organs, the microvasculature has unique architectural and structural characteristics.

Examples of exceedingly intricate and extremely convoluted microcirculation are found in the lung, hoof, and claw (Fig. 7-11).

Arterioles

The tunica interna of arterioles consists of endothelium, a thin subendothelial layer of collagen and elastic fibers (which is absent in the smallest arterioles), and an internal elastic membrane. The internal elastic membrane is fenestrated and eventually disappears in the smallest arterioles, allowing basal processes of the endothelial cells to establish direct contact with the underlying smooth muscle cells of the tunica media. In addition to one to three layers of smooth muscle cells, the tunica media may also contain collagen fibers (Fig. 7-12). An external elastic membrane is absent. The tunica externa is loose connective tissue.

Capillaries

Capillaries are tubules of uniform diameter that are approximately 8 μm wide (ranging from 5 to 10 μm). The walls of capillaries are composed of endothelial cells, an associated basal lamina, pericytes, and a thin adventitial connective-tissue layer that is lacking around brain capillaries (Figs. 7-13 and 7-14). A tunica media is absent.

Pericytes of capillaries and postcapillary venules are basal lamina–enclosed cells with numerous processes. They are considered to be undifferentiated mesenchymal cells that can be readily stimulated to divide mitotically and to migrate around or away from the vessels. Pericytes may play a critical role in blood vessel development and maturation. These cells are believed to transform into other cell types, especially fibroblasts and smooth muscle cells. Apparently a capillary can transform by this means into other types of vascular tubes if the internal flow characteristics change. Indeed, this description is compatible with the method by which arteries and veins develop during embryogenesis. All blood vessels start as simple, endothelium-lined capillarylike tubes during **vasculogenesis,** which is the de novo

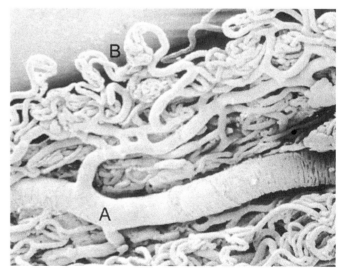

FIGURE 7-11 Scanning electron micrograph of microcorrosion cast of bovine pododermal arteriole (A) with branching convoluted capillaries (B) (×70). *(Courtesy of Dr. R. Hirschberg, Berlin.)*

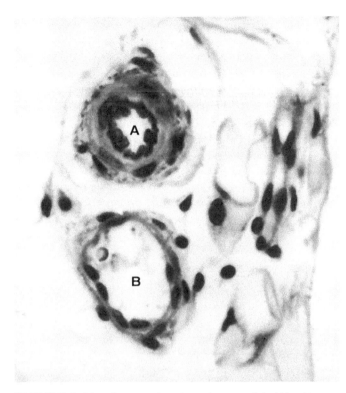

FIGURE 7-12 Cross sections through an arteriole (A), with two layers of smooth muscle in the tunica media, and a venule (B), classified as intermediate between pericytic and muscular because of the presence of one incomplete layer of smooth muscle. Hematoxylin and eosin (×400). *(From Dellmann HD, Carithers JR. Cytology and Microscopic Anatomy. Philadelphia: Williams & Wilkins, 1996.)*

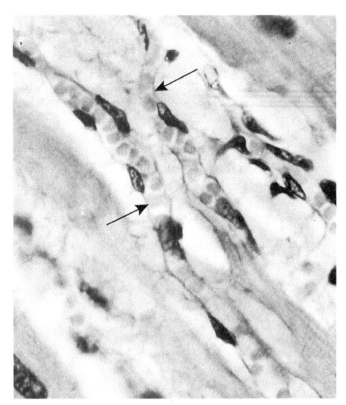

FIGURE 7-14 Capillaries (arrows) in the canine myocardium. Note that the variable widths of the capillaries may be barely greater than or slightly smaller than the diameter of an erythrocyte. It is not always possible to distinguish clearly between the nuclei of endothelial cells and pericytes. Hematoxylin and eosin (×750).

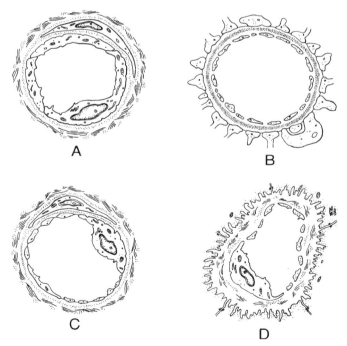

FIGURE 7-13 Drawing of the fine structural characteristics of the four types of capillaries: continuous capillary (**A**), porous capillary (**B**), fenestrated capillary (**C**), and sinusoid (**D**). The fine dots around the endothelial cells and pericytes (in **A** and **C** only) indicate the basal lamina, which is particularly thick in porous capillaries and discontinuous in sinusoids.

differentiation of blood vessels from mesodermal precursor cells, or during **angiogenesis,** which is the formation of new blood vessels by migration and proliferation of endothelial cells from preexisting vessels. Recent studies have shown that, in the presence of various soluble factors, it is possible to activate or inhibit capillary growth in certain tissues.

Capillaries form networks called **capillary beds,** the density of which is a reflection of the metabolic requirements of different organs. For example, capillary beds are most dense in cardiac and skeletal muscle and relatively less dense in tendons. Capillaries are absent in most epithelia, dental enamel, dentin, cementum, most cartilage, cornea, vitreous body, and lens. Vascular as well as avascular zones have also been identified in fibrocartilaginous articular menisci.

Within the capillary beds, exchange takes place between the circulating blood and interstitial fluid with water and water-soluble substances leaving the arterial end of the capillaries. Fluids then reenter at the venous end of the capillary as well as into post-capillary venules further downstream. Plasma molecules may leave the capillary lumen by transcytosis, through temporary transendothelial channels, across monolayered diaphragms, or by free diffusion (e.g., lipid-soluble substances).

Continuous capillaries, fenestrated capillaries, porous capillaries, and sinusoids are distinguished by fine-structural characteristics of the capillary wall. The structural differences correspond to measurable differences in capillary permeability. Fenestrated and porous capillaries have the highest permeability, continuous neural capillaries have the least permeability, and the permeability of continuous muscular capillaries lies between these limits.

Continuous capillaries are virtually ubiquitous in the organism. Individual endothelial cells are held together by tight junctions (Figs. 7-13A, 7-15, and 7-16). Usually, these cells contain only a few mitochondria and ribosomes, little endoplasmic reticulum, and small Golgi complexes. Transcytotic vesicles may be either numerous, as in muscular capillaries (Fig. 7-15), or scarce to nonexistent, as in neural capillaries.

Fenestrated capillaries (visceral capillaries) commonly occur in the gastrointestinal tract (Fig. 7-13C and 7-17). They have a large diameter and their shape is adapted to the surrounding parenchymal cells from which they are separated by a basal lamina and small amount of adventitial connective tissue. In these capillaries, portions of the endothelial cells are attenuated and have circular fenestrae that are 60 to 80 nm in diameter. The fenestrae are closed by monolayered **diaphragms** that are thinner than the cell membrane (Fig. 7-17). Diaphragms are absent in the kidney where the capillary wall is porous (Figs. 7-13B and 7-18). Fenestrations facilitate the passage of substances across the endothelium.

Sinusoids are present in the liver, bone marrow, and certain endocrine glands (Fig. 7-13D). They are larger than other capillaries, lack uniformity in diameter, and shape themselves to fill the space within the confines of the surrounding parenchyma. Large intercellular openings and pores through the endothelial

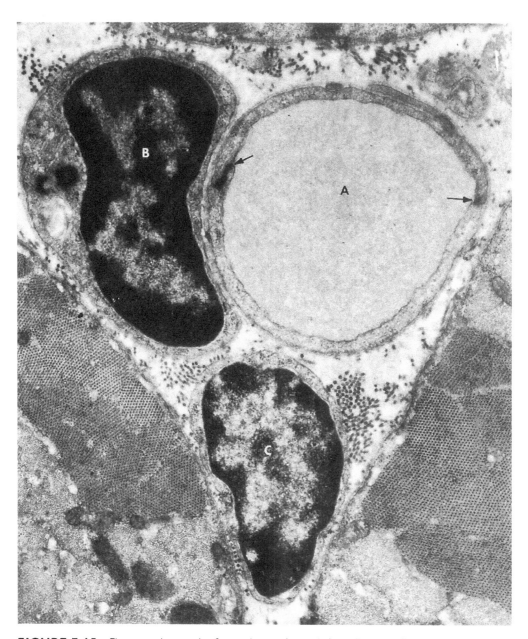

FIGURE 7-15   Electron micrograph of a continuous (muscular) capillary (A). Tight junctions are present between the endothelial cells (arrows). The basal lamina of the endothelium continues around the adjacent pericyte (B). The cell labeled C is either a fibrocyte or another pericyte. Black dots between the cells are cross sections of collagen fibrils (×16,000).

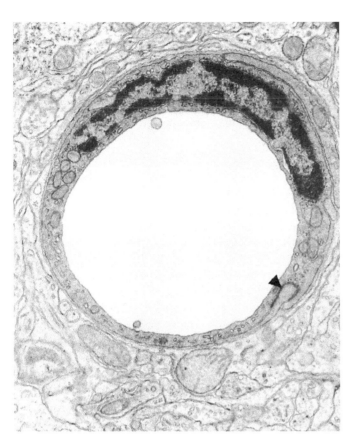

FIGURE 7-16 Electron micrograph of a continuous (neural) capillary. Tight junctions (arrowhead) are present between adjacent endothelial cells (×21,000).

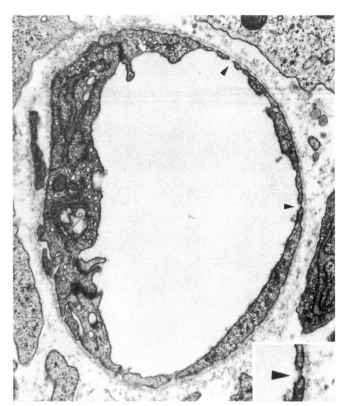

FIGURE 7-17 Electron micrograph of a fenestrated capillary in the lamina propria of the small intestine (rat). The fenestrations (arrowheads) are closed by a monolayered diaphragm (×15,600). Insert (lower right) shows detail of a pore with a diaphragm (×45,000).

cells, along with a concomitant discontinuity or absence of the surrounding basal lamina, provide for a maximum exchange between blood and surrounding parenchyma. Phagocytic cells often span the lumen of sinusoids or lie just outside the endothelium.

Arterioles continue into capillary beds (Fig. 7-19). Each capillary bed has a wide **central channel** through which blood flows continuously. Capillaries that branch from the central channel have more intermittent blood flow. The proximal portion of the central channel, the **metarteriole**, is a narrow vessel surrounded by large, isolated bundles of smooth muscle. The initial portion of the metarteriole is surrounded by additional smooth muscle cells, which form a **precapillary sphincter** that regulates the blood flow through the capillary bed. The distal portion of the central channel is similar in structure to other capillaries but lacks smooth muscle found in the wall of the metarteriole. This portion of the central channel empties into the venule.

Venules

Immediate **postcapillary venules** are similar in structure to capillaries but are larger in diameter (10 to 30 µm) (Fig. 7-19). The tunica interna is formed by either continuous or fenestrated endothelial cells connected by incomplete tight junctions, a basal lamina, and a thin subendothelial layer of longitudinal collagen fibers. Occasional pericytes are present.

Postcapillary venules have a functional significance that is not evident with simple morphologic studies. The junctions be-

tween the endothelial cells are more permeable than those in capillaries and are more sensitive to leakage induced by such agents as serotonin and histamine. These compounds play a role in the inflammatory reaction, resulting in the accumulation of excessive extravascular fluid, soluble substances, and blood cells. Immediate postcapillary venules, referred to as **high endothelial venules,** are found in most lymphoid tissue and are characterized by specialized endothelial cells involved in the migration of lymphocytes (see Chapter 8).

As the venules increase in diameter (30 to 50 µm), they are called **pericytic venules** or **collecting venules** in which pericytes form a continuous layer (Fig. 7-19). Fibrocytes and collagen fibers form a thin tunica externa. As venules increase further in diameter (50 to 100 µm), the pericytes are gradually replaced by circularly arranged muscle cells (Fig. 7-19). When these cells form one to two complete layers, the venule is referred to as a **muscular venule** (Fig. 7-19). The tunica externa, containing elastic and collagen fibers and scattered fibrocytes, becomes more prominent. Pericytic venules are a definite site for large molecular exchange between the vascular and connective tissue spaces.

Arteriovenous Anastomoses

Direct connections between arterioles and venules without an intervening capillary bed are called **arteriovenous anastomoses.** These anastomoses are short, usually nonbranched, and often coiled vessels. They possess a thick smooth muscle layer

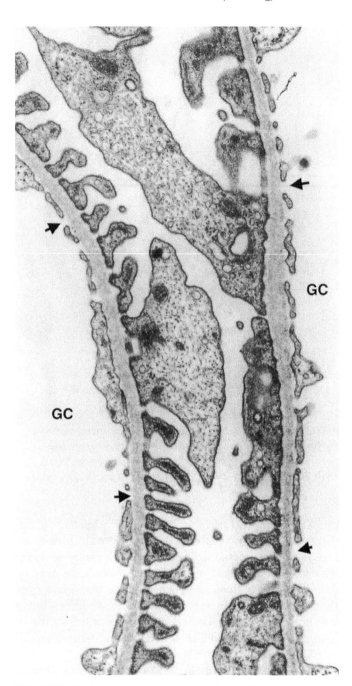

FIGURE 7-18 Electron micrograph of part of the walls of two glomerular capillaries (GC) of the kidney. The endothelial cells have pores (arrowheads) (×27,600).

in the subendothelium that receives a dense vasomotor nerve supply. Often, longitudinally oriented smooth muscle fibers form cushions or sleeves. When arteriovenous anastomoses are open, the blood essentially bypasses capillary beds and is shunted directly into the venous system; when they are closed, the blood flow to capillary beds is increased. Arteriovenous anastomoses are particularly numerous in the skin, lips, intestine, salivary glands, nasal mucosa, and male and female reproductive tracts. They function in the regulation of blood pressure and blood flow into capillary beds, thermoregulation, and erection.

A highly convoluted arteriovenous anastomosis surrounded by a thick connective-tissue capsule is called a **glomus**. The vessel of the glomus is characterized by numerous longitudinal, subendothelial epithelioid muscle cells surrounded by circularly arranged muscle cells in the media. An internal elastic membrane is absent. Glomera are particularly numerous in digital pads and the external ear and have a thermoregulatory function.

Veins

Blood courses through venous trees in a direction opposite to that in arterial trees. The structure of veins varies widely and is apparently determined by differing local mechanical conditions. Consequently, classification of veins is difficult, especially because layers in their walls are often absent or difficult to distinguish.

The terms **small, medium,** and **large veins** have only relative meaning in any one animal. The large veins of a cat may be smaller than the medium-sized veins of a cow. Small veins are the continuation of muscular venules. The medium-sized veins are actually collecting veins and correspond in function and location to the medium or muscular arteries. Veins corresponding to the aorta are referred to as the great veins or large veins, or simply by their gross anatomic names such as the vena cava.

All types of veins that carry blood against gravity, ranging from venules to small and medium veins of the extremities, are equipped with flaplike, semilunar **valves**. Venous valves are paired folds of the interna that are composed of endothelium covering a core of collagen fibers (Fig. 7-20). Proximal to the attachment of the valves, the wall of the vein is slightly distended to form a valve sinus. Free margins of the valves are oriented toward the heart. When closed, the valves prevent the backflow of blood.

Small Veins

As venules further increase in diameter, they become **small veins.** Endothelium and the associated basal lamina lining a small vein are surrounded by a distinct media. The media has two to four continuous layers of circularly oriented smooth muscle cells interspersed with a varying amount of connective tissue that blends with the surrounding tunica externa.

Medium Veins

The wall structure of the **medium veins** reflects the physical stresses of gravity and the centrifugal forces of locomotion that they must withstand. Because the variation in position and orientation of smooth muscle components is considerable in different veins within the various species, inclusive descriptions are difficult.

The tunica interna consists of an endothelial lining and a thin subendothelial layer of collagen and elastic fibers. An internal elastic membrane may be present in the larger vessels. Usually, the tunica media consists of several layers of smooth muscle with associated collagen and elastic networks, which are commonly arranged in circular or spiral fashion. In the outer tunica media, smooth muscle cells may be longitudinally oriented. The tunica externa is composed predominantly of collagen networks an-

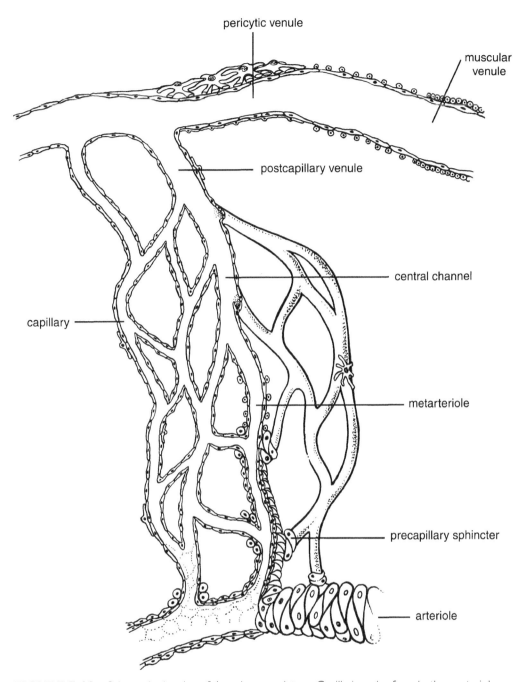

FIGURE 7-19 Schematic drawing of the microvasculature. Capillaries arise from both an arteriole and a metarteriole; precapillary sphincters are present. The metarteriole continues into a central channel, followed by a postcapillary venule, pericytic venule, and muscular venule, linked by a venule with an incomplete layer of smooth muscle.

chored to both the tunica media and the surrounding connective tissue. Longitudinally oriented elastic fibers are also present in the externa.

Large Veins

The tunica interna of **large veins** has essentially the same structure as that of medium veins. However, the endothelium is often slightly thicker and blocklike, smooth muscle cells are present occasionally, and the internal elastic membrane is more prominent.

The tunica media is thin when compared to the relative size of the vessel or the diameter of the lumen. It consists of collagen, elastic fibers, and smooth muscle cells in varying proportions (Fig. 7-21). In most large veins, the amount of smooth muscle is insignificant.

Conversely, the tunica externa is prominent and composed of longitudinally or spirally oriented bundles of smooth muscle cells, together with collagen and elastic fibers that maintain the proper tension of the wall. The thickness of this layer depends on the location of the vein and is more pronounced in veins under

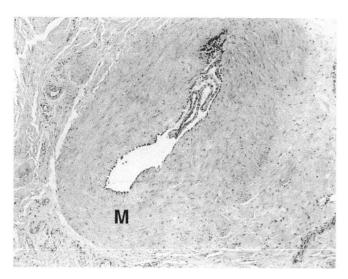

FIGURE 7-20 Cross section through a vein with a thick muscular tunica media (M) in the ovine teat. Hematoxylin and eosin (×200).

greater pressure exerted by the surrounding environment (e.g., in the thoracic and abdominal cavities) (Fig. 7-21).

Specialized Blood Vessels

Many blood vessels have special structural features that fulfill specific functions in the regulation of blood flow. An increase in the thickness of the wall is observed in vessels subjected to unusual blood pressures such as arteries and veins of the teat (Fig. 7-20), veins of the glans penis, and coronary arteries. Conversely, a decrease in the wall thickness occurs in protected, low-pressure areas such as the skull (e.g., arteries of the brain, dural venous sinuses), bones, and lungs. Longitudinal muscle bundles that can stop blood flow through the vessel occur in the tunica interna in both arteries and veins of the penis, ovary, and uterus. Circular,

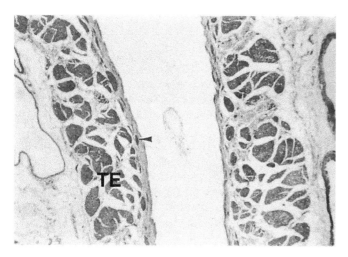

FIGURE 7-21 Cross section through part of the ovine vena cava. The thin tunica media consists of a few bundles of smooth muscle cells (arrowhead). The tunica externa (TE) is the most prominent layer and contains many bundles of longitudinally oriented smooth muscle. Hematoxylin and eosin (×40).

sphincterlike thickenings of the tunica media of veins perform similar functions in the large intestine, liver, and skin.

Sensory Receptors

Sensory receptors are present at the bifurcation of the common carotid artery. They include the carotid body and the carotid sinus, which monitor changes in blood chemical composition (chemoreceptors) and blood pressure (baroreceptors), respectively.

Carotid Body

The carotid body is enclosed by a connective tissue capsule and consists of a dense sinusoidal capillary network surrounding clusters of cells. Two cell types are present within these clusters: **granular endocrine cells** (type I cells or chemoreceptor cells), which contain many granules rich in catecholamines and serotonin, and **sustentacular cells** (type II cells), which have few or no granules. The sustentacular cells incompletely invest several granular endocrine cells (Fig. 7-22). Nonmyelinated afferent and efferent nerve terminals synapse on granular endocrine cells. Changes in oxygen and carbon dioxide tension and the blood pH generate action potentials in afferent nerve fibers, which then travel to the central nervous system and trigger responses primarily in the respiratory and cardiovascular systems.

Carotid Sinus

The baroreceptor area of the **carotid sinus** is a dilation of the internal carotid artery, where it originates from the common

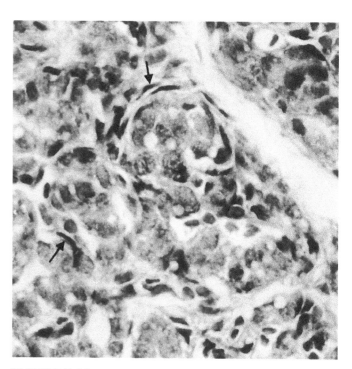

FIGURE 7-22 Ovine carotid body. Groups of large type I cells are invested by flatter type II cells (arrows). Hematoxylin and eosin (×350). *(Preparation courtesy of J. H. Riley.)*

carotid artery. At this point, the tunica media of the artery is thin and surrounded by a thick tunica externa that contains many terminals from the carotid sinus branch of the glossopharyngeal nerve. The terminals are mechanoreceptors that cause reflex bradycardia (a decrease in heart rate) and dilation of the splanchnic blood vessels when stimulated by increased blood pressure.

HEART

The thick wall of the heart is primarily composed of cardiac muscle cells capable of spontaneous rhythmic contractions that pump blood into the vascular system. The inner layer of the heart is referred to as **endocardium** and is continuous with the tunica interna of the large blood vessels entering and leaving the heart. The middle contractile muscular layer is called the **myocardium** and is by far the thickest layer of the organ. The outermost layer is the **epicardium.**

Endocardium

The **endocardium** lines the ventricles and atria completely and covers the cardiac valves and associated structures. The endocardium usually consists of three layers (Fig. 7-23). A continuous **endothelium** forms the innermost layer. The **subendothelial layer,** located beneath the endothelium is composed of dense irregular connective tissue with collagen and elastic fibers and occasional smooth muscle cells. Elastic fibers are particularly abundant in the atrial walls and are usually arranged parallel to the endocardial surface.

The **subendocardial layer** is predominantly composed of loosely arranged collagen and elastic fibers. Adipose cells may be present, along with a rich supply of blood and lymph vessels and connective tissue that is continuous with that of the myocardium. In some locations, modified cardiac muscle cells of the cardiac impulse conduction system are present in the subendocardial layer (Fig. 7-23).

The **cardiac valves** are endocardial folds covered by endothelium. The subendothelial layer is rich in elastic and collagen fibers. The **atrioventricular valves** consist of a **stratum spongiosum** located toward the atrial side and a **stratum fibrosum** on the ventricular side (Fig. 7-24). In the stratum spongiosum, elastic and collagen fibers are loosely arranged. Blood vessels are located in the stratum spongiosum exclusively. In the stratum fibrosum, collagen fibers predominate and connect with the fibrous rings surrounding the atrioventricular openings. The fibers are also continuous with collagen fibers of the fibrous cords (**chordae tendineae**) that arise from the endomysium of the papillary muscles. In the **semilunar valves** of the aorta and the pulmonary trunk, the central collagen fibers have a predominantly circular arrangement and are reinforced by a thin layer of elastic fibers near the vessel and a thicker layer of elastic fibers on the ventricular side. The thickening of the free edge of the semilunar valves is caused by the presence of loose connective and cartilaginous tissues.

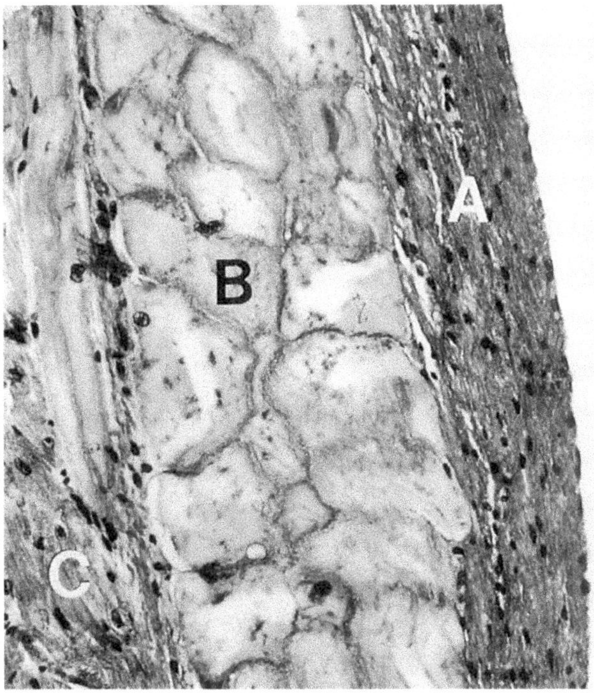

Myocardium

The middle and thickest layer of the heart is the **myocardium,** which is composed of bundles of cardiac muscle cells, branches

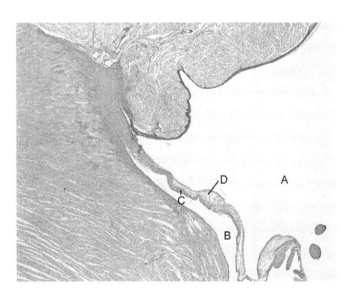

FIGURE 7-23 Horizontal section through part of the bovine heart wall. Peripheral to the subendothelial layer (A) is the subendocardial layer, with large impulse-conducting muscle fibers (B), and the myocardium (C). Trichrome (×200).

FIGURE 7-24 Sagittal section through the heart of a rabbit. The atrioventricular valve (bicuspid valve), which is located between the left atrium (A) and ventricle (B), is covered by endothelium and consists of a stratum fibrosum (C) and stratum spongiosum (D). Elastica-Domagk stain (×50).

of cardiac conduction fibers, an extensive capillary network, and the cardiac skeleton.

Bundles of cardiac muscle cells are embedded in loose connective tissue that contains a dense capillary network, lymph vessels, and autonomic nerve fibers. The amount of interstitial connective tissue is subject to local variations and is greater in the myocardium of the right ventricle when compared to that of the left ventricle. The atrial cardiac muscle cells are usually smaller than the ventricular cardiac muscle cells. In atrial cardiac muscle cells, numerous specific **atrial granules** containing atrial natriuretic peptide (ANP) are present. ANP plays an important role in fluid homeostasis (e.g., diuresis, natriuresis, vasodilation).

The musculature of the atrial and ventricular walls is inserted into the **cardiac skeleton,** which is made up of three parts: (1) the fibrous rings (annuli fibrosi), (2) the fibrous triangles (trigona fibrosa cordis), and (3) the fibrous (or membranous) part of the interventricular septum. The **fibrous rings** are composed of intermingling bundles of collagen and a few elastic fibers that surround the atrioventricular, aortic, and pulmonary trunk openings. The **fibrous triangles** are small areas of connective tissue that fill the spaces between the atrioventricular openings and the base of the aorta. The nature of this connective tissue is species- and age-dependent. The triangles may be predominantly dense, irregular connective tissue (in pigs, cats, and rabbits), fibrocartilage (in dogs) (Fig. 7-25), hyaline cartilage (in horses), or bone (in large ruminants). The **fibrous part of the interventricular septum** consists of collagen fiber bundles.

Epicardium and Pericardium

The myocardium is covered externally by the **epicardium** (visceral serous pericardium). The outermost layer is mesothelial cells, which line the pericardial cavity. Under this epithelium is a loose connective-tissue layer rich in elastic fibers that forms protective sheaths around blood vessels and nerves. The connective tissue, which is often rich in adipocytes, is particularly abundant around the large coronary blood vessels.

The epicardium reflects off the surface of the heart to form the **parietal serous pericardium.** The parietal pericardium consists of an innermost mesothelial cell layer resting on a thin layer of loose connective tissue, which fuses with the **fibrous pericardium,** a thick layer of collagen fiber bundles and elastic fibers. Located between the visceral and parietal serous pericardium, the **pericardial cavity** contains serous fluid that lubricates the mesothelial surfaces, allowing frictionless cardiac movement.

The pericardium can readily adapt to normal continual changes in the size of the heart and can also limit overfilling of the heart. However, cardiac tamponade (compression of the heart) may result if the pericardial cavity fills with excessive fluid.

Cardiac Conduction System

The electrical impulse for cardiac contraction is generated in the sinoatrial node, subsequently spreads to the atrioventricular node,

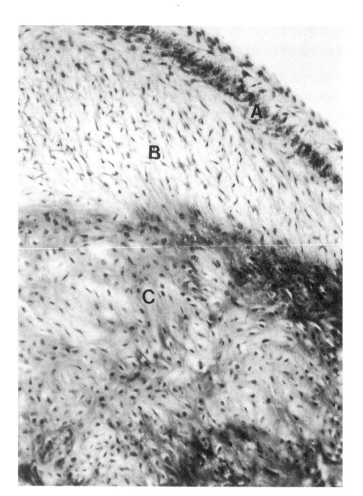

FIGURE 7-25 Horizontal section through a canine fibrous ring and adjacent fibrous triangle of the heart. The ring is lined by a layer of endothelium followed by an inner subendothelial layer of dense irregular connective tissue (A) and an outer layer of loose connective tissue (B). The fibrous triangle (C) is highly cellular fibrocartilage. Hematoxylin and eosin (×130).

and continues in the atrioventricular bundle. The **sinoatrial node** is composed of a network of thin, branching nodal muscle cells that contain scarce myofibrils and lack intercalated disks. The nodal fibers are continuous with ordinary cardiac muscle fibers of the atrial myocardium. Individual fibers are separated by relatively large amounts of highly vascularized connective tissue containing many autonomic nerve fibers and occasional ganglion cells (vagus nerve).

The **atrioventricular node** is composed of irregularly arranged, small, branching nodal muscle fibers, the morphology of which is similar to those of the sinoatrial node. Nodal muscle fibers are interposed between atrial myocardial fibers and the impulse-conducting fibers, which form the atrioventricular bundle.

Fibers in the **atrioventricular bundle** are also known as **cardiac conduction fibers** (Purkinje fibers). These fibers are readily identified by their large diameter, large central spherical nucleus, and scarce peripheral myofibrils. The central area of the cytoplasm is rich in glycogen and creates a light-staining halo around the nucleus (Fig. 7-23). In longitudinal sections, characteristic cross-striations and intercalated disks typical of cardiac muscle cells are visible. The conducting fibers connect with smaller transitional cells that lack intercalated disks and in turn connect with ordinary myocardial cells.

Cardiac Blood Vessels, Lymph Vessels, and Nerves

The coronary arteries are thick muscular arteries that often contain bundles of longitudinal smooth muscle and epithelioid muscle cells in the interna. The muscle component regulates the blood flow within these vessels. From the coronary arteries, a dense capillary network supplies the myocardium, epicardium, cardiac skeleton, and peripheral portions of cardiac valves. Blood flowing from the cardiac capillary beds is collected by venules and veins that open into the right atrium either through the coronary sinus or through direct openings in the endocardium (venae cordis minimae).

Lymph capillaries form a network in the cardiac connective tissue. The small lymphatics are continuous with larger lymph vessels, especially in the subendocardial layer and the subepithelial connective tissue of the epicardium.

Both sympathetic and parasympathetic nerves innervate the heart. They are numerous in the atria but scarce in the ventricles, where mainly sympathetic fibers are represented. The nerves form extensive plexuses that are particularly dense around the sinoatrial and atrioventricular nodes. The parasympathetic (vagus) fibers terminate on ganglion cells, which in turn contribute fibers to the aforementioned plexuses. Both the myocardium and epicardium receive sensory fibers that terminate with club-shaped or platelike enlargements.

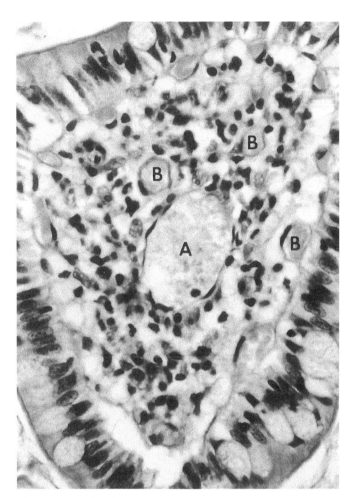

FIGURE 7-26 Cross section through a canine intestinal villus. Lymph capillary (A); blood capillaries (B). Hematoxylin and eosin (×435).

LYMPH VESSELS

The lymph vascular system is an integral part of both the circulatory system and the defense system. It originates as a network of anastomosing lymph capillaries in the connective tissue of the organism. The capillaries are continuous with larger lymph vessels that pass through at least one lymph node on their way to larger collecting ducts that drain the lymph into the venous system.

Lymph Capillaries

Lymph capillaries are endothelium-lined tubes that are usually larger in diameter than blood capillaries and variable in shape (Fig. 7-26). It is often difficult to distinguish between lymph and blood capillaries in histologic sections; however, recently described histochemical markers that discriminate between vascular and lymphatic endothelium may allow this distinction. The endothelial lining of lymph capillaries is usually thin. Adjacent endothelial cells are joined by intimate interdigitations, simple overlapping,

or adhering junctions. Frequently, variably sized gaps are observed between adjacent cells. These gaps are probably temporary as they appear or disappear continuously.

The basal lamina around lymph capillaries is either discontinuous or absent (Fig. 7-27). Fine, extracellular matrix-anchoring filaments link the outer surface of the endothelial cells to pericapillary collagen fibrils and elastic fibers. These filaments are responsible for keeping the lumina of the capillaries open, especially when the tissues are edematous.

Valves may be occasionally present in lymph capillaries and are a constant feature of all other lymph vessels (Fig. 7-28). They are composed of an endothelial fold with little intervening connective tissue, except at the junction with the vessel wall, where it is more abundant. Occasional smooth muscle fibers are found in the valves of the larger lymph vessels.

As a general rule, lymph capillaries are found in conjunction with loose connective tissue where they drain excess interstitial fluid that contains fat, proteins, cells, and particulate matter. They are absent in the central nervous system, certain structures within the eye, bone marrow, cartilage, red pulp of the spleen, and liver lobules.

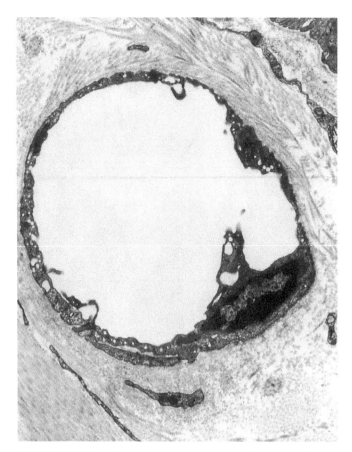

FIGURE 7-27   Electron micrograph of a lymph capillary. The thin endothelium contains numerous pinocytotic vesicles and lacks a basal lamina (×16,000).

Small and Medium Lymph Vessels

The structure of the wall of small and medium lymph vessels is subject to great variability according to location and the species

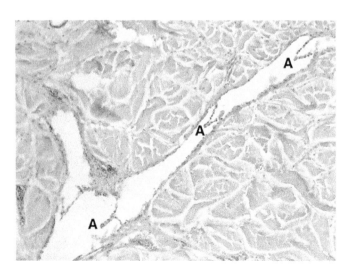

FIGURE 7-28   Lymphatic vessels of the bovine dermis cut longitudinally. Lymphatic vessels have valves (A) and display very large caliber lumina compared with the thickness of the wall. Hematoxylin and eosin (×100).

involved. These vessels differ from lymph capillaries by their larger diameter and the presence of a continuous basal lamina. With increasing vessel diameter, a thin subendothelial connective tissue layer appears. One or two layers of smooth muscle and elastic fibers are subsequently added in larger vessels. A tunica externa is not distinguishable from connective tissue surrounding the lymph vessel.

Large Lymph Vessels and Collecting Ducts

As in blood vessels, the walls of these large lymph vessels (ducts) comprise three tunics; however, the layers are not always well delineated (Fig. 7-29). The tunica interna consists of endothelium and a layer of longitudinal, interlacing collagen and elastic fibers. An internal elastic membrane is usually absent. The tunica media contains smooth muscle cells, surrounded by many elastic and collagen fibers, the number and orientation of which vary with the location and species. The tunica externa is composed of collagen and elastic fibers and may contain muscle cells.

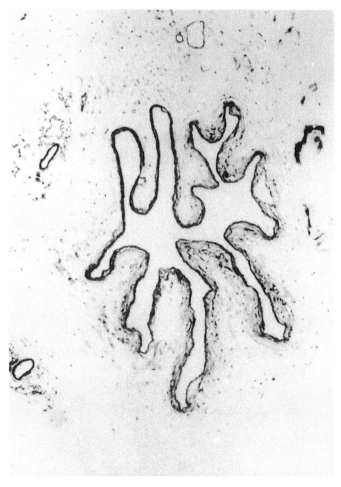

FIGURE 7-29   Cross section through the canine thoracic duct. The wall consists of an endothelium and a thin tunica media with sparse muscle cells; a distinct tunica externa is absent. Hematoxylin and eosin (×110). *(From Dellmann HD, Carithers JR. Cytology and Microscopic Anatomy. Philadelphia: Williams & Wilkins, 1996.)*

SUGGESTED READINGS

Bagshaw RJ, Fisher GM. Morphology of the carotid sinus in the dog. J Appl Physiol 1971;31:198–202.

Biscoe TJ. Carotid body: structure and function. Physiol Rev 1971; 51:437–495.

Egginton S, Zhou AL, Brown MD, et al. The role of pericytes in controlling angiogenesis in vivo. Adv Exp Med Biol. 2000;476:81–99.

Johansson BR. Size and distribution of endothelial plasmalemmal vesicles in consecutive segments of the microvasculature of cat skeletal muscle. Microvasc Res 1979;17:107–117.

Kaley G, Altura BM, eds. Microcirculation. Baltimore: University Park Press, 1977, 1978;1–3.

Leak LV. Lymphatic capillary ultrastructure and permeability. Eur J Physiol 1972;336:S46.

Majno G, Joris I. Endothelium 1977: a review. Adv Exp Med Biol 1978;104:169–225, 481–526.

Marais J, Fossum TW. Ultrastructural morphology of the canine thoracic duct and cisterna chyli. Acta Anat 1988;133:309–312.

Maul GG. Structure and function of pores in fenestrated capillaries. J Ultrastruct Res 1971;36:768–782.

Opthof T, de Jonge B, Masson-Pevet M, et al. Functional and morphological organization of the cat sinoatrial node. J Mol Cell Cardiol 1986;18:1015–1031.

Patan S. Vasculogenesis and angiogenesis as mechanisms of vascular network formation, growth and remodeling. Review. J Neurooncol 2000;50:1–15.

Racker DK. Atrioventricular node and input pathways: a correlated gross anatomical and histological study of the canine atrioventricular junctional region. Anat Rec 1989;224:336–354.

Ribatti D, Nico B, Vacca A, et al. Endothelial cell heterogeneity and organ specificity. J Hematother Stem Cell Res 2002;11: 81–90.

Simionescu N, Simionescu M, Palade GE. Structural basis of permeability in sequential segments of the microvasculature. Microvasc Res 1978:15:17–36.

Stone EA, Stewart GJ. Architecture and structure of canine veins with special reference to confluences. Anat Rec 1988;222:154–163.

Thaemert JC. Atrioventricular node innervation in ultrastructural three dimensions. Am J Anat 1970;128:239–263.

van Breemen C, Skarsgard P, Laher I, et al. Endothelium-smooth muscle interactions in blood vessels. Arterioscler Thromb Vasc Biol 1997;17:1203.

Verna A. Ultrastructure of the carotid body in mammals. Int Rev Cytol 1979;60:271–330.

Viragh S, Challice CE. The impulse generation and conduction system of the heart. In: Dalton AJ, Challice CE, eds. Ultrastructure in Biological Systems. New York: Academic Press, 1973.

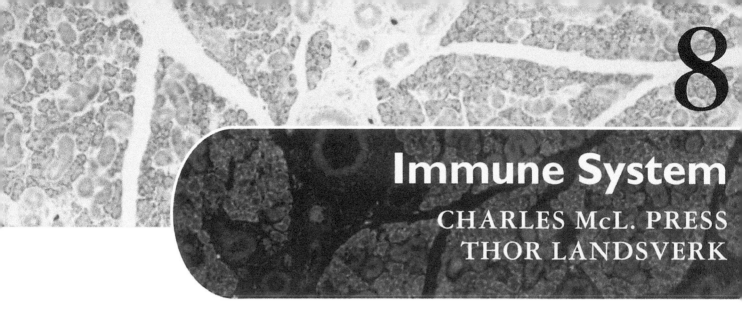

8

Immune System
CHARLES McL. PRESS
THOR LANDSVERK

Cells of the Immune System
  Lymphocytes
  Stromal Cells
    Reticular cells
    Epithelial reticular cells
  Antigen-Presenting Cells
    Dendritic cells
      Follicular dendritic cells
      Interdigitating dendritic cells
    Macrophages
    B cells
Organization of Cells to Form Lymphatic Tissues and Organs
  Diffuse Lymphatic Tissue
  Lymphatic Nodules
    Primary lymphatic nodules
    Secondary lymphatic nodules
Primary Lymphatic Organs
  Bone Marrow
  Aggregated Lymphatic Nodules in the Distal Small
    Intestine
  Cloacal Bursa of Birds
  Thymus
    Cortex

    Medulla
    Blood vessels, lymph vessels, and nerves
Secondary Lymphatic Tissues and Organs
  Mucosa-Associated Lymphatic Tissue
    Tonsils
    Bronchus-associated lymphatic tissue
    Gut-associated lymphatic tissue
  Lymph Nodes
    Lymph vessels and sinuses
    Cortex
    Medulla
    Blood vessels and nerves
    Species differences
  Spleen
    Capsule and supportive tissue
    Red pulp
    White pulp
    Marginal zone
    Blood vessels
    Lymph vessels and nerves
    Species differences
  Hemal Nodes and "Milk Spots"

The immune system comprises organs, aggregated lymphatic tissue, and cells that work to maintain the integrity of the body. Cells and tissues of the immune system identify and protect against pathogenic organisms and ensure that the body's response to foreign substances is appropriate. The system has innate components that act rapidly but nonspecifically and adaptive components that act specifically but need a period of time to respond. Threats to the integrity of the individual are not limited to ex-

trinsic sources. The processes of wear and tear and pathologic changes in tissues also result in an immune response.

CELLS OF THE IMMUNE SYSTEM

The cellular participants of the immune response can be categorized as either migratory cells or fixed cells. Lymphocytes are the principal **migratory cells** that are free to move anywhere in the body. Recirculation through the lymph or blood is a prominent feature of these leukocytes, ensuring effective surveillance of the tissues. The **fixed cells** are either mesenchymal or epithelial cells that form a scaffold for the stromal matrix in lymphatic tissue. These cells create a supportive framework that sustains the lymphocytes during different phases of development and function. The remarkable diversity of both migratory and fixed cells creates the unique character of lymphatic tissue.

Lymphocytes

The histology of lymphocytes is described in detail in Chapter 4. Lymphocytes are migratory cells of the immune system that control adaptive immunity by initiating a specific response after encountering antigens. **Antigens** are molecular components of **exogenous agents,** such as bacteria, viruses, protozoa, or toxins, and **endogenous agents,** such as tumor cells and virus-infected cells. The lymphocytic lineage gives rise to two major cell types: **B cells** (*bone* marrow–dependent) and **T cells** (*thymus-*dependent). B cells and T cells and their subpopulations are distinguished by different surface molecules that recognize antigens (i.e., **antigen receptors** [Fig. 8-1]) and are involved in signal transduction and cell cooperation (e.g., major histocompatibility markers). B and T cells cannot be identified using standard histologic stains such as hematoxylin and eosin.

B cells and T cells also differ in the way that they effect an immune response. After antigen stimulation, both lymphocyte types undergo proliferation and differentiation to become either memory cells or effector cells. **Memory cells** are long-lived cells that have the ability to mount an enhanced response upon a reencounter with antigen. **Effector B-cell** function is mediated by the secreted antigen receptor (immunoglobulin, also known as antibodies). In their active secretory phase, B effector cells typically are manifest as **plasma cells** (see Chapter 3 for the histology of plasma cells). Since antibodies circulate in the extracellular fluids ("humors"), B cells are said to be responsible for the **humoral immune response.** Antigen with attached antibody is more easily recognized by phagocytes and eliminated. The antigen–antibody complex also triggers a collection of plasma proteins, called the **complement system.** The complement system is an important component of innate defense with wide-ranging effects that include the ability to kill microorganisms.

Effector T cells, on the other hand, act more directly on adjacent cells within tissues. The two major subsets of effector T cells mediate their effects in different ways. **T helper cells** act through the secretion of soluble, local-acting molecules called **cytokines,** whereas the **T cytotoxic cells** attach to antigens on target cells to kill them (Fig. 8-2). Since these cell-killing actions require close cell-to-cell contact, T cells are said to be responsible for the **cell-mediated immune response.**

A third category of lymphocyte, the **natural killer (NK) cell,** lacks an antigen receptor that is typical for either B or T cells. NK cells appear to rely on an antigen recognition system that is less specific than that used by B cells and T cells; however, cell-mediated killing by NK cells is similar to the mechanism of T cytotoxic cells. NK cells participate in the elimination of tumors and virus-infected cells or other cells that show altered expression of "self" molecules. In some species, these cells appear as large granular lymphocytes.

Lymphocytes circulate continuously from the blood through lymphatic and nonlymphatic tissues and subsequently return to the blood either directly or via the lymph. This process, called **lymphocyte recirculation,** facilitates the dissemination of an immune response throughout the body and enables effective immune surveillance for foreign invaders and alterations in the body's own cells. Most lymphocytes enter organs such as the lungs, liver, and bone marrow and return to the blood via venules, whereas some lymphocytes leave these organs via the lymph and drain to lymph nodes via afferent lymph vessels. Tissue fluid from large peripheral areas also drains into regional lymph nodes, further enhancing the likelihood of an encounter between a lymphocyte and its target antigen. A proportion of lymphocytes migrates from blood directly into lymphatic tissues through specialized postcapillary venules called **high endothelial venules** (see Lymph Node section below [Fig. 8-18]). High endothelial venules have lining cells that are cuboidal, in contrast to the flattened endothelial cells of other blood vessels. These specialized venules are abundant in lymphatic tissue and serve as the sites of entry for both T cells and B cells from the blood circulation. The spleen is an exception, because it does not possess specialized postcapillary venules or afferent lymphatics. Lymphocytes migrate into the spleen via

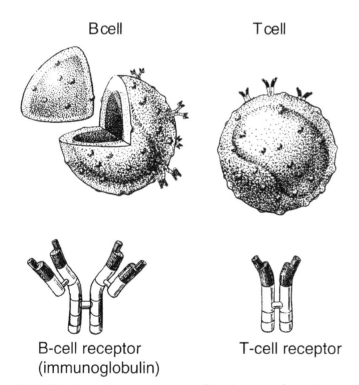

B cell **T cell**

B-cell receptor (immunoglobulin) **T-cell receptor**

FIGURE 8-1 Schematic drawing of lymphocyte surface antigen receptors. The B-cell receptor is an immunoglobulin (antibody) molecule that has two antigen-binding sites (dark segments), whereas the T-cell receptor has a single antigen-binding site.

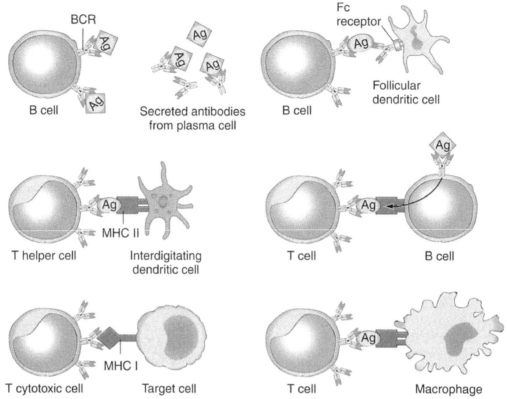

FIGURE 8-2   Schematic drawing of antigen–antigen receptor interaction. The B-cell receptor (BCR) can interact directly with native antigen (Ag), either while bound to the plasma membrane of a B cell or as secreted antibody. The B-cell receptor also recognizes antigen presented by the follicular dendritic cell. The T-cell receptor recognizes processed antigen presented by a major histocompatibility complex (MHC-II) molecule on the surface of the interdigitating dendritic cell. The B cell can present antigen to T cells by binding the antigen, processing it, and presenting it in the context of MHC II (black arrow). Macrophages are also capable of presenting antigen to T cells.

blood capillaries in the marginal zone (see Spleen section below). Normally, relatively few lymphocytes migrate into organs such as the skin, synovia, muscle, and brain; however, during acute and chronic inflammation, an influx of large numbers of lymphocytes can occur.

Stromal Cells

Stromal cells are fixed cells of the lymphatic system that form a tissue reticulum and support the immune response. Either mesenchymal reticular cells or epithelial reticular cells form a supportive mesh or stroma for the lymphocytes that constitute the parenchyma of lymphatic organs.

Reticular Cells

Reticular cells of mesenchymal origin and fibroblastlike structure form a reticulum in all lymphatic organs except the thymus and cloacal bursa (see Lymph Node section below [Fig. 8-16]). Because of their numerous long and branching processes, reticular cells have a stellate appearance. These cells synthesize reticular fibers that are closely associated with or invaginated into their cell surface.

Epithelial Reticular Cells

In the thymus and cloacal bursa, stellate **epithelial reticular cells** form a reticulum that supports developing lymphocytes and macrophages (see Thymus section below [Fig. 8-8]). Unlike reticular cells, epithelial reticular cells do not produce reticular fibers.

Antigen-Presenting Cells

For antigen recognition and the initiation of an immune response to occur, B cells recognize antigen either directly or as complexes presented by an **antigen-presenting cell** such as the follicular dendritic cell (Fig. 8-2). T cells require antigen to be presented on the surface of an antigen-presenting cell, such as the interdigitating dendritic cell, in association with a **major histocompatibility complex (MHC) molecule**.

Dendritic Cells

Most **dendritic cells** (DCs), including the interstitial dendritic cell, interdigitating dendritic cell, veiled cell, and intraepidermal macrophage, are derived from hematopoietic stem cells. The origin of follicular dendritic cells is unclear. Typical dendritic cells have numerous long cytoplasmic processes (Fig. 8-2). Functionally, dendritic cells bind antigens and cluster lymphocytes on their surface in tissues throughout the body. Once antigens are bound and processed, the dendritic cell then becomes an antigen-presenting cell. In the stratified squamous epithelia, dendritic cells localize in the upper spinous layer and are termed **intra-epidermal macrophages** (Langerhans cells) (see Chapter 16). When they are in lymph and blood, dendritic cells possess prominent surface folds and have been called **veiled cells. Interstitial dendritic cells** are located in the heart, kidney, gut and lung. Follicular dendritic cells and interdigitating dendritic cells are found in lymphatic tissues.

Follicular dendritic cells

Follicular dendritic cells are specialized stromal cells localized within the B-cell areas of lymphatic tissue. Receptors on the follicular dendritic cell surface bind to antigen and present it to B cells that induce a humoral immune response (Fig. 8-2). In contrast to other dendritic cells, follicular dendritic cells can trap and maintain antigen in a complex for long periods of time. Follicular dendritic cells lack the MHC-II surface molecules found in interdigitating dendritic cells.

Interdigitating dendritic cells

Interdigitating dendritic cells are found in lymph nodes, thymic medulla, and spleen. Cytoplasmic granules are characteristic features of these dendritic cells, which also have numerous MHC-II molecules on their surface that are associated with antigen presentation (Fig. 8-2). The interdigitating dendritic cell presents antigen to T lymphocytes (helper cells), which induce a cellular immune response.

Macrophages

Macrophages, also known as mononuclear phagocytes, exist in various tissues and are active in the phagocytosis and degradation of foreign substances (see Chapter 3 for the histology of macrophages). The processing of foreign substances into short peptides is essential for presentation of antigen to T cells in the peptide-binding groove of the MHC-II molecule (Fig. 8-2).

B Cells

B cells express MHC-II molecules and are very efficient in the presentation of antigen to T helper cells. In contrast to macrophages, which will ingest most foreign substances, B cells bind a specific single antigen through surface immunoglobulin. The bound molecule is then endocytosed, fragmented, and presented by MHC-II molecules.

ORGANIZATION OF CELLS TO FORM LYMPHATIC TISSUES AND ORGANS

As the fetus develops, the immune system is molded into two principal types of tissues: the diffuse and the organized lym-

phatic tissues. **Diffuse lymphatic tissues** are found scattered throughout loose connective tissues of the gut, respiratory tract, urogenital system, and skin and in extranodular areas of lymphatic organs. The **organized lymphatic tissues** include encapsulated organs such as the lymph nodes and spleen.

Diffuse Lymphatic Tissue

Diffuse lymphatic tissue contains a variable number of small lymphocytes, mingled with lymphoblasts (often seen in mitosis) and macrophages. The stroma of diffuse lymphatic tissue consists of a three-dimensional network of dendritic cells and connective tissue.

Lymphatic Nodules

Primary Lymphatic Nodules

Primary lymphatic nodules consist of a stromal network of connective tissue and immature follicular dendritic cells (Fig. 8-3). Small, tightly packed lymphocytes and some medium lymphocytes are distributed throughout the stromal network and represent predominantly naive recirculating B cells. Primary nodules do not contain germinal centers.

Secondary Lymphatic Nodules

Secondary lymphatic nodules are characterized by a light-staining **germinal center** within the nodule (Fig. 8-4). Formation of the germinal center begins in a primary nodule with an accumulation of large, euchromatic lymphoblasts and tingible body macrophages. Differentiated follicular dendritic cells form the stroma of the secondary nodules. An established germinal center consists of a central light zone and an adjacent dark zone. The **light zone** is populated by B lymphocytes with euchromatic, light-staining nuclei. Along the periphery of the light zone is a thin layer of small heterochromatic lymphocytes that often form a thicker cap, called the **mantle,** over the apex of the germinal center. The **dark zone** is composed of B-cell lymphoblasts engaged in intense mitotic activity. The germinal center is usually oriented such that the light zone is closest and the dark zone is farthest from the subcapsular sinus in lymph nodes, the surface epithelium in mucosal nodules, or the marginal zone in the spleen. The germinal center regresses when cellular activity declines late in an immune response.

PRIMARY LYMPHATIC ORGANS

During the development of the fetus, the unique identity of T and B lymphocytes first becomes established within **primary lymphatic organs**. The primary lymphatic organs include the bone marrow (mammals), aggregated lymphatic nodules of the distal small intestine (sheep, cattle), cloacal bursa (birds), and thymus (both mammals and birds). Stem cells in these organs are located in a specialized environment that is isolated from antigen and suitable for cellular differentiation and development. Intense cell proliferation is accompanied by random rearrangement of the

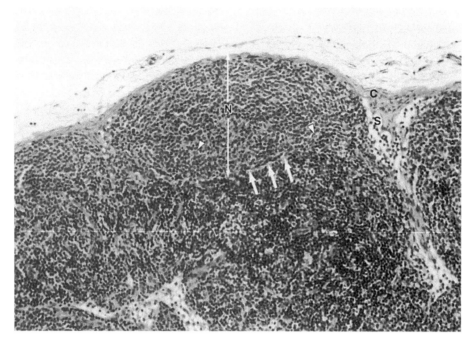

FIGURE 8-3 Lymph node (fetal lamb 140 days of gestation). Primary lymphatic nodule (N) in the outer cortex consists of an aggregate of small to medium-sized lymphocytes and some follicular dendritic cells (arrowheads). Note the presence of a capillary network outlining the primary nodule (arrows). Subcapsular sinus (S); capsule (C). Hematoxylin and eosin.

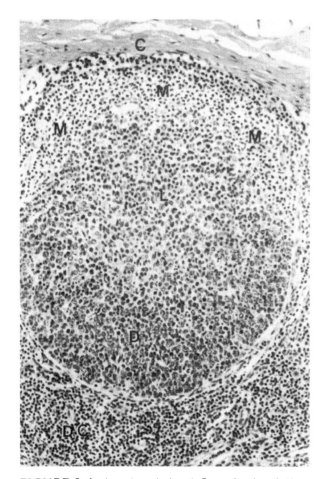

FIGURE 8-4 Lymph node (goat). Secondary lymphatic nodule with germinal center. Dark area (D); light area (L); mantle (M); capsule (C); deep cortex (DC). Hematoxylin and eosin. (×150).

genes responsible for the antigen receptor and expression of accessory molecules that allow interaction with other cells and that also confer effector functions. Lymphocytes leaving a primary lymphatic organ are classified as naive or virgin cells because they have not been exposed to antigen. Scrutiny of the emerging lymphocytes is followed by elimination of more than 90% of the cells that are identified as unsuitable, largely because of their reaction with the body's own molecules (autoreactivity). These lymphocytes are eliminated by apoptosis, a mechanism that involves activation of a genetic pathway ensuring rapid disintegration of the selected cells with minimal harm to the surrounding tissues.

Even with the elimination of most of their cells, primary lymphatic organs still produce vast numbers of B and T cells that have a diverse repertoire of antigen specificities. The released cells are disseminated throughout the body to diffuse lymphatic tissue, secondary lymphatic tissue (i.e., mucosa-associated lymphoid tissue), and secondary lymphatic organs (e.g., lymph nodes), where they will encounter antigen.

Bone Marrow

The structure and major hematopoietic functions of the bone marrow are presented in Chapter 4. In mammals, the bone marrow is the source of pluripotent stem cells (e.g., B-cell and T-cell precursors) and B-cell differentiation. B cells are located adjacent to the endosteum of bone and undergo differentiation and selection as they migrate centrally toward the venous sinuses in the hematopoietic space. B-cell maturation occurs in close association with stromal reticular cells and macrophages of the bone marrow.

Aggregated Lymphatic Nodules in the Distal Small Intestine

Most organized lymphatic tissue associated with the gut has been attributed with functions related to mucosal and systemic immunity (see Gut-Associated Lymphoid Tissue below). In young ruminants, pigs, and carnivores, a single large aggregate of lym-

phatic nodules (the ileal Peyer's patch) is present in the distal jejunum/ileum. A specific role for the ileal Peyer's patch in the diversification of the preimmune antigen-receptor repertoire and expansion of early B-cell populations has recently been defined in sheep and cattle (Fig. 8-5).

Removal of the ovine ileal Peyer's patch before birth results in a marked decline in the number of mature, circulating B cells.

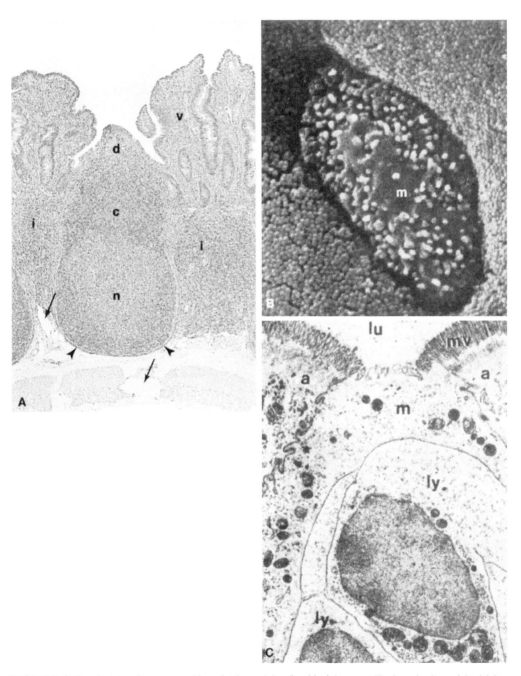

FIGURE 8-5 **A.** Jejunal aggregated lymphatic nodules (lamb). A large saclike lymphatic nodule (n) is separated from other nodules in the submucosa by wide internodular (T-cell) regions (i). A prominent corona (c) is interposed between the nodule and a broad dome region (d) that extends into the gut lumen. Villus (v); lymphatic sinuses (arrows); capsule of nodule (arrowheads). Hematoxylin and eosin. **B.** Jejunal Peyer's patch (3-week-old calf). Short microfolds are present on an M cell (m) at the dome surface; adjacent absorptive cells have densely packed microvilli (×10,000). **C.** Jejunal Peyer's patch (3-week-old calf). An M cell (m) with microfolds is wedged between two microvilli-bearing (mv) absorptive cells (a) and envelops lymphocytes (ly). Lumen (lu) (×7500).

At 2 months of age, the weight of the ileal Peyer's patch is more than twice that of the thymus.

The intense cell division in the aggregated nodules is independent of foreign antigen. Similar to the avian bursa described below, the processes of positive and negative lymphocyte selection likely occur, ensuring the suitability of the lymphocytes that are permitted to exit into the blood and lymphatic circulations.

It should be noted that the earliest immigrants to both the single large aggregate of lymphatic nodules in the distal small intestine of sheep and the avian bursa are already committed to the B-cell lineage. Thus, neither organ is strictly a primary lymphatic organ; that is, B cells do not develop de novo from uncommitted precursors.

Cloacal Bursa of Birds

The dichotomy of the T- and B-cell lineages was first revealed in birds. B cells were discovered in association with the avian cloacal bursa. The **cloacal bursa** (bursa of Fabricius) is a lymphatic organ located in the dorsal wall of the cloaca (Fig. 8-6). The bursa is considered to be functionally equivalent to the mammalian bone marrow in regard to the differentiation of B cells.

From day 8 to day 15 of chicken embryo development, precursor cells committed to the B-cell lineage migrate into the developing organ. Lymphatic nodules develop as invaginations of the cloacal epithelium into underlying tissues of the cloaca at approximately day 12 of incubation. Longitudinal folds containing the nodules and a stroma of epithelial reticular cells then protrude into the bursal lumen, followed by the formation of light central and dark peripheral zones and the initiation of lymphocyte differentiation within the nodules. Simple columnar or pseudostratified epithelium overlying the nodules within the folds has

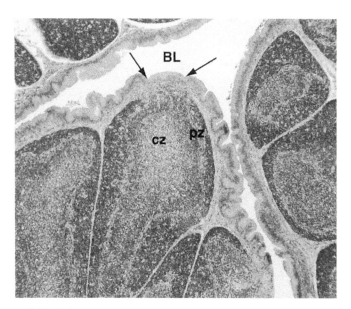

FIGURE 8-6 Cloacal bursa (chicken). A modified epithelium (between arrows) overlies a lymphatic nodule that contains a dark peripheral zone (pz) and a light central zone (cz). Bursal lumen (BL). Hematoxylin and eosin.

a remarkable capacity for transcytosis of macromolecules, including antigens, from the bursal lumen into the nodules.

Thymus

The thymus originates as a solid outgrowth from the epithelium (endoderm) of the third pharyngeal pouch. The spreading of epithelial cells gives rise to a thymic epithelial reticulum, which is invaded by blood vessels from the surrounding mesenchyme. Migration of lymphocytic stem cells from the bone marrow into the thymus occurs early in ontogeny and is probably associated with chemotactic signals produced by the thymic anlage. The lymphocytic stem cells invade the interstices, filling the spaces between the epithelial cells. The thymus is therefore often referred to as a "lymphoepithelial organ." Within the thymus, lymphocytic stem cells develop into T cells.

The thymus consists of right and left lobes, each of which is surrounded by a capsule of connective tissue continuous with thin septa that subdivide the lobes into partially separated lobules. The central medulla of each lobule is a branch of tissue that arises from a central stalk in the lobe and is surrounded by a cortex (Fig. 8-7).

Cortex

The thymic cortex consists mainly of an epithelial reticulum and lymphocytes (Fig. 8-8). The stellate **epithelial reticular cells** have large, pale, ovoid nuclei and long, branching cytoplasmic processes that contain numerous intermediate filaments; their cellular organelles are inconspicuous. Adjacent epithelial reticular cells are connected to each other by desmosomes, thus forming a cellular stromal network. At the periphery of the lobules and around the perivascular spaces, a single layer of long, flattened epithelial cells forms a continuous lining. Lymphoblasts and medium-sized lymphocytes predominate in the meshes of the peripheral epithelial reticulum, where they undergo mitotic divisions producing small lymphocytes that differentiate in the deep cortex. **Tingible body macrophages,** which are frequent near the medulla, phagocytize and eliminate dead T lymphocytes and often contain lymphocyte remnants. The thymic cortex stains much darker than the medulla because it contains a greater number of lymphocytes (Fig. 8-9).

Medulla

Many of the epithelial reticular cells in the medulla have the same structure as those in the cortex; however, others are much larger and their epithelial nature is thus more obvious. These larger cells contain more mitochondria, an extensive rough endoplasmic reticulum, well-developed Golgi complex, and granules when compared to cortical epithelial reticular cells.

Some medullary epithelial reticular cells form **thymic corpuscles,** also called Hassall's corpuscles (Fig. 8-10). The corpuscles consist of one to several calcified or degenerated large central cells, which are surrounded by flat keratinized cells in a concentric arrangement. Corpuscle cells are connected by desmosomes and contain bundles of intermediate filaments.

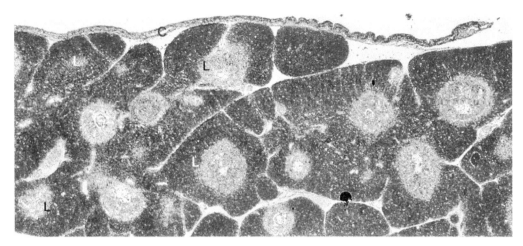

FIGURE 8-7   Thymus (cat). The thymic lobules (L), each consisting of a light medulla surrounded by a dark cortex, are partially separated by thin septa of connective tissue. Capsule (C). Hematoxylin and eosin (×20).

Interdigitating dendritic cells, similar to those present in the T-cell areas of secondary lymphatic organs, are also present in the medulla. The cells within the meshes of the epithelial reticular network are predominantly small lymphocytes, along with a few macrophages.

Blood Vessels, Lymph Vessels, and Nerves

The blood supply of the thymus is derived from arteries that penetrate the parenchyma at the corticomedullary junction by way of the connective tissue septa. The arteries divide into

arterioles that course along the junction and give rise to a capillary network in the cortex. Capillaries then drain into postcapillary venules located either at the corticomedullary junction or in the medulla; the postcapillary venules join veins in the connective tissue septa. Cortical capillaries are characterized by a continuous endothelium, perivascular connective tissue, and a

FIGURE 8-8   Schematic drawing of a portion of a thymic lobule. The lobule consists of a cortex and medulla and has a border of flattened epithelial cells. The epithelial reticulum of the cortex is heavily infiltrated by lymphocytes undergoing cell division and differentiation. The epithelial cells of the medulla may form concentric arrangements called thymic corpuscles or Hassall's corpuscles. Blood vessels supply the lobule via the capsule and thin connective tissue septa to reach the corticomedullary junction.

capsule
epithelial reticular cells
macrophages
lymphocytes
continuous lining of epithelial cells
interdigitating cell
septal artery
thymic corpuscle

cortex
medulla

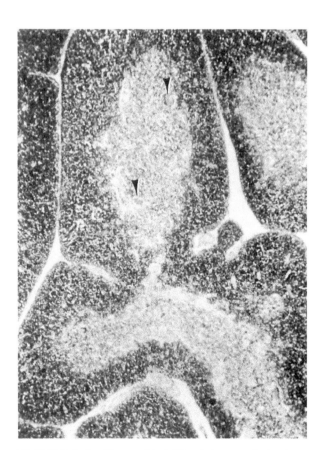

FIGURE 8-9   Thymus (dog). The dark cortex is clearly distinguishable from the light medulla, in which thymic corpuscles (arrowheads) are readily identified. Hematoxylin and eosin (×40).

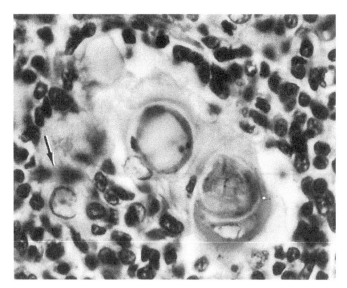

FIGURE 8-10 Thymic corpuscles, thymus (dog). Notice the arrangement of the cells in concentric layers and an enlarged epithelial reticular cell (arrow), which is probably the point of origin of a new thymic corpuscle. Hematoxylin and eosin (×735).

sheath of epithelial reticular cell processes. Together, these layers form the **blood-thymus barrier,** which decreases the access of circulating antigens that could interfere with the positive selection of lymphocytes in the cortical tissue. The absence of such a barrier at the corticomedullary junction allows circulating antigens to contribute to the negative lymphocyte selection processes.

T cells enter the blood by migrating through the endothelium of postcapillary venules at the corticomedullary junction. The T cells released from the thymus settle within the T-cell areas of diffuse lymphatic tissue, secondary lymphatic tissue, and organs.

The thymus is particularly active in young animals, with normal involution of the organ occurring after sexual maturity. Involution of the thymus is characterized by a gradual depletion of lymphocytes (especially from the cortex), enlargement of the epithelial reticular cells, and invasion of the parenchyma by white adipocytes originating from the interlobular connective tissue. In adult animals, the thymus consists of narrow cords of lymphocytes, in which enlarged epithelial reticular cells predominate, surrounded by adipose tissue.

SECONDARY LYMPHATIC TISSUES AND ORGANS

Secondary lymphatic tissues and organs are strategically situated at sites of antigen entry and are equipped with specialized microenvironments populated by the antigen-presenting cells necessary to induce an immune response. Secondary lymphatic tissues and organs are routinely exposed to antigen, in distinct contrast to the primary lymphatic organs where exposure to antigen is strictly controlled. Antigens are transported from their site of entry into the body to the secondary lymphatic tissues, via blood or lymph, either free or associated with cells such as dendritic cells and/or macrophages. The secondary lymphatic tissues are associated with mucosal surfaces, and thus are termed mucosa-associated lymphatic tissue (MALT). The secondary lymphatic organs include lymph nodes, spleen, and hemal nodes.

Mucosa-Associated Lymphatic Tissue

Cells of the immune system are present either within or adjoining the mucosa of the respiratory, alimentary and urogenital tracts and the mammary gland and are collectively referred to as **MALT (mucosa-associated lymphatic tissue)**. These lymphatic tissues function as an integrated mucosal immune system to augment the mechanical and chemical barriers of surface mucosal epithelia. Solitary lymphatic nodules, as well as aggregates of nodules, are common in the subepithelial connective tissue of most mucous membranes. Lymphatic nodules are especially numerous in the digestive and respiratory systems and are also present in the urogenital tract and around the eye. Aggregated lymphatic nodules in the pharynx are referred to as tonsils.

Tonsils

The **tonsils** are often the site of an early encounter with infectious agents and other antigens. Local production of antibodies by tonsillar cells is important in a rapid initial immune response and a subsequent more generalized response.

The tonsils are located adjacent to the lumen of the host organ and are covered by either a stratified squamous (oropharynx) or pseudostratified columnar (nasopharynx) epithelium. The tonsillar surface may be relatively smooth (e.g., palatine tonsil of dogs and cats) (Fig. 8-11A), or it may have surface invaginations, referred to as tonsillar fossulae, that continue as deep, penetrating crypts (e.g., lingual tonsil in horses, palatine tonsil in horses and ruminants) (Fig. 8-11B). These invaginations allow a high concentration of lymphatic tissue in a given area.

The epithelium is usually infiltrated to a variable degree with lymphocytes, neutrophils, and macrophages. This infiltration is particularly pronounced in the tonsils of the oropharynx. Leukocytes that reach the lumen form **salivary corpuscles** (Fig. 8-11B). When they are not washed out of the fossulae by secretions from the surrounding salivary glands, these cells, along with microorganisms, may obstruct the fossulae and cause inflammation.

Beneath the epithelium, diffuse lymphatic tissue with plasma cells surrounds lymphatic nodules, which frequently have a germinal center and a cap (mantle) of small lymphocytes adjacent to the epithelium. The tonsil is separated from the surrounding tissue by a distinct connective tissue capsule, which makes the "enucleation" of the tonsil possible (e.g., palatine tonsil of the dog). Tonsillar blood vessels have essentially the same distribution and character as those of lymph nodes (see Lymph Node section below). Afferent lymph vessels are lacking. A plexus of lymph cap-

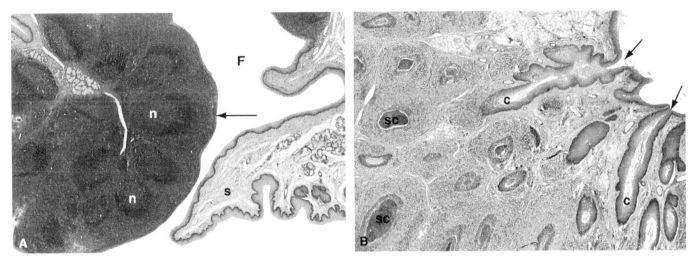

FIGURE 8-11 Palatine tonsil. **A.** Dog. The lymphatic tissue is embedded in a fossa (F) and is partly covered by a semilunar fold (s). The smooth tonsillar surface (arrow) is a stratified squamous epithelium and overlies many lymphatic nodules (n). **B.** Calf. The stratified squamous epithelium invaginates forming tonsillar fossulae (arrows) that continue as blind epithelial tubes or crypts (c) surrounded by lymphatic tissue. Salivary corpuscles (sc). Hematoxylin and eosin.

illaries is present in the deep layers of the tonsil and drains into the larger efferent lymph vessels in the tonsillar capsule.

Bronchus-Associated Lymphatic Tissue

BALT is the acronym for **bronchus-associated lymphatic tissue,** which includes clusters of lymphocytes present in the walls of bronchi and bronchioles. Both T cells and B cells are present, primarily at sites between an arteriole and bronchus epithelium, but these cells are not organized into nodules like intestinal aggregated lymphatic nodules. The development of BALT is antigen-dependent, and BALT is not a constitutive structure in all species. The presence of BALT varies widely from 100% in rabbits and rats, 50% in guinea pigs, and 33% in pigs, to its absence in normal cat and human lungs. BALT is not well developed in sheep and cattle.

Gut-Associated Lymphatic Tissue

GALT is the acronym for **gut-associated lymphatic tissue,** which includes solitary and aggregated lymphatic nodules, intraepithelial lymphocytes, subepithelial lymphocytes, plasma cells, and macrophages. **Aggregated lymphatic nodules** (Peyer's patches) occurring in the small intestine are visible as elevations in the mucosa (Figs. 8-5, 8-12 and 8-13). These lymphatic areas are most conspicuous in the ileum, appearing in ruminants, pigs, and carnivores as a single large patch that involutes in young age and may have a function different from that of smaller patches. The numerous discrete small-intestinal aggregated lymphatic nodules and scattered aggregated or solitary nodules of the colon and rectum persist into adulthood.

Aggregated lymphatic tissue of the intestine contains (a) submucosal lymphatic nodules with high mitotic activity (Fig. 8-13), (b) a zone of small lymphocytes that caps the sub-mucosal lymphatic nodule (the corona), (c) an internodular region rich in T cells and postcapillary venules through which lymphocytes recirculate, (d) an elevated region overlying lymphatic nodules (the dome), and (e) a nodule-associated epithelium. The domes are located between typical small intestinal villi and crypts. The nodule-associated epithelium covering the dome lacks goblet cells but includes **M cells** that have numerous microfolds of their luminal surface (Fig. 8-13). M cells typically enfold groups of lymphocytes and occasionally surround macrophages and dendritic cells.

Lymph Nodes

Lymph nodes, situated along the extensive drainage system of lymph vessels, filter antigens from the lymph before returning it to the bloodstream. Lymph nodes are the only lymphatic organ with both afferent and efferent lymph vessels and sinuses. These organs usually have a slight indentation, the **hilus,** where blood and lymph vessels enter or leave the lymph node. The parenchyma is organized into a cortex of lymphatic nodules and diffuse lymphatic tissue, and a medulla of lymphatic tissue arranged in cords (Fig. 8-14).

Lymph nodes are surrounded by a capsule composed primarily of dense irregular connective tissue. In ruminants, smooth muscle cells are also present. Trabeculae extend from the capsule into the parenchyma as irregular septa that are distributed throughout the cortex and medulla (Fig. 8-15). The trabeculae provide support for the entire node, carry blood vessels and nerves, and are surrounded by sinuses. The stroma of the lymph node is composed of reticular cells and fibers. Lymphocytes, macrophages, and plasma cells are supported by this reticular meshwork.

Lymph Vessels and Sinuses

Afferent lymph vessels penetrate the capsule at several different sites and open into the **subcapsular sinus** (Fig. 8-14). Valves are

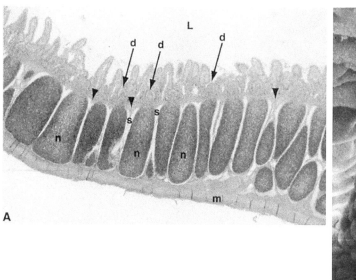
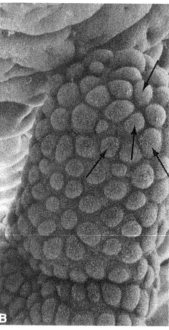

FIGURE 8-12 Ileal aggregated lymphatic nodules. **A.** Goat kid. The submucosa contains many closely apposed large lymphatic nodules (n) that are separated by lymphatic sinuses (s) and small triangular internodular (T-cell) regions (arrowheads). Small conical domes (d) protrude through the tunica mucosa to come in contact with the gut lumen (L.) Tunica muscularis (m). Hematoxylin and eosin. **B.** Calf. Nodule-associated epithelium. A homogenous population of modified epithelial cells possessing surface folds (arrows) overlies the dome.

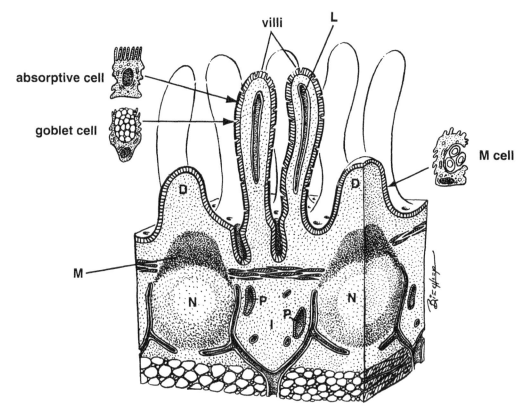

FIGURE 8-13 Schematic drawing of part of aggregated lymphatic nodules in the small intestine. Submucosal lymphatic nodules (N) are capped by a mantle (M) and lie beneath the dome (D). The nodule-associated epithelium overlying the dome contains many M cells interspersed among absorptive cells but lacks goblet cells. Postcapillary venules (P) and T lymphocytes are present in the internodular region (I), which, along with the lamina propria of the villi, is drained by lymphatic vessels (L).

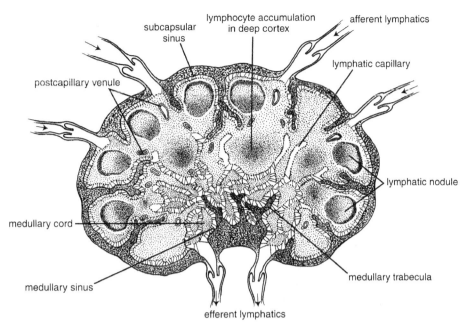

FIGURE 8-14 Schematic drawing of a lymph node. The direction of lymph flow is shown with arrows.

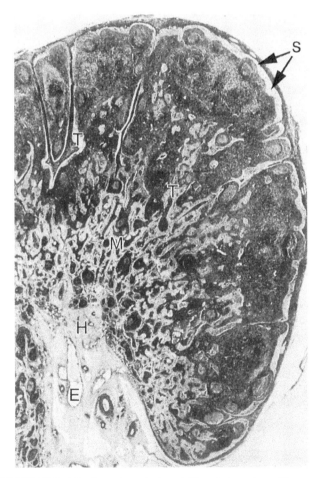

FIGURE 8-15 Lymph node (cow). The dark cortex with lymphatic nodules lies adjacent to the lighter-appearing medulla. Subcapsular (S) and trabecular (T) sinuses are continuous with medullary sinuses (M) that drain toward the hilus (H) containing efferent lymph vessels (E). Hematoxylin and eosin (×10). *(Courtesy of A. Hansen.)*

present in both the afferent and the efferent lymph vessels, thereby ensuring a one-way flow of lymph. **Cortical sinuses** arise from the subcapsular sinus to accompany the connective tissue trabeculae and continue into **medullary sinuses**. These sinuses form a network of branching and anastomosing channels that converge toward the hilus to open into the efferent lymph vessels. All lymph leaves the node through the efferent lymph vessels (Fig. 8-14).

The sinuses are lined by flattened endothelial-like reticular cells that form a continuous lining in the proximal portion of the sinus adjacent to the capsule and trabeculae. Near the parenchyma, the sinus lining becomes more discontinuous. The lumina of the sinuses are traversed by a dense network of interconnected reticular cells attached to the sinus walls through numerous slender processes (Fig. 8-16). Many macrophages are attached to this network. Lymphocytes, macrophages, and dendritic cells lie free within the stromal mesh and also in the sinus lumen. The reticular cells probably function as a baffle to slow lymph flow within the sinuses to facilitate both antigen–cell interactions and phagocytic activities of macrophages. Lymph then percolates into the parenchyma through gaps in the sinus walls, thereby giving the parenchymal cells access to lymphborne antigens, cells, and particulate matter.

Cortex

Most of the outer cortex of the lymph node consists of primary and secondary lymphatic nodules separated by diffuse lymphatic tissue (Fig. 8-15). The deep cortex is composed of diffuse lymphatic tissue and is drained by lymphatics (Fig. 8-15). Because most lymphocytes in the deep cortex originate from the thymus, this area is referred to as a T-cell area or thymus-dependent zone. The term paracortex has been applied variously to the deep cortex or to the diffuse lymphatic tissue of both the deep and outer regions of cortex.

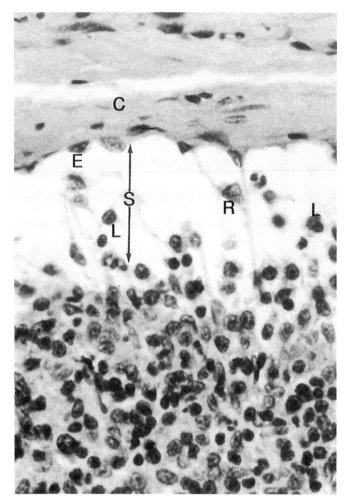

FIGURE 8-16 Lymph node (dog). Beneath the connective-tissue capsule (C) is the subcapsular sinus (S) lined by flattened endothelial-like reticular cells (E). Reticular cells (R) and lymphocytes (L) are present in the sinus. Crossman's trichrome (×600).

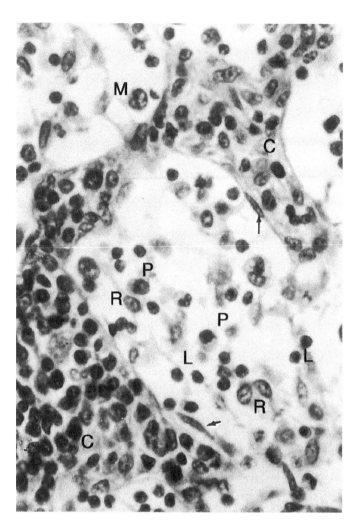

FIGURE 8-17 Lymph node, medulla (dog). Flattened endothelial-like reticular cells (arrows) line the medullary sinus containing lymphocytes (L), macrophages (M), plasma cells (P), and reticular cells (R). Medullary cords (C) are composed of lymphocytes, macrophages, and plasma cells. Crossman's trichrome (×600).

Medulla

The medulla of the lymph node is much less organized than the cortex. The lymphatic tissue extends from the cortical T-cell areas as **medullary cords,** which branch and anastomose throughout the medulla (Fig. 8-14). The medullary cords are separated by a network of sinuses and connective-tissue trabeculae. Plasma cells are prominent in the stromal mesh of the medullary cords, which also contain lymphocytes and macrophages (Fig. 8-17).

Blood Vessels and Nerves

The major arteries enter the lymph node at the hilus, whereas smaller vessels penetrate the capsule at various sites. Upon entering the hilus, some arteries branch to supply the medullary cords directly while other branches enter the trabeculae to supply the connective tissue and capsule. Vessels supplying the medullary cords distribute capillaries along their course, and the main vessels continue into the cortex where branches feed capillary networks between and within the nodules. The internodular branches form capillary arcades below the subcapsular

sinus and then continue inward to the deep cortex to form post-capillary venules lined by a cuboidal endothelium in most species (Fig. 8-18). The postcapillary venules join veins in the medullary trabeculae, which in turn empty into veins that leave at the hilus.

Nerve fibers supply the capsule and trabeculae, and vasomotor nerves form perivascular networks throughout the lymph node.

Species Differences

Porcine lymph nodes are different from those of most other mammals (Fig. 8-19). The majority of nodules occupy a deep position in the center of the node along trabecular sinuses. Areas similar to the deep cortex in conventional lymph nodes, with many postcapillary venules, are seen near the groups of nodules, but the periphery of the node is occupied primarily by loose lymphoreticular tissue containing macrophages and only a few plasma cells. Afferent lymph vessels enter the capsule at one or more sites and penetrate via the trabeculae deep into the

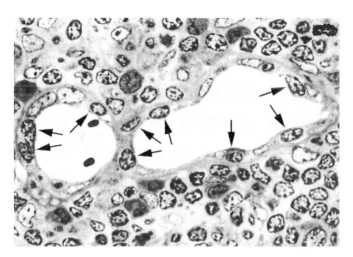

FIGURE 8-18 Lymph node (goat). High endothelium in postcapillary venules with many migrating lymphocytes (arrows). Vascular perfusion. Epon. Toluidine blue (×1000).

area occupied by the lymphatic nodules, where they join the trabecular sinuses. The lymph then filters into the peripheral sinuses that converge and form several efferent vessels at the periphery of the node. Functionally, the flow of the lymph in the porcine lymph node is identical to that in other animals because the incoming lymph first reaches the area of the node that is rich in lymphatic nodules. The efferent lymph, however, is poor in lymphocytes compared with that of other species, and recirculating lymphocytes are believed to leave the porcine lymph node via the blood.

Arteries enter the porcine lymph node with the afferent lymph vessels and veins exit with the efferent lymph vessels. As a result, a definitive hilus may not always be seen; instead, microscopic hiluslike indentations are apparent wherever af-

ferent lymph vessels enter. Many small lymph nodes may fuse, thereby forming a large cluster of nodes, which often contributes to the difficulty in locating a hilus in porcine lymph nodes.

Spleen

The spleen is the major secondary lymphatic organ involved in filtering the blood and mounting immune responses against blood-borne antigens. Erythrocytes are stored in the red pulp of the spleen, and platelets are stored in the splenic cords. The major hemopoietic activity of the spleen in adult animals is lymphopoiesis. In contrast, erythropoiesis is a major function of the fetal spleen, and splenic erythropoiesis persists in newborn horses and ruminants for several weeks postpartum.

Erythrocyte cell membrane elasticity declines with age. Old erythrocytes are identified when they can no longer pass through the narrow spaces of the splenic cords and the interendothelial slits of venous sinuses or venules in the red pulp. Macrophages then remove the damaged erythrocytes from circulation.

The ability of the spleen to filter the blood is enhanced by a reticular fiber network filled with reticular cells and macrophages. Almost any section of red pulp contains numerous macrophages filled with engulfed red blood cell fragments and an iron pigment called **hemosiderin**.

Capsule and Supportive Tissue

The spleen is surrounded by a thick connective tissue capsule invested by the peritoneum. The capsule consists of two layers: a layer of dense irregular connective tissue and a layer of smooth muscle. The total thickness and relative amount of smooth muscle vary with the species. Trabeculae composed of collagen and elastic fibers and smooth muscle cells extend from the capsule and the hilus into the parenchyma. The trabeculae contain arteries, veins, lymph vessels, and nerves. The capsule, trabeculae, and

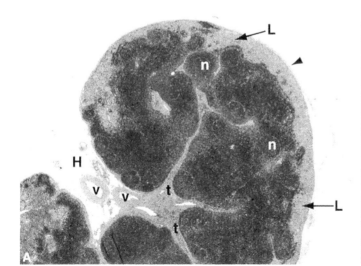

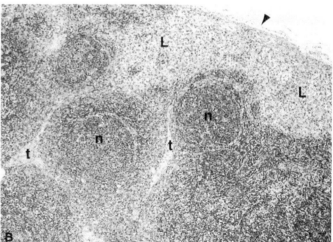

FIGURE 8-19 Lymph node (pig). **A.** Afferent lymphatic vessels (v) enter the node at a hilus (H) and accompany trabeculae (t) to penetrate deeply into the parenchyma to reach central tissue containing lymphatic nodules (n). Capsule (arrowhead). Loose peripheral tissue (L). Hematoxylin and eosin. **B.** Higher magnification showing arrangement of lymphatic nodules (n) along trabeculae (t). Loose peripheral tissue (L). Capsule (arrowhead). Hematoxylin and eosin.

reticular fibers support the splenic parenchyma composed of a red pulp involved in the storage of red blood cells and a white pulp rich in lymphocytes and active in immune responses.

Red Pulp

Most of the splenic parenchyma is **red pulp,** owing its name to the vast amount of blood held within the reticular network (Fig. 8-20). The red pulp is composed of venous sinuses or venules and **splenic cords.** Two main types of red pulp are present in mammalian spleens, depending on the type of postcapillary vessels: sinusal or nonsinusal. Among the domestic animals, only dogs have typical venous sinuses, similar to those in human and rat spleens.

The **splenic sinuses** are wide vascular channels lined with elongated, longitudinally oriented endothelial cells that contain contractile microfilaments aligned in bands parallel and adjacent to the lateral cell margins. Gaps or slits in the sinus wall are created upon contraction of these filaments, thus allowing erythrocytes to migrate from the surrounding splenic cords into the sinus lumen. The lining cells rest on a fenestrated basal lamina and are supported by reticular fibers, some of which form hooplike structures encircling the sinus at right angles to the long axis. In most domestic mammals, venules rather than venous sinuses are pres-ent. Their wide lumina are lined by a thin endothelium with a discontinuous basal lamina supported by reticular cells and fibers. Openings between endothelial cells in this wall are common (Fig. 8-21).

The narrow **splenic cords** situated between the sinuses form a vast three-dimensional network composed of reticular fibers with enmeshed reticular cells, erythrocytes, macrophages, lymphocytes, plasma cells, and other leukocytes. The membranous processes of the reticular cells tend to form channel-like structures that may function to conduct blood toward the endothelial slits in the sinus walls. In nonsinusal spleens, the splenic cords are wider than in sinusal spleens. The red pulp of ruminant and porcine spleens contains numerous smooth muscle cells, whereas that of horses and dogs has myofibroblasts, which are cells that resemble fibroblasts but have some features of smooth muscle (e.g., actin filaments and dense bodies).

White Pulp

White pulp is lymphatic tissue that is distributed throughout the spleen and is comprised of lymphatic nodules and diffuse lymphatic tissue called **periarterial lymphatic sheaths (PALS)** (Figs. 8-22 and 8-23). **Nodules** of the white pulp are B-cell zones

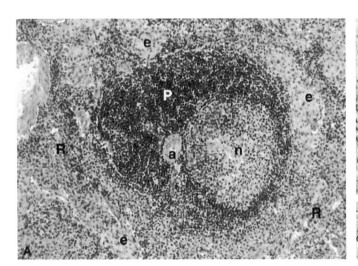
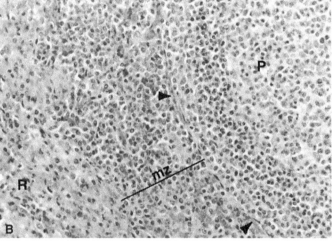
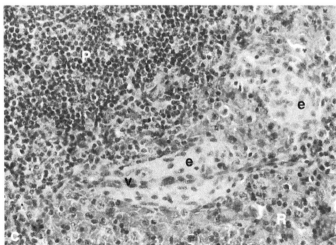

FIGURE 8-20   A. Spleen (sheep). An artery of the white pulp (a) is ensheathed with lymphocytes that constitute the periarterial lymphatic sheath (PALS; P). A nodule (n) is embedded within the PALS. Sheathed capillaries, or ellipsoids, are surrounded by a wide macrophage sheath (e). Red pulp (R). Hematoxylin and eosin. **B.** Spleen (horse). A line has been drawn to indicate the extent of the marginal zone (mz), which lies between the white pulp (P) and the red pulp (R). A marginal sinus (arrowheads) is immediately adjacent to the PALS. **C.** Spleen (dog). A narrow vessel (v) courses through a wide macrophage sheath (e). Periarterial lymphatic sheath (P); red pulp (R). Hematoxylin and eosin.

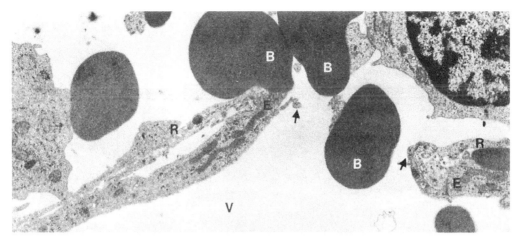

FIGURE 8-21 Spleen (sheep). Electron micrograph of a venule with erythrocytes (B) passing through an opening in the wall. Lumen (V); endothelium (E); reticular cells (R); lymphocyte (L). Arrows indicate the edges of the endothelial opening (×8000).

and may or may not have germinal centers, depending on their functional state. The PALS are organized along the artery of the white pulp. Within the PALS, T cells are concentrated adjacent to the tunica media of the artery, whereas the peripheral region of the sheaths contains a more diverse mixture of T cells and B cells, macrophages, and dendritic cells. Throughout the white pulp, reticular cells and associated reticular fibers form a three-

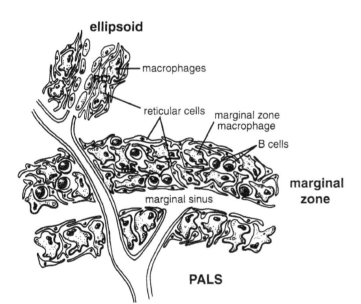

FIGURE 8-22 Schematic drawing of the marginal zone and an ellipsoid. Blood vessels leave the periarterial lymphatic sheath (PALS) to pass through a rim of macrophages and empty into the marginal sinus, which represents the inner limit of the marginal zone. The marginal zone is composed of reticular cells, B cells, and marginal zone macrophages. Some blood vessels pass through the marginal zone and terminate in the red pulp as sheathed capillaries or ellipsoids. These structures are surrounded by a meshwork of reticular cells and macrophages.

dimensional stroma containing lymphocytes, macrophages, and dendritic cells similar to those seen in lymph nodes.

Marginal Zone

The **marginal zone** lies between the white pulp and the red pulp. The periphery of the white pulp is bounded by a circumferential reticulum, the reticular cells of which branch into the marginal zone. The marginal zone blends into the splenic cords of the red pulp (Figs. 8-22 and 8-23). The reticular network of the marginal zone receives capillaries from the white pulp and some terminal capillaries of the red pulp. The capillaries empty into a **marginal sinus,** which is a series of anastomosing channels, not equally apparent in all species (Fig. 8-23). From here, the blood is drained slowly toward the venous sinuses or venules of the red pulp. Many macrophages and B cells are in the marginal zone. All elements of the blood, as well as antigens and particles, are brought into contact with the local macrophages and lymphocytes, facilitating phagocytosis and the initiation of an immune response. Bloodborne antigens trapped within the marginal zone are transported by marginal zone macrophages to the PALS, an environment rich in recirculating lymphocytes and dendritic cells.

Blood Vessels

The circulation of blood through the spleen has important functional implications, particularly with respect to antigenic stimulation and the extraction of hemoglobin and iron from red blood cells (Fig. 8-23). Branches of the splenic artery enter the capsule and extend into the large trabeculae as **trabecular arteries.** As the artery leaves the trabecula, it is called the **artery of the white pulp.** As the artery of the white pulp becomes smaller, the PALS and marginal zone attenuate and eventually the surrounding reticulum disappears. Strands of white pulp stretch across the attenuated marginal zone to the red pulp, forming bridging channels. Branches of the white pulp artery continue to feed capillary

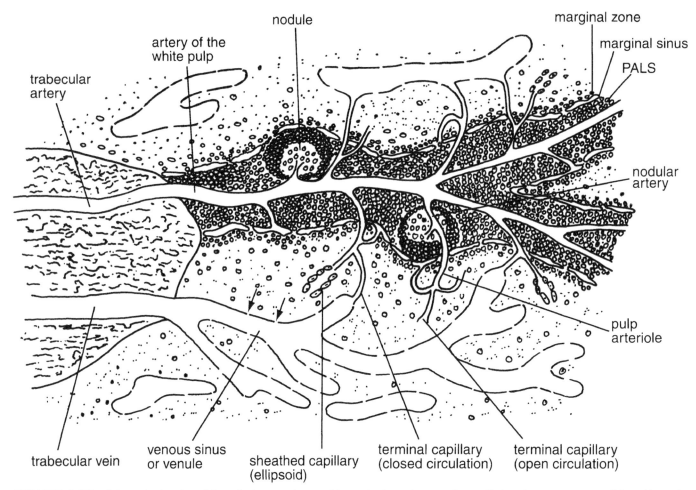

FIGURE 8-23 Schematic drawing of the splenic parenchyma with emphasis on the vasculature. Trabecular artery; artery of the white pulp with lymphatic sheath; nodular artery; pulp arteriole; sheathed capillary (ellipsoid); terminal capillaries emptying into reticular mesh (open circulation); terminal capillaries emptying into venous sinus or venule (closed circulation); venous sinus or venule; trabecular vein. Arrows indicate openings in the wall of sinuses or venules. Periarterial lymphatic sheath (PALS).

beds in the nodule and terminate in the marginal zone or enter the red pulp, forming a **penicillar artery** (brushlike tuft). Each branch of the penicillar artery continues into the red pulp as a **pulp arteriole.** Each pulp arteriole continues into a distinctive structure called a **sheathed capillary** or **ellipsoid** (Fig. 8-23). Here, the vessel lumen narrows, and the endothelium is cuboidal, with permeable junctions and a discontinuous basal lamina. The vessel is surrounded by a sheath of macrophages sequestered in a meshwork of reticular cells and fibers, called a **pericapillary macrophage sheath.** The sheathed capillary continues as an unsheathed **terminal capillary.**

The junction of the terminal capillaries with the venous system is controversial, and currently, three theories exist regarding the type of connection. The first theory is that the terminal capillaries expand, form an ampulla, and open directly into the splenic sinuses or venules. This is called the "closed" theory because the connection forms a continuous tubular structure. The second theory, or "open" theory, suggests that the capillaries open into the spaces between the reticular cells of the red pulp and the blood, then enters the venous sinuses through the slits in

their walls. The third theory proposes the existence of both an "open" and "closed" circulation, depending on the physiologic state. When the spleen is distended, the spaces between the endothelial cells lining the sinuses or venules are pulled apart, and the blood leaks through the open meshwork from the terminal capillaries to the sinuses or venules. In a contracted spleen, the cells in the venous sinuses or venules are pushed together to form a continuous uninterrupted connection with the terminal capillaries. Thus, the circulatory flow is closed. The third theory is widely accepted for sinusal spleens, but nonsinusal spleens seem to have an open circulatory flow. Whatever the exact nature of the capillary–venous junction, the blood in the small vessels eventually drains into the trabecular veins and leaves by the splenic vein.

Lymph Vessels and Nerves

The spleen has no afferent lymph vessels. Efferent capsular and trabecular lymph vessels originate in the white pulp and are an exit route from the white pulp for some lymphocytes. The efferent lymph vessels drain into the splenic lymph nodes.

Species Differences

The spleens of horses, dogs, and pigs have abundant lymphatic nodules and periarterial lymphatic sheaths. In the cat and ruminant spleens, lymphatic tissue is less abundant and occurs mainly as lymphatic nodules; the periarterial lymphatic sheaths are short.

The size and number of the sheathed capillaries also vary considerably among the domestic animals. In pigs and cats, the pericapillary macrophage sheaths are large and abundant and often particularly numerous near the white pulp. The pericapillary macrophage sheaths are smaller in horses and dogs than in other domestic animals, and small and narrow in ruminants.

The ability to mobilize rapidly the reservoir of erythrocytes stored in the spleen differs between and within species, as evidenced by the large increases in hematocrit following physical activity in thoroughbred horses and greyhounds. Only moderate or small changes in hematocrit occur in other domestic animal species such as sheep.

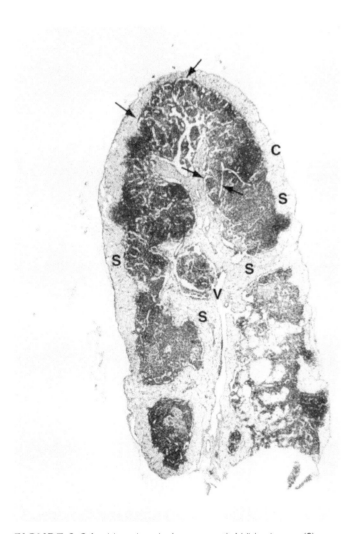

FIGURE 8-24 Hemal node (young goat). Wide sinuses (S) under capsule (C) and around central veins (V). There are many small venules (arrows) in the lymphatic tissue. Vascular perfusion. Hematoxylin and eosin (×35).

Hemal Nodes and "Milk Spots"

Hemal nodes are only described in ruminants, where they are prevalent in the sublumbar area along the vena cava and abdominal aorta. They are generally small, brown to dark red organs, but their size, number, and histologic characteristics vary within wide limits. Hemal nodes develop during fetal life from lymph node primordia that lose their lymph vessels. Therefore, hemal nodes receive all their cells and antigens from the blood. The functional significance of hemal nodes is not clear, although it is probable that they respond to bloodborne antigens.

In young animals, the lymphocytes in hemal nodes accumulate in a distinct region resembling the deep cortex of a lymph node, but few nodules are present (Fig. 8-24). In healthy adults, the entire node is generally filled with red blood cells. As a result of antigenic stimulation, many nodules may form, and only a few red blood cells are present. The sinuses are wide, with few macrophages and few lymphocytes. The diffuse lymphatic tissue contains relatively few lymphocytes but has many macrophages that digest erythrocytes and granulocytes. A typical medulla is lacking.

The vascular supply to hemal nodes is similar to that of lymph nodes, but all venules have a thin endothelium. Many lymphocytes and erythrocytes pass through this endothelium.

So-called **"milk spots"** are small aggregations of lymphocytes and macrophages that occur along the blood vessels of the omentum.

SUGGESTED READINGS

Bélisle C, Sainte-Marie G. Topography of the deep cortex of the lymph nodes of various mammalian species. Anat Rec 1981;201: 553–561.

Blue J, Weiss L. Electron microscopy of the red pulp of dog spleen including vascular arrangements, periarterial macrophage sheaths (ellipsoids), and the contractile, innervated reticular meshwork. Am J Anat 1981;161:189–218.

Griebel P, Hein W. Expanding the role of Peyer's patches in B-cell ontogeny. Immunol Today 1996;17:30–39.

Halleraker M, Landsverk T, Press C. Development and cell phenotypes of primary follicles in sheep fetal lymph nodes. Cell Tissue Res 1994; 275:51.

Janeway CA, Travers P, Walport M, et al. Immunobiology: The Immune System in Health and Disease. 4th Ed. New York: Elsevier Science Ltd/Garland Publishing, 1999.

Kraal G. Cells in the marginal zone of the spleen. Int Rev Cytol 1992; 132:31–74.

Landsverk T, Halleraker M, Aleksandersen M, et al. The intestinal habitat for organized lymphoid tissues in ruminants; comparative aspects of structure, function and development. Vet Immunol Immunopathol 1991;28:1–16.

Lanzavecchia A, Sallusto F. Regulation of T cell immunity by dendritic cells. Cell 2001;106:263–266.

Morris B. The ontogeny and comportment of lymphoid cells in fetal and neonatal sheep. Immunol Rev 1986;91:219–233.

Nicander L, Halleraker M, Landsverk T. Ontogeny of reticular cells in the ileal Peyer's patch of sheep and goats. Am J Anat 1991; 191:237–249.

Nicander L, Nafstad P, Landsverk T, et al. A study of modified lymphatics in the deep cortex of ruminant lymph nodes. J Anat 1991;178:203–212.

Pabst R, Gehrke I. Is the bronchus-associated lymphoid tissue (BALT) an integral structure of the lung in normal mammals, including humans? Am J Respir Cell Mol Biol 1990;3:131–135.

Pastoret P-P, Griebel P, Bazin H, et al. Handbook of Vertebrate Immunology. San Diego: Academic Press, 1998.

Rajewsky K. Clonal selection and learning in the antibody system. Nature 1996;381:751–758.

Reynaud C, Weill J. Postrearrangement diversification processes in gut-associated lymphoid tissues. Curr Top Microbiol Immunol 1996; 212:7–15.

Rothkotter HJ, Pabst R, Bailey M. Lymphocyte migration in the intestinal mucosa: entry, transit and emigration of lymphoid cells and the influence of antigen. Vet Immunol Immunopathol 1999;72: 157–165.

Tizard IR. Veterinary Immunology. An Introduction. 6th Ed. Philadelphia: WB Saunders, 2000.

Van Rooijen N, Claassen E, Kraal G, et al. Cytological basis of immune functions of the spleen. Immunocytochemical characterization of lymphoid and non-lymphoid cells involved in the 'in situ' immune response. Prog Histochem Cytochem 1989;19:1–71.

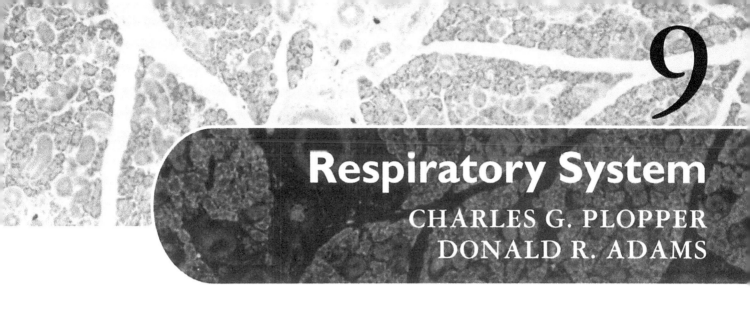

Respiratory System

CHARLES G. PLOPPER
DONALD R. ADAMS

Nasal Cavity, Vomeronasal Organ, and Paranasal Sinuses
    Nasal Cavity
        Cutaneous region
        Respiratory region
        Olfactory region
    Vomeronasal Organ
    Paranasal Sinuses
Nasopharynx
Larynx
Trachea and Extrapulmonary Bronchi
Lung

Intrapulmonary Conducting Airways
    Bronchi
    Bronchioles
Gas Exchange Area
    Respiratory bronchioles
    Alveolar ducts and alveolar sacs
    Alveoli
Pleura
Blood Vessels and Lymphatics
Innervation
Avian Respiratory System

The primary function of the respiratory system is to provide for the exchange of respiratory gases (oxygen and carbon dioxide) between the organism and the environment. The conducting airways provide a series of air passages for moving air to and from the gas exchange area in the lungs. The conducting airways also serve a protective function by conditioning incoming (inspired) air. This conditioning includes heating the air to body temperature, saturating it to 100% relative humidity, and filtering out noxious gases and particulates. The conducting airways also conserve body heat and water by extracting them from the air during expiration. The mucociliary blanket, which covers the mucosal surface of conducting airways, serves to trap inhaled particles and conveys them and cellular debris out of the system. Other structures, such as the nasolacrimal duct, vomeronasal organ, paranasal recesses and sinuses, auditory tube, and equine guttural pouch, connect to the conducting airways.

The distal, smallest conducting airways connect to the gas exchange area, which includes the respiratory bronchioles, alveolar ducts, and alveolar sacs. Gas exchange occurs in alveoli, where only a thin blood-air barrier is present between pulmonary capillary blood and respired air. An extensive pulmonary capillary bed receives the entire output of the right ventricle of the heart.

NASAL CAVITY, VOMERONASAL ORGAN, AND PARANASAL SINUSES

Nasal Cavity

Each **nasal cavity** is divided into a cutaneous region, a respiratory region, and an olfactory region. The skin of the nasal apex is continuous through a tissue gradient with the mucous membrane of the caudal nasal cavity proper.

Cutaneous Region

Rostrally, the **cutaneous region** (nasal vestibule) is lined by a relatively thick keratinized stratified squamous epithelium (Fig. 9-1). At midvestibule, the epithelium is thinner and nonkeratinized. Superficial cells have microridges on their free surface. The caudal portion of the cutaneous region and the rostral third of the nasal

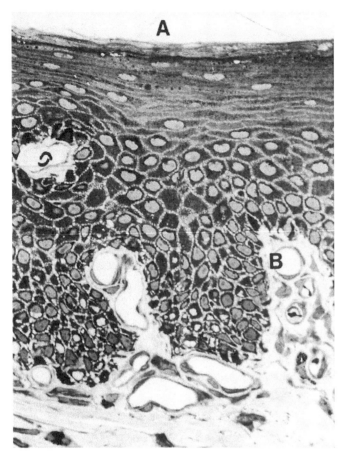

FIGURE 9-1   Stratified squamous epithelium in the cutaneous region of the canine nasal cavity. Airway lumen (A); dermal papilla (B). 1 μm. Azure II (×385). *(With permission from Adams DR, Hotchkiss DK. The canine nasal mucosa. Zentralbl Veterinarmed C Anat Histol Embryol 1983;12:111.)*

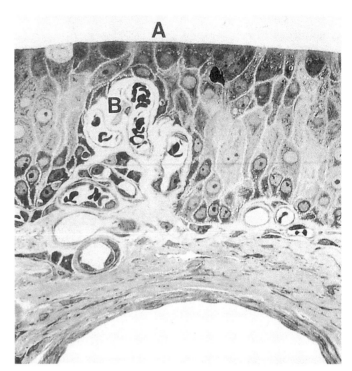

FIGURE 9-2   Stratified cuboidal epithelium in the transitional zone of the canine nasal cavity. Airway lumen (A); connective-tissue papilla (B). 1 μm. Azure II (×385). *(With permission from Adams DR, Hotchkiss DK. The canine nasal mucosa. Zentralbl Veterinarmed C Anat Histol Embryol 1983;12:113.)*

cavity proper are a **transitional zone** lined by an epithelium that varies from stratified cuboidal to nonciliated pseudostratified columnar. Surface epithelial cells in the transitional zone contain multilobated nuclei, have microvilli on their free surface, and are frequently spherical (Fig. 9-2).

The propria-submucosa of the cutaneous region interdigitates via papillae with the epithelium. The papillae contain small vessels, nerves, and numerous migratory cells, including mast cells, plasma cells, lymphocytes, macrophages, and granulocytes. Lymphocytes and other migratory cells are also frequently observed in the basal portion of the epithelium. Bundles of collagen fibers, larger blood vessels and nerves, and serous glands are located deep in the propria-submucosa.

In horses, a nasal diverticulum lined with skin opens into the cutaneous region of the nasal vestibule; this region is lined by an integument containing vibrissae, sebaceous glands, and sweat glands. The papillary layer of the vestibular propria-submucosa in dogs has particularly numerous papillae and capillary loops.

Respiratory Region

Epithelium lining the caudal two thirds of the nasal cavity proper, with the exception of the olfactory region, is classified as **respi-**

ratory epithelium (i.e., ciliated pseudostratified columnar); that lining the middle nasal meatus is thinner and contains fewer ciliated and goblet cells. The ciliated pseudostratified epithelium of the nasal cavity contains several cell types, including ciliated, secretory, brush, and basal cells (Figs. 9-3, 9-4, and 9-5).

Individual **ciliated cells** are columnar and have 200 to 300 motile cilia and numerous microvilli projecting into the nasal lumen. The supranuclear portion of the cell contains basal bodies, a Golgi complex, and numerous mitochondria; small strands of rough endoplasmic reticulum (rER) are scattered throughout the cell. Defects in the fine structure of cilia may result in ineffective ciliary beat or immotility. Immotile cilia syndrome is a condition associated with congenital ciliary abnormality, resulting in respiratory tract infections.

Secretory cells of the respiratory epithelium extend from the basal lamina to the epithelial surface. Their luminal surface bears microvilli. The morphologic and histochemical appearance of these cells is both species and regionally variable. Their description as mucous or serous is based on their glycoprotein content. Granules of **mucous epithelial cells** are relatively electron-lucent and contain sialated or sulfated acid glycoproteins. The supranuclear portion of mucous epithelial cells varies in appearance with the secretory phase from tall and slender with few granules to wide and globular with numerous mucous granules. Globular mucous cells, known as **goblet cells,** have nuclei pressed to the base of the cell by the supranuclear mass of large mucous granules. Organelles usually present in the perinuclear region of the goblet cell include a Golgi complex, rER, and mitochondria. Goblet cells of most

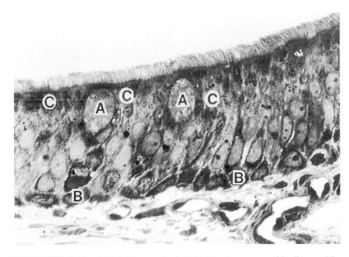

FIGURE 9-3 Ciliated pseudostratified columnar epithelium with goblet cells lining the respiratory region of the nasal cavity. Goblet cells (A); basal cells (B); ciliated cells (C). 1 μm. Azure II (×590).

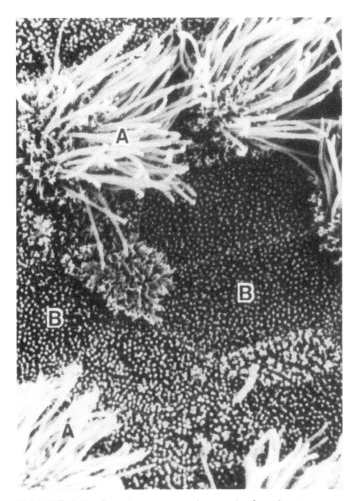

FIGURE 9-4 Scanning electron micrograph of respiratory epithelium (ciliated pseudostratified columnar epithelium). Ciliated cells with cilia and microvilli (A); secretory cells with apical microvilli (B) (×3500).

species secrete primarily sulfated glycoprotein as a major component of mucus.

Granules of **serous epithelial cells** have electron-dense cores, contain neutral glycoproteins, and are smaller than those of mucous cells.

Brush cells have long, thick microvilli and a cytoplasm containing mitochondria and many filaments. These cells may be sensory receptors associated with endings of the trigeminal nerve.

Basal cells are small polyhedral cells located along the basal lamina. The cytoplasm of basal cells contains numerous bundles of tonofilaments and free ribosomes. Basal cells are characterized by anchoring attachments (desmosomes) to other cell types and to the basal lamina (hemidesmosomes). While basal cells appear to have some role in replacing other cell types, the rate of cell proliferation is very low and most of the replacement cells are derived from the other cell types in the epithelium.

Another unnamed cell in the nasal mucosa has surface microvilli and contains much smooth endoplasmic reticulum (sER) and little secretory material; this cell type is believed to function in the metabolism of xenobiotic compounds (see below).

The respiratory mucosa (respiratory epithelium plus underlying propria-submucosa) of the nasal cavity is more vascular than the mucosae of the cutaneous, transitional, or olfactory regions. The highly vascular propria-submucosa, in which arteries and large, thin-walled veins are oriented rostrocaudally, is called the **cavernous stratum** (Fig. 9-6). The veins anastomose profusely and are referred to as **capacitance vessels** because they determine the degree of mucosal congestion and, inversely, nasal patency. Constriction of nasal blood vessels is effected by α-adrenergic stimulation via the sympathetic nervous system. Periods of vascular engorgement varying from 30 minutes to 4 hours followed by periods of decongestion normally occur in the cavernous stratum of mammals; during this nasal cycle, the vascular activity in one side of the nose alternates with that in the other side.

Serous or mixed nasal glands are present between the numerous veins of this stratum (Fig. 9-7). Acini of nasal glands also secrete secretory immunoglobulin A, lysozyme, and odorant-binding protein.

Nerves in the nasal mucosa include sensory fibers arising from the terminal, olfactory, vomeronasal, and maxillary division of the trigeminal nerves and efferent fibers of the autonomic nervous system. Nerves are distributed throughout all compartments of the nasal mucosa, including within epithelium.

Lymphatic nodules are commonly present in the caudal part of the nasal cavity, adjacent to the choana, the opening between the nasal cavity and nasopharynx.

Metabolically active exogenous compounds (xenobiotics) that reach nasal tissues via air or blood pathways may remain firmly bound to tissue elements unless degraded. Cytochrome P-450-dependent monooxygenase enzymes in surface epithelium and in acinar cells of the lateral nasal gland (see below) actively metabolize endogenous compounds (e.g., progesterone and testosterone) and exogenous compounds. These enzymes convert lipid-soluble exogenous compounds, some of which are highly toxic (e.g., formaldehyde and acetaldehyde), to water-soluble metabolites.

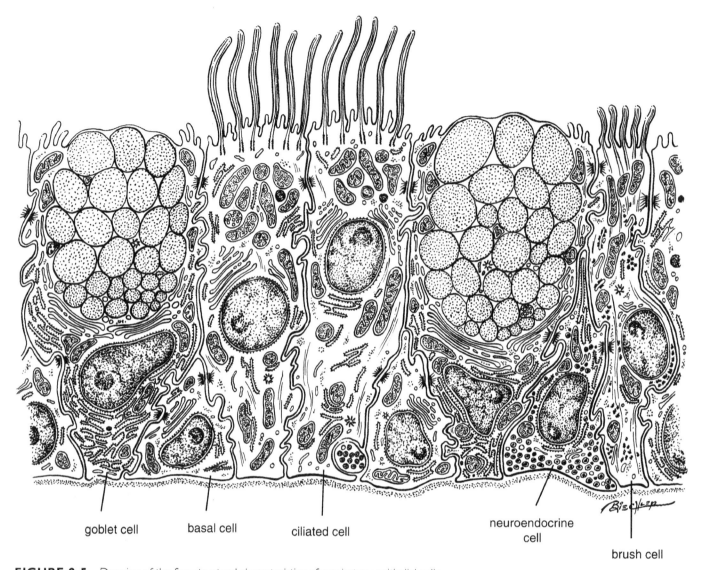

FIGURE 9-5   Drawing of the fine structural characteristics of respiratory epithelial cells.

goblet cell   basal cell   ciliated cell   neuroendocrine cell   brush cell

Olfactory Region

The olfactory region comprises the dorsocaudal portion of the nasal cavity, including some of the surfaces of the ethmoid conchae, dorsal nasal meatus, and nasal septum. Olfactory mucosa may be discerned from adjacent respiratory mucosa because it has a thicker epithelium, numerous tubular glands, and many bundles of nonmyelinated nerve fibers in the lamina propria.

The olfactory mucosa is lined by a ciliated pseudostratified columnar epithelium, the **olfactory epithelium,** consisting of three primary cell types: neurosensory, sustentacular, and basal (Fig. 9-8).

Neurosensory olfactory cells are bipolar neurons with perikarya in a wide basal zone of the epithelium, dendrites extending to the lumen, and axons reaching the olfactory bulb of the brain. A club-shaped apex, the **dendritic bulb,** protrudes from each dendrite into the lumen (Fig. 9-9), from which 10 to 30 cilia emanate. Each cilium is 50- to 80-μm long and consists of a wide, short basal portion and a long, thin, tapering distal portion. The number of microtubules decreases from the typical nine periph-

eral doublets (fused pairs of microtubules) plus two single central microtubules in the basal portion to singlets of one to four microtubules distally. The perikaryon has typical neuronal structural characteristics. Individual axons converge as they pass into the lamina propria, thereby forming bundles of nonmyelinated nerve fibers. Neurosensory cells are continuously replaced during the life of the animal by cells derived from basal cells.

Sustentacular cells are columnar cells with a narrow base and a wide apical portion. Their oval nuclei form the most superficial nuclear layer in the epithelium. Microvilli, often branched, cover the luminal surface of sustentacular cells. Juxtaluminal junctional complexes occur between sustentacular cells and the adjacent dendrites of neurosensory cells. Pigment granules are present in the infranuclear cytoplasm. Sustentacular cells are also replaced by basal cells.

Basal cells of the olfactory mucosa are similar in structure to those of the nonolfactory epithelium.

Olfactory glands, the cells of which contain pigment granules, are located in the propria-submucosa. The intraepithelial

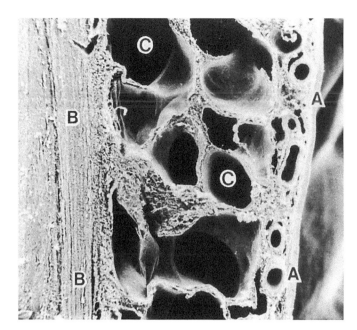

FIGURE 9-6 Scanning electron micrograph of a section of the respiratory mucosa of the bovine nasal cavity. Epithelium (A); perichondrium (B); lumina of blood vessels (C) in the cavernous stratum (×40).

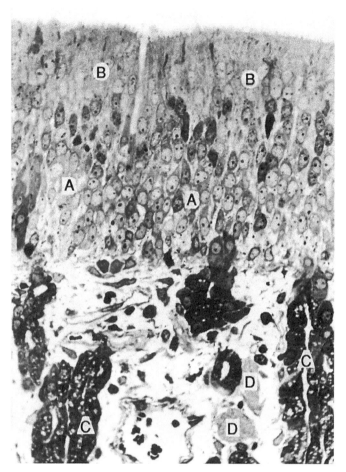

FIGURE 9-8 Mucosa of the canine olfactory region. Nuclei of neurosensory cells (A); nuclei of sustentacular cells (B); olfactory glands (C); olfactory nerves (D). 1 μm. Azure II (×410).

portion of their ducts is lined by squamous cells. The glands secrete a watery product, which may serve to enhance the solubility of airborne odorants and cleanse the cilia, facilitating access for new odorants.

The olfactory mucosa also has very high levels of cytochrome P-450-monooxygenase activity and is the primary site for chemically induced nasal tumors.

Vomeronasal Organ

Located in the mucosa of the ventral portion of the nasal septum, the tubular, blind-ended bilateral **vomeronasal organ** consists of an internal epithelial duct (vomeronasal duct), a middle propria-submucosa, and an external cartilaginous support. Rostrally, the vomeronasal duct joins the **incisive duct,** which connects the nasal cavity with the oral cavity, except in horses, in which the ventral end is blind.

The **vomeronasal duct** is crescent-shaped in transverse section with a lateral convex and a medial concave mucosal wall. The epithelium transitions from a stratified cuboidal lining rostrally near the incisive duct to a ciliated pseudostratified columnar epithelium over much of the caudal portion of the vomeronasal duct.

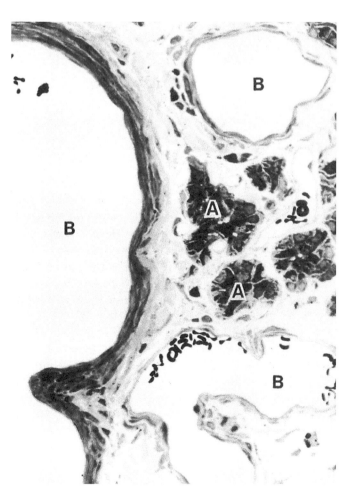

FIGURE 9-7 Nasal gland acini (A) occupy the connective tissue between the veins of the cavernous stratum (B) of the respiratory mucosa. 1 μm. Azure II (×425).

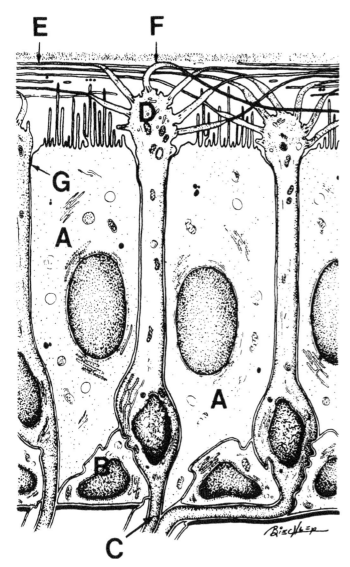

FIGURE 9-9 Schematic drawing of the olfactory epithelium. Sustentacular cells (A); basal cell (B); axon of the receptor cell (C); dendritic bulb (D); thin distal portion of cilium (E); thick proximal portion of cilium (F); junctional complex between receptor and sustentacular cells (G).

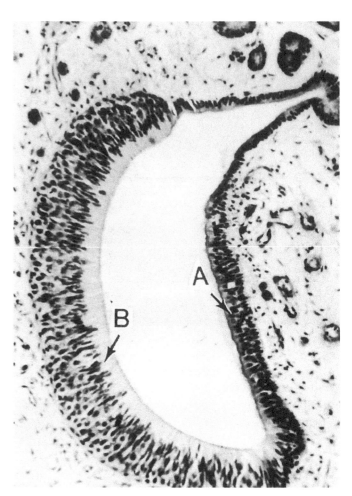

FIGURE 9-10 Canine vomeronasal duct. The lateral epithelium (A) includes ciliated and nonciliated cells, whereas the medial epithelium (B) contains neurosensory and sustentacular epithelial cells (×158). *(Courtesy of A. W. Stinson.)*

The medial pseudostratified columnar epithelium has neurosensory, sustentacular, and basal cells (Fig. 9-10). The dendritic portions of vomeronasal neurosensory cells lack dendritic bulbs and, with the exception of those in dogs, have microvilli instead of cilia on their apical surfaces. Neurosensory cells are periodically replaced in the adult mammal. The lateral pseudostratified columnar epithelium has ciliated and nonciliated columnar, goblet, and basal cells.

Vomeronasal glands, located in the highly vascular propria-submucosa, secrete into the vomeronasal duct most commonly through the commissures between lateral and medial mucosal walls. Secretory granules of the acinar cells contain neutral glycoproteins. The hyaline **vomeronasal cartilage** is J-shaped, enclosing all but the dorsolateral portion of the organ.

The vomeronasal organ functions in the chemoreception of liquidborne compounds of low volatility. Sensing of these com-

pounds is believed to function in sexual behavior of both the female and the male, in maternal behavior, and in the interaction of the fetus with its amniotic environment. In several mammals, vomeronasal detection of the odor of a female results in an elevation of plasma testosterone in the male. The vomeronasal organ is associated with the lip-curl type of facial grimace (Flehmen response) used by some male mammals to sample substances in the urine of the female; odorant particles may reach the incisive duct with inhaled air, through contact with the tongue, or during passage through the mouth with food or water. These substances, dissolved in fluid in the incisive duct, are sucked into the vomeronasal duct by constriction of blood vessels within the propria-submucosa of the vomeronasal organ. Upon dilation of these vessels, the dissolved substances are expelled from the vomeronasal lumen.

Paranasal Sinuses

The mucosae of the paranasal sinuses are thinner than those of the respiratory region of the nasal cavity with which they are continuous. Glands and blood vessels in the propria-submucosa are scant. The epithelium is ciliated pseudostratified columnar, containing a few goblet cells. The ciliary beat carries mucus toward openings connecting the sinuses with the nasal cavity.

The **lateral nasal gland** (Fig. 9-11) is a relatively large compound gland that secretes neutral glycoproteins via a long duct into the nasal vestibule. The lateral nasal gland is present in the maxillary recess of carnivores, in the maxillary sinus of pigs, and at the nasomaxillary aperture in horses and small ruminants; it is absent in cattle. In addition, separate maxillary recess glands are present in carnivores.

NASOPHARYNX

The **nasopharynx** is the portion of the pharynx located dorsal to the soft palate, extending from the nasal cavity to the laryngopharynx. The lining of the nasopharynx consists mostly of respiratory epithelium, but stratified squamous epithelium over the caudodorsal portion of the soft palate makes contact either with the dorsal wall of the nasopharynx during deglutition or with the epiglottis. The propria-submucosa is loose connective tissue containing mixed glands. Lymphatic nodules are prominent in the dorsal portion of the nasopharynx, where they aggregate as the pharyngeal tonsil.

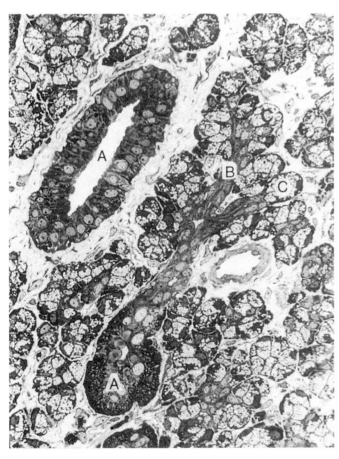

FIGURE 9-11 Two striated ducts (A), an intercalated duct (B), and acinar cells (C) in the canine lateral nasal gland. I µm. Azure II (×425).

LARYNX

The **larynx** opens rostrally into the laryngopharynx and is continuous caudally with the trachea (Fig. 9-12). It is lined by mucosa and supported by cartilage.

The epithelium lining the epiglottis, laryngeal vestibule, and vocal folds is nonkeratinized stratified squamous; the laryngeal epithelium caudal to the vocal fold gradually changes into respiratory epithelium (Fig. 9-3). Respiratory epithelium also lines the equine laryngeal ventricle. The epithelium on the laryngeal surface of the epiglottis, aryepiglottic folds, and arytenoid cartilages may contain taste buds in all species except horses. Sensory receptors of the cranial laryngeal nerve in the epithelium respond to the presence of fluids, such as water, milk, gastric fluid, and saliva; stimulation of these receptors results in reflex apnea.

The propria-submucosa beneath the stratified squamous epithelium is a dense, irregular connective tissue; the propria-submucosa beneath the respiratory epithelium is a loose connective tissue rich in elastic fibers, leukocytes, plasma cells, and mast cells. Diffuse lymphatic tissue or solitary lymphatic nodules are frequently observed. In pigs and small ruminants, a paraepiglottic tonsil is present on either side of the base of the epiglottis; this tonsil occurs occasionally in cats. Mixed glands (Fig. 9-13) occur in the propria-submucosa but are absent in the vestibular and vocal folds. Numerous elastic fibers are present in the vocal ligament and, to a lesser extent, in the vestibular ligament.

The laryngeal cartilages are connected to each other, to the trachea, and to the hyoid apparatus by ligaments. Extrinsic skeletal muscles move the larynx during swallowing; intrinsic skeletal muscles move individual laryngeal cartilages during respiration and phonation. Most of the laryngeal cartilages are of the hyaline type. The epiglottis, the cuneiform and corniculate cartilages or processes, and the vocal process of the arytenoid cartilage contain elastic cartilage. The epiglottis of carnivores often consists of a peripheral cartilaginous wall enclosing white adipose tissue,

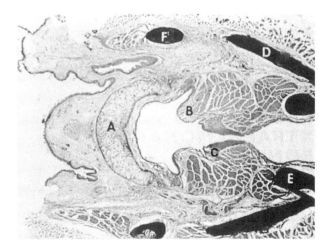

FIGURE 9-12 Horizontal section through a feline larynx. Epiglottis cartilage (A); vestibular fold (B); vocal ligament (C), thyroid cartilage (D); cricoid cartilage (E); thyrohyoid bone (F). Hematoxylin and eosin (×8.3). *(From Dellmann HD. Veterinary Histology: An Outline Text–Atlas. Philadelphia: Lea & Febiger, 1971.)*

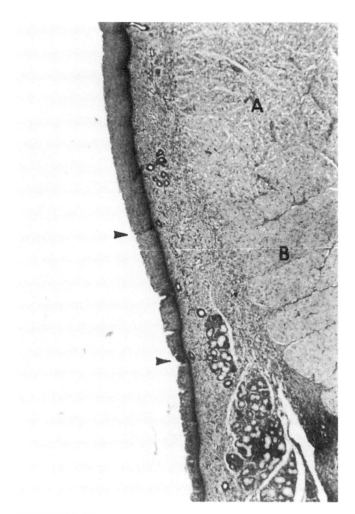

FIGURE 9-13 Horizontal section through the caudal portion of a feline vocal fold. Vocal ligament (A); vocal muscle (B). Note the thick stratified squamous epithelium on the vocal fold and its gradual decrease in height toward the trachea. After a short transitional zone (between arrowheads), the epithelium becomes respiratory in nature. Hematoxylin and eosin (×39).

strands of elastic fibers, and small areas of elastic cartilage. A loose connective tissue forms the tunica adventitia surrounding the laryngeal cartilages and muscles.

TRACHEA AND EXTRAPULMONARY BRONCHI

Distal to the larynx, the respiratory system consists of a series of branching tubes (Fig. 9-14), the tracheobronchial airways, which open into the large (approximately 25 times the body surface) alveolar gas exchange area. The **trachea,** the largest in diameter and length of these tubes, provides the air passageway between the larynx and the bronchi. It is a semiflexible and semicollapsible tube that extends from the larynx into the thoracic cavity.

The lining epithelium of the tracheobronchial tree is respiratory epithelium (Fig. 9-15), containing ciliated cells, brush

cells, secretory cells, bronchiolar exocrine cells, basal cells, and neuroendocrine cells. Ciliated cells, brush cells, and secretory cells of the trachea are similar to those of the upper respiratory system (see Respiratory Region earlier in this chapter). **Goblet cells** are the predominant secretory cell type in domestic mammals. Bronchiolar exocrine cells are relatively scarce or even absent in the larger airways; they are described on page 162. **Neuroendocrine cells** are APUD cells; that is, they are characterized by amine precursor uptake and decarboxylation. They are typically pyramid-shaped with their bases on the basal lamina. The neuroendocrine cells are identified with histochemical methods and, at the fine-structural level, contain dense-cored, argyrophilic granules, abundant ER, Golgi complex, ribosomes, and many filaments. These cells are most abundant in young animals and are sometimes associated with nerves.

A variety of **migratory cells** are also observed in the epithelium. These include lymphocytes, globule leukocytes, and mast cells. **Globule leukocytes** are cells of unknown function that contain relatively large acidophilic, metachromatic granules.

The tracheal propria-submucosa consists of loose connective tissue and a subepithelial layer of longitudinally oriented elastic fibers; cells include fibrocytes, lymphocytes, plasma cells, globule leukocytes, and mast cells. The propria-submucosa contains tubuloacinar seromucous glands that open into the lumen via ducts that are lined with ciliated cells, mucus-secreting cells, and various intermediate cells. The tubular portions of the **tracheal glands** are lined by mucus-secreting cells, and their acinar portions are lined primarily by serous secretory cells. The mucus-secreting cells generally secrete sulfated acid glycoproteins. Serous cells are the major secretory cells of the glands in most species; their secretory product is a neutral glycoprotein that is sometimes sulfated. Tracheal glands provide most of the secretory material that covers the ciliated surface in the trachea. These glands are abundant in the proximal portions of the trachea of virtually all domestic mammalian species.

The most distinctive feature of the trachea is hyaline cartilage (Fig. 9-15), which in most species occurs as roughly C- or U-shaped separate pieces. In some individuals, however, the cartilage is fused in places to form a continuum. The dorsal free ends of the cartilages are bridged by the **trachealis muscle,** a band of smooth muscle. In most species, the muscle attaches to the perichondrium on the internal side of the cartilage. In carnivores, this attachment is on the external surface of the cartilage. Nerves and large blood vessels are generally associated with the smooth muscle band. The external perichondrium is surrounded by the loose connective tissue of the adventitia.

Within the thoracic cavity, the trachea terminates by bifurcating into two **primary bronchi.** Distal to the bifurcation, the primary bronchi provide branches that enter the lungs. The structural characteristics of primary bronchi are the same as those of the trachea, except that cartilage is in the form of irregular plates.

LUNG

Most of the thoracic cavity is occupied by right and left lungs. The lung of mammals may be divided into intrapulmonary conducting

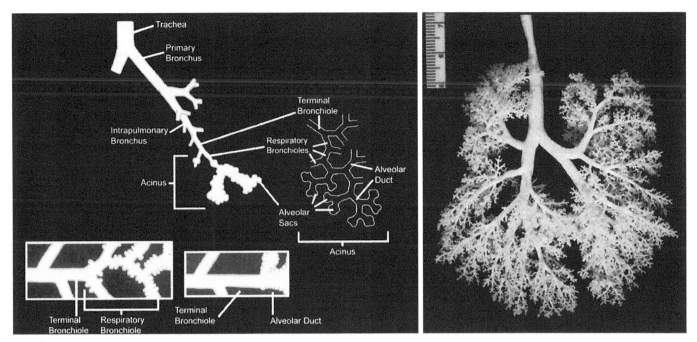

FIGURE 9-14 Comparison of a schematic drawing of the organization of the tracheobronchial airways and gas exchange area (left) and a cast of the air space in the tracheobronchial airways (right). In many species, terminal bronchioles have a very short transition to alveolar ducts (inset, lower right), while in other species the transition is extensive with many generations of bronchioles containing alveolar outpocketings and called respiratory bronchioles (inset, lower left).

airways, gas exchange area (parenchyma), and pleura. The intrapulmonary conducting airways (bronchi and bronchioles) compose approximately 6% of the lung. The gas exchange area, consisting of respiratory bronchioles (also referred to as transition zone), alveolar ducts, alveolar sacs, and alveoli, comprises approximately 85% of the lung. The lung is encapsulated by a layer of connective tissue covered by mesothelial cells termed the **visceral (pulmonary) pleura.** Along with the pleura, the intrapulmonary nervous and vascular tissue (pulmonary arteries, pulmonary veins, and bronchial arteries) comprise the remaining 9 to 10% of the lung.

Intrapulmonary Conducting Airways

Bronchi

The bronchial tree is formed by a primary bronchus and the various orders of airways that it supplies (Fig. 9-14). The largest segments of the intrapulmonary conducting airways are called **lobar bronchi,** each of which enters a lobe of the lung at its hilum. The lobar bronchi divide into two smaller branches, which divide again, and this process continues until the gas exchange area is reached. The first two or three generations of branching from a

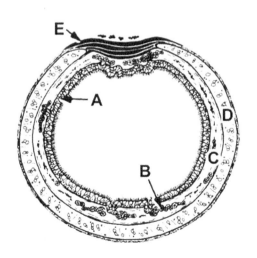

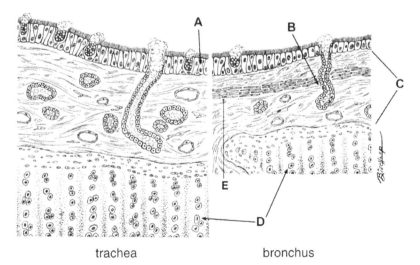

trachea   bronchus

FIGURE 9-15 Schematic drawing of a cross section of the trachea and detailed sections through parts of the wall of the trachea and a bronchus. Note the differences in the height of the epithelium (A), the glandular density (B), the thickness of the soft tissue in the propria-submucosa (C), the presence of hyaline cartilage as rings in the trachea versus plates in the bronchus (D), and the location of smooth muscle (E).

lobar bronchus supply portions of the lung lobe called **bronchopulmonary segments**. Each succeeding generation of branching is made of a greater number of airways and has a larger total cross-sectional area than the generation before it.

The histologic appearance of a bronchus is generally similar to that of the trachea, except that the various layers are thinner (Fig. 9-15). Bronchi are lined by a respiratory epithelium composed primarily of ciliated cells, secretory cells, and basal cells. Proximodistally, the composition of the epithelium changes; mucous cells and basal cells decrease and bronchiolar exocrine cells increase in number. At the same time, the epithelial height and the thickness of the propria-submucosa progressively decrease.

The propria-submucosa is loose connective tissue containing mixed glands (**bronchial glands**) in all species except goats; bronchial glands are less abundant in distal bronchi. The hyaline cartilage of the proximal bronchi is in the form of irregular plates, and the smooth muscle is interspersed either between or on the luminal side of the plates. The muscle cells are generally arranged in a circular fashion, perpendicular to the long axis of the airway. The amount of cartilage decreases proximodistally, whereas smooth muscle becomes relatively more abundant. The adventitial connective tissue is primarily loose, with many collagen fibers and variable numbers of elastic fibers. Many of the fibers are oriented longitudinally, whereas others are oriented perpendicularly to the long axis of the airway. Adventitial and submucosal nerve plexuses and intraepithelial nerve endings are present. In most domestic species, the extensive vascular supply derives from the systemic circulation via the bronchial artery.

Bronchioles

Bronchioles arise from bronchi, branch into several generations, and terminate as terminal bronchioles (Fig. 9-14). Several generations of **terminal bronchioles** are present in horses, cattle, and sheep, whereas generally only one or two generations are present in carnivores.

Bronchioles have roughly circular cross-sectional profiles and are lined with simple columnar or cuboidal epithelium (Fig. 9-16) composed of ciliated cells and **bronchiolar exocrine cells** (Clara cells). These cells have characteristics of both secretory cells and cells capable of metabolizing xenobiotic compounds. The secretory granules contain either neutral glycoprotein or low-molecular-weight protein. Smooth endoplasmic reticulum is abundant in cells from horses and sheep but is minimally present in those from carnivores, cattle, and pigs. Glycogen is the predominant feature of bronchiolar exocrine cells in carnivores and cattle and is rarely observed in most other species. In carnivores, the epithelium of terminal bronchioles consists primarily of bronchiolar exocrine cells.

The propria-submucosa is sparse loose connective tissue; glands and cartilage are absent. The smooth muscle is arranged in separate circular and oblique fascicles. Numerous nerve fibers occur in the area immediately below the epithelium and interspersed between muscle fascicles.

The adventitia is loose connective tissue, including elastic fibers oriented circularly or obliquely. The outer border of the ad-

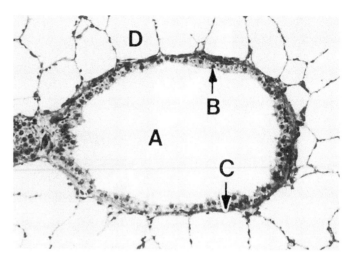

FIGURE 9-16   Cross section of a bronchiole. The airway lumen (A) is lined by simple cuboidal epithelium (B) followed by a thin layer of smooth muscle (C). Alveoli (D) surround the bronchiole. Toluidine blue (×135).

ventitia is attached to the alveolar gas exchange area and is lined by alveolar epithelial cells and a pulmonary capillary bed.

Gas Exchange Area

The gas exchange area, also referred to as parenchyma, can be organized into either functional or structural units. The functional unit of the gas exchange area is called the **acinus,** or terminal respiratory unit (Figs. 9-14 and 9-17). The acinus includes all air spaces distal to a single terminal bronchiole, including branching respiratory bronchioles, alveolar ducts, alveolar sacs, and alveoli.

The **lobule** is a structural unit rather than a functional unit. It comprises a cluster of acini that is separated from adjacent clusters by connective-tissue septa. These connective-tissue septa are termed **interlobular septa** and are composed of collagen and elastic fibers and blood vessels. Both bronchial arteries and pulmonary veins are located in interlobular septa. The lungs of cattle, sheep, and pigs are highly lobulated and have complete septa. The lungs of horses have incomplete septa and are considered poorly lobulated. Carnivores do not have interlobular septa.

Respiratory Bronchioles

Bronchioles in which the walls possess outpocketings of gas exchange tissue (i.e., alveoli) are termed **respiratory bronchioles**. They are also called the **transition zone,** which is the focus of most lung disorders. The histologic appearance of respiratory bronchioles is similar to that of terminal bronchioles, with the exception that the epithelium is interrupted by alveoli (Figs. 9-17 and 9-18). The smooth muscle is arranged in fascicles that underlie the simple columnar or cuboidal epithelium. The alveoli open between these muscle bundles.

In respiratory bronchioles of carnivores, extensive alveolarization occurs (Fig. 9-18); generally, there are fewer alveoli in the proximal generation of branching. The epithelium consists almost

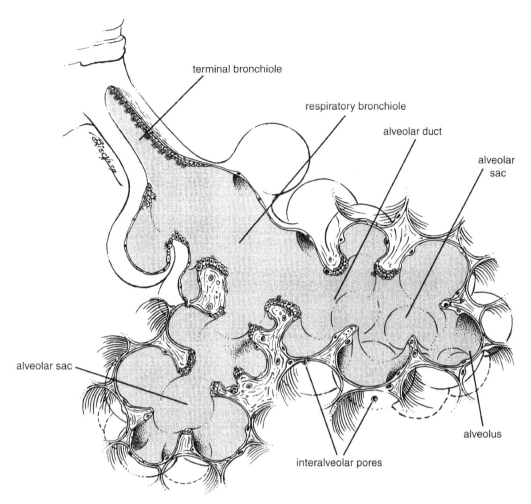

FIGURE 9-17 Schematic illustration of the gas exchange area originating from a terminal bronchiole.

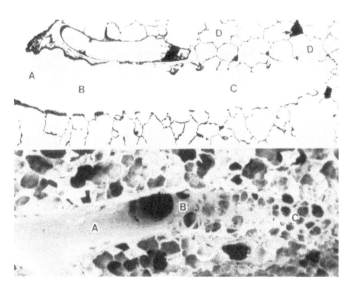

FIGURE 9-18 Light microscopic and scanning electron microscopic appearance of a terminal bronchiole and gas exchange area in the feline lung. Terminal bronchiole (A), respiratory bronchiole into which open a few alveoli (B), alveolar duct completely surrounded by alveoli (C), alveoli (D). Methylene blue–Azure II (top: ×55; bottom: ×70).

entirely of bronchiolar exocrine cells. In horses, cattle, sheep, and pigs, respiratory bronchioles are short or absent (Fig. 9-19).

Alveolar Ducts and Alveolar Sacs

Respiratory bronchioles branch into tubular structures termed **alveolar ducts** (Figs. 9-14, 9-17, 9-18, and 9-19). The ducts are comparable to hallways lined by doorless rooms on all sides. Each of these doorless rooms is an alveolus. Between one and five generations of alveolar ducts are supplied by a single respiratory bronchiole. The walls of an alveolar duct are composed of the open sides of alveolar air spaces and the terminations of the interalveolar septa that separate these alveoli. Spiraling bands of smooth muscle and elastic fibers oriented perpendicular to the long axis of the alveolar ducts lie underneath the epithelium at the terminations of the interalveolar septa.

The alveolar ducts terminate in clusters of alveoli called **alveolar sacs** (Figs. 9-14 and 9-17). A shared space into which several alveolar sacs open is called an **atrium.**

Alveoli

The basic unit for gas exchange in the pulmonary parenchyma is the **alveolus** (Figs. 9-14, 9-20, and 9-21). Alveoli are epithelium-lined

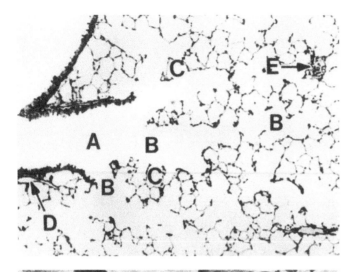

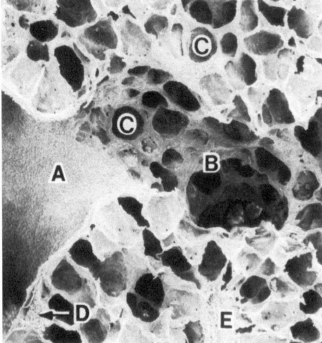

FIGURE 9-19 Light microscopic and scanning electron microscopic appearance of the terminal air spaces of the mouse (top) and the rat (bottom). Terminal bronchiole (A); alveolar duct that is completely surrounded by alveoli (B); alveoli (C); pulmonary arteriole (D); pulmonary venule (E). Toluidine blue (top: ×85; bottom: ×110).

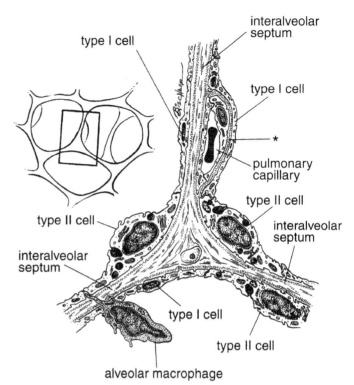

FIGURE 9-20 Schematic illustration of parts of three adjacent alveoli, as outlined in the rectangle (inset): type I alveolar epithelial cell; type II alveolar epithelial cell; interalveolar septum; pulmonary capillary; alveolar macrophage. Note the merger of the basal laminae of the pulmonary capillary and adjacent alveolus (*).

spheroid air spaces that open into an alveolar sac, alveolar duct, or respiratory bronchiole; they are separated by interalveolar septa.

The alveolar epithelial lining, located adjacent to the air space, comprises two epithelial cell types: type I and type II alveolar epithelial cells. The **type I** or **squamous alveolar epithelial cell** (respiratory epithelial cell) is flat with a central nucleus and rests on a continuous basal lamina (Fig. 9-20). The thin cytoplasm has few mitochondria, minimal amounts of rER, and a moderate number of endocytotic vesicles. This cell type covers approximately 97% of the interalveolar septal surface in all the species studied thus far. The average surface area of a type I cell ranges from 5000 to 7000 μm².

The **type II** or **granular (great) alveolar epithelial cell** (Fig. 9-22) is a cuboidal cell with a central nucleus. This cell type covers the remainder of the interalveolar septal surface area (approximately 3%). Its alveolar surface bears microvilli and ranges from 100 to 280 μm² per cell. This cell contains mitochondria, rER, microvesicles, a Golgi complex, and multiple characteristic osmiophilic vesicles called **lamellar bodies.** These lamellar bodies are believed to be primarily phospholipid and are the source of phospholipids in pulmonary surfactant that lines the air spaces. The type II alveolar cell is the progenitor cell for both type I and type II cells.

Pulmonary **alveolar macrophages** are likewise present on the air side of the interalveolar septa (Fig. 9-23). As active phagocytic cells, they are part of the mononuclear phagocyte system distributed throughout the body.

Interalveolar septa are thin sheets of connective tissue containing a capillary plexus (Fig. 9-20). The interalveolar **interstitial connective tissue** contains collagen and elastic fibers and fibrocytes; pericytes, macrophages, lymphocytes, and plasma cells may also be present.

The capillary bed of the interalveolar septa is an intermeshed network of short, branching vessels. Individual capillary beds traverse the walls of three to seven alveoli when passing from a pulmonary arteriole to a pulmonary venule. Most endothelial cells have attenuated cytoplasm in the region adjacent to type I alveolar epithelial cells. In these attenuated areas, the basal laminae of

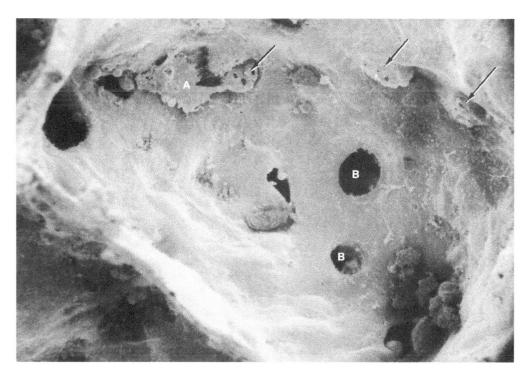

FIGURE 9-21 Scanning electron micrograph of portion of an alveolus in the equine lung. Type II (granular) alveolar epithelial cells bulge into the lumen (arrows). On the left is a pulmonary alveolar macrophage (A). Note the pores in the interalveolar septum (B) (×1232). *(Courtesy of W. S. Tyler.)*

alveolar epithelial cells and endothelial cells fuse. Capillary endothelial cells (Fig. 9-20) are characterized by few organelles and relatively numerous endocytotic vesicles. The intercellular junctions tend to be loose or leaky; the tight junctions have few anastomosing ridges. The surface area of the gas exchange capillary bed is between 66 and 75% of the surface area of the air side of the interalveolar septa.

The alveoli contain a small amount of fluid, consisting of a biphasic layer of plasma filtrates overlaid by a thin layer of phospholipids. This phospholipid layer or **pulmonary surfactant** reduces the intraalveolar surface tension, preventing alveolar collapse.

The **blood-air barrier** consists of the surface-lining layer of pulmonary surfactant and fluid, the alveolar type I cell, fused basal laminae of the alveolar epithelial cell and the underlying capillary endothelial cell, the capillary endothelial cell, and the plasmalemma of a red blood cell (Fig. 9-20). The average thickness of this barrier is 1.5 μm in most species, with the thinnest areas ranging from 0.2 to 0.7 μm. At its thickest, this barrier consists of the above-mentioned layers and interstitial connective tissue and cells between the basal laminae of epithelial and endothelial cells. The blood-air barrier prevents the massive release of fluid filtrate from capillaries into the air space while permitting diffusion of oxygen and carbon dioxide between blood capillaries and alveoli (Figs. 9-20 and 9-23).

Openings in the interalveolar septa interconnect adjacent alveoli. These openings, called **septal pores** (alveolar pores) (Figs. 9-21 and 9-23), are lined by epithelial cells and permit air and alveolar macrophages to pass from one alveolus to another.

Pleura

The visceral, or pulmonary, pleura is a serous membrane that completely covers both lungs, except at the hilum and pulmonary ligament. This covering layer consists of squamous to cuboidal mesothelial cells overlaying varying amounts of elastic fibers and dense irregular connective tissue. Pleural mesothelial cells contain large amounts of rER and mitochondria; their free surfaces are covered by microvilli. At its thickest, the connective-tissue elements of the pleura consist of two or more layers of elastic laminae, many dense irregular bundles of collagen fibers, pulmonary capillaries, and two additional sets of vessels. These two sets of vessels include capillaries and small arterioles from the bronchial circulatory system and lymph vessels. The pulmonary capillaries supply the superficial portion of the gas exchange area. The connective tissue of the pulmonary pleura is continuous with that of the interalveolar septa. The thickness of the pulmonary pleura varies from species to species and within different regions of the same species. The pleura is thinnest in the dog and cat. In these species, the submesothelial connective tissue is minimal, and the only blood supply is derived from the pulmonary artery. The pleura is thick in large domestic mammals.

Blood Vessels and Lymphatics

Blood is supplied to the lungs through two different circulatory systems: **pulmonary** and **bronchial**. **Pulmonary arteries** carry the entire output of unoxygenated blood from the right ventricle. Pulmonary arteries and their branches are under low pressure;

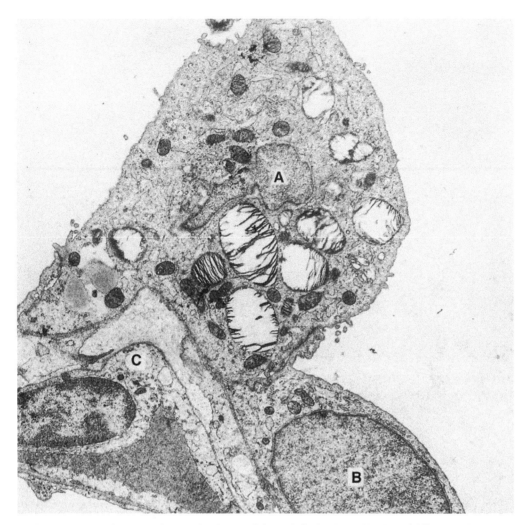

FIGURE 9-22 Electron micrograph of a type II (granular) alveolar epithelial cell (A) containing numerous characteristic lamellar bodies, and a type I (squamous) alveolar epithelial cell (B). Capillary endothelial cell (C) (×8200). (From Tyler WS, Gillespie JR, Nowell JA. Modern functional morphology of the equine lung. Equine Vet J 1971;3:84–94.)

thus, their walls have fewer elastic and collagen fibers and fewer smooth muscle cells than vessels of comparable size in the systemic circulatory system. Pulmonary arteries and the tracheobronchial tree have a common adventitia.

The **bronchial arteries** are under high pressure as a part of the systemic arterial circulatory system. The blood vessels in this system have the same wall structure as those of other systemic arteries of the same size. In all species, the bronchial artery supplies blood to the large bronchi, the major pulmonary vessels, and the pulmonary lymph nodes. Anastomoses between bronchial and pulmonary arterial circulatory systems have been identified in the walls of medium-sized bronchi and bronchioles of horses, cattle, and sheep.

All blood from the lungs is carried back to the heart by **pulmonary veins,** a low-pressure system. The pulmonary veins have thin walls with little smooth muscle in dogs, cats, horses, and goats. Pulmonary veins with large muscle bundles are present in cattle and pigs. In most species, the pulmonary veins are located at the periphery of lobules and course to the hilum in interlobu-

lar septa. In cattle, horses, pigs, and sheep, the pulmonary veins accompany the bronchial tree on the side opposite that of pulmonary arteries.

The **pulmonary lymphatics** begin as lymph capillaries, located throughout the interstitium, except for the interstitium of interalveolar septa. Collecting lymph vessels are found throughout the connective tissue of the lung, with the exception of that surrounding alveoli, alveolar sacs and ducts, and respiratory bronchioles.

Innervation

The innervation is from two sources: the parasympathetic system (via the vagus nerve) and the sympathetic system (via the middle cervical and cervicothoracic ganglia). General visceral afferent sensory fibers from pulmonary tissue are also contained in the vagus nerve. Fibers from vagus nerves intermingle to form a plexus along the walls of the airway tree and the pulmonary vasculature, with ganglia present in the adventitia of large air-

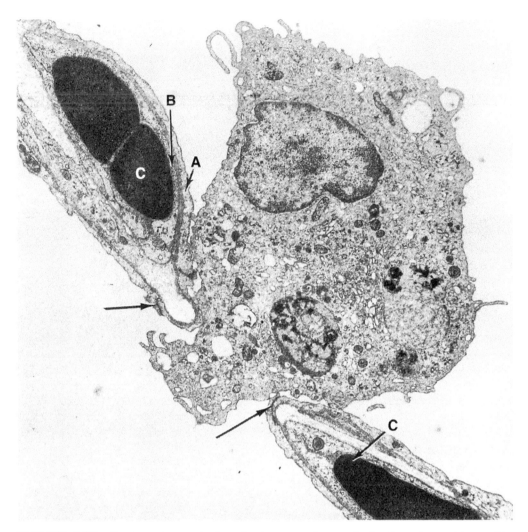

FIGURE 9-23   Electron micrograph of an alveolar macrophage projecting through a septal pore. The macrophage has numerous filopodia, phagosomes, and phagolysosomes. The thin layer of cytoplasm of the type I (squamous) alveolar epithelial cells (A) is separated by a basal lamina from the capillary endothelium (B). Erythrocytes (C) are in the capillary lumen. The dark lines (arrows) are tight junctions between adjacent squamous alveolar epithelial cells (×8100). *(From Tyler WS, Gillespie JR, Nowell JA. Modern functional morphology of the equine lung. Equine Vet J 1971;3:84–94.)*

ways. Individual nerve fibers are distributed irregularly over the wall of arteries, veins, and airways. Free nerve endings are present near glands, within smooth muscle bundles, and in the interalveolar septa.

AVIAN RESPIRATORY SYSTEM

In contrast to the mammalian respiratory system, the respiratory system of birds contains a simpler larynx, a syrinx, only four orders or generations of conducting airways, a compact spongy lung, and air sacs. The highly efficient avian respiratory system comprises lung tissue positioned between conducting airways and air sacs. During inspiration, air is drawn into the nasal cavity and through the lung tissue to the air sacs; during expiration, the reverse occurs. Birds breathe more slowly and deeply than mammals, and unlike that of mammals, the lung volume

of birds remains relatively constant while the volume of their air sacs changes during ventilation.

The nasal cavity is lined by epithelia similar to those of mammals, with stratified squamous epithelium rostrally, olfactory epithelium dorsocaudally, and respiratory epithelium lining most of the remaining areas. In the respiratory epithelium, groups of goblet cells form intraepithelial glands. Large air spaces, the paired infraorbital sinuses, are often clinically involved in respiratory infections; these sinuses, which drain into the nasal cavity, are lined by respiratory epithelium.

The larynx, devoid of vocal folds, produces little sound. The trachea is similar in structure to that in mammals, except that the tracheal cartilages form complete rings encircling the airway; the cartilage rings overlap and interlock with adjacent rings. The trachealis muscle is absent, and intraepithelial mucous glands are numerous (Fig. 9-24). As a result of differences in cartilage structure and smooth muscle content, the trachea of birds, unlike that

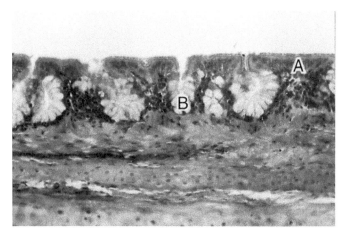

FIGURE 9-24 Epithelium from the trachea of a chicken. Most epithelial cells (A) that line the surface of the conducting airways of birds are ciliated. Intraepithelial mucous glands (B) that open onto the luminal surface. Hematoxylin and eosin (×270).

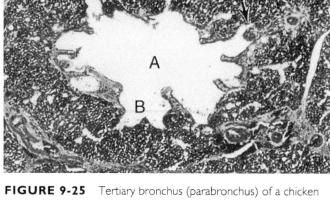

FIGURE 9-25 Tertiary bronchus (parabronchus) of a chicken lung. An atrium (B) opens into the lumen (A) of the tertiary bronchus. Air capillaries (C) open into the atria. Hematoxylin and eosin (×110).

of mammals, does not undergo phasic changes in diameter during breathing.

Vocalization occurs in the avian **syrinx,** a specialized region of the tracheobronchial junction with considerable species-dependent structural variation. The intrasyringeal (tympaniform) membranes, which vibrate during production of sound, are lined by stratified squamous epithelium.

The lungs comprise primary, secondary, and tertiary bronchi, atria, and air capillaries. Extrapulmonary primary bronchi continue as intrapulmonary **primary bronchi** or **mesobronchi,** each of which terminates by opening into an abdominal air sac. Epithelium of the primary bronchi is similar to that of the trachea. The bronchial cartilages are incomplete medially in the proximal portion of the bronchi and are patchlike more distally. **Secondary bronchi** arise from each intrapulmonary primary bronchus, and many open into other air sacs. **Tertiary bronchi** or **parabronchi,** approximately 100 to 150 μm in diameter, interconnect the secondary bronchi. The epithelium varies from respiratory epithelium in the secondary bronchi to simple cuboidal or squamous epithelium in the tertiary bronchi. A network of spiraling bundles of smooth muscle occurs in the lamina propria of the secondary and tertiary bronchi. Numerous small air spaces, or **atria,** open into tertiary bronchi; the projecting tips of the **interatrial septa** contain smooth muscle and are lined by squamous cells (Fig. 9-25).

Gas exchange in the avian lung occurs between blood and **air capillaries.** These capillaries, 5 to 15 μm in diameter, open into the atria. Simple squamous epithelium lines the greater portion of the atria and air capillaries. The epithelial portion of the gas exchange area consists of both type I and type II cells similar to those of mammals; a biphasic fluid lining layer, similar to surfactant of mammals, is also observed in birds.

The terminal **air sacs** are lined by a simple squamous to cuboidal epithelium; epithelial surfaces adjacent to ostia of bronchi are ciliated.

SUGGESTED READINGS

Adams DR, Hotchkiss DK. The canine nasal mucosa. Zentralbl Veterinärmed C Anat Histol Embryol 1983;12:109–125.

Adams DR, Wiekamp MD. The canine vomeronasal organ. J Anat 1984;138:771–787.

Berendsen PB, Ritter AB, DeFouw DO. An ultrastructural morphometric comparison of the peripheral with the hilar air-blood barrier of dog lung. Anat Rec 1984;209:535–540.

Frasca JM, Auerbach O, Parks VR, et al. Electron microscopic observations of the bronchial epithelium of dogs. I. Control dogs. Exp Mol Pathol 1968;9:363–379.

Gladysheva O, Martynova G. The morphofunctional organization of the bovine olfactory epithelium. Gegenbaurs Morphol Jahrb 1982; 128:78.

Gross EA, Morgan KT. Architecture of nasal passages and larynx. In: Parent RA, ed. Comparative Biology of the Normal Lung. Boca Raton: CRC Press, 1991.

Harkema JR. Epithelial cells of the nasal passages. In: Parent RA, ed. Comparative Biology of the Normal Lung. Boca Raton: CRC Press, 1991.

Jacobs VL, Sis RF, Chenoweth PJ, et al. Structure of the bovine vomeronasal complex and its relationships to the palate: tongue manipulation. Acta Anat 1981;110:48–58.

Kay JM. Blood vessels of the lung. In: Parent RA, ed. Comparative Biology of the Normal Lung. Boca Raton: CRC Press, 1991.

Mariassy AT. Epithelial cells of trachea and bronchi. In: Parent RA, ed. Comparative Biology of the Normal Lung. Boca Raton: CRC Press, 1991.

Mariassy AT, Plopper CG. Tracheobronchial epithelium of the sheep. I. Quantitative light microscopic study of epithelial cell abundance and distribution. Anat Rec 1983;205:263–275.

Mariassy AT, Plopper CG. Tracheobronchial epithelium of the sheep. II. Ultrastructural and morphometric analysis of the epithelial secretory types. Anat Rec 1984;209:523–534.

Mariassy AT, Plopper CG, Dungworth DL. Characteristics of bovine lung as observed by scanning electron microscopy. Anat Rec 1975; 183:13–26.

McBride JT. Architecture of the tracheobronchial tree. In: Parent RA, ed. Comparative Biology of the Normal Lung. Boca Raton: CRC Press, 1991.

Mercer RR, Crapo JD. Architecture of the acinus. In: Parent RA, ed. Comparative Biology of the Normal Lung. Boca Raton: CRC Press, 1991.

Pinkerton KE, Gehr P, Crapo JD. Architecture and cellular composition of the air-blood barrier. In: Parent RA, ed. Comparative Biology of the Normal Lung. Boca Raton: CRC Press, 1991.

Plopper CG, Hyde DM. Epithelial cells of bronchioles. In: Parent RA, ed. Comparative Biology of the Normal Lung. Boca Raton: CRC Press, 1991.

Plopper CG, Mariassy AT, Wilson DW, et al. Comparison of nonciliated tracheal epithelial cells in six mammalian species: ultrastructure and population densities. Exp Lung Res 1983;5:281–294.

Reid L, Jones R. Bronchial mucosal cells. Fed Proc 1979;38:191–196.

Robertson B, Van Golds LMG, Batenberg JJ, eds. Pulmonary Surfactant. Amsterdam: Elsevier Science Publishers, 1984.

Tandler B, Sherman JM, Boat TF. Surface architecture of the mucosal epithelium of the cat trachea. I. Cartilaginous portion. Am J Anat 1983;168:119–131.

Tandler B, Sherman JM, Boat TF, et al. Surface architecture of the mucosal epithelium of the cat trachea. II. Structure and dynamics of the membranous portion. Am J Anat 1983;168:133 144.

Tyler WS, Julian MD. Subgross anatomy of lungs, pleura, connective tissue septa, distal airways and structural units. In: Parent RA, ed. Comparative Biology of the Normal Lung. Boca Raton: CRC Press, 1991.

Wysocki CJ. Neurobehavioral evidence for the involvement of the vomeronasal system in mammalian reproduction. Neurosci Biobehav Rev 1979;3:301–341.

Zorychta E, Richardson JB. Innervation of the lung. In: Parent RA, ed. Comparative Biology of the Normal Lung. Boca Raton: CRC Press, 1991.

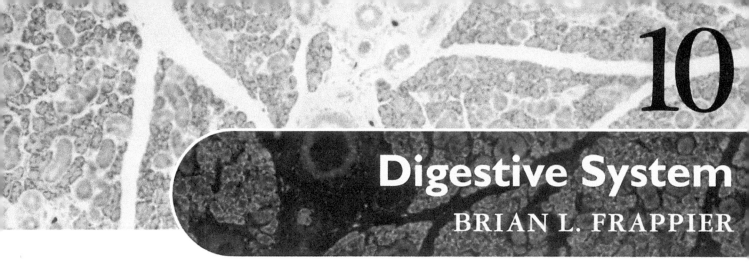

10

Digestive System

BRIAN L. FRAPPIER

General Structure of Tubular Organs
  Tunica Mucosa
  Tela Submucosa
  Tunica Muscularis
  Tunica Serosa/Adventitia
Oral Cavity
  Lips
  Cheeks
  Hard Palate
  Soft Palate
  Tongue
    Special lingual structures
  Teeth
    Brachydont and hypsodont teeth
    Structure
    Development
Salivary Glands
  General Characteristics
  Parotid Salivary Gland
  Mandibular Salivary Gland
  Sublingual Salivary Gland
  Minor Salivary Glands
Pharynx
Esophagus
  Esophagus–Stomach Junction
Stomach
  Nonglandular Region of the Tunica Mucosa
  Glandular Region of the Tunica Mucosa
    Cardiac gland region
    Proper gastric (fundic) gland region
    Pyloric gland region

Species Differences
  Ruminant Stomach
    Rumen
    Reticulum and reticular sulcus
    Omasum
    Abomasum
Small Intestine
  Tunica Mucosa
  Tela Submucosa
  Tunica Muscularis
  Tunica Serosa
  Blood Supply
  General Identifying Features
Large Intestine
  Cecum
  Colon
  Rectum
  Anal Canal
Liver
  Capsule and Stroma
  Parenchyma
  Bile Canaliculi and Bile Ducts
  Blood Supply
  Lymph and Lymph Vessels
  The Classic Liver Lobule—The Anatomic Unit of the Liver
  The Portal Lobule and the Liver Acinus—Functional Units
    of the Liver
Gallbladder
Pancreas
Avian Digestive System

The digestive system consists of a series of tubular organs and associated glands, the main function of which is to break down the ingested food into smaller units that can be absorbed into the circulation and used for the maintenance of the organism.

Morphologic adaptations for specialized functions are characteristic of the digestive systems of the domestic species. Considerable variations in the teeth, stomachs, and large intestines result mainly from the variety of food consumed. For example, the teeth of carnivores are adapted for tearing flesh, whereas those of herbivores are specialized for grinding roughage. The forestomach of ruminants and the cecum and colon of horses reflect structural variations that facilitate the microbial digestion of rough, fibrous food.

Although the large accessory digestive glands—salivary glands, liver, and pancreas—are located outside the tubular portion of the digestive system, they originate as epithelial evaginations from the digestive tube. Their ducts penetrate the walls of the tubular organs and discharge their secretory products into the lumina.

GENERAL STRUCTURE OF TUBULAR ORGANS

A general structural pattern exists for all tubular organs of the digestive, respiratory, urinary, and reproductive systems (Fig. 10-1). Familiarity with this general pattern is helpful in understanding the specific characteristics of each organ. The wall of a typical tubular organ is composed of four coats. Each coat is called either a tunic or a tela. A tela has a delicate weblike structure while a tunic is comprised of denser tissue.

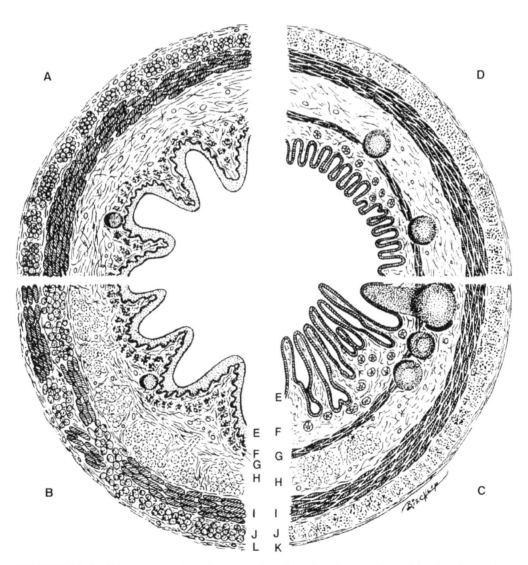

FIGURE 10-1 Schematic drawing of cross sections through various portions of the digestive tract. Esophagus without submucosal glands (**A**). Esophagus with submucosal glands (**B**). Small intestine with and without submucosal glands and with aggregated lymphatic nodules (**C**). Large intestine (**D**). Tunica mucosa: epithelium (E), lamina propria (F), lamina muscularis (G). Tela submucosa (H). Tunica muscularis: circular layer (I), longitudinal layer (J). Tunica serosa (K). Tunica adventitia (L).

Tunica Mucosa

The tunic next to the lumen is the **tunica mucosa**. The tunica mucosa is also referred to as a mucous membrane or simply, the mucosa. A mucosa lines all organs that communicate to the outside of the body and is protected by a layer of **mucus**, a viscous material containing cast-off epithelial cells and leukocytes, in addition to **mucin**, a product of specialized glands. Structures associated with, or located within, the oral cavity, such as the lips, cheeks, and tongue, have a mucosa, even though they are not typical tubular organs. The mucosa is composed of three layers or laminae: an epithelium, a lamina propria, and a lamina muscularis.

The mucosal **epithelium** is constantly present and may consist of any of the types of surface epithelia, depending on the function of the specific organ. The epithelium rests on a basement membrane.

The **lamina propria** is a layer of connective tissue immediately beneath the epithelium. In most organs, this is a loose connective tissue containing fine collagen, elastic, and reticular fibers as well as all of the cells typical of loose connective tissue (see Chapter 3). The lamina propria is also classified as diffuse lymphatic tissue because it contains immunocompetent T and B lymphocytes. The lymphocytes initiate the immune response to injurious agents that have penetrated the epithelium. Blood vessels essential for the nourishment of the epithelium, along with lymph capillaries and nerves, are also present in the lamina propria. In some organs, the lamina propria contains glands that are referred to as **mucosal glands** because they are confined to the mucosa.

The **lamina muscularis** is inconstantly present. It consists of one to three layers of smooth muscle. The lamina muscularis allows independent movement of the mucosa, possibly to facilitate the movement of luminal contents or to assist in the expression of secretions from mucosal glands.

Tela Submucosa

The **tela submucosa**, or simply **submucosa**, is a layer of connective tissue that may contain glands (**submucosal glands**). In most organs, the connective tissue of the submucosa is more dense than that of the lamina propria. Also present are blood vessels, lymph vessels, and the **submucosal (Meissner's) plexus**, a ganglionic nerve plexus of the autonomic nervous system. In organs without a lamina muscularis, the lamina propria and submucosa blend without a clear line of demarcation, forming a propria-submucosa.

Tunica Muscularis

The **tunica muscularis** is the coat of smooth muscle or skeletal muscle responsible for moving the ingesta through the tract and for mixing the ingesta with glandular secretions. Usually, two layers of muscle are present in the tunica muscularis of the tubular organs of the digestive system. The muscle fibers of the inner layer are oriented circularly or in a tightly coiled pattern, whereas those of the outer layer are arranged longitudinally or in a loosely coiled pattern. Between these two layers is a ganglionic nerve plexus of the autonomic nervous system, the **myenteric (Auerbach's) plexus**.

Tunica Serosa/Adventitia

The outermost tunic may be either a tunica serosa or tunica adventitia. The **tunica serosa** (serosa or serous membrane) is composed of a layer of connective tissue with a covering of mesothelium. Organs that border the pleural, pericardial, and peritoneal cavities are covered by a serosa. In each of these locations, the serosa is given a special name: pleura, epicardium, and peritoneum, respectively. All organs not bordering these cavities, such as the cervical part of the esophagus, lack a mesothelium. They have a layer of connective tissue, called a **tunica adventitia**, or simply **adventitia**, which blends with the surrounding fascia (Fig. 10-1).

ORAL CAVITY

Lips

The junction between the integument and the digestive system occurs on the lips, which are covered on the outside by skin and on the inside by a mucosa. Near the **mucocutaneous junction**, the skin is devoid of hair follicles and the epidermis is thicker, with a more elaborate interdigitation with the underlying connective tissue (Fig. 10-2). The mucosa of the lips is covered by stratified squamous epithelium that is keratinized in ruminants and horses, but nonkeratinized in carnivores and pigs. The lamina propria and submucosa blend without a clear line of demarcation. Aggregates of serous or seromucous minor salivary glands, referred to as **labial glands**, are distributed throughout the propria-submucosa. The tunica muscularis consists of skeletal muscle fibers of the orbicularis oris muscle.

Cheeks

The cheeks, like the lips, are composed of an external covering of skin, a middle muscular layer (the buccinator muscle), and an

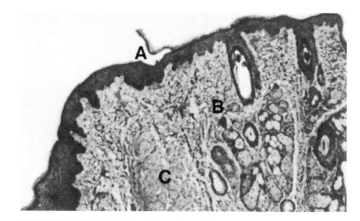

FIGURE 10-2 Lip (cat). Junction of keratinized stratified squamous epithelium of skin and mucosa (A); junction of dermis and lamina propria of lip (B); orbicularis oris muscle (skeletal) of lip (C). Hematoxylin and eosin (×45).

internal mucosa lined by stratified squamous epithelium that may or may not be keratinized, depending on the particular area or species. In ruminants, the mucosa is studded with macroscopic, caudally directed, conical **buccal papillae** that facilitate the prehension and mastication of food (Fig. 10-3). The **buccal glands** are minor salivary glands located in the propria-submucosa and among the skeletal muscle bundles of the cheek, with some secretory units extending into the dermis. The glands are compound tubuloacinar glands and may be serous, mucous, or seromucous, depending on the location and the species.

Hard Palate

The bones of the hard palate are covered by a mucosa, which exhibits a series of transverse ridges called **rugae.** The mucosa is covered by a keratinized stratified squamous epithelium, which is particularly thick in ruminants (Fig. 10-4). The lamina propria has a well-developed papillary layer that blends with the submucosa

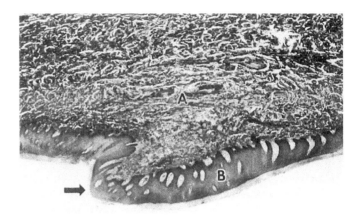

FIGURE 10-4 Hard-palate mucosa (large ruminant). Propria-submucosa (A); keratinized stratified squamous epithelium (B); caudal surface of ruga (arrow). Hematoxylin and eosin (×22).

without an intervening lamina muscularis, forming a propria-submucosa. The propria-submucosa is composed of a dense network of collagen and reticular fibers and blends with the adjacent periosteum. A dense network of capillaries and veins, especially well developed in horses, permeates the propria-submucosa. Branched tubuloacinar mucous and seromucous minor salivary glands (**palatine glands**) are located in the caudal part of the hard palate in all domestic mammals, except pigs. The rostral portion of the mucosa of the hard palate is especially thick in ruminants and forms the dental pad (**pulvinus dentalis**). The dental pad consists of a heavily keratinized stratified squamous epithelium overlying a thick layer of dense irregular connective tissue (Fig. 10-5). The lower (inferior) incisor teeth press against the pad, forming a tight grip on forage during grazing.

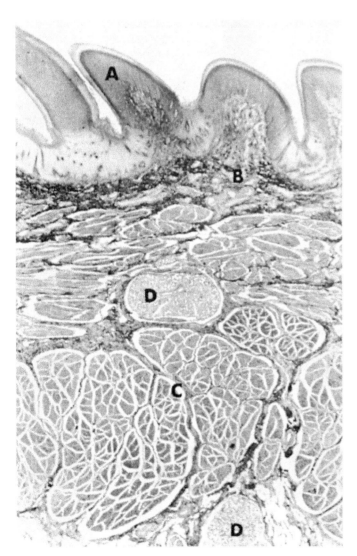

FIGURE 10-3 Cheek (large ruminant). Conical buccal papilla covered with keratinized stratified squamous epithelium (A); lamina propria (B); skeletal muscle (C); buccal glands (D). Hematoxylin and eosin (×12).

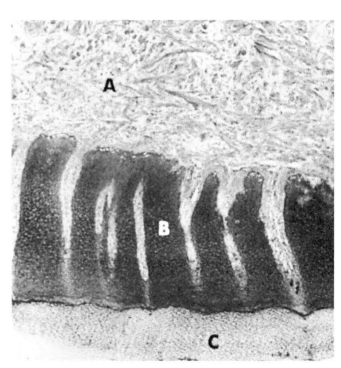

FIGURE 10-5 Dental pad (sheep). Propria-submucosa (A) with papillae interdigitating with stratified squamous epithelium (B); stratum corneum (C). Trichrome (×48).

Soft Palate

The soft palate consists of a core of skeletal muscle fibers with a mucosa covering both surfaces. The oropharyngeal (ventral) surface is covered by a stratified squamous epithelium. The nasopharyngeal (dorsal) surface is covered by a stratified squamous epithelium caudally and a ciliated, pseudostratified columnar epithelium rostrally. Between the two types of epithelium, a narrow transition zone consisting of transitional epithelium is present. The propria-submucosa contains branched tubuloacinar mucous and seromucous **palatine glands.** Lymphatic tissue occurs in the mucosa of both the oropharyngeal and the nasopharyngeal surfaces; in pigs and horses, a macroscopically visible **tonsil** is present on the oropharyngeal surface. Longitudinally oriented skeletal muscle fibers (the palatinus muscle) and connective tissue are located between the two mucous membranes.

Tongue

The tongue is a muscular organ covered by a mucosa. It is important in the prehension, mastication, and deglutition of food.

The epithelium covering the tongue is stratified squamous. It is keratinized and thick on the dorsum, and nonkeratinized and thin on the ventral surface. The dorsum bears numerous macroscopic **lingual papillae.** These papillae differ somewhat in shape, are named according to their morphologic characteristics, and serve either a mechanical or a gustatory function. The filiform, conical, and lenticular papillae are purely mechanical; they facilitate the movement of ingesta within the oral cavity. The fungiform, vallate, and foliate papillae are gustatory; that is, they contain the taste buds, which are responsible for perception of the sense of taste.

The **filiform papillae** are the most numerous type. They are slender, threadlike structures that project above the surface of the tongue and are covered by a keratinized stratified squamous epithelium with a thick stratum corneum. They are supported by a highly vascularized connective tissue core. Equine filiform papillae consist of very fine keratinized threads projecting above the surface (Fig. 10-6). The connective tissue core ends at the base of the thread. In ruminants, a keratinized cone projects above the surface, and the connective tissue core has several secondary papillae. Cats have large papillae with two prominences of unequal size (Fig. 10-7). The caudal prominence is especially large and gives rise to a caudally directed keratinized spine, supported by a more rounded rostral papilla with a thinner stratum corneum. The filiform papillae of dogs may have two or more apices; the caudal apex is largest and has a stratum corneum thicker than that of the other(s) (Fig. 10-8).

Conical papillae occur on the root of the tongue in dogs, cats, and pigs, and on the **torus linguae** of ruminants (see Special Lingual Structures section below). They are larger than the filiform papillae and usually are not highly keratinized. They contain both primary and secondary connective tissue papillae. In pigs, the conical papillae are more correctly referred to as **tonsillar papillae,** because they contain a core of lymphatic tissue and, therefore, collectively constitute the **lingual tonsil.**

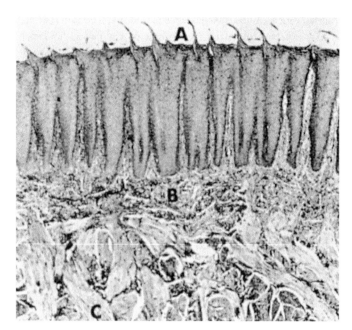

FIGURE 10-6 Tongue (horse). Filiform papillae are keratinized threads extending from the surface of the stratified squamous epithelium on the dorsum of the tongue (A); submucosa propria (B); skeletal muscle (C). Hematoxylin and eosin (×26).

Lenticular papillae are flattened, lens-shaped projections that are found on the torus linguae of ruminants. They are covered by keratinized stratified squamous epithelium and have a core of dense irregular connective tissue.

The **fungiform papillae** are scattered among the filiform papillae and have a dome-shaped upper surface in horses and pigs (Fig. 10-9). The shape is suggestive of a mushroom, and thus the name fungiform. The papillae are covered by a nonkeratinized stratified squamous epithelium containing one or more taste buds on the upper surface. The taste buds are sparse in these papillae in the tongues of horses and cattle, more numerous in those of sheep and pigs, and abundant in those of carnivores and goats. The connective tissue core is rich in blood vessels and nerves.

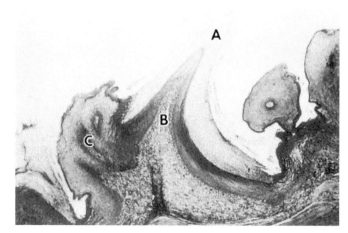

FIGURE 10-7 Tongue (cat). Filiform papilla with a caudally directed keratinized spine arising from the caudal prominence (A); lamina propria (B); supporting rostral papilla (C). Hematoxylin and eosin (×35).

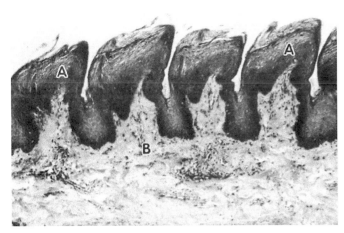

FIGURE 10-8 Tongue (dog). Filiform papillae with caudally directed apices (A); lamina propria (B). Hematoxylin and eosin (×75).

The **vallate papillae** are located on the dorsum of the tongue, just rostral to the root. They are large, flattened structures completely surrounded by an epithelium-lined sulcus (Fig. 10-10). They extend only slightly, if at all, above the lingual surface and are covered by a stratified squamous epithelium. The epithelium on the papillary side of the sulcus contains many taste buds. Groups of serous **gustatory glands** are located deep to the sulcus and have ducts that open into the sulcus at various levels (Fig. 10-10). Mucous glands may also be found beneath the papillae, but their secretory products are emptied directly onto the lingual surface. The connective tissue core is rich in blood vessels and nerves. The number of vallate papillae varies with the species; horses and pigs typically have one pair, carnivores have four to six pairs, and ruminants have eight to 24 pairs.

The **foliate papillae** are parallel folds of the lingual mucosa located on the margin of the tongue just rostral to the palatoglossal arch. Taste buds are located in the epithelium on the sides of the folds. The folds are separated by gustatory sulci (Figs. 10-11 and 10-12). Deep to the sulci lie serous gustatory glands, the ducts of which empty into the sulci. Foliate papillae are absent in ruminants; they are rudimentary and lack taste buds in cats.

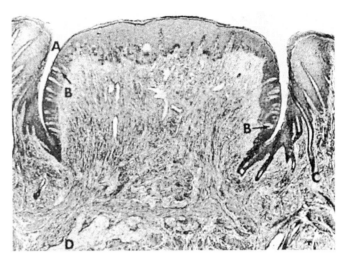

FIGURE 10-10 Tongue (large ruminant). Vertical section of a vallate papilla with a surrounding sulcus (A); taste buds in the epithelium (B); a gustatory gland duct opening into the sulcus (C); gustatory gland (D). Hematoxylin and eosin (×30). *(From Stinson AW, Brown EM. Veterinary histology slide sets. East Lansing, MI: Michigan State University, Instructional Media Center, 1970.)*

The **taste buds** are ellipsoid clusters of specialized epithelial cells embedded in the stratified squamous epithelium of the fungiform, vallate, and foliate papillae of the tongue (Fig. 10-12). They also occur widely dispersed in the soft palate, epiglottis, or other areas of the oral cavity and pharynx. The taste bud consists of a cluster of spindle-shaped epithelial cells that extend from the basement membrane to a small opening, the **taste pore**, at the epithelial surface (Fig. 10-12). In most mammalian species, three cell types have been identified. They are referred to as type I cells, type II cells, and type III cells. Type I and type II cells

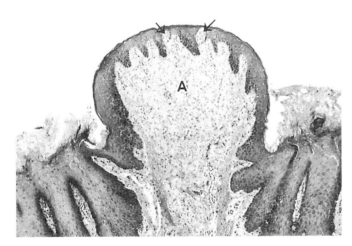

FIGURE 10-9 Tongue (pig). Fungiform papilla (A) with taste buds (arrows). Hematoxylin and eosin (×75).

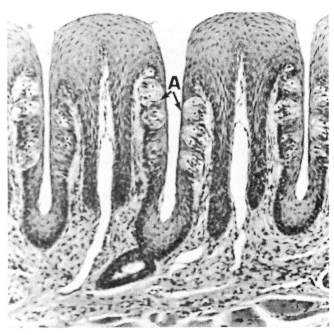

FIGURE 10-11 Tongue (rabbit). Foliate papillae with prominent taste buds (A). Hematoxylin and eosin (×110).

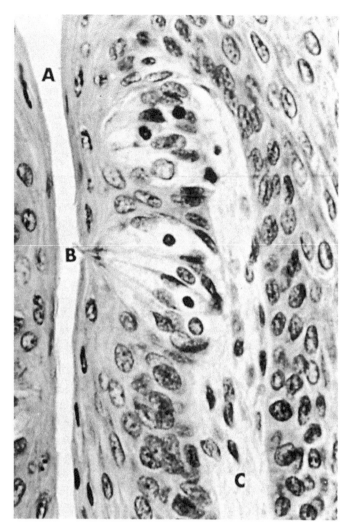

FIGURE 10-12 Taste buds (rabbit). Gustatory sulcus (A); taste pore (B); nonmyelinated nerve fibers (C). Hematoxylin and eosin (×615).

Scattered among the muscle fibers and in the propria-submucosa of the tongue are clusters of seromucous minor salivary glands, which are collectively referred to as the **lingual glands.**

Special Lingual Structures

The **lyssa** of the tongue of carnivores is a cordlike structure enclosed in a dense irregular connective tissue capsule and extends longitudinally, in the midline, near the ventral surface of the apex of the tongue. The lyssa of dogs is filled with white adipose tissue, skeletal muscle, blood vessels, and nerves, but that of cats contains mainly white adipose tissue (Fig. 10-13). The tongue of pigs contains a similar structure. A middorsal fibroelastic cord with hyaline cartilage, skeletal muscle, and white adipose tissue is present in the tongue of horses. It is termed the **dorsal lingual cartilage.**

The ruminant tongue has a large prominence, the **torus linguae,** covering the caudal portion of the dorsum and character-

have apical microvilli that project into the taste pore; type III cells have a club-shaped apex that also projects into the taste pore. The type III cell is characterized by clusters of cytoplasmic vesicles, resembling synaptic vesicles, adjacent to intraepithelial nonmyelinated afferent nerve fibers. Therefore, the type III cell is considered to be the **chemoreceptor (taste) cell,** whereas the type I and type II cells are believed to serve a **sustentacular (supportive)** role. The average life span of the cells is approximately 10 days. New cells are recruited from mitotically dividing cells in the perigemmal region (Latin *gemma,* meaning "bud").

The proper (intrinsic) lingual muscles consist of longitudinally, transversely, and perpendicularly arranged bundles of skeletal muscle (Fig. 10-6). Because of the diverse arrangement of these muscle fibers, the tongue has extensive mobility to facilitate movement of food into and within the oral cavity.

The ventral surface of the tongue is covered by nonkeratinized stratified squamous epithelium. The mucosa contains an abundance of capillaries, arteriovenous anastomoses, and branches of the lingual artery and vein. They participate in thermoregulation.

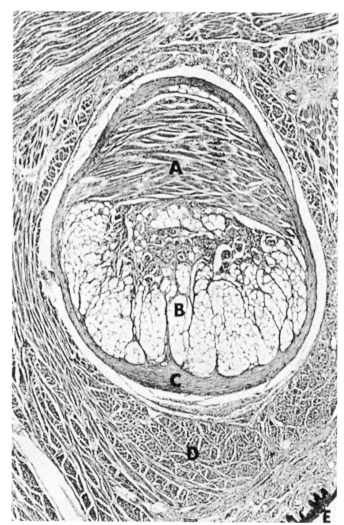

FIGURE 10-13 Lyssa (dog). Skeletal muscle (A); white adipose tissue (B); dense irregular connective tissue capsule (C); intrinsic lingual muscles (D); ventral surface of tongue (E). Hematoxylin and eosin (×28).

ized by a thickened mucosa. Connective tissue papillae extend almost to the surface of the epithelium, which is thicker than that on other regions of the tongue. Lenticular papillae and conical papillae are scattered over the surface of this area.

Teeth

Teeth are highly mineralized structures in the oral cavity that serve domestic mammals during the procuring, cutting, and crushing of food and as weapons of offense and defense. The tooth consists of a highly mineralized outer part surrounding the **pulp cavity,** which contains the **dental pulp,** a core of connective tissue, blood vessels, lymph vessels, and nerves (Fig. 10-14).

Brachydont and Hypsodont Teeth

Two types of teeth occur in the domestic mammals: **brachydont** and **hypsodont.** These teeth differ in their rates of growth and in the arrangement of the layers of mineralized tissue.

Brachydont teeth are short and cease to grow after eruption is completed (Fig. 10-14). They have a **crown** (the portion above the gingiva), a **neck** (the constricted region just below the gingival line), and one or more **roots** embedded in a bony socket called the **alveolus.** Brachydont teeth include all those of carnivores (and human beings), the incisor teeth of ruminants, and the teeth of pigs, except for the canine teeth.

Hypsodont teeth are much longer than brachydont teeth and continue their growth throughout a portion, if not all, of the adult life of the animal (Fig. 10-15). They do not have a crown and neck but, instead, have an elongated **body;** in some species, the roots and neck form only after a delayed period. The tusks of the boar continue to grow throughout life and never develop roots. Hypsodont teeth include all those of horses, the cheek teeth of ruminants, and the canine teeth of pigs.

Structure

The mineralized tissues of the teeth are enamel, dentin, and cementum. Each of these has a separate origin and differs morphologically and in degree of mineralization.

Enamel covers the external surface of the crown of brachydont teeth and lies beneath a layer of cementum in hypsodont teeth. It is the hardest substance in the body, composed of 99% mineral (**hydroxyapatite**) and 1% organic matrix by weight. Histologically, enamel is composed of long, slender rods, **enamel prisms,** held together by **interrod enamel.** Parallel bundles of rods pursue a wavy or oblique course from the inner to the outer surface of the enamel layer (Fig. 10-16). Curved lines (**incremental lines**) appear where these bundles change directions. Enamel

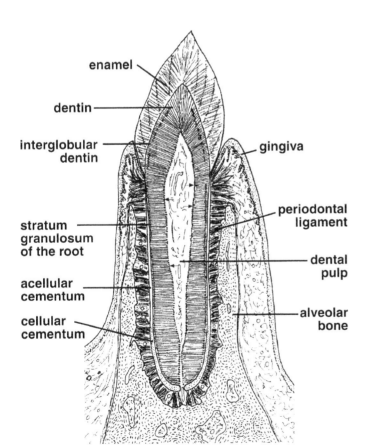

FIGURE 10-14 Schematic drawing of a longitudinal section through a brachydont tooth in situ. The dental pulp fills the pulp cavity of the tooth. The location of the odontoblasts, at the periphery of the dental pulp, is indicated by arrows. (From Dellmann HD. Veterinary Histology: An Outline Text—Atlas. Philadelphia: Lea & Febiger, 1971.)

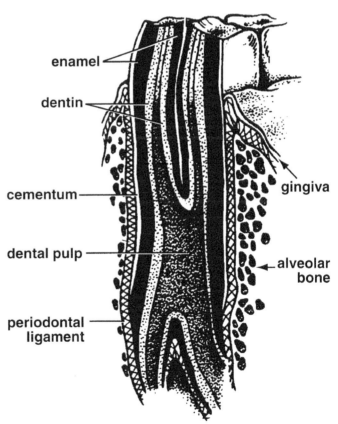

FIGURE 10-15 Schematic drawing of a longitudinal section through a hypsodont tooth in situ.

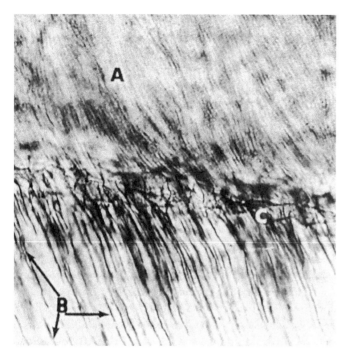

FIGURE 10-16   Ground tooth (human). Junction of enamel (A) and dentin (B) with the odontoblastic processes penetrating the dentinal tubules; interglobular dentin (C). Unstained (×235).

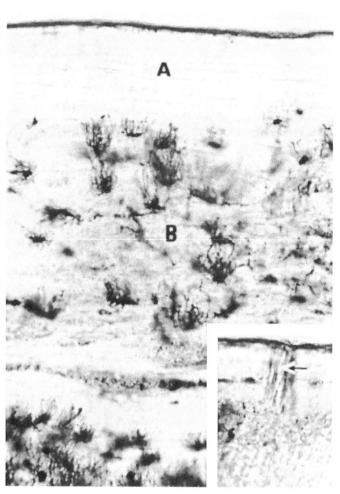

FIGURE 10-17   Ground tooth (human). Lamellae of acellular cementum (A) oriented parallel to the surface of the root. Cellular cementum with cementocytes (B) (×185). Inset: cementoalveolar (Sharpey's) fibers (arrow) embedded in the cementum. Unstained (×185).

is produced by **ameloblasts** that differentiate from the inner enamel epithelium of the enamel organ (see Development section below). Ameloblasts disappear from the fully developed brachydont tooth, but a small population of columnar cells remains at the base of the hypsodont tooth to continue enamel production.

   Cementum resembles bone in all its structural features. **Acellular cementum** is composed of lamellae oriented parallel to the surface of the tooth (Fig. 10-17). **Cellular cementum** has **cementocytes,** which occupy lacunae and canaliculi similar to those of bone. Bundles of collagen fibers, called **cementoalveolar (Sharpey's) fibers,** extend from the alveolar bone into the cementum of the tooth (Fig. 10-17). Collectively, these fibers form the **periodontal ligament,** which anchors the tooth in the alveolus. **Cementoblasts** at the junction of the cementum and the periodontal ligament produce the fibrous matrix of the cementum, and then later mineralize the cementum by depositing hydroxyapatite crystals within the matrix. Once the cementoblasts are surrounded by matrix, they are known as **cementocytes.** The roots of brachydont teeth are covered by a layer of cementum that may slightly overlap the enamel on the neck. Cementum covers the outside surface of equine and ruminant hypsodont teeth, both above and below the gingiva. It begins just above the area at the base of the tooth where the ameloblasts produce enamel. Equine cementum has cementocytes throughout and lacks the brachydont equivalent of acellular cementum. Equine cementum is also unique in that it is vascular and innervated.

   Dentin is a highly mineralized tissue that constitutes the major part of the tooth. It underlies the enamel of the crown and the cementum of the root in brachydont teeth, and also underlies

the enamel of the body in hypsodont teeth. Dentin also forms the wall of the **pulp cavity.** It consists of a matrix of organic material, mainly randomly oriented collagen fibrils and glycoproteins, upon which is deposited minerals including primarily hydroxyapatite with some carbonate, magnesium, and fluoride. The composition is approximately 70% mineral and 30% organic matter. Dentin is produced by a columnar layer of cells, called **odontoblasts,** which are located adjacent to the interior surface of the dentin in the outer layer of the dental pulp. **Odontoblast processes** lie in roughly parallel anastomotic channels, the **dentinal tubules,** that extend from the inner to the outer surface of the dentin. **Peritubular dentin** immediately surrounds the odontoblast processes and is more highly mineralized than **intertubular dentin,** which constitutes the remainder of the dentin. Unmineralized organic material, termed **predentin,** lies between the apex of the cell body of the odontoblasts and the mineralized dentin. **Interglobular dentin** is composed of small, unmineralized or incompletely mineralized areas within the dentin at its periphery, immediately adjacent to the enamel or cementum. These areas are more numerous in the root of the tooth and form the stratum granulosum of the dental root at the dentinocementum junction (Fig. 10-18). The odontoblasts continue to produce dentin throughout the life of the tooth, although at a slower rate after the tooth erupts.

Unlike brachydont teeth, the hypsodont cementum and enamel layers invaginate into the dentin. The invaginations that extend from the occlusal surface down into the tooth are known as **infundibula,** whereas similar invaginations along the sides of the tooth form **enamel plicae.** These invaginations are common in the cheek teeth (premolars and molars) of horses and ruminants. Because enamel is the hardest of the mineralized tissues, it is most resistant to wear and projects above the occlusal surface as sharp **enamel crests;** dentin and cementum are less resistant and wear away more readily. The uneven wearing of the mineralized tissues creates a corrugated surface, which is highly effective for grinding food.

Dental pulp occupies the pulp cavity of the tooth. It is composed of connective-tissue cells and fibers, amorphous ground substance, numerous blood and lymph vessels, and nerves. It resembles embryonic connective tissue in texture, with delicate collagen fibers coursing through the amorphous ground sub-

stance. The most peripheral part of the pulp is the layer of odontoblasts, from which the odontoblast processes extend into the dentinal tubules. Basal processes from the odontoblasts extend into the amorphous ground substance or unite with similar processes from neighboring cells. Because dentin is continuously deposited on the inside of the tooth, the size of the pulp cavity is gradually reduced as the animal ages.

Development

In the embryo, an invagination of the oral ectoderm into the underlying mesenchyme forms the **dental lamina** (Fig. 10-19), a continuous, arch-shaped sheet of epithelial cells extending along the future site of the gingiva in both the upper and lower jaws. Isolated thickenings arise on the labial side of the dental lamina, where

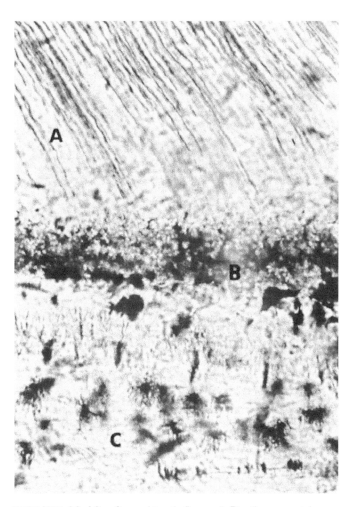

FIGURE 10-18 Ground tooth (human). Dentinocemental junction. Dentin (A) containing dentinal tubules (the dark lines); stratum granulosum of the root (B); cementum (C) with lacunae. Unstained (×185).

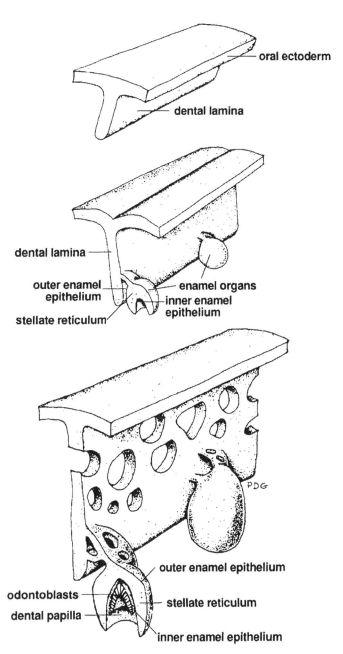

FIGURE 10-19 Stages in the development of the tooth. The dental lamina degenerates (holes) as the teeth mature.

each deciduous and permanent tooth develops. These thickenings are the primordia of the **enamel organ,** which eventually gives rise to the enamel. As the enamel organ develops, it takes on the appearance of an inverted cup, attached to the dental lamina by a thin stem (Figs. 10-19 and 10-20). The epithelial cells lining the inside of the cup form the **inner enamel epithelium,** and those covering the outside form the **outer enamel epithelium.** The epithelial cells between these two layers become stellate and take on the appearance of connective tissue, thus forming the **stellate reticulum** of the enamel organ. The mesenchyme (derived from neural crest ectoderm) enclosed by the cup of the enamel organ condenses to form the **dental papilla,** the future dental pulp. The internal contour of the cup is a replica of the shape of the tooth crown to be produced (Fig. 10-21).

As the enamel organ enlarges, the cells of the inner enamel epithelium take on a distinct columnar shape and differentiate into ameloblasts, which later produce the enamel. The neural crest-derived mesenchymal cells of the dental papilla immediately ad-

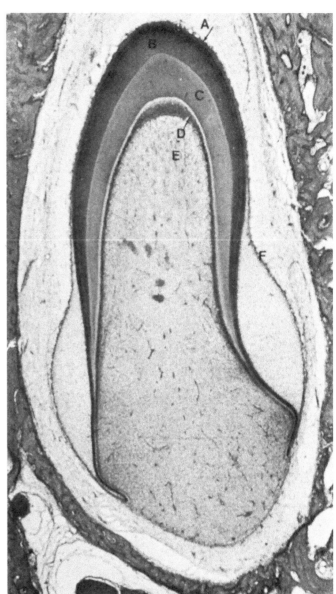

FIGURE 10-21 Developing permanent tooth (dog). Ameloblasts (A); enamel (B); dentin (C); odontoblasts (D); dental pulp (E); outer enamel epithelium (F) (×25). *(Courtesy of A. Hansen.)*

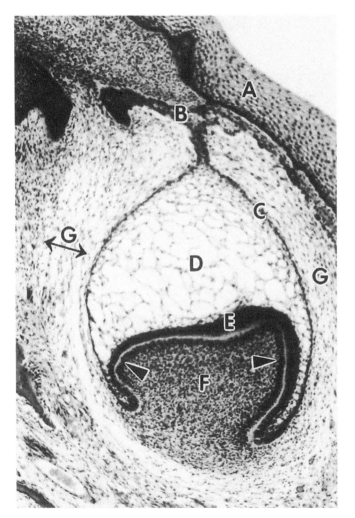

FIGURE 10-20 Developing tooth (dog). Oral ectoderm (A); dental lamina (B); outer enamel epithelium of enamel organ (C); stellate reticulum of enamel organ (D); inner enamel epithelium of enamel organ (E); dental papilla (F) with peripheral odontoblasts (arrowheads); developing dental sac (G). Hematoxylin and eosin (×85).

jacent to the ameloblasts differentiate into odontoblasts, which produce dentin. Dentin is deposited as sheaths of mineralized material around the odontoblast processes that are anchored to the basement membrane of the inner enamel epithelium. As more dentin is produced, the cell body of the odontoblast recedes toward the developing pulp cavity. Shortly after the first dentin is deposited, the ameloblasts begin to produce the enamel matrix (Figs. 10-21 and 10-22). The deposition of the dentin and enamel begins at the apex of the crown and continues down the sides of the crown to the neck of the tooth.

The formation of the root of the tooth begins shortly before eruption. The root is formed by a downward growth of a sheet of cells originating from the enamel organ at the junction of the inner and outer enamel epithelia. This downward-growing sheet of cells, the **epithelial sheath of Hertwig,** surrounds the connective tis-

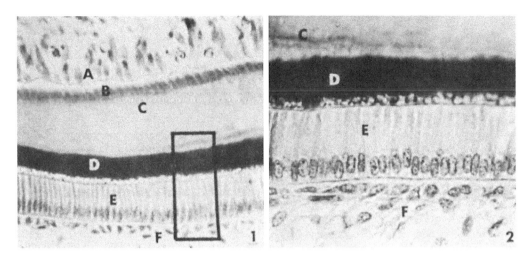

FIGURE 10-22 Developing tooth (dog). **1.** Odontoblasts (A); predentin (B); dentin (C); enamel (D); ameloblasts (E); stellate reticulum (F) (×200). **2.** Area marked in **1.** Trichrome (×300).

sue of the dental papilla and induces the formation of odontoblasts. The dentin of the root is produced by these odontoblasts.

The entire enamel organ and developing tooth are enclosed by the **dental sac,** a thickened connective tissue layer that completely surrounds the developing tooth (Fig. 10-20). In brachydont teeth, the crown erupts through the dental sac, which then collapses against the dentin of the root. The cells of the collapsed dental sac then differentiate into cementoblasts, which deposit a covering of cementum over the roots. In hypsodont teeth, the dental sac collapses before the tooth erupts, and therefore, cementum covers the entire tooth.

SALIVARY GLANDS

General Characteristics

The salivary glands comprise a series of secretory units (glandular epithelium) that originate from the oral ectoderm and grow into the underlying mesoderm as large aggregates of compound glands (see Chapter 2). The **major salivary glands** include the parotid, mandibular, and sublingual glands. The **minor salivary glands** are named according to their location, for example, labial, lingual, buccal, palatine, molar (cats), and zygomatic (carnivores).

Saliva is a mixture of both serous and mucous secretory products of salivary glands. It is important in the moistening of the ingested food and the lubrication of the surface of the upper digestive organs, thus enhancing the flow of ingesta into the stomach. Saliva dissolves water-soluble components of food, thereby facilitating access to the taste buds. Consequently, the sense of taste is somewhat dependent on the saliva. Saliva in domestic mammals is considered to play only a minor role in the digestion of food before it reaches the stomach. Ruminants, however, produce a large volume of saliva, which is an important source of fluids in the rumen.

Parotid Salivary Gland

The parotid salivary gland in domestic mammals is predominantly serous, although occasional isolated mucous secretory

units may occur in dogs and cats. Structurally, it is a compound acinar gland composed of numerous lobules separated by thin connective tissue septa. The lobule consists of acini formed by pyramid-shaped cells with basal nuclei surrounded by basophilic cytoplasm (Fig. 10-23). The apex of each cell is filled with secretory granules, referred to as **zymogen granules,** containing precursors of digestive enzymes. Myoepithelial cells are located between the secretory cells and the basement membrane.

The narrow lumen of the acinus opens into a short **intercalated duct** lined by low cuboidal epithelium (see Fig. 2-18). The intercalated duct joins a large **striated or salivary duct** lined by simple columnar epithelium that is characterized by striations in the basal portion of the cells (see Figs. 2-18 and 10-24). This appearance results from perpendicularly oriented mitochondria within numerous cytoplasmic compartments formed by deep infoldings of the basal cell membrane. This arrangement creates a large basal membrane surface area containing energy-requiring ion pumps located near energy-producing mitochondria, thus facilitating active transport of substances between the cells and the underlying tissue. The striated ducts are easily recognized as the largest structures within the lobule and participate in the secretory process. The striated ducts extend to the edge of the lobule, where they join **interlobular ducts** located in the connective tissue septa between lobules (see Fig. 2-18).

Interlobular ducts are lined by simple columnar epithelium, which changes to stratified columnar epithelium as the ducts become larger and fuse with similar ducts draining other lobules. The interlobular ducts converge to form the parotid duct. The epithelium changes from stratified columnar to stratified squamous where the parotid duct opens into the vestibule of the oral cavity.

Mandibular Salivary Gland

The mandibular salivary gland is a seromucous (mixed) compound tubuloacinar gland. The morphologic structure of the secretory unit is somewhat variable from one species to another but generally consists of a tubular unit with an enlarged terminal acinus. Mucus-secreting cells border the lumen of the tubule and acinus,

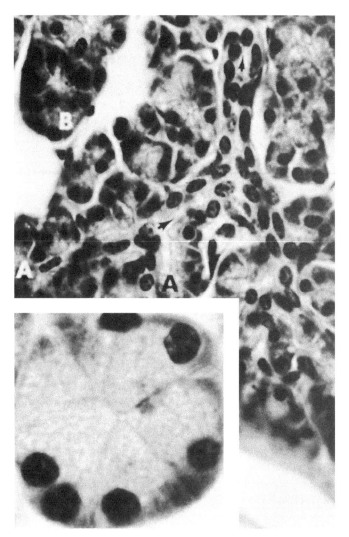

and serous demilunes occur at the periphery (Fig. 10-25). The serous secretory product reaches the lumen through intercellular canaliculi between the mucous cells. Variations in this basic pattern may include separate serous and mucous acini or mucous tubular units with enlarged, serous, acinar end pieces. In dogs and cats, the mucous elements predominate. **Myoepithelial cells** are present around the secretory units (see Fig. 2-19). The duct system is like that of the parotid salivary gland. In the epithelium of the main duct, goblet cells may occur.

Sublingual Salivary Gland

Like the mandibular salivary gland, the sublingual salivary gland is also a seromucous (mixed) compound tubuloacinar gland (Fig. 10-26). The number of mucous acini and serous demilunes and the seromucous nature of their secretory product vary among species. Sublingual glands of cattle, sheep, and pigs are almost entirely mucous, with relatively few serous demilunes. In addition to the typical mucous acini and demilunes, the glands of dogs

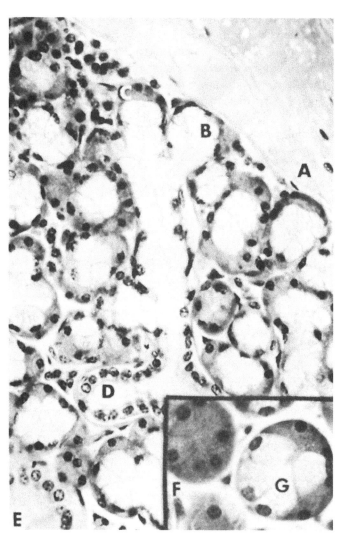

FIGURE 10-23 Parotid salivary gland (horse). Serous acini (A) opening into intercalated ducts (arrows); serous acinus (B). Hematoxylin and eosin (×440). Inset: serous acinus. Hematoxylin and eosin (×1382).

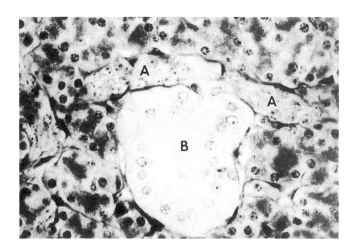

FIGURE 10-24 Parotid salivary gland (horse). Intercalated ducts (A) joining striated duct (B). Hematoxylin and eosin (×425).

FIGURE 10-25 Mandibular salivary gland (horse). Capsule (A); mucous acinus (B) and serous demilunes (C); intercalated duct (D); striated duct (E). Hematoxylin and eosin (×384). Inset: serous acinus (F); mixed acinus (G). Hematoxylin and eosin (×530).

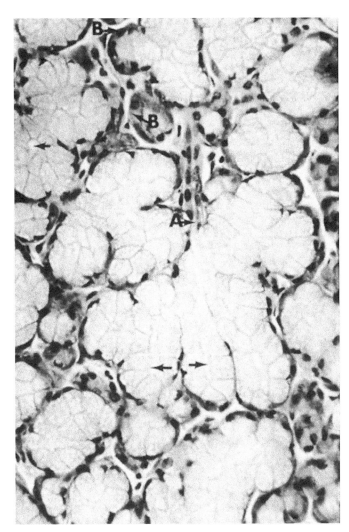

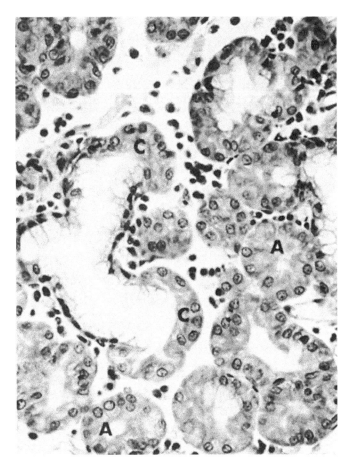

FIGURE 10-27 Sublingual salivary gland (dog). Serous acini (A); serous demilunes (C) on tubular mucous secretory unit. Hematoxylin and eosin (×275).

FIGURE 10-26 Sublingual salivary gland (dog). Mucous acini with lumina (arrows) emptying into intercalated duct (A); serous demilunes (B). Hematoxylin and eosin (×280).

and cats contain clusters of serous acini with periodic acid-Schiff (PAS)–positive granules in their basal portion (Fig. 10-27). The mucous cells form tubular secretory units that connect the serous acini with intercalated ducts. Striated and intercalated ducts are present, but not prominent, in cats and dogs. In horses, ruminants, and pigs, however, they are well developed. The interlobular ducts have, at their origin, a low simple columnar epithelium that increases in height and becomes two-layered in larger ducts. The main duct is lined with stratified cuboidal epithelium, and goblet cells occur in cattle and pigs.

Minor Salivary Glands

Clusters of serous, seromucous, or mucous minor salivary glands, occurring throughout the oral cavity, are generally named according to their location. The **lingual glands** are located in the propria-submucosa and between the intrinsic muscle bundles of the tongue. The **gustatory glands,** associated with the vallate and foliate papillae (Fig. 10-10), are entirely serous and their ducts

open into the sulcus at the base of the papillae. The **labial, buccal, palatine,** and **pharyngeal glands** also contribute mucous and serous secretory products to the saliva. Histologically, the secretory units resemble those of the major salivary glands and occur in a variety of forms (i.e., acinar, tubuloacinar, or tubular). Mucous tubules and acini frequently have serous demilunes associated with them; however, striated ducts are not characteristic of the minor salivary glands. The duct system is lined with simple cuboidal epithelium within the lobules and two-layered cuboidal epithelium in the larger interlobular ducts. The stratification of the duct epithelium increases as it reaches the oral cavity, where it changes to a stratified squamous type.

Among the domestic species, the **zygomatic salivary gland** is present only in carnivores. The parenchyma is composed of long, branched tubuloacinar secretory units that are predominantly mucus-secreting (Fig. 10-28). Intercalated and striated ducts are almost nonexistent. The interlobular and main ducts are similar to those of the other glands.

The **molar salivary gland** of cats is histologically similar to the zygomatic salivary gland. It is a compound tubuloacinar gland that is predominantly mucus-secreting. Intercalated and striated ducts are not present, and the interlobular ducts have a two-layered cuboidal epithelium. Several main ducts empty into the vestibule of the oral cavity opposite the molar teeth.

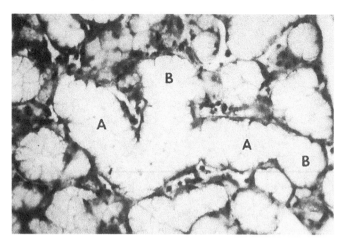

FIGURE 10-28 Zygomatic salivary gland (dog). Mucous tubules (A); mucous acini (B). Hematoxylin and eosin (×300).

PHARYNX

The pharynx connects the oral cavity with the esophagus and the nasal cavity with the larynx. It contains openings to the oral cavity (**oropharynx**), nasal cavity and auditory tubes (**nasopharynx**), and the larynx and esophagus (**laryngopharynx**). A mucosa, a tunica muscularis of skeletal muscle, and an adventitia form the wall. The mucosa is lined by a stratified squamous epithelium, except for a portion of the nasopharynx, which is lined by a ciliated, pseudostratified columnar epithelium. A lamina muscularis is absent. The propria-submucosa contains collagen and elastic fibers intermingled with lymphatic tissue and mucous glands. The tunica muscularis consists entirely of skeletal muscle. The adventitia is dense irregular connective tissue that attaches the pharynx to the surrounding tissue.

ESOPHAGUS

The esophagus (Table 10-1) joins the laryngopharynx with the stomach and contains all the layers of a typical tubular organ of the digestive system (Fig. 10-1). An internal annular fold, the **pharyngoesophageal limen,** marks the junction of the laryngopharynx and esophagus in carnivores.

The mucosa is composed of three layers: a stratified squamous epithelium, a lamina propria, and a lamina muscularis. The degree of keratinization of the stratified squamous epithelium varies with the species. It is usually nonkeratinized in carnivores, slightly keratinized in pigs, more so in horses, and keratinized to a high degree in ruminants. The lamina propria consists largely of a dense feltwork of fine collagen fibers with an abundance of evenly distributed elastic fibers; the esophagus is atypical in that the connective tissue of the lamina propria is more dense than the connective tissue of the submucosa (Fig. 10-29). The lamina muscularis contains only longitudinally oriented smooth muscle bundles. It is absent in the cranial end of the esophagus of pigs and dogs, but cats, horses, and ruminants have isolated smooth muscle bundles near the pharynx that increase in number and become confluent toward the stomach. In pigs, the lamina muscularis is especially well developed in the caudal end, where it is as thick as the outer layer of the tunica muscularis.

TABLE 10-1 Characteristics of the Esophagus

	Horses	Pigs	Cattle	Goats	Sheep	Dogs	Cats
Stratified squamous epithelium[a]	Keratinized	Keratinized	Keratinized	Keratinized	Keratinized	Nonkeratinized	Nonkeratinized
Lamina muscularis	[b]	Absent in cranial part / Highly developed in caudal part	[b]	[b]	[b]	Absent in cranial part / Interrupted in middle part	[b]
Submucosal glands	[c]	Present only in cranial half	[c]	[c]	[c]	Present throughout and extend into stomach	[c]
Tunica muscularis[d]	Cranial two thirds striated / Caudal one third smooth	Cranial part striated / Middle part mixed / Caudal part smooth	Striated throughout and extends into the reticular sulcus			Striated throughout	Cranial part striated / Caudal one third to one fifth smooth
Tunica adventitia	Loose connective tissue cells and fibers with blood and lymph vessels and nerves surround the esophagus. A tunica serosa may be present in the thoracic cavity (mediastinal pleura) or near the stomach (visceral peritoneum).						

[a]Related to character of food: coarse food, highly keratinized; soft food, slightly keratinized to nonkeratinized.
[b]Isolated bundles of smooth muscle near pharynx, increases in thickness near stomach.
[c]Present only at the pharyngoesophageal junction.
[d]Inner circular muscle layer becomes thicker at the cardiac ostium of the stomach (forming the cardiac sphincter muscle), especially in horses.

The tunica muscularis of the esophagus consists of two layers of muscle. In ruminants and dogs, the tunica muscularis consists entirely of skeletal muscle (Fig. 10-29). In horses, skeletal muscle comprises the cranial two thirds of the tunica muscularis but gradually changes to smooth muscle in the caudal third. The tunica muscularis of pigs is similar to that of horses except that the middle third has mixed smooth and skeletal muscle. In cats, the skeletal muscle may extend four fifths of the length of the esophagus before changing to smooth muscle. At the cranial end of the esophagus, there is some interdigitation and spiraling of the two muscle layers, but more caudally, these layers change orientation to inner circular and outer longitudinal. The inner circular muscle layer thickens at the cardiac ostium of the stomach in all domestic mammals, forming the **cardiac sphincter muscle.** This muscle is especially prominent in horses, where it is 10 to 15 mm thick. In ruminants, skeletal muscle extends from the esophagus into the wall of the **reticular sulcus (groove).**

In the cervical part of the esophagus, the tunica muscularis is surrounded by an adventitia, a loose connective tissue containing blood vessels, lymph vessels, and nerves (Fig. 10-29). The thoracic part of the esophagus is largely invested by a serosa (the mediastinal pleura) in most species. In horses, the abdominal part of the esophagus is approximately 2.5 cm in length and is also covered by a serosa (visceral peritoneum). In carnivores, the abdominal part is shorter but is also covered by visceral peritoneum, whereas in other species, the esophagus–stomach junction is at or near the diaphragm, and a mesothelial covering is lacking.

Esophagus–Stomach Junction

The morphologic characteristics of this junction vary considerably among species. In the carnivores, the junction of the stratified squamous epithelium of the esophagus with the simple columnar epithelium of the cardiac gland region is abrupt (Fig. 10-30). In cats, the junction is 3 to 5 mm cranial to the cardiac part (cardia)

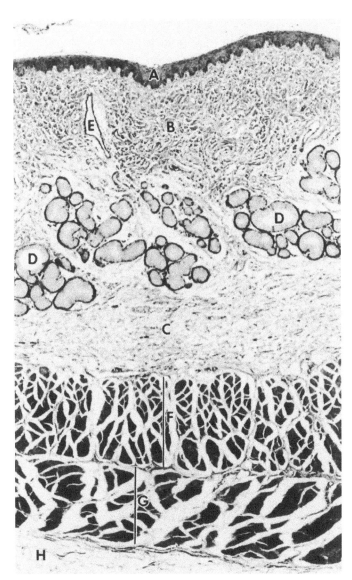

FIGURE 10-29 Esophagus, midcervical region (dog). Nonkeratinized stratified squamous epithelium of the tunica mucosa (A); lamina propria of the tunica mucosa (B); submucosa (C); submucosal glands (D); submucosal gland duct (E); inner circular layer of the tunica muscularis (F); outer longitudinal layer of the tunica muscularis (G); adventitia (H). Note that a lamina muscularis is absent in this region of the canine esophagus. Hematoxylin and eosin (×88).

The submucosa is loose connective tissue containing large, longitudinally oriented arteries, veins, large lymph vessels, and nerves. Seromucous glands containing mucous acini with serous demilunes are present in this layer in pigs and dogs (Fig. 10-29). In pigs, the glands are abundant in the cranial half but do not extend into the caudal half, whereas in dogs, they are present throughout, extending into the cardiac gland region of the stomach. Density of the glands may be as much as four times greater near the stomach (caudally) than at the beginning of the organ (cranially). Glands are present only at the pharyngoesophageal junction in horses, cats, and ruminants. Mixed acini with serous demilunes occur in cattle. The loose nature of the submucosa allows the mucosa of the relaxed esophagus to form longitudinal folds.

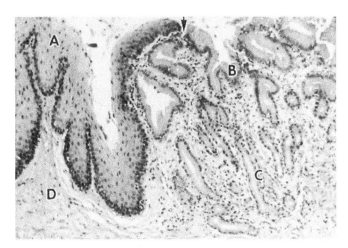

FIGURE 10-30 Esophagus—stomach junction (dog). Epithelium of esophagus (A); epithelium of stomach (B); junction of nonkeratinized stratified squamous epithelium with simple columnar epithelium (arrowhead); cardiac glands (C); lamina propria (D). Hematoxylin and eosin (×180).

of the stomach, whereas in dogs, it is 1 to 2 cm cranial to the cardiac part. In horses and pigs, the stratified squamous epithelium extends throughout the nonglandular portion of the mucosa of the stomach, whereas in ruminants, it lines the entire forestomach. The glands of the esophagus may extend a short distance into the submucosa of the stomach in species in which they are present throughout the length of the esophagus. In species in which the skeletal muscle of the esophagus extends to the stomach (carnivores and ruminants), a gradual change from skeletal to smooth muscle occurs.

STOMACH

The stomach is an enlarged part of the digestive tube specialized for initiating the enzymatic and hydrolytic breakdown of food into digestible nutrients. The tunica muscularis aids in mixing the ingesta with gastric secretions. The stomach is lined exclusively by a glandular mucosa in carnivores, whereas herbivorous animals have, in addition to a glandular region, a nonglandular region of the mucosa lined with stratified squamous epithelium.

The wall of the stomach has all the layers of a typical tubular organ (Fig. 10-31). The mucosa is composed of an epithelium, a lamina propria (of typical loose connective tissue), and a lamina

muscularis. The submucosa contains collagen fibers, white adipose tissue, blood vessels, and the submucosal nerve plexus. The tunica muscularis has three layers: inner oblique, middle circular, and outer longitudinal. The myenteric plexus is located between the middle and outer muscle layers. The serosa is composed of mesothelium overlying a layer of loose connective tissue.

Nonglandular Region of the Tunica Mucosa

The nonglandular region of the mucosa is absent in carnivores and is small in pigs. In horses, the nonglandular region extends a considerable distance from the esophagus and ends at the **margo plicatus**. The nonglandular region reaches its greatest development in the ruminant stomach, where it lines the entire **forestomach** (rumen, reticulum, and omasum) (Fig. 10-32). These parts are described in detail later in this chapter.

The lining epithelium of the nonglandular region of the mucosa is stratified squamous and may be keratinized, depending on species and diet. The lamina propria is composed of typical loose connective tissue. The lamina muscularis is distinct. The junction between the epithelial linings of the nonglandular and glandular regions of the mucosa is abrupt, with stratified squamous epithelium joining simple columnar epithelium.

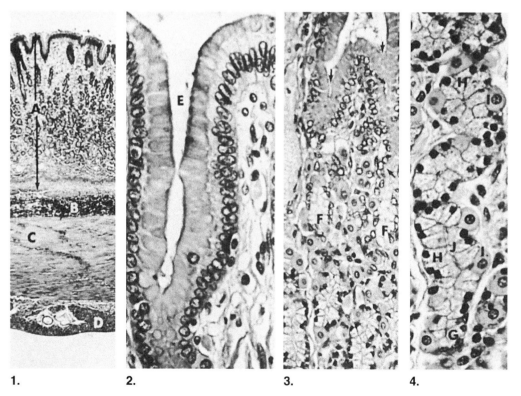

1.   **2.**   **3.**   **4.**

FIGURE 10-31 Proper gastric (fundic) gland region of tunica mucosa, stomach (dog). **1.** Section through proper gastric gland region. Trichrome (×48). **2.** Gastric pit. Hematoxylin and eosin (×450). **3.** Neck of proper gastric gland with mucous neck cells. Hematoxylin and eosin (×210). **4.** Fundus of proper gastric gland with chief and parietal cells. Hematoxylin and eosin (×480). Tunica mucosa (A); tela submucosa (B); circular (C) and longitudinal (D) layers of tunica muscularis; gastric pit (E); gastric gland lumen opening into gastric pit (arrows); mucous neck cells (F); fundus of gastric gland (G); chief cells (H); parietal cells (I); gland lumen (J).

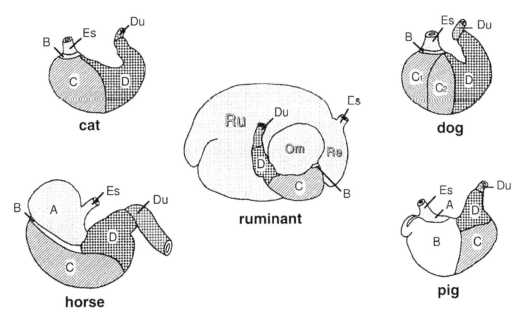

FIGURE 10-32 Schematic drawing illustrating the regions of the gastric tunica mucosa. Nonglandular region of the mucosa lined by stratified squamous epithelium (A), including the rumen (Ru), reticulum (Re), and omasum (Om); cardiac gland region (B); fundic gland region (C), with light (C1) and dark (C2) zones in the dog; pyloric gland region (D); esophagus (Es); duodenum (Du).

Glandular Region of the Tunica Mucosa

The structure of the glandular region of the mucosa conforms to the general pattern described earlier. The mucosa has extensive folds (**gastric folds**), which flatten as the stomach fills. The surface is covered with small invaginations called **gastric pits,** which are continuous with the **gastric glands** and receive their secretory products (Figs. 10-31[2], 10-31[3], and 10-33). The mucosal surface, including the gastric pits, is lined with tall simple columnar epithelial cells, the mucous secretory product of which is released continuously and serves as a protective coat that prevents digestion of the mucosa. The surface epithelial cells have a rapid turnover rate; within approximately 3 to 4 days, they are replaced by cells originating from mitosis in the gastric pit. The gastric glands are densely packed within the lamina propria (Figs. 10-31[3] and 10-33). The loose connective tissue in this area is often difficult to visualize because of the large amount of glandular epithelium. In carnivores, a layer of densely packed collagen fibers called the **stratum compactum** may be interposed between the bases of the gastric glands and the lamina muscularis (Fig. 10-34). The function of this layer may be to limit penetration of the stomach wall by sharp bones in the gastric contents.

The lamina muscularis is relatively thick, usually comprising three layers (Fig. 10-34). Small bundles of smooth muscle cells extend into the lamina propria, coursing between the gastric glands (Fig. 10-33).

The glandular region of the mucosa of the stomach is divided into three distinct smaller regions named according to the various glandular types present: **cardiac, proper gastric (fundic),** and **pyloric.** The extent of the various glandular regions of the mucosa in the domestic mammals is illustrated in Figure 10-32.

Cardiac Gland Region

The cardiac gland region of the mucosa occupies a narrow strip at the junction of the glandular and nonglandular mucosae in all domestic mammals except pigs, in which it covers nearly half the stomach, including most of the **diverticulum ventriculi** (Fig. 10-32). The **cardiac glands** are relatively short, simple, branched, coiled tubular glands that release a mucous secretory product (Fig. 10-35). The cells of the cardiac glands are cuboidal, and the nuclei are located in the basal portion of the cells. The cardiac glands empty into relatively shallow gastric pits (Fig. 10-35). Parietal cells (described below) may occur at the junction of the cardiac and proper gastric (fundic) gland regions.

Proper Gastric (Fundic) Gland Region

The proper gastric (fundic) gland region of the mucosa is well developed in all domestic mammals (Fig. 10-32). In carnivores, it occupies more than one half of the stomach mucosa; in horses, it occupies more than one third; and in pigs, it occupies approximately one fourth. Two thirds of the mucosa of the abomasum in ruminants is occupied by proper gastric glands. Also note in Figure 10-32 that this gland region actually occupies the fundus of the stomach only in dogs and cats, as in human beings; therefore, the term **proper gastric** is used to eliminate confusion as to location within the stomach.

Proper gastric glands are simple, branched, straight tubular glands that extend to the lamina muscularis (Figs. 10-31[4] and 10-33). The gland consists of a short **neck,** a long **body,** and a slightly dilated blind end, the **fundus.** Four structurally and functionally distinct cell types comprise the secretory epithelium of the proper gastric gland: mucous neck cells, chief cells, parietal cells, and endocrine cells.

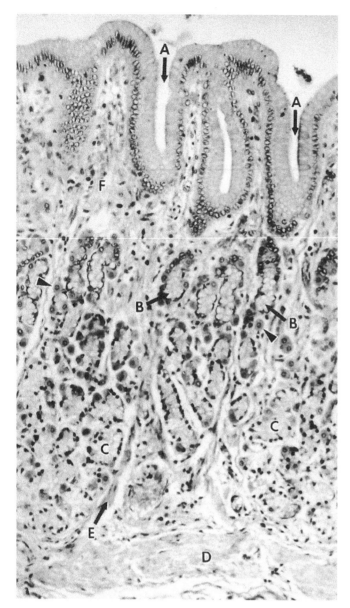

FIGURE 10-33 Proper gastric gland region of tunica mucosa, stomach (dog). Gastric pits (A); mucous neck cells (B); chief cells (C); lamina muscularis (D); smooth muscle cells entering lamina propria (E); lamina propria (F); parietal cells (arrowheads). Hematoxylin and eosin (×180).

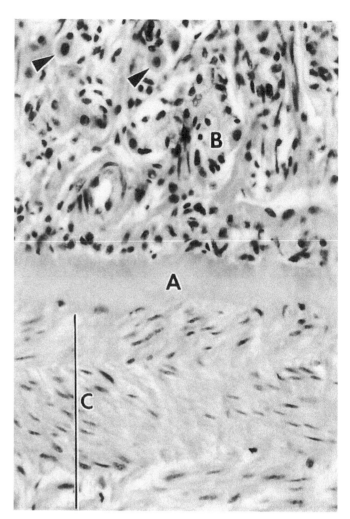

FIGURE 10-34 Proper gastric gland region of tunica mucosa, stomach (cat). Stratum compactum of lamina propria (A); fundus of proper gastric gland (B); lamina muscularis (C); parietal cells (arrowheads). Hematoxylin and eosin (×355).

The **mucous neck cells** occupy the neck of the proper gastric gland (Figs. 10-31[3] and 10-33). They are typical mucous cells, with a flat nucleus located toward the cell base. They appear similar to the mucus-producing surface epithelial cells but have cytoplasm that is more basophilic. In addition, when treated with PAS, the mucous neck cells are intensely positive throughout, whereas the surface cells have PAS-positive material only in the upper two thirds of the cell.

The **chief cells** are the most numerous of the gastric gland cells (Figs. 10-31[4] and 10-33). They are cuboidal or pyramidal, with a spherical nucleus near the base of the cell. The area between the nucleus and the free surface appears lacy owing to clear spaces that remain after fixation. In the living state, zymo-

gen granules occupy these vacuoles and are demonstrable with special fixation and staining. Thus, chief cells are also referred to as zymogen cells. The basal area of the chief cell has an extensive rough endoplasmic reticulum (rER), resulting in a basophilic staining reaction. Chief cells secrete **pepsinogen**, which is transformed into pepsin by hydrochloric acid.

The **parietal cells** are larger and less numerous than the chief cells. They have a tendency to occur singly and are peripheral to the chief cells (Figs. 10-31[4] and 10-33). Usually, only a narrow apex of the cell borders the gland lumen. Frequently, the base of the cell bulges outward from the external surface of the gland. The parietal cell has a spherical nucleus. The cytoplasm stains deeply with eosin and has a granular appearance due to the presence of numerous mitochondria. At the apex, the cell membrane invaginates to form a branching **intracellular canaliculus** that extends toward the center of the cell and communicates with the lumen of the gastric gland. Numerous microvilli of varying lengths project into the canaliculus, thereby providing an extensive surface area associated with the active transport system necessary for the production of free hydrochloric acid. Parietal cells form car-

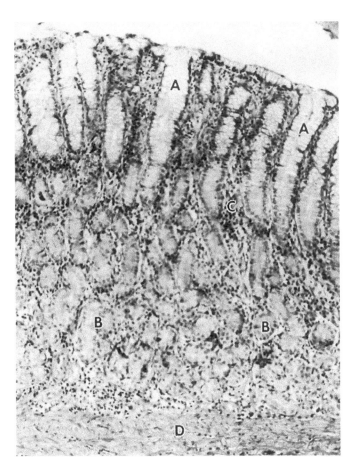

FIGURE 10-35 Cardiac gland region of tunica mucosa, stomach (pig). Gastric pits (A); cardiac glands (B); lamina propria (C); lamina muscularis (D). Hematoxylin and eosin (×80).

bonic acid through the action of the enzyme, carbonic anhydrase. Carbonic acid dissociates into bicarbonate ions, which remain in the cell, and hydrogen ions, which are transported across the cell membrane into the intracellular canaliculus, where they combine with chloride ions. Thus, free hydrochloric acid is formed within the canaliculus and lumen of the gastric gland.

Throughout the glandular regions of the gastric mucosa and continuing into the small and large intestines is a series of **endocrine cells (enteroendocrine cells)** responsible for the production of gastrointestinal hormones, such as gastrin, secretin, cholecystokinin, and gastric inhibitory polypeptide. The hormone is released either into the blood or lymph vascular systems, where it circulates throughout the body or diffuses locally to its target cells (i.e., a paracrine mode of secretion). These cells are difficult to identify in routine hematoxylin and eosin sections and generally appear clear or poorly stained. Many of these cells demonstrate an affinity for silver stains and therefore have been referred to as **argentaffin cells** or **argyrophilic cells** (see Fig. 10-53). Some of these cells can also be demonstrated with potassium dichromate solutions and are therefore referred to as **enterochromaffin cells.** Most frequently, these cells are wedged between the basement membrane and the chief cells and do not reach the surface of the epithelium. Some of these cells, however, do extend to the lumen and are believed to monitor the luminal contents and respond with

the release of hormones. At least 12 different endocrine cell types have been identified by electron microscopy in the gastrointestinal tract. They all have numerous small membrane-bounded granules, mostly within the basal cytoplasm, and also contain relatively little rER and small Golgi complexes. The endocrine cells of the gastrointestinal tract are part of a larger group of cells designated as the **diffuse neuroendocrine system (DNES)** (see Chapter 15).

Pyloric Gland Region

The pyloric gland region occupies approximately one half of the gastric mucosa in carnivores, but only one third of the gastric mucosa in horses and one third of the abomasal mucosa in ruminants. In pigs, the pyloric gland region is small, representing approximately one fourth of the mucosa (Fig. 10-32).

Pyloric glands are simple, branched, coiled tubular glands that are relatively short compared to the other gastric glands (Fig. 10-36). The gastric pits are considerably deeper than those in the cardiac and proper gastric gland regions. The cells of the pyloric glands have the appearance of typical mucus-secreting cells with flat nuclei located at the base of the cell and a lightly stained apical cytoplasm.

At the pylorus–duodenum junction, **submucosal intestinal glands** extend into the submucosa of the pyloric gland region from the duodenum. The middle circular layer of the tunica muscularis thickens at the pylorus to form the **pyloric sphincter muscle,** which causes the submucosa and mucosa to bulge into the lumen. In ruminants and pigs, this protuberance, called the **torus pyloricus,** is especially prominent (Fig. 10-37).

Species Differences

In carnivores, the cardiac gland region is a relatively narrow area, with the proper gastric and pyloric gland regions occupying the remainder of the stomach. In dogs, the proper gastric gland region is divided into two zones. The light zone has a thinner mucosa with deep gastric pits and short tortuous glands that appear in groups and do not reach the lamina muscularis. The dark zone is adjacent to the pyloric gland region and has a thicker mucosa, shallow gastric pits, and proper gastric glands that more closely resemble those of the other species (Fig. 10-32).

The stomach of the pig has a very large cardiac gland region that contains numerous lymphatic nodules in the lamina propria. The parietal cells in the proper gastric gland region tend to occur in clusters.

The stomach of the horse has an extensive nonglandular region of the mucosa that terminates abruptly, forming the **margo plicatus.** The cardiac gland region is almost nonexistent, whereas the proper gastric and pyloric gland regions follow the normal pattern.

Ruminant Stomach

The stomach of ruminants is composed of four structurally distinct parts. The first three parts (the rumen, reticulum, and omasum) are collectively called the **forestomach** or **proventriculus**

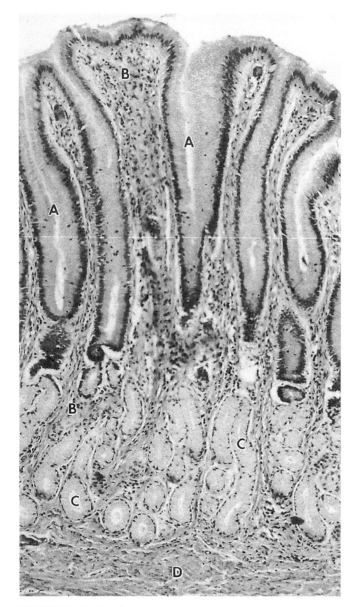

FIGURE 10-36   Pyloric gland region of tunica mucosa, stomach (pig). Gastric pits (A); lamina propria (B); pyloric glands (C); lamina muscularis (D). Hematoxylin and eosin (×80).

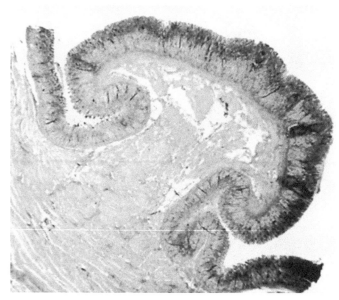

FIGURE 10-37   Torus pyloricus, stomach (pig). Hematoxylin and eosin (×3.7). *(From Dellmann HD. Veterinary Histology: An Outline Text—Atlas. Philadelphia: Lea & Febiger, 1971.)*

masum further degrade the ingesta, along with accompanying microorganisms, to such substances as glucose and amino acids in a manner similar to that of the stomach of nonruminants.

Rumen

The mucosa of the rumen is characterized by small tongue-shaped **papillae** (Figs. 10-38 and 10-39), the size and shape of which vary considerably from one region of the rumen to another. The papillae develop prenatally and remain small as long as the animal is on a milk diet. When roughage is included in the diet and fermentation begins in the rumen, the papillae increase rapidly in size (Fig. 10-39).

The ruminal epithelium is keratinized stratified squamous and performs at least three important functions: protection, metabolism, and absorption (Figs. 10-40 and 10-41). The stratum corneum forms a protective shield against the rough, fibrous ingesta, whereas the deeper strata metabolize short-chain, volatile fatty acids, particularly butyric, acetic, and propionic acids, the chief products of fermentation. Sodium, potassium, ammonia, urea, and many other products are also absorbed from the ruminal contents.

The **stratum corneum** varies in thickness from one to two cells to as many as 10 to 20 cells. Stainable nuclei may or may not be present. The **stratum granulosum** is usually one to three cells thick. The cells are distinctly flattened, and keratohyalin granules are present in the cytoplasm. Cells of the stratum granulosum near the stratum corneum are frequently swollen and are characterized by a pyknotic nucleus surrounded by clear, electron-lucent cytoplasm. The peripheral cytoplasm of these cells contains keratohyalin granules, tonofilaments, and numerous membrane-bounded, electron-dense granules (Fig. 10-41). The **stratum spinosum** consists of polyhedral cells that are slightly larger than the basal cells (Fig. 10-41). The thickness of this layer varies

(Fig. 10-32). The forestomach is lined entirely by a nonglandular mucosa having a keratinized stratified squamous epithelium. The fourth part of the ruminant stomach (the **abomasum**) is lined by a glandular mucosa that is similar to the stomach of other species.

The forestomach is effective in breaking down the coarse, fibrous ingesta into absorbable nutrients by both mechanical and chemical action. The rumen acts as a fermentation vat where a large population of bacteria and protozoa act on the ingesta, thereby producing short-chain, volatile fatty acids, which are then absorbed through the mucosa into the blood. The reticulum and omasum exert a mechanical action on the ingesta that reduces the mass to fine particles. The wall of the omasum is especially well adapted for this function. In addition to fermentation and mechanical activities, considerable absorption occurs across the keratinized stratified squamous epithelium of all three portions of the forestomach. The enzymatic digestive processes in the abo-

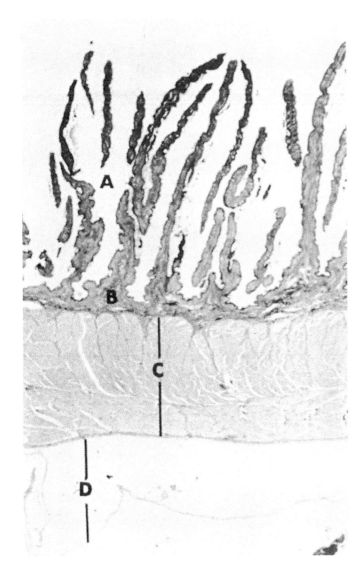

FIGURE 10-38 Rumen (large ruminant). Papillae (A); propria-submucosa (B); tunica muscularis (C); tunica serosa (D). Hematoxylin and eosin (×7). *(From Stinson AW, Brown EM. Veterinary Histology Slide Sets. East Lansing, MI: Michigan State University, Instructional Media Center, 1970.)*

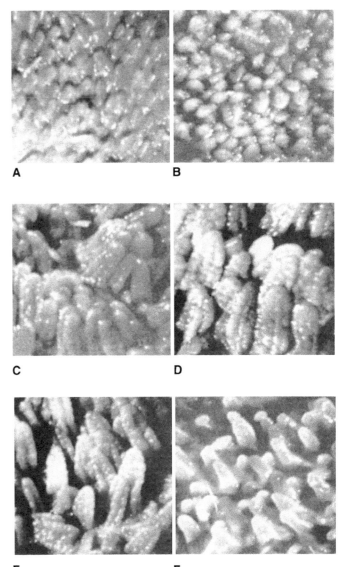

FIGURE 10-39 Changes in ruminal papillae caused by age and diet (same steer) (×2). **A.** Six months of age, milk since birth. Papillae are rudimentary. **B.** Hay and grain for 3 weeks. Papillae are enlarged. **C.** Hay and grain for 2 months. **D.** Hay and grain for 3 months. Papillae have reached maximal length. **E.** After return to milk diet for 3 days. Papillae are smaller. **F.** After return to milk diet for 10 days. Papillae are strikingly reduced. *(From Stinson AW, Brown EM. Veterinary Histology Slide Sets. East Lansing, MI: Michigan State University, Instructional Media Center, 1970.)*

from one to 10 cells. Cytologic features of these cells include numerous mitochondria and ribosomes distributed throughout the cytoplasm. Adjacent cells are connected through numerous desmosomes (Fig. 10-41). The cells of the **stratum basale** are columnar and extend numerous processes to the basement membrane, which greatly increases the basal cell membrane surface area. The cytologic features of the basal cells are similar to those of the stratum spinosum.

The intercellular spaces throughout the entire epithelium are distended to varying degrees. The spaces may be wide and contain flocculent material that is passing through the epithelium (Fig. 10-41), or in other areas, they may be collapsed with no flocculent material present, thus reflecting a period of little or no movement of material across the epithelium.

A lamina muscularis is absent; thus, the lamina propria blends with the submucosa, forming a propria-submucosa. Each

papilla has a core (an extension of the propria-submucosa) containing a dense feltwork of collagen, elastic, and reticular fibers. A dense network of fenestrated capillaries lies just beneath the basement membrane of the epithelium. Near the tunica muscularis, the connective tissue of the propria-submucosa is more loosely arranged. A network of blood vessels and the submucosal nerve plexus is located within this layer.

The tunica muscularis is composed of inner circular and outer longitudinal layers of smooth muscle. The myenteric plexus is located between the layers.

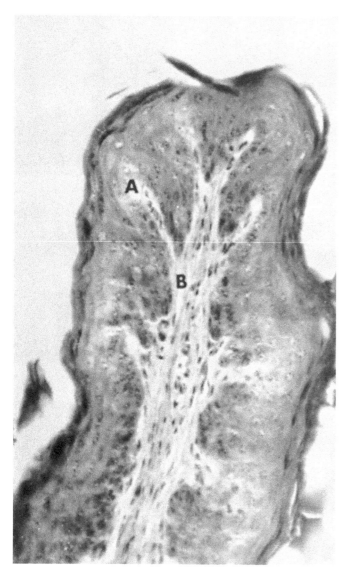

FIGURE 10-40   Tip of ruminal papilla (large ruminant). Keratinized stratified squamous epithelium (A); lamina propria (B). Hematoxylin and eosin (×250). *(From Stinson AW, Brown EM. Veterinary Histology Slide Sets. East Lansing, MI: Michigan State University, Instructional Media Center, 1970.)*

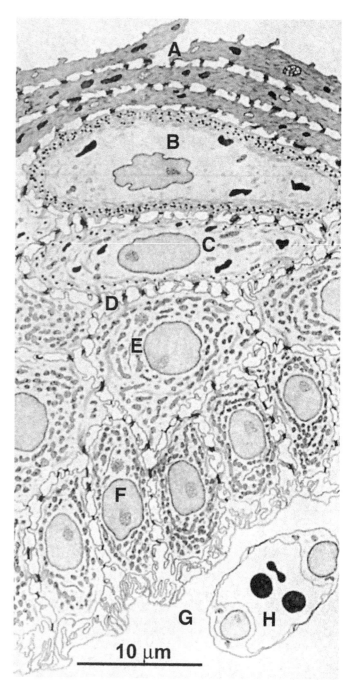

FIGURE 10-41   Drawing from an electron micrograph of ruminal epithelium. Stratum corneum (A); swollen cells of the stratum granulosum (B); flat cells of the stratum granulosum (C); intercellular canaliculi (D); stratum spinosum with desmosomes (E); stratum basale (F); lamina propria (G); capillary in lamina propria (H). *(From Stinson AW, Brown EM. Veterinary Histology Slide Sets. East Lansing, MI: Michigan State University, Instructional Media Center, 1970.)*

The serosa of the rumen is a loose connective tissue covered by a mesothelium. Varying amounts of white adipose tissue, as well as blood vessels, lymph vessels, and nerves, are located in the loose connective tissue of the serosa.

Reticulum and Reticular Sulcus

The reticulum has a mucosa with permanent interconnecting folds, the **reticular crests,** giving it the appearance of a honeycomb (Fig. 10-42). These crests are of two different heights. The taller crests separate the mucosal surface into shallow compartments, the **reticular cells,** which are further divided into smaller areas by the shorter crests. The sides of the crests have vertical ridges, and the mucosa between the crests is covered by conical **reticular papillae** that project into the lumen.

The keratinized stratified squamous epithelium resembles that of the rumen. The propria-submucosa consists predominantly of a feltwork of collagen and elastic fibers. A lamina muscularis is located only in the upper part of the larger reticular crests; therefore, the lamina propria and the submucosa blend imperceptibly (Fig. 10-43). The lamina muscularis is continuous

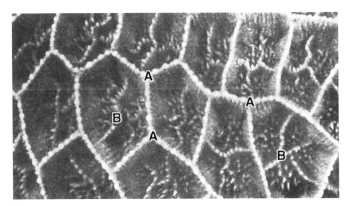

FIGURE 10-42 Surface view of the reticulum mucosa. Primary crests (A) delineating the reticular cells; secondary crests (B). *(Courtesy of A. Hansen.)*

with that of the esophagus. The smooth muscle bundles pass from one crest into another where the crests intersect, thus forming a continuous network of smooth muscle throughout the reticular mucosa.

The tunica muscularis consists of two layers of smooth muscle cells that follow an oblique course and cross at right angles. The serosa is like that of the rumen.

The **reticular sulcus** (groove) begins at the cardiac ostium and passes ventrally on the medial wall of the reticulum to end at the reticulo-omasal ostium. The sulcus is bordered by two thick folds, the labia (lips). The entire sulcus is lined by keratinized stratified squamous epithelium (Fig. 10-44). The propria-submucosa consists predominantly of collagen and elastic fibers. The lamina muscularis, an extension of the esophageal lamina muscularis, is incomplete and is most conspicuous in the labia of the sulcus. It forms a complete layer near the omasum.

The tunica muscularis of the reticular sulcus is composed largely of smooth muscle fibers. Skeletal muscle fibers from the tunica muscularis of the esophagus are present near the cardiac ostium but fade out rapidly in the sulcus. Both longitudinally and transversely oriented smooth muscle fibers are found in the floor of the sulcus, whereas the labia contain mainly longitudinally oriented smooth muscle fibers. The longitudinal muscle fibers in the labia form a loop around the cardiac ostium corresponding to the cardiac loop of animals with simple stomachs. At the ventral end of the reticular sulcus, the muscle fibers pass into the sphincter of the reticulo-omasal ostium. In the young animal, the smooth muscle layers of the labia contract reflexly during suckling. As a result, the edges of the labia come together to create a channel that allows milk to bypass the reticulum and rumen. The milk passes through a very short omasal groove directly into the abomasum.

Omasum

The omasum is nearly filled with approximately 100 longitudinal folds, the **laminae,** that arise from the internal surface of the greater curvature and sides of the organ (Fig. 10-45). The largest laminae, approximately 12 in number, have a thick, concave, free edge that reaches to within a short distance of the lesser curvature.

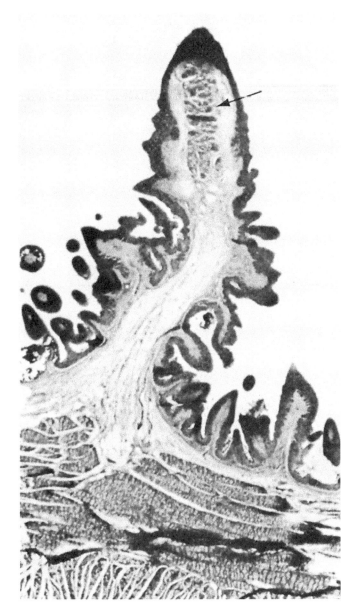

FIGURE 10-43 Reticulum (large ruminant). Cross section through a primary crest with condensed lamina muscularis (arrow) in the upper portion. Hematoxylin and eosin (×9.5). *(From Dellmann HD. Veterinary Histology: An Outline Text—Atlas. Philadelphia: Lea & Febiger, 1971.)*

Second, third, fourth, and fifth orders of shorter laminae progressively decrease in length. The omasal contents are pressed into thin layers in the narrow spaces between the laminae (**interlaminar recesses**) and are reduced to a fine pulp by the numerous rounded, horny **omasal papillae** that stud the surface of the mucosa. The papillae are directed so that the movement of the laminae works the solid contents from the reticulo-omasal ostium into the interlaminar recesses and out at the omaso-abomasal ostium.

The lining is keratinized stratified squamous epithelium, and the aglandular lamina propria contains a dense subepithelial capillary network. A lamina muscularis forms a thick layer just beneath the lamina propria on both sides of the laminae. The submucosa is very thin.

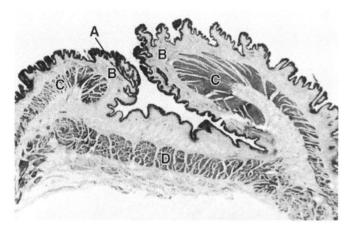

FIGURE 10-44 Cross section of the reticular sulcus (large ruminant). Keratinized stratified squamous epithelium covering the reticular papillae (A); lamina propria blending with the submucosa between scattered small bundles of the lamina muscularis (B); longitudinal musculature of the labia (C); transverse musculature of the floor (D). Hematoxylin and eosin (×12). *(From Dellmann HD. Veterinary Histology: An Outline Text—Atlas. Philadelphia: Lea & Febiger, 1971.)*

The tunica muscularis is composed of a thin, outer longitudinal layer and a thicker, inner circular layer of smooth muscle. The innermost fibers of the circular layer are continued into the large omasal laminae (first through third orders) as the intermediate muscle sheet (Fig. 10-46).

Abomasum

The omaso-abomasal ostium is marked by two mucosal folds, the **vela abomasica,** where the epithelium changes abruptly from keratinized stratified squamous to simple columnar. In cattle, this change is on the apex of the folds, whereas in small ruminants, the change occurs on the omasal side. The lamina propria becomes less dense on the abomasal side of the folds and frequently exhibits a lymphatic nodule beneath the epithelial junction. The mucosa of the abomasum has all the characteristic glandular regions of the stomach described previously (Fig. 10-32).

SMALL INTESTINE

The small intestine is divided into three parts: the **duodenum, jejunum,** and **ileum.** Intestinal digestion, or reduction of food to an absorbable form, begins when the contents from the stomach are acted on by the pancreatic secretions, bile, and intestinal secretions, and it continues throughout the length of the small intestine.

The digestive and absorptive functions of the small intestine are facilitated by several specialized structures. The digestive functions require voluminous amounts of digestive enzymes in addition to a copious supply of mucus to protect the lining cells from mechanical injury and irritating compounds. The enzymes originate from the columnar absorptive cells and the pancreas. The enzymes

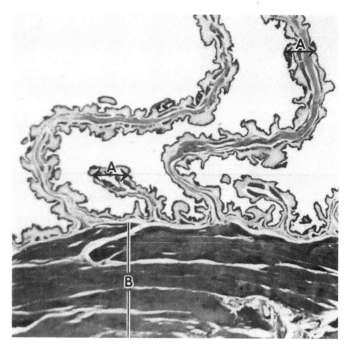

FIGURE 10-45 Omasum (large ruminant). Portion of the wall including laminae of different sizes (A); tunica muscularis (B). Large laminae are penetrated by an extension of the tunica muscularis, whereas the smaller laminae have muscle originating from the lamina muscularis only. Hematoxylin and eosin (×6.5).

produced by the columnar absorptive cells are membrane-bound at the microvillous luminal surface, while those produced by the pancreas mix freely with the luminal contents. Mucus is produced by submucosal glands in the small intestine (Figs. 10-47 and 10-48) and by goblet cells, which are intermingled with the columnar absorptive cells throughout the entire intestine (Figs. 10-49 and 10-50).

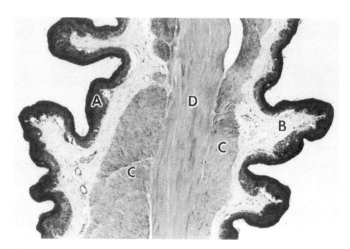

FIGURE 10-46 Omasum (large ruminant). Portion of a large lamina containing three layers of muscle. Keratinized stratified squamous epithelium (A); lamina propria (B); lamina muscularis (C); extension of inner circular layer of tunica muscularis (D). Hematoxylin and eosin (×47).

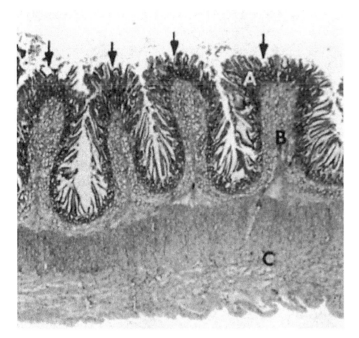

FIGURE 10-47 Longitudinal section of the duodenum, large ruminant. Circular folds (plicae circulares) (arrows). Mucosa (A); submucosal glands (B); tunica muscularis (C). Hematoxylin and eosin (×42).

The efficiency of the absorptive function is enhanced by three structural features that increase the surface area exposed to the intestinal contents: (1) the upper two thirds of the small intestine has circularly disposed mucosal folds (**plicae circulares**) extending approximately two thirds of the way around the lumen. In ruminants, these folds are permanent, but in all other domestic mammals, they disappear when the organ is distended (Fig. 10-47); (2) the surface of the mucosa is covered with finger-like projections, the intestinal **villi** (Figs. 10-49 and 10-51). The villi vary in length, depending on the region of the small intestine and the species. They are long and slender in carnivores and short and wide in cattle; and (3) microvilli are present on the free surface of the simple columnar epithelial cells of the villi (Fig. 10-50).

Tunica Mucosa

The mucosa includes the lining epithelium, a lamina propria with glands, and a lamina muscularis. The villi are mucosal projections and are the most characteristic feature of the small intestine. The **intestinal glands (crypts of Lieberkühn),** which open between the bases of the villi, penetrate the mucosa as far as the lamina muscularis. These simple tubular glands are sometimes referred to simply as mucosal glands (Fig. 10-48).

The lumen of the small intestine is lined by a simple columnar epithelium containing numerous goblet cells interspersed among columnar absorptive cells (Fig. 10-50). Junctional complexes, located between the epithelial cells at the luminal surface, prevent the fluid of the intestinal contents from diffusing into

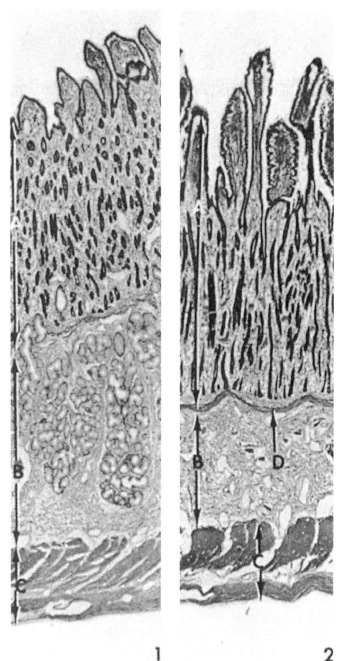

1 **2**

FIGURE 10-48 Duodenum (dog). **1.** Area near pylorus with submucosal glands. **2.** More caudal area without submucosal glands. Tunica mucosa with villi and intestinal (mucosal) glands (A); tela submucosa (B); tunica muscularis (C); lamina muscularis (D). Hematoxylin and eosin (×28). *(From Adam WS, Calhoun ML, Smith EM, et al. Microscopic Anatomy of the Dog: A Photographic Atlas. Springfield, IL: Charles C. Thomas, 1970.)*

the lamina propria without going through the cells. The columnar **absorptive cells** have ovoid nuclei situated near the cell base and prominent microvilli that form a striated border. In electron micrographs, mitochondria are seen near the nucleus and in the basal region (Fig. 10-50). The apical cytoplasm contains a terminal web and extensive smooth endoplasmic reticulum (sER) necessary for the synthesis of triglycerides. A prominent supranuclear

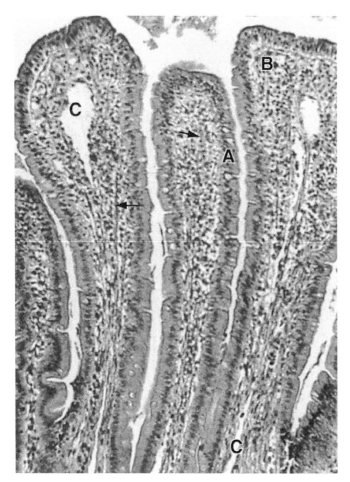

FIGURE 10-49 Villi of the small intestine (dog). Simple columnar epithelium with goblet cells (A); lamina propria (B); lymphatic capillary (lacteal) (C); smooth muscle (arrows). Hematoxylin and eosin (×115). *(From Titkemeyer CW, Calhoun ML. A comparative study of the structure of the small intestine of domestic animals. Am J Vet Res 1955;16:152.)*

Golgi complex functions in digestive enzyme secretion as well as in the transformation of emulsified fats into chylomicrons, small droplets of fat transported by the blood. Free ribosomes and rER are located in the basal part of the cell.

Goblet cells are dispersed among the columnar absorptive cells (Fig. 10-50). As **mucinogen** is produced within the cell, the apical portion of the cell becomes distended, mucinogen droplets accumulate, and the nucleus and remaining cytoplasm are pushed into the narrow cell base that rests on the basement membrane (Fig. 10-50). (For more details, see Chapter 2.) The number of goblet cells is decreased at the tips of the villi; however, the density of the goblet cells is two to three times greater in the ileum than in the duodenum.

The simple tubular **intestinal glands (crypts of Lieberkühn)** are lined by a variety of cell types. The principal cell type of the intestinal glands is the **undifferentiated columnar cell.** These cells multiply, differentiate, and migrate onto the villus, giving rise to the columnar absorptive cells and the goblet cells. They are pushed toward the tip of the villus by succeeding cells, where

they slough off into the lumen. Because of this continuous cell renewal, many mitotic figures occur among the cells lining the glands. The mitotic activity is constant and bears no relation to the amount of ingesta or enzyme activity. The epithelium is renewed approximately every 2 to 3 days.

Near the base of the intestinal glands, **acidophilic granular cells (of Paneth)** are present in ruminants and horses (Fig. 10-52). They are pyramid-shaped cells with prominent spherical, acidophilic granules located between the nucleus and the cell apex. The acidophilic granular cells have all the characteristics of enzyme-producing cells, and substantial evidence shows that they produce **peptidases,** which hydrolyze peptide bonds, and **lysozyme,** an antibacterial compound. These cells also contain zinc, which has been reported to be important in the activation of peptidases. **Enteroendocrine cells** are also present in the intestinal glands and were described earlier in the Proper Gastric (Fundic) Gland Region section (Fig. 10-53).

The lamina propria forms the cores of the villi and surrounds the intestinal glands. It is composed of loose connective tissue with a prominent reticular fiber framework. Within this extensive fiber network are blood and lymph vessels, leukocytes, fibrocytes, smooth muscle cells, plasma cells, and mast cells. **Globule leukocytes** are found in the intestinal mucosa of most domestic species. They contain large eosinophilic globular material surrounding a small nucleus. Their function is unknown. Diffuse lymphatic tissue and solitary lymphatic nodules are present throughout the lamina propria of the small intestine. The number of lymphatic nodules increases toward the ileum. A **stratum compactum** similar to that found in the stomach may be found between the bases of the intestinal glands and the lamina muscularis of carnivores.

A single lymphatic capillary, the **lacteal,** is located in the center of the lamina propria within the villus (Fig. 10-49). This vessel has a blind terminal end at the tip of the villus and is the origin of the lymph vessels that form a plexus at the bases of the villi. This basal plexus gives rise to a larger plexus surrounding the intestinal glands and the lymphatic nodules. Longitudinally oriented smooth muscle cells that originate from the lamina muscularis extend to the tip of the villus (Fig. 10-49). Contraction of these muscle cells causes the villus to shorten and undoubtedly is responsible for lateral movements as well. Muscle contraction also aids in pumping the lymph out of the lacteal into the plexus below. A single arteriole from an arterial plexus in the submucosa penetrates the lamina muscularis and courses into the villus, where it forms an arteriovenular loop and a capillary network immediately beneath the surface epithelium. As a result of digestive activity, the vascular network becomes engorged with blood, causing the villus to lengthen. During muscular contraction, the blood is pumped out as the villus shortens. Thus, the villi act as pumping stations for moving blood and lymph into the general circulation.

The lamina muscularis is composed of inner circular and outer longitudinal layers of smooth muscle that tend to be thin and incomplete, except in dogs. The lamina muscularis may vary with the species, the individual animal, and the region.

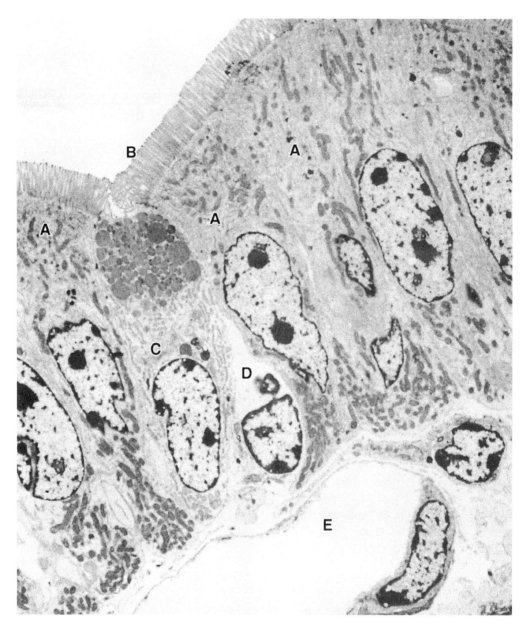

FIGURE 10-50 Transmission electron micrograph of jejunum surface epithelium (calf). Simple columnar epithelial cells (A) with microvilli (B). One goblet cell (C) and a migrating lymphocyte (D) are also present. Immediately below the epithelium is a capillary (E) (×5000). *(Courtesy of J. F. Pohlenz.)*

Tela Submucosa

The submucosa is a layer of connective tissue that is more dense than that of the lamina propria. Tubuloalveolar **submucosal glands (Brunner's glands),** located within this connective tissue, open into the base of the intestinal mucosal glands (Fig. 10-48). The submucosal glands are mucous in dogs and ruminants, serous in pigs and horses, and seromucous in cats. The serous (protein-aceous) or mucous secretory product of these glands lubricates the surface epithelium and provides protection from the acidic gastric chyme. The glands are present in all domestic mammals, but their distribution varies with the species. For example, they are confined to the proximal portion of the duodenum in dogs, whereas in horses, they extend well into the jejunum.

Solitary (isolated) lymphatic nodules are present in the submucosa throughout the small intestine. Large **aggregated lymphatic nodules (Peyer's patches)** occur in all three segments of the small intestine, but they are usually considered to be more characteristic of the ileum (Figs. 10-54 and 10-55). These masses of lymphatic tissue can be located grossly, except in cats, because they create well-delineated elevations of the mucosal surface. Aggregated lymphatic nodules are largest in cattle and most numerous in horses. The intestinal glands may extend into the submucosa in areas of the small intestine where the lamina muscularis is disrupted by the aggregated lymphatic nodules. (See Chapter 8 for details on this gut-associated lymphatic tissue.)

The submucosa also contains the submucosal nerve plexus. Nerve fibers from this plexus extend into the villi.

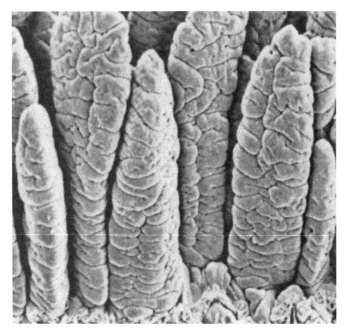

FIGURE 10-51   Scanning electron micrograph of intestinal villi, ileum (calf). These villi are in a contracted state (×85). *(Courtesy of J. F. Pohlenz.)*

Tunica Muscularis

In all species, the tunica muscularis of the small intestine consists of inner circular and outer longitudinal smooth muscle layers. The tunica muscularis is thickest in horses, in which the two layers are nearly equal in thickness. The connective tissue between the two muscle layers contains the myenteric plexus.

Tunica Serosa

A serosa covers the entire small intestine. It consists of a layer of loose connective tissue covered by mesothelium.

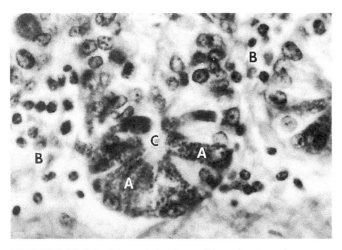

FIGURE 10-52   Mucosal glands, small intestine (horse). Acidophilic granular cells (of Paneth) (A) in the base of an intestinal mucosal gland; lamina propria (B); lumen of intestinal mucosal gland (C). Hematoxylin and eosin (×560).

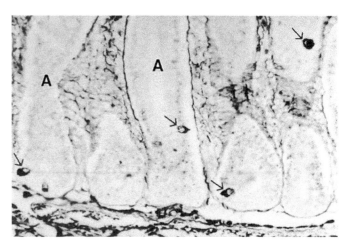

FIGURE 10-53   Mucosal glands, small intestine (cat). Lumen of intestinal mucosal gland (A); enteroendocrine cells (arrows). Silver stain (×320).

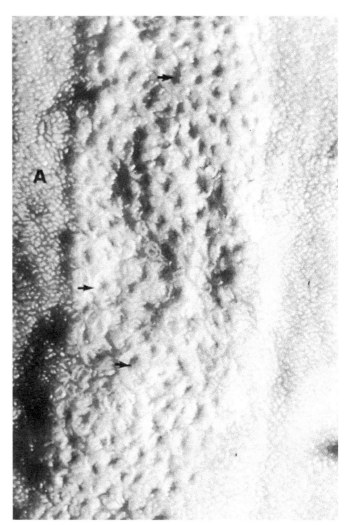

FIGURE 10-54   Mucosa of small intestine with aggregated lymphatic nodules (pig). Villi (A); surface depressions over lymphatic nodules (arrows) (×6). *(From Titkemeyer CW, Calhoun ML. A comparative study of the structure of the small intestine of domestic animals. Am J Vet Res 1955;16:152.)*

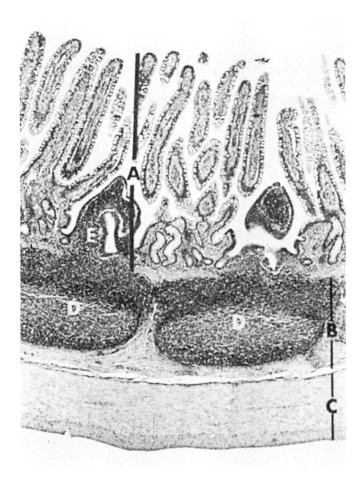

FIGURE 10-55 Ileum (cat). Tunica mucosa (A); submucosa (B); tunica muscularis (C); aggregated lymphatic nodules (D); dome (E) (see Chapter 8). Hematoxylin and eosin (×48).

digestive process is inactive, these AV anastomoses are open and a partial bypass of the villus circulation is created.

General Identifying Features

The various regions of the small intestine in the domestic mammals are not clearly defined microscopically, as they are in human beings. For example, the submucosal glands do not extend the full length of the duodenum in sheep, goats, and carnivores, whereas in horses, cattle, and pigs, these glands extend into the jejunum. Likewise, the aggregated lymphatic nodules (Peyer's patches), often considered an identifying feature of the ileum, may be seen anywhere along the small intestine of domestic mammals.

Because the length of the villi varies with physiologic activities and with species, it is not a reliable characteristic for the identification of the various segments.

LARGE INTESTINE

The large intestine is composed of the cecum, colon, rectum, and anal canal. It is a site for microbial action on the ingesta; absorption of water, vitamins, and electrolytes; and secretion of mucus. Many gross and functional variations in the large intestine relate to the necessity of breaking down the large masses of cellulose-containing material consumed by the herbivores. However, despite gross anatomic differences, the cecum, colon, and rectum are difficult to differentiate in histologic sections. Characteristics common to these three segments of the large intestine are the absence of villi; longer, less-coiled, simple tubular intestinal glands with many goblet cells (Fig. 10-56); the absence of acidophilic

Blood Supply

Branches of the celiac and cranial mesenteric arteries, coursing in the mesoduodenum and mesentery (mesojejunum and mesoileum), penetrate the tunica muscularis along the line of mesenteric attachment. These arteries give off branches to supply the tunica muscularis and continue into the submucosa, where they form a submucosal arterial plexus. The plexus gives rise to short arterioles, which supply capillary beds around the lamina muscularis and intestinal (mucosal) glands, and long arterioles, which extend to the tips of the villi. In the villus, the single arteriole supplies a capillary network and continues to the tip of the villus, where it is continuous with a venule, forming an arteriovenular loop. Venules from the villi and the periglandular capillary bed combine to form a submucosal venous plexus. This plexus gives rise to veins that traverse the tunica muscularis parallel to the arterial supply and drain into the portal vein. The circulatory system in the small intestine of horses, carnivores, and pigs differs from the previously described pattern in that these animals lack arteriovenular loops in the villi but have arteriovenous (AV) anastomoses in the submucosa preceding the villous circulation. During digestion, circularly arranged smooth muscle cells in the AV anastomoses contract, shunting blood to the villi. When the

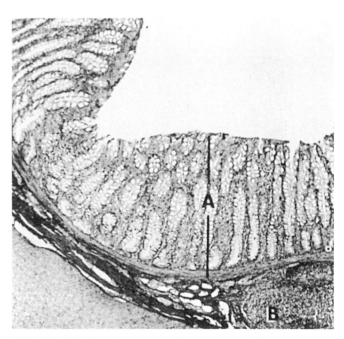

FIGURE 10-56 Cecum (cat). Tunica mucosa (A) containing simple tubular glands; lymphatic nodule in submucosa (B). Trichrome (×45).

granular (Paneth) cells; and an increased number of lymphatic nodules. Plicae circulares are absent in the large intestine, but longitudinal folds are present. Animals fattened for slaughter tend to accumulate white adipose tissue in the submucosa (Fig. 10-57).

Cecum

The **cecum** varies in size among the different species. In herbivores with simple stomachs (e.g., horses), the cecum is large and is an important bacterial fermentation reservoir, but in carnivores, it is small. In all domestic mammals, the cecum has a substantial number of lymphatic nodules scattered throughout its length (Fig. 10-56). Lymphatic nodules are especially numerous around the ileal ostium (the opening of the ileum into the cecum or colon) in pigs, ruminants, and dogs; however, in horses and cats, lymphatic nodules are concentrated near the apex of the cecum.

Colon

The mucosa of the **colon** is substantially thicker than that of the small intestine because of the increased length of the intestinal glands. Because villi are absent, the mucosal surface is smooth (Fig. 10-58). The number of goblet cells is increased compared to the small intestine. The submucosa is often distended by lymphatic tissue, which also disrupts the lamina muscularis. In such instances, intestinal glands may extend into the submucosa.

In pigs and horses, the outer longitudinal layer of the tunica muscularis of the cecum and colon forms large, flat muscle bands containing numerous elastic fibers, the **taenia ceci** and **taenia coli**. Those of the cecum and ventral colon of horses have more elastic fibers than smooth muscle cells.

Rectum

Like that of the cecum and colon, the mucosa of the **rectum** is smooth, and except for the increased number of goblet cells, the

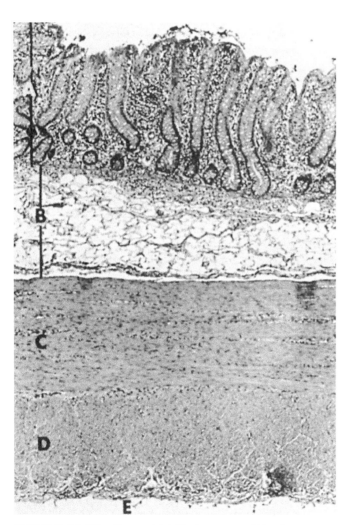

FIGURE 10-57   Cecum (pig). Tunica mucosa (A); submucosa filled with white adipose tissue (B); inner circular (C) and outer longitudinal (D) layers of the tunica muscularis; serosa (E). Hematoxylin and eosin (×48).

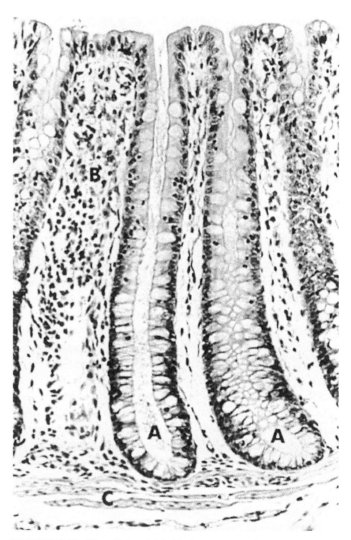

FIGURE 10-58   Colon (pig). Tunica mucosa with intestinal glands containing numerous goblet cells (A); lamina propria (B); lamina muscularis (C). Hematoxylin and eosin (×200).

basic structures are similar as well. In horses and cattle, the rectal wall is thicker than the wall of the colon. In carnivores, the outer longitudinal layer of the tunica muscularis is thickened. Elastic fibers are most prominent in the rectum of horses and cattle and least prominent in the rectum of sheep and goats. The outer longitudinal layer of the tunica muscularis contains more elastic fibers than does the inner circular layer. The cranial portion of the rectum is covered by a serosa, whereas the retroperitoneal portion is surrounded by an adventitia, which blends with the pelvic fascia.

Near its junction with the anal canal, the rectal mucosa in ruminants is thrown into longitudinal folds, the **rectal columns (columnae rectales).** All domestic mammals have an extensive venous plexus in the lamina propria of this region of the rectum. In dogs, approximately 100 solitary lymphatic nodules are a prominent feature of the rectum. They are visible grossly because of pitlike depressions, **rectal pits,** in the mucosa overlying the lymphatic nodules.

Anal Canal

The **anal canal** is the terminal segment of the digestive tract, and at the **anorectal line,** the simple columnar epithelium of the rectum changes abruptly to nonkeratinized stratified squamous epithelium (Fig. 10-59). Also at the anorectal junction, the lamina muscularis of the rectum terminates.

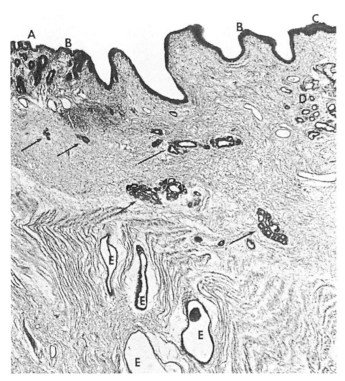

FIGURE 10-59 Rectum and anal canal (dog). Rectum (A); anal canal (B); skin (C) with sweat and sebaceous glands (D); veins (E); anal glands (arrows). Hematoxylin and eosin (×66). *(From Adam WS, Calhoun ML, Smith EM, et al. Microscopic Anatomy of the Dog: A Photographic Atlas. Springfield, IL: Charles C. Thomas, 1970.)*

The mucosa of the anal canal is smooth and lacks glands in ruminants and horses. In pigs and carnivores, the anal mucosa is divided into three distinct zones: (1) columnar zone (zona columnaris ani), (2) intermediate zone (zona intermedia), and (3) cutaneous zone (zona cutanea). The **columnar zone** contains longitudinal folds, the **anal columns,** between which are grooves, the **anal sinuses.** The **intermediate zone** is a narrow strip between the columnar zone and the cutaneous zone. The mucosa of both the columnar and intermediate zones is lined with nonkeratinized stratified squamous epithelium, and modified tubuloalveolar sweat glands, the **anal glands,** occupy the propria-submucosa. The anal glands produce a lipid secretion in cats and dogs (Fig. 10-59) and a mucous secretion in pigs. The **cutaneous zone** begins at the **anocutaneous line,** at which the nonkeratinized stratified squamous epithelium of the intermediate zone changes abruptly to a keratinized form, marking the beginning of the cutaneous zone. The cutaneous zone is lined by keratinized stratified squamous epithelium. In carnivores, the ducts from the **anal sacs (paranal sinuses)** open at the junction of the intermediate and cutaneous zones. The anal sacs and ducts are bilateral evaginations of the anal mucosa. In dogs, the mucosa of the outermost part of the cutaneous zone, near the junction with the skin, contains large, modified sebaceous glands, the **circumanal glands.** The anal sacs and their associated glands and the circumanal glands are discussed with the integument in Chapter 16.

The outer longitudinal layer of the tunica muscularis of the rectum terminates at the anorectal junction. The inner circular layer continues into the anal canal and terminates as the internal anal sphincter muscle. The external anal sphincter muscle, which is circularly disposed skeletal muscle, covers the internal anal sphincter muscle.

LIVER

The liver is the largest gland in the body and is characterized by multiple, complex functions: excretion (waste products), secretion (bile), storage (lipids, vitamins A and B, glycogen), synthesis (fibrinogen, globulins, albumin, clotting factors), phagocytosis (foreign particulate matter), detoxification (lipid-soluble drugs), conjugation (toxic substances, steroid hormones), esterification (free fatty acids to triglycerides), metabolism (proteins, carbohydrates, lipids, hemoglobin, drugs), and hemopoiesis (in the embryo and potentially in the adult). An understanding of the structure of the liver is vital to the interpretation of these processes.

Capsule and Stroma

Each lobe of the liver is covered by a typical serosa (visceral peritoneum) overlying a thin connective-tissue capsule. Connective tissue from the capsule extends into the liver lobes, as interlobular connective tissue, to surround individual liver lobules and support the vascular and bile duct systems. A fine network of reticular fibers surrounds the cells and sinusoids. Smooth muscle cells may be present in the capsule and interlobular connective tissue.

Interlobular connective tissue is scant and difficult to see (Fig. 10-60), except in pigs, which have distinct interlobular connective tissue septa (Fig. 10-61). This difference accounts for the tougher nature of pork liver as a food, as opposed to beef liver.

Expanded areas of interlobular connective tissue supporting (a) a **lymph vessel,** (b) branches of the **hepatic artery,** (c) branches of the **portal vein,** and (d) a **bile duct** appear throughout any section of liver. These groups of vessels and ducts, together with the supportive connective tissue, are called **portal canals** or **portal areas** (Figs. 10-60 and 10-62).

Parenchyma

The hepatic laminae consist of rows of **hepatocytes.** Hepatocytes have six or more surfaces that are of three different types: (1) microvillous surfaces that face the perisinusoidal space; (2) canalicular surfaces that border the bile canaliculi; and (3) contact surfaces between adjacent hepatocytes where apposed cell membranes may

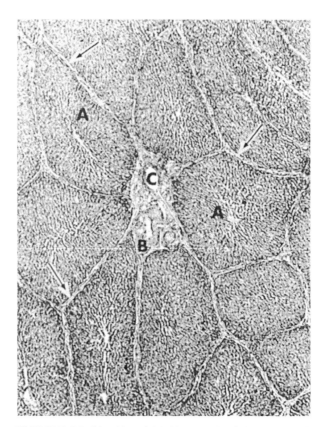

FIGURE 10-61 Liver (pig). Liver lobules (A); portal canal (B); branch of the portal vein (C); interlobular connective tissue (arrows). Trichrome (×30). *(From Stinson AW, Brown EM. Veterinary Histology Slide Sets. East Lansing, MI: Michigan State University, Instructional Media Center, 1970.)*

have tight junctions and desmosomes (Fig. 10-63). Hepatocytes are further characterized by a centrally located spherical nucleus with one or more prominent nucleoli and scattered clumps of heterochromatin. Occasionally, binucleated cells are seen. The appearance of the cytoplasm of hepatocytes varies within wide limits, depending on nutritional and functional changes. Mito-

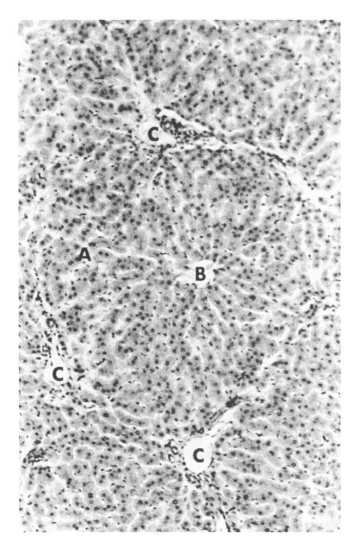

FIGURE 10-60 Liver (calf). Lobule (A) with central vein (B) is not separated from adjacent lobules by connective tissue as is that of the pig in Figure 10-61. Interlobular portal venules (C) in portal canals (areas). Hematoxylin and eosin (×80).

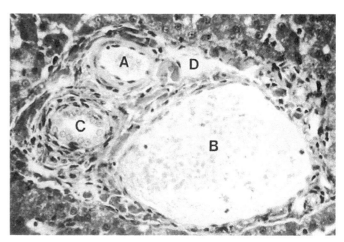

FIGURE 10-62 Liver (pig). Portal canal (area). Branch of the hepatic artery (A); branch of the portal vein (B); bile duct (C); lymph capillary (D). Hematoxylin and eosin (×200).

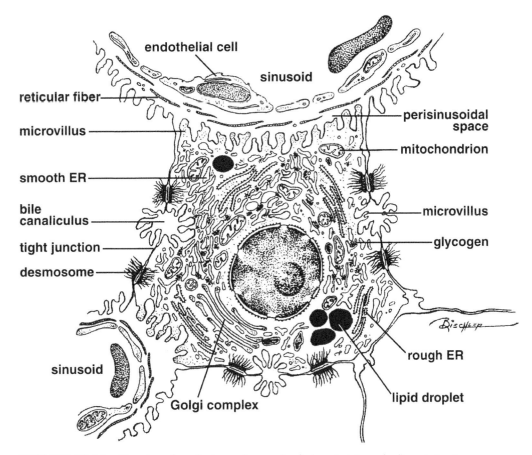

FIGURE 10-63 Drawing of an electron micrograph of a hepatocyte and adjacent structures.

chondria are abundant and the Golgi complex is usually near the bile canaliculus but may be juxtanuclear. There are numerous lysosomes, clusters of free ribosomes, and well-developed rER and sER, which are often continuous with each other. At the ultrastructural level, glycogen is seen as dense granules in a rosette configuration. In ordinary histologic preparations, glycogen-rich areas appear grainy or as irregularly shaped empty spaces, whereas sites occupied by lipids appear as round vacuoles. Bile pigments may be seen as fine yellow granules throughout the cytoplasm of normal hepatocytes. In cytology preparations stained with Wright's stain, bile pigments are blue-green granules located both inside and outside the hepatocytes.

Considerable evidence indicates that all hepatocytes may not be functionally identical, but instead, certain enzyme patterns and metabolic systems may be related to the position of the cell within the lobule. Although metabolic activity of the hepatocytes is generally believed to be closely associated with blood supply, the extent to which hepatocytes are similar or dissimilar with respect to metabolic systems, susceptibility to insults, and nutritional needs remains to be resolved.

Bile Canaliculi and Bile Ducts

Hepatocytes absorb bilirubin (the principal bile pigment) from the blood, conjugate it, and secrete it as one component of bile. Bile salts, protein, and cholesterol are the other components.

Bile is secreted into **bile canaliculi,** which are minute canals (0.5 to 1.0 μm in diameter) between apposed hepatocytes (Figs. 10-63 and 10-64). The canaliculi are expanded intercellular spaces bordered by cell membranes with short microvilli that project into the lumen. Tight junctions prevent bile from escaping into the narrow intercellular space adjacent to the canaliculus.

Bile flows in the bile canaliculi toward the periphery of the classic lobule, where it enters small **bile ductules** lined by low simple cuboidal epithelium. The bile ductules join **interlobular bile ducts** located in the portal canals. These ducts are lined by a simple cuboidal or simple columnar epithelium. Interlobular bile ducts converge to form progressively larger **intrahepatic ducts,** which finally leave the liver lobes through the **hepatic ducts.** The extrahepatic biliary passages are composed of the hepatic ducts, the cystic duct, the bile duct, and the gallbladder. Hepatic ducts drain the individual liver lobes. The **cystic duct** drains the gallbladder (absent in horses). The hepatic ducts and the cystic duct unite to form the **bile duct,** which empties into the duodenum. All of the extrahepatic biliary passages are lined by a tall simple columnar epithelium.

Blood Supply

The vascularity of the liver is directly related to its multiple functions. The liver has a dual blood supply. The **portal vein** brings blood from the intestines and associated organs, and the **hepatic**

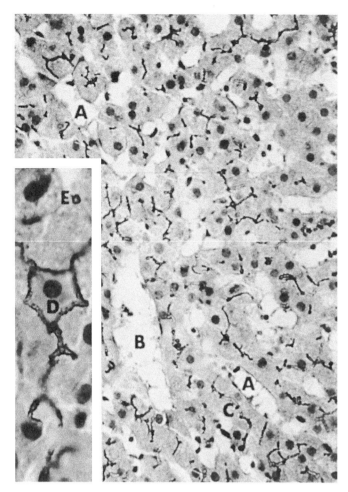

FIGURE 10-64 Liver (pig). Sinusoids (A); central vein (B); liver laminae with bile canaliculi between the cells (C). Silver stain (×300). Inset: bile canaliculi surrounding a hepatocyte (D) and a cross section of a bile canaliculus (E). Silver stain (×768)

artery supplies the liver cells with oxygenated blood. These vessels enter the liver at a hilus, called the porta, on its visceral surface. Branches (rami) of these two vessels enter the lobes, where they ramify and follow the interlobular connective tissue. The small branches within the portal canal are termed the **interlobular portal venule** and the **interlobular hepatic arteriole** (Fig. 10-62).

The interlobular portal venules give rise to small branches, sometimes referred to as distributing venules, which form the axis of the liver acinus. Short terminal venules arise from the distributing venules and end directly in the sinusoids. Most of the blood from the interlobular hepatic arterioles enters a capillary plexus within the portal canal and interlobular connective tissue; only a small portion of the blood reaches the sinusoids directly by way of terminal arterioles.

The **hepatic sinusoids** are blood capillaries, located between hepatic laminae, that course through the lobule carrying blood from terminal branches of the interlobular hepatic arteriole and interlobular portal venule to the central vein. The sinusoids often communicate with each other via interruptions in the laminae. This ramifying arrangement ensures that hepatocytes

have at least one surface adjacent to a sinusoid. Sinusoids are lined by two types of cells: endothelial cells and **stellate macrophages (Kupffer cells)** (Fig. 10-65).

The porous sinusoidal endothelium rests on a discontinuous basal lamina (Fig. 10-63). The endothelial cells contain small pores that lack diaphragms. The pores are too small to allow the passage of blood cells, but blood plasma can flow through them freely. The endothelium is separated from the hepatocytes by a space, the **perisinusoidal space (of Disse)**. Hepatocyte microvilli extend into the perisinusoidal space, where they are bathed in plasma, allowing a direct exchange of substances between blood and hepatocytes. The sinusoids of the ruminant liver differ from those described above in that the endothelium is nonporous and the basal lamina is continuous.

Stellate macrophages are scattered among the sinusoidal endothelial cells, often sending long pseudopodia through the endothelial pores or between the cells. These highly phagocytic

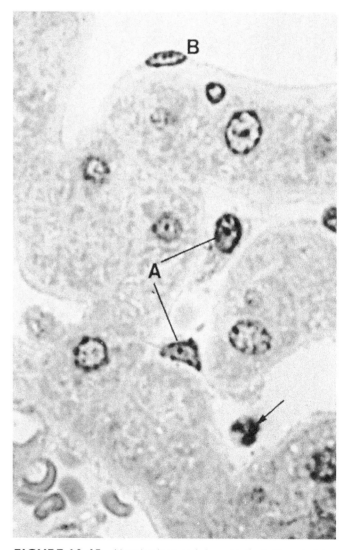

FIGURE 10-65 Liver laminae and sinusoids (cat). Two stellate macrophages (Kupffer cells) (A) and one endothelial cell (B) comprise the sinusoidal lining cells. Notice the erythrocytes (lower left) and one neutrophil (arrow). Epon. Toluidine blue (×1600).

cells are derivatives of blood monocytes and, as such, are components of the monocyte–macrophage system.

In addition to the hepatocyte microvilli, the perisinusoidal space contains reticular fibers as well as **perisinusoidal adipocytes.** These cells are believed to store vitamin A and synthesize type III collagen after injury to the liver.

Blood in the sinusoids leaves the lobule via the **central vein** (Figs. 10-60 and 10-66). Central veins are lined by endothelium resting on a thin adventitia. The central veins connect with **sublobular veins** at the periphery of the lobules. Sublobular veins join to form progressively larger veins that eventually form the **hepatic veins,** which drain directly into the caudal vena cava.

Lymph and Lymph Vessels

Lymph in the liver is formed in the perisinusoidal space. It flows toward the periphery of the lobule and enters the intercellular spaces of the portal canal and interlobular connective tissue.

Here, it diffuses into lymph capillaries within the portal canals. The lymph is carried from the portal canals by larger lymph vessels that ultimately leave the liver at the porta. These lymph vessels drain to the hepatic lymph nodes.

The Classic Liver Lobule—The Anatomic Unit of the Liver

The clear delineation afforded by abundant interlobular connective tissue in the liver of pigs has led to the recognition of **hepatic lobules (classic liver lobules).** This morphologic unit is organized around the central vein (Figs. 10-60, 10-61, and 10-67). The lobule consists of a polyhedral prism of hepatic tissue measuring approximately 2 mm long and approximately 1 mm wide. Cross-sectional profiles of this lobule are roughly hexagon-shaped, with the sinusoids converging from the periphery to the central vein, into which they empty. Portal canals are present at approximately three of the six angles of the lobule. The parenchyma located between the portal canals and the central vein consists of cells arranged in branching plates or laminae (Fig. 10-66). The laminae are one cell thick and the free surfaces of the cells face the sinusoids. An anastomosing network of bile canaliculi, formed by the apposed cell membranes of hepatocytes, is present throughout the laminae (Fig. 10-64).

The Portal Lobule and the Liver Acinus— Functional Units of the Liver

The **portal lobule** is a functional unit developed to emphasize the exocrine function (bile secretion) of the liver. The portal lobule is defined as a triangular area consisting of the parenchyma

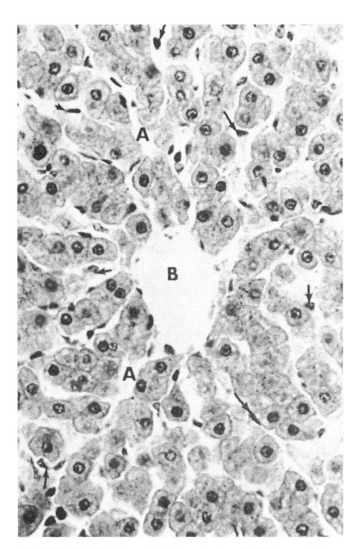

FIGURE 10-66 Liver (calf). Hepatic sinusoids (A); central vein (B); stellate macrophages (Kupffer cells) (arrows). Hematoxylin and eosin (×384).

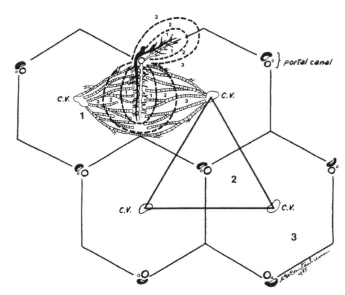

FIGURE 10-67 Schematic drawing of the functional units of the liver in relation to the anatomic unit (classic lobule). **1.** Liver acinus with three zones on each side of the vascular backbone. **2.** Portal lobule with an interlobular bile ductule (in the portal area) as the axis and one central vein at each point of the triangle. **3.** Classic hepatic lobule (anatomic unit) with the central vein as its axis.

of three adjacent classic lobules that is drained by the bile ductule in the portal canal. Thus, the axis (center) of the portal lobule is the interlobular bile ductule in the portal canal and the peripheral angles are the central veins of the three adjacent lobules (Fig. 10-67)

The **liver acinus** is a functional unit that describes the vascular supply to the parenchyma. The liver acinus is a roughly diamond-shaped area made of parts of two classic lobules supplied by terminal branches of the interlobular portal venule and interlobular hepatic arteriole. The blood vessels course at right angles from a portal canal between two hepatic lobules to form the axis of the acinus, and the two central veins are at the two opposing points of the diamond (Fig. 10-67). Three ill-defined zones have been identified in the liver acinus. **Zone 1** is the nearest to the vascular axis of the acinus. In this zone, hepatocytes receive an excellent nutrient and oxygen supply and are metabolically most active. Cells in this zone may also be the first to be exposed to toxic substances entering the liver. **Zone 2** is one of intermediate activity, whereas **zone 3** borders the central vein and is the least favorably situated with respect to oxygen and nutrient supply.

GALLBLADDER

Bile produced by the liver is *stored* in the gallbladder and *concentrated* by the reabsorption of water and inorganic salts. In the contracted (empty) state, the gallbladder mucosa is thrown into numerous folds (**plicae**). As it fills and expands, the folds have a tendency to flatten, resulting in a smoother mucosal surface. A tall simple columnar epithelium lines the luminal surface of the gallbladder and extends into mucosal **crypts**, which are small epithelial diverticula that sometimes give the impression of being glands (Fig. 10-68). Two types of columnar cells are located in the gallbladder epithelium. The most numerous type is the "light" cell, which has a pale cytoplasm of uniform density. The cytoplasm of the apical region contains vesicles but is devoid of organelles. Electron-dense bodies with smooth outlines occur in the subapical and supranuclear cytoplasm. The less numerous "dark" cells are scattered among the light cells. They have a narrow profile and contain a dark, dense cytoplasm with few organelles and a nucleus that is more heterochromatic than that of the light cells. The epithelial cell surface is covered with microvilli, and tight junctions (zonulae occludens) between adjacent cells prevent the intercellular passage of fluids from the lumen of the organ. Goblet cells are characteristic of the epithelium of some species, such as cattle, and globule leukocytes may be found in the epithelium of cats. Endocrine cells, possibly of the APUD system (characterized by amine precursor uptake and decarboxylation), have been described in the epithelium of the gallbladder of cattle.

The propria-submucosa (a lamina muscularis is absent) is composed of loose connective tissue. Lymphatic tissue, either diffuse or nodular, is often present. In some species, particularly ruminants, glands are present in the propria-submucosa. They may be serous or mucous, depending on the species, individual, or location in the mucosa (Fig. 10-69). The tunica muscularis consists of thin bundles of smooth muscle cells that generally course in a

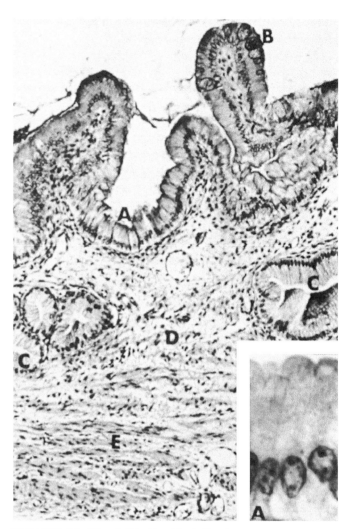

FIGURE 10-68   Gallbladder (dog). Simple columnar epithelium (A); goblet cells (B); cross sections of mucosal crypts (C); propria-submucosa (D); tunica muscularis (E). Hematoxylin and eosin (×120). Inset: simple columnar epithelial lining. Hematoxylin and eosin (×768).

circular direction. The muscle is supplied by both sympathetic and parasympathetic axons.

The walls of the hepatic, cystic, and bile ducts are composed of the same tunics as the gallbladder.

PANCREAS

The pancreas is an encapsulated, lobulated, compound tubuloacinar gland containing both exocrine and endocrine parts (Fig. 10-70). The function of the exocrine part is to produce a variety of enzymes, including amylase, lipase, and trypsin, which act on the products of gastric digestion as they reach the duodenum. The endocrine part, pancreatic islets (Fig. 10-71), produces mainly insulin and glucagon. The histologic structure of the islets is discussed in Chapter 15.

The parenchyma of the pancreas is separated into distinct lobules by a connective tissue stroma. Each lobule is composed of secretory units and intralobular ducts.

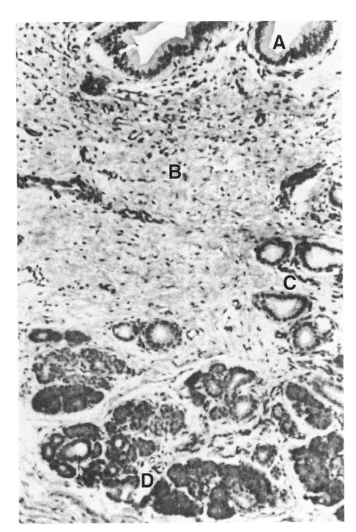

FIGURE 10-69 Gallbladder (large ruminant). Simple columnar epithelium (A); propria-submucosa (B); mucous glands (C); serous glands (D). Hematoxylin and eosin (×120).

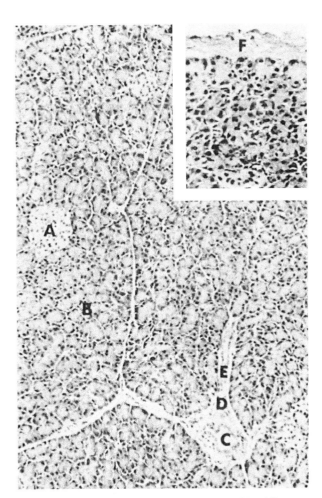

FIGURE 10-70 Pancreas (pig). Pancreatic islet (A); pancreatic acini (B); interlobular duct (C) in interlobular connective tissue (D); intralobular duct (E). Hematoxylin and eosin (×120). Inset: capsule of sheep pancreas (F). Hematoxylin and eosin (×192).

The secretory units of the pancreas are tubuloacinar, with a small lumen. The tubular portion is more prominent in ruminants. The glandular epithelial cells are generally pyramid-shaped, with a spherical nucleus near the base of the cells (Figs. 10-72 and 10-73). The cytoplasm surrounding the nucleus is intensely basophilic and contains an extensive rER and numerous mitochondria. The apical region of the cells contains eosinophilic, membrane-bounded zymogen granules, which are filled with the proenzymes synthesized in the rER. An extensive Golgi complex is located between the nucleus and the zymogen granules. The acinar cells have receptors for **cholecystokinin,** which is produced by endocrine cells in the small intestine and stimulates the release of pancreatic enzymes as well as the contraction of the tunica muscularis of the gallbladder.

The tubuloacinar secretory unit is continuous with a short **intercalated duct.** This duct begins with flattened cells that extend into the lumen of the acinus; therefore, they are referred to as **centroacinar cells** (Fig. 10-73). Centroacinar cells and intercalated duct cells secrete bicarbonate and water when stimulated by the polypeptide, **secretin.** Bicarbonate raises the pH of the

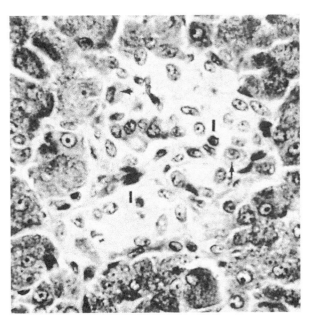

FIGURE 10-71 Pancreatic islet surrounded by pancreatic acini (dog). A cells (arrows); B cells (I). Trichrome (×450).

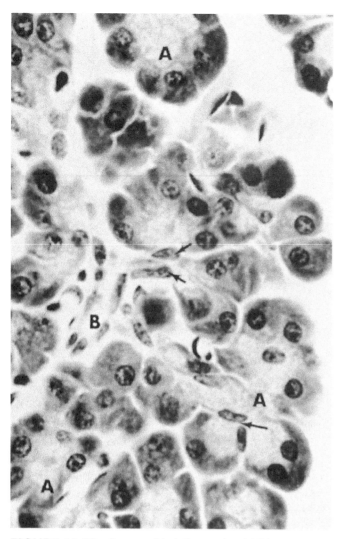

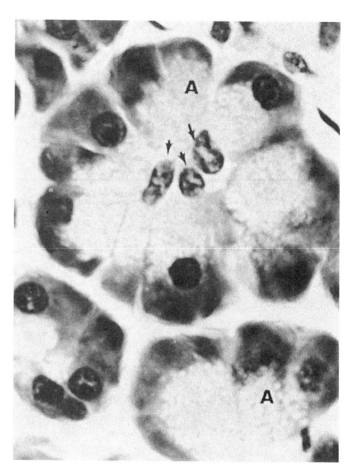

FIGURE 10-73   Pancreatic acinus with three centroacinar cells at arrows. Zymogen granules (A). Hematoxylin and eosin (×1200).

FIGURE 10-72   Pancreas (dog). Pancreatic acini (A); intercalated duct (B); centroacinar cells (arrows). Hematoxylin and eosin (×768).

intestinal contents, thereby facilitating the action of intestinal digestive enzymes. Intercalated ducts join **intralobular ducts,** which are lined by low simple cuboidal epithelium. The intralobular ducts of the pancreas are not "striated," as are the intralobular ducts of the parotid salivary gland. The intralobular ducts continue into **interlobular ducts** that are lined by simple columnar epithelium (Fig. 10-74). Interlobular ducts converge to eventually form the **pancreatic duct** and the **accessory pancreatic duct,** both of which empty into the duodenum. Goblet cells may be present in the epithelium of larger ducts.

The stroma of the pancreas consists of a thin capsule that gives rise to delicate connective tissue septa separating the lobules. Frequently, **lamellar (Pacini's) corpuscles** are present in the interlobular connective tissue of the pancreas of cats.

AVIAN DIGESTIVE SYSTEM

The oral cavity is lined throughout by a keratinized stratified squamous epithelium. The propria-submucosa contains consid-

erable diffuse lymphatic tissue and salivary glands. The tongue is covered by a keratinized stratified squamous epithelium and contains bundles of skeletal muscle, lingual salivary glands, and a bone, the **entoglossal bone.** Taste buds are found only on the base of the tongue and the floor of the oral cavity. All salivary glands are branched tubular mucous glands with openings into a common cavity from which an excretory duct leads to the oral cavity.

The esophagus is similar in structure both cranial and caudal to the crop. It is characterized by a thick keratinized stratified squamous epithelium. The lamina propria is a loose connective tissue containing large mucous glands. The lamina muscularis consists of longitudinally arranged smooth muscle fibers. The submucosa consists of a thin layer of loose connective tissue. The tunica muscularis is composed of a thick inner circular layer and a thin outer longitudinal layer of smooth muscle (Fig. 10-75).

The **crop** is a saclike diverticulum of the esophagus. It is a storage organ where the ingested food is moistened by the mucous secretions of the esophageal glands. The histologic structure of the crop is similar to that of the esophagus, except that glands are restricted to an area near its junction with the esophagus.

The bird does not have a glandular stomach similar to that of mammals, but instead has two separate organs between the esoph-

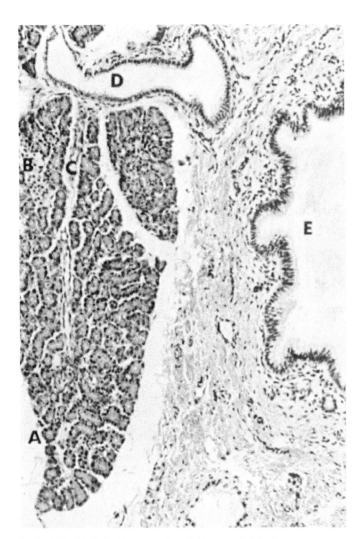

FIGURE 10-74 Pancreas (goat). Pancreatic lobule (A); pancreatic islet (B); intralobular duct (C); interlobular duct (D); pancreatic duct (E). Hematoxylin and eosin (×145).

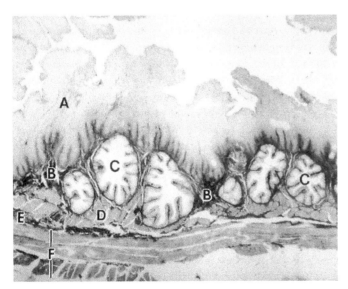

FIGURE 10-75 Esophagus (chicken). Keratinized stratified squamous epithelium (A); lamina propria (B); mucous glands (C); lamina muscularis (D); submucosa (E); tunica muscularis (F). Hematoxylin and eosin (×45).

agus and the duodenum. The **proventriculus,** or "glandular" stomach, and the **ventriculus,** or "muscular" stomach, perform many of the functions of the mammalian stomach.

The mucosa of the **proventriculus** is characterized by macroscopic papillae with numerous microscopic folds (plicae) of varying height that are arranged concentrically around the single duct opening at the apex of each papilla (Fig. 10-76). Simple columnar epithelium covers the plicae and continues into three generations of ducts of the **proventricular glands** (Fig. 10-76). The glands are lined by a simple cuboidal to low columnar epithelium in which the adjacent cells are in direct contact only on their basal half, thereby giving a serrated appearance to the luminal surface. Only one cell type is identifiable (**oxynticopeptic cells**), and this type produces both pepsinogen and hydrochloric acid. The lamina propria is typical loose connective tissue. The lamina muscularis is split into a very thin inner layer and a thick outer layer inner by the proventricular glands. A typical two-layered tunica muscularis consisting entirely of smooth muscle underlies the loose connective tissue of the very thin submucosa (Fig. 10-76). The proventriculus is covered by a typical **serosa.**

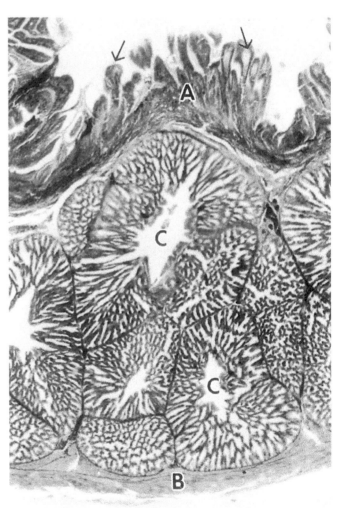

FIGURE 10-76 Proventriculus (chicken). Papilla (A) with plicae (arrows); tunica muscularis (B); proventricular glands (C). Hematoxylin and eosin (×23).

The **ventriculus (gizzard)** is a highly muscular organ responsible for grinding and macerating the ingesta (Figs. 10-77 and 10-78). The lining of the ventriculus is referred to as the **cuticle** or **koilin membrane.** Koilin is a secretory product produced by mucosal glands and surface epithelial cells; it is not a stratum corneum. The glands form hard koilin rod clusters, which enter the membrane and are separated by soft koilin produced by the surface epithelial cells. The surface epithelium is simple columnar while that of the simple, branched tubular mucosal glands is simple cuboidal. The lumina of the glands are filled with secretory product, which stains bright red with keratohyalin stains. The lamina propria and submucosa are both composed of loose connective tissue. The lamina muscularis is very discontinuous. The tunica muscularis is a single thick layer of parallel smooth muscle cells that spreads from two aponeuroses at the center of the organ. It is crisscrossed by bands of dense connective tissue. The outermost tunic is a typical serosa.

The histologic structure of the **small intestine** is similar to that of the mammalian small intestine. The lamina propria and submucosa contain large amounts of diffuse and nodular lym-

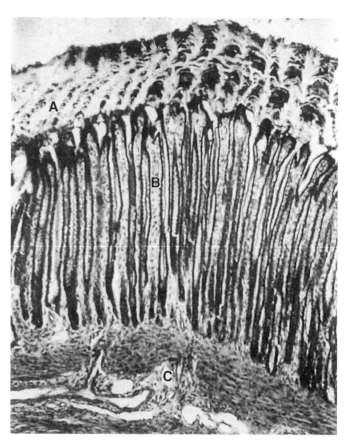

FIGURE 10-78 Ventriculus, gizzard (chicken). Cuticle (A); lamina propria between the ventricular glands (B); submucosa (C). Trichrome (×88).

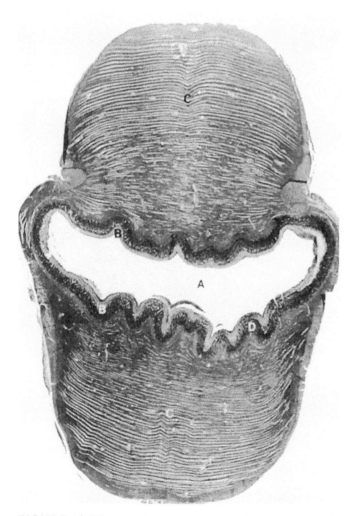

FIGURE 10-77 Ventriculus, gizzard (chicken). Lumen (A); cuticle (B); smooth muscle of tunica muscularis (C); simple branched tubular ventricular glands (D). Hematoxylin and eosin (×10).

phatic tissue. Submucosal glands of the duodenum are generally absent. The tunica muscularis is composed of inner circular and outer longitudinal layers of smooth muscle. The outermost tunic is a typical serosa.

Two **ceca** open into the digestive tract at the junction of the ileum and rectum. Three regions of this organ present slightly different histologic features. The proximal portion contains prominent villi. In the adult bird, large masses of diffuse and nodular lymphatic tissue infiltrate the lamina propria and submucosa of this portion, forming grossly visible **cecal tonsils.** In the midportion, the villi are shorter and broader and mucosal folds are present. The distal ceca are devoid of villi. The surface epithelium of the mucosa is simple columnar with goblet cells.

The **rectum,** a part of the large intestine, extends from the ileum to the coprodeum of the cloaca. It resembles the small intestine in that villi are present. Scattered diffuse and nodular lymphatic tissues occur in the lamina propria and submucosa.

The **cloaca** is divided into three parts—the **coprodeum, urodeum,** and **proctodeum**—by transverse folds. All three parts have a similar structure. Villi are present and the epithelium of the mucosa is simple columnar. The **cloacal bursa** opens into the proctodeum.

Histologic features of the liver, gallbladder, and exocrine pancreas of the bird are not significantly different from those of the same organs in mammals.

SUGGESTED READINGS

Adam WS, Calhoun ML, Smith EM, et al. Microscopic Anatomy of the Dog: A Photographic Atlas. Springfield, IL: Charles C. Thomas, 1970:102.

Akester AR. Structure of the glandular layer and koilin membrane in the gizzard of the adult domestic fowl (Gallus gallus domesticus). J Anat 1986;147:1–25.

Boshell JL, Wilborn WH. Histology and ultrastructure of the pig parotid gland. Am J Anat 1978;152:447–465.

Budsberg SC, Spurgeon TL. Microscopic anatomy and enzyme histochemistry of the canine anal canal. Anat Histol Embryol 1983; 12:295–316.

Chu RM, Glock RD, Ross RF. Gut-associated lymphoid tissue of young swine with emphasis on some epithelium of aggregated lymph nodules (Peyer's patches) of the small intestine. Am J Vet Res 1979; 40:1720.

Dyce KM, Sack WO, Wensing CJG. Textbook of Veterinary Anatomy. 3rd Ed. Philadelphia: WB Saunders Company, 2002.

Gemmell RT, Heath T. Fine structure of sinusoids and portal capillaries in the liver of adult sheep and the newborn lamb. Anat Rec 1972;172:57–70.

Gershon MD, Kirchgessner AL, Wade PR. Functional anatomy of the enteric nervous system. In: Johnson LR, ed. Physiology of the Gastrointestinal Tract. 3rd Ed. New York: Raven Press, 1994;1:381

Herdt T. Regulation of gastrointestinal function. In: Cunningham JG, ed. Textbook of Veterinary Physiology. 3rd Ed. Philadelphia: WB Saunders Company, 2002.

International Committee on Veterinary Gross Anatomical Nomenclature. Nomina Anatomica Veterinaria. 4th Ed. Ithaca, NY: International Committee on Veterinary Gross Anatomical Nomenclature, 1994.

International Committee on Veterinary Histological Nomenclature. Nomina Histologica, 2nd Ed. revised. Ithaca, NY: International Committee on Veterinary Histological Nomenclature, 1994.

Krstić RV. General histology of the mammal. New York: Springer-Verlag, 1985.

Krstić RV. Ultrastructure of the mammalian cell. New York: Springer-Verlag, 1979.

Madara JL, Trier JS. The functional morphology of the mucosa of the small intestine. In: Johnson LR, ed. Physiology of the Gastrointestinal Tract. 3rd Ed. New York: Raven Press, 1994;2:1577.

McLelland J. A Color Atlas of Avian Anatomy. Philadelphia: WB Saunders Company, 1991.

Noden DM, deLahunta A. The Embryology of Domestic Animals. Baltimore: Williams & Wilkins, 1985.

Titkemeyer CW, Calhoun ML. A comparative study of the structure of the small intestines of domestic animals. Am J Vet Res 1955;16: 152–157.

Wünsche A. Anatomy of the liver lobule of pig. Anat Histol Embryol 1981;10:342.

11

Urinary System

JILL W. VERLANDER

Kidney
   General Organization
      Superficial anatomic features
      Cortex and medulla
      Parts of the renal corpuscle and the renal tubule
      Nephron
   Renal Corpuscle
      General structure
      Glomerular capillaries
      Mesangium
      Glomerular capsule
   Renal Tubule
      Proximal tubule
      The loop of Henle
         Thin limbs of the loop of Henle
         Thick ascending limb of the loop of Henle

      Distal convoluted tubule
      Connecting segment
      Collecting ducts
   Vasculature of the Kidney
   Interstitium, Lymphatics, and Nerves
   Juxtaglomerular Apparatus
   Structure–Function Relationships in the Kidney
      General function
      Filtration and regulation of blood pressure
      Tubule function
      Proximal tubule
      Thin limbs and thick ascending limb of the loop of
         Henle
      Distal convoluted tubule
      Collecting duct
Urinary Passages

The urinary system is composed of two kidneys, two ureters, a urinary bladder, and a urethra. The kidneys excrete nitrogenous wastes and regulate the volume and composition of body fluids by filtration of the blood, reabsorption of filtered solutes and water, and secretion of electrolytes. The ureters conduct urine from the kidneys to the urinary bladder, which stores the urine and expels it via the urethra.

KIDNEY

General Organization

Superficial Anatomic Features

In all species, the two kidneys are retroperitoneal and positioned either flat against the lumbar muscles or suspended from the dorsal abdomen. The right kidney is usually slightly more cranial than the left. The renal artery and vein, lymphatics, nerves, and the ureter pass through a single indentation or hilus. The surface of the kidney is covered by a fibrous capsule, which is composed primarily of collagen fibers, but which also may contain smooth muscle and blood vessels.

The kidneys of domesticated animals have various shapes (Fig. 11-1). In dogs, cats, sheep, and goats, the external surface of the kidney is smooth and bean-shaped. In pigs, the kidneys are smooth, elongated, and flattened. In horses, the kidneys are smooth, but only the left kidney is bean-shaped whereas the right kidney is heart-shaped. In large ruminants, the overall shape is oval, but multiple lobes are visible on the surface.

The simplest form of the mammalian kidney is the **unipapillary kidney,** with a single renal pyramid that includes the base next to the cortex and an apex or papilla. The unipapillary kidney is common in laboratory animals and represents the basic unit of more complex kidneys, which are formed of multiple lobes that are fused to a variable extent. Cats, dogs, horses, sheep, and goats have **unilobar kidneys** with papillae that are fused to form a sin-

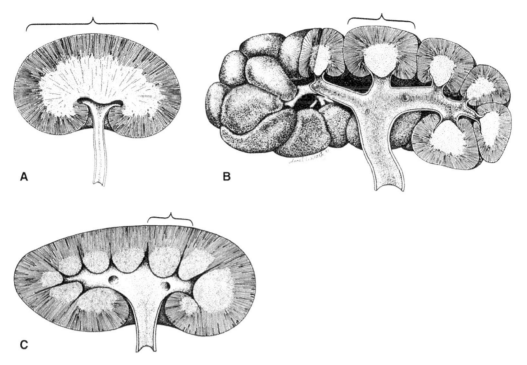

FIGURE 11-1 Schematic drawing of the gross structure and lobation pattern in three different kidneys. **A.** Unilobar kidney typical of carnivores. **B.** Multilobar kidney typical of large ruminants. On the surface of the kidney, each lobe is distinctly outlined by deep grooves. Note that this kidney lacks a renal pelvis. **C.** Multilobar kidney of the pig. Note the smooth surface. In the bovine kidney, the lobes are clearly demarcated (bracket in **B.**), while in the porcine kidney, cortical portions of the lobes fuse (bracket in **C.**). In the carnivore kidney (as well as in equine and small ruminant kidneys), lobes fuse extensively (bracket in **A.**) to give the appearance of a single lobe ("unilobar"). *(Redrawn from Dellmann H-D, Brown EM. Textbook of Veterinary Histology. Philadelphia: Lea & Febiger, 1987.)*

gle renal crest that empties into the renal pelvis (Fig. 11-1). Pigs, large ruminants, and humans have a **multilobar** (multipyramidal) **kidney** with numerous medullary pyramids and papillae. The papillae discharge into extensions of the renal pelvis or ureter called **calices** (minor or major) or into the pelvis directly.

Cortex and Medulla

A longitudinal or transverse section through the kidney reveals the parenchyma, which is divided into the outer, dark red **cortex** and the inner, lighter-colored **medulla** (Figs. 11-1 and 11-2). The structures within the renal cortex are arranged in **medullary rays** and the **cortical labyrinth** (Figs. 11-2 and 11-3). These terms arose because, unlike the medulla, which is composed entirely of straight tubule segments, the renal cortex contains both straight tubule segments and convoluted tubule segments. In a transverse section, the medulla appears striated throughout and the straight segments in the cortex, which are aligned more or less in parallel bundles, appear to radiate from the medulla out toward the fibrous capsule, thus "medullary rays." The medullary rays contain the cortical collecting ducts, cortical thick ascending limbs of the loop of Henle, and the proximal straight tubule. Sections of the cortical labyrinth contain irregular profiles of convoluted tubules including proximal convoluted tubule, distal convoluted tubule and connecting segment, as well as renal corpuscles, the

distal thick ascending limb (which diverges from the medullary ray to contact the juxtaglomerular apparatus of the glomerulus), and initial collecting tubule.

The **outer medulla** is located deep to the cortex; the arcuate blood vessels mark the border between the cortex and the outer medulla (Fig. 11-4). The outer medulla is subdivided into **outer** and **inner stripes.** The outer stripe is the outermost region of the outer medulla and contains proximal straight tubules (S_3 segments), thick ascending limbs, and collecting ducts. The inner stripe is the inner portion of the outer medulla. The inner stripe contains no proximal tubules; the transition from proximal straight tubules to thin descending limbs of Henle's loop marks the border between the outer and inner stripes. Thus, the inner stripe contains the collecting ducts, thick ascending limbs, and thin descending limbs of Henle's loop.

The **inner medulla** is located deep to the outer medulla. Transitions between the thin limbs and thick ascending limbs of Henle's loop mark the border between the inner and outer medulla. Thus, the inner medulla contains no thick ascending limb segments, only collecting ducts and descending and ascending thin limbs of Henle's loop in addition to capillaries and lymphatics. Macroscopically, the inner medulla can be subdivided into the **base** and the **papilla** or **renal crest.** The base is adjacent to the outer medulla. The papilla, or renal crest, is the terminal portion of the inner medulla, which extends into the renal pelvis or calices.

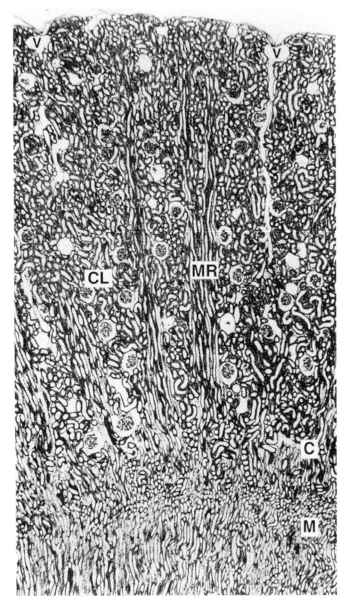

FIGURE 11-2 Kidney (cat). Cortex (C) and small part of medulla (M). The cortex is composed of the cortical labyrinth (CL) and medullary rays (MR). The renal corpuscles and convoluted tubules are in the cortical labyrinth. The medullary rays contain long straight tubules, including proximal straight tubules, thick ascending limbs of Henle's loop, and cortical collecting ducts. Note the capsular veins (V) at the surface of the kidney. Hematoxylin and eosin (×30).

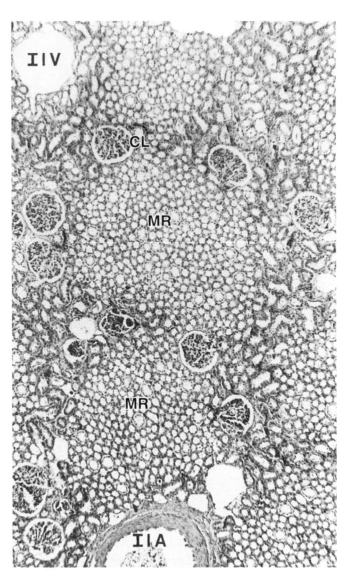

FIGURE 11-3 Kidney (horse). Section cut parallel to the surface of the kidney, deep in the cortex. The medullary rays (MR) are cut in cross section and contain roughly circular profiles of straight tubules. The cortical labyrinth (CL) surrounds the medullary rays. Note the interlobular artery (IIA) and vein (IIV) in the cortical labyrinth. Hematoxylin and eosin (×55).

Parts of the Renal Corpuscle and the Renal Tubule

The following lists the components of the renal corpuscle and the segments of the renal tubule in sequence from where the filtrate is formed to where it is released as urine:

- I. Nephron
  - A. Renal corpuscle
    - 1. Glomerulus
      - a. Glomerular capillaries
      - b. Mesangium
    - 2. Glomerular capsule (Bowman's capsule)
  - B. Proximal tubule
    - 1. Proximal convoluted tubule, including both S_1 and S_2 epithelia
    - 2. Proximal straight tubule, including both S_2 and S_3 epithelia
  - C. Thin limbs of Henle's loop
    - 1. Descending portion
    - 2. Ascending portion
  - D. Thick ascending limb of Henle's loop
  - E. Distal convoluted tubule
  - F. Connecting segment
- II. Collecting duct
  - A. Arcade—initial collecting tubule

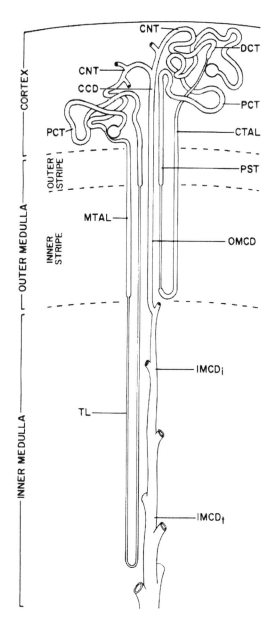

FIGURE 11-4 Schematic drawing of the relationships between various segments of the nephron and collecting duct and regions of the kidney. Long-looped (left) and short-looped (right) nephrons are illustrated. Cortical collecting duct (CCD); connecting segment (CNT); cortical thick ascending limb (CTAL); distal convoluted tubule (DCT); initial inner medullary collecting duct (IMCD$_i$); terminal inner medullary collecting duct (IMCD$_t$); medullary thick ascending limb (MTAL); outer medullary collecting duct (OMCD); proximal convoluted tubule (PCT); proximal straight tubule (PST); thin limb of the loop of Henle (TL). Glomeruli, PCT, DCT, terminal segments of the CTAL, and CNT are located in the cortical labyrinth; PST, CTAL, and CCD are located in the medullary rays in the cortex. *(From Madsen KM, Verlander JW. Renal structure in relation to function. In: Wilcox CS, Tisher CC, eds. Handbook of Nephrology and Hypertension. 5th Ed. Philadelphia: Lippincott Williams and Wilkins, 2004.)*

B. Straight portions
    1. Cortical collecting duct
    2. Outer medullary collecting duct
    3. Inner medullary collecting duct

Nephron

Traditionally, the **nephron** is considered the structural and functional unit of the kidney and includes the glomerulus and all renal tubule segments through the connecting segment. The number of nephrons varies among species. Dogs have approximately 400,000 per kidney, whereas cats have approximately 200,000 per kidney. In carnivores and pigs, species in which the young are fairly immature when born, the formation of nephrons may continue for several weeks after birth. After renal maturity, no new nephrons can be formed.

Nephrons can be classified either by the location of their glomeruli in the cortex as **superficial** (near the capsule), **midcortical**, or **juxtamedullary** (near the medulla), or by the length of their loop of Henle as **short-looped** or **long-looped** (Fig. 11-4). **Short-looped nephrons** generally have superficial or midcortical glomeruli and tubules that extend only into the outer medulla before reflecting back into the cortex. In pigs, the loops turn in the medullary ray in the cortex. **Long-looped nephrons** have juxtamedullary glomeruli and tubules that extend into the inner medulla before reflecting back into the cortex. Most species have both short- and long-looped nephrons. However, cats, dogs, and many species native to arid climates have only long-looped nephrons, which conserve water more efficiently than short-looped nephrons. Conversely, beavers, which live in fresh water, have only short-looped nephrons.

Renal Corpuscle

General Structure

The **renal corpuscle** is composed of the glomerular capillary tuft, the mesangium, and the glomerular capsule, also known as Bowman's capsule (Figs. 11-5 and 11-6). Although the term **glomerulus** formerly referred to only the glomerular capillary tuft and mesangium, the term is now widely used to refer to the entire renal corpuscle. The renal corpuscle is spherical and varies in size among species. Larger animals tend to have larger corpuscles. For example, horse corpuscles average 220 μm in diameter, whereas cat corpuscles average 120 μm in diameter. Blood vessels enter and exit the glomerulus at the **vascular pole**. The **urinary pole** is opposite the vascular pole where the glomerular capsule opens into the proximal convoluted tubule.

Glomerular Capillaries

The **glomerular capillary tuft,** or glomerular rete, is a network of branching and anastomosing capillaries. These capillaries are lined by an extremely thin layer of fenestrated endothelium; the diameter of the endothelial fenestrations or pores ranges from 50 to 150 nm (Fig. 11-7). Blood enters via the afferent arteriole and leaves via the efferent arteriole at the vascular pole (Fig. 11-6).

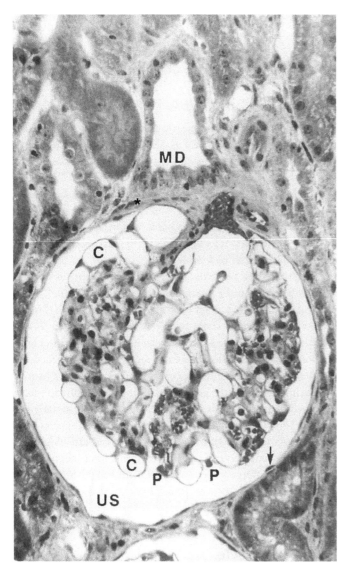

FIGURE 11-5 Renal corpuscle (horse). The glomerulus, composed of numerous capillary loops (C) and mesangial cells (not easily distinguished here), is surrounded by the glomerular capsule made up of a visceral layer of podocytes (P) and a parietal layer of squamous cells (arrow). The glomerular filtrate collects in the urinary space (US) of the glomerular capsule. The macula densa (MD) of the juxtaglomerular apparatus is located in the thick ascending limb of the vascular pole of the renal corpuscle. JB-4 plastic. Hematoxylin and eosin and phloxine (×335).

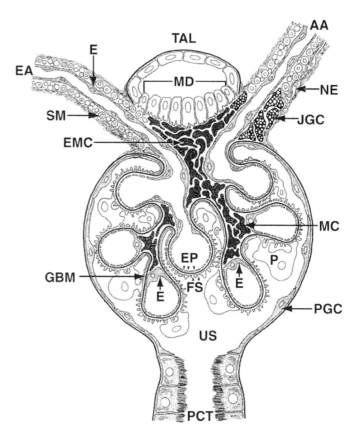

FIGURE 11-6 Schematic drawing of the renal corpuscle and juxtaglomerular apparatus. The afferent arteriole (AA) supplies the glomerulus, and the efferent arteriole (EA) carries blood away. The endothelial cells (E) lining the arterioles are not porous, whereas those of the glomerulus have endothelial pores (EP). The mesangial cells (MC) of the glomerulus are on the same side of the glomerular basement membrane (GBM) as the endothelial cells. The glomerular capsule surrounds the glomerulus; the complex podocytes (P) cover the capillaries and form the visceral layer that reflects at the vascular pole and is continuous with the parietal layer of simple, squamous epithelial cells (PGC). The podocyte foot processes contact the GBM; the spaces between the foot processes are the filtration slits (FS). The urinary space (US) is continuous with the lumen of the proximal convoluted tubule (PCT). The juxtaglomerular apparatus includes the macula densa (MD) within the thick ascending limb (TAL), the extraglomerular mesangial cells (EMC), the juxtaglomerular cells (JGC), and the afferent and efferent arterioles which contain smooth muscle (SM) in the tunica media. Nerve endings (NE) are found near the juxtaglomerular cells. *(Redrawn from Koushanpour E, Kriz W. Renal Physiology. Principles, Structure and Function. New York: Springer-Verlag, 1986.)*

The **glomerular basement membrane (GBM)** separates the endothelial cells on its inner surface from the visceral epithelial cells, or podocytes, which cover its outer surface (Fig. 11-7). The GBM is composed of three layers: the **lamina rara interna,** the layer adjacent to the endothelium; the **lamina rara externa,** the layer adjacent to the podocytes; and the **lamina densa,** the layer between the laminae rara. The terms lamina rara and lamina densa refer to the electron density of the layers when viewed with a transmission electron microscope, lamina rara being electron-lucent and thus pale, and lamina densa being electron-dense, and thus dark on electron micrographs. The GBM is 100- to 250-nm

thick in dogs and is composed largely of type IV collagen, heparan sulfate proteoglycans, and the glycoproteins laminin, fibronectin, and entactin. The GBM is stained by the periodic acid-Schiff (PAS) reaction, which facilitates the microscopic evaluation of the glomeruli in renal biopsies.

Mesangium

The **mesangium** forms the core of the glomerulus and is composed of specialized contractile cells embedded in an acellular

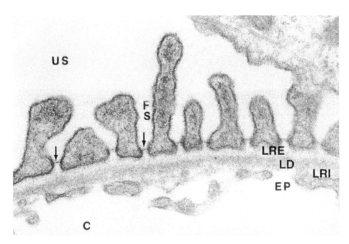

FIGURE 11-7   Transmission electron micrograph of glomerular basement membrane (rat). The blood within the glomerular capillary (C) is selectively filtered as it passes through the endothelial pores (EP), the three layers of the glomerular basement membrane (lamina rara interna [LRI], lamina densa [LD], and lamina rara externa [LRE]) and the filtration slits (FS) between the podocytic foot processes to enter the urinary space (US). Note the filtration diaphragms (arrows), which bridge adjacent foot processes (×67,000).

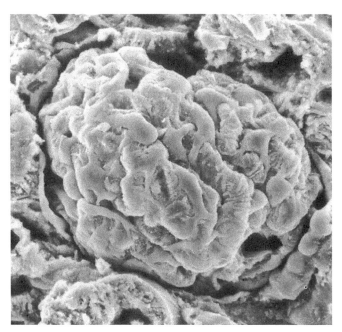

FIGURE 11-8   Scanning electron micrograph of glomerulus (rat) as seen from the urinary space. The parietal layer of the glomerular capsule has been removed, revealing the visceral layer of podocytes embracing the glomerular capillaries. The large, smooth-surfaced cell bodies of the podocytes extend primary processes that branch into secondary and tertiary processes (pedicels). (×1300).

matrix (Fig. 11-6). Mesangial cells have elongated, irregular cell processes, contain bundles of microfilaments made up of contractile proteins, and are joined to adjacent mesangial cells by gap junctions. The functions of mesangial cells include phagocytosis, production of the mesangial matrix, maintenance of the coherence of the capillary loops, and regulation of glomerular blood flow through regulation of capillary resistance. The mesangial matrix is characterized by a dense network of microfibrils surrounded by an amorphous material that is similar to the GBM.

Glomerular Capsule

The **glomerular capsule** (Bowman's capsule) surrounds the glomerulus (Figs. 11-5 and 11-6). The relationship of the glomerular capillary tuft to the glomerular capsule has been compared to a fist pushed into a partially inflated balloon. The fist represents the glomerular capillary tuft, the part of the balloon directly covering the fist represents the visceral epithelium, and the outer layer of the balloon not touching the fist represents the parietal epithelium. The space between the visceral and parietal layers is the **urinary space** (Bowman's space) (Figs. 11-6 and 11-7).

The visceral epithelial cells, or **podocytes,** cover the outer surface of the glomerular capillaries (Figs. 11-8, 11-9, and 11-10). The visceral epithelial cell body contains the nucleus and is the origin of several large, primary processes from which smaller secondary and tertiary processes emanate. The smallest of these are called **foot processes** or **pedicels.** The secondary and tertiary foot processes of one cell interdigitate with those of adjacent cells. The narrow spaces (25 to 60 nm) between the foot processes are called **filtration slits,** which are bridged by the **slit diaphragm** (Fig. 11-7). The **parietal epithelium,** a layer of simple squamous epithelium that lines the capsule, makes an abrupt

transition at the urinary pole to the cuboidal proximal tubule epithelium (Fig. 11-11).

An additional epithelial cell in Bowman's capsule is the **peripolar cell.** Peripolar cells are located at the vascular pole of the glomerulus at the junction between the parietal and visceral epithelia facing the urinary space and are largest and most

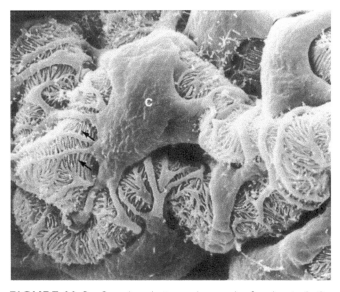

FIGURE 11-9   Scanning electron micrograph of podocyte (rat). The cell body (C) of one podocyte is in the center of the field. Numerous processes of varying size extend from the cell body, wrap around the glomerular capillaries, and interdigitate with secondary and tertiary processes of other podocytes (×4100).

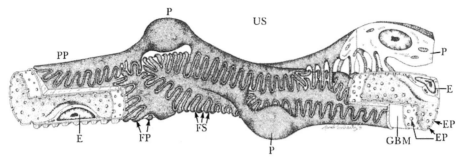

FIGURE 11-10 Schematic drawing of the components of the filtration barrier of the kidney. The capillaries consist of the glomerular basement membrane (GBM) lined by the endothelium (E), which contains numerous endothelial pores (EP) or fenestrations. Podocytes (P) cover the outer side of the GBM; the primary processes (PP) branch into secondary and tertiary processes, forming small foot processes (FP). Components of the plasma pass through the endothelial pores, the GBM, and the filtration slits (FS) and form the glomerular filtrate in the urinary space (US).

numerous in sheep and goats. Peripolar cells contain dark-staining, membrane-bounded granules that contain albumin, transthyretin, immunoglobulins, neuron-specific enolase, and kallikrein, but not renin. The cells also contain adseverin, a protein involved in exocytosis in secretory cells. Thus, it is believed that the peripolar cell is a secretory cell, but its specific function is unknown.

Renal Tubule

Proximal Tubule

The **proximal tubule** begins at the urinary pole of the renal corpuscle (Figs. 11-11 and 11-12 and Table 11-1). The proximal tubule is by far the longest cortical tubule segment and

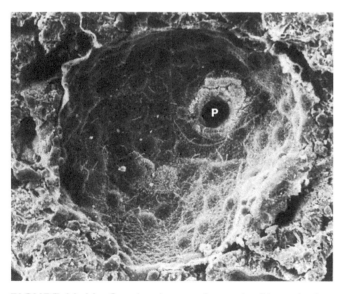

FIGURE 11-11 Scanning electron micrograph of the parietal layer of the glomerular capsule (rat). All the components of the renal corpuscle have been removed except the parietal layer. Each squamous cell of the parietal layer is distinctly outlined and projects a single, centrally located cilium. The opening into the proximal convoluted tubule (P) is surrounded by cells with a brush border, demonstrating the abrupt transition from the parietal epithelium to proximal tubule epithelium (×1200).

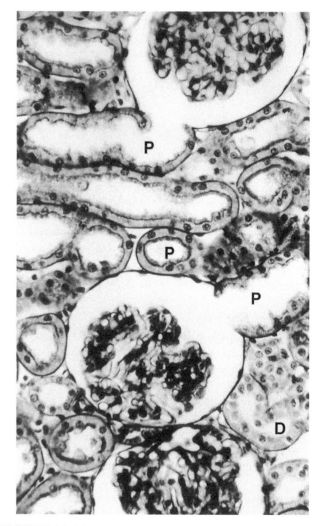

FIGURE 11-12 Cortical labyrinth (perfused rat kidney). The cortical labyrinth contains the renal corpuscles, proximal convoluted tubules (P), distal convoluted tubules (D), connecting segments, initial collecting tubules, and the terminal segment of the thick ascending limb. Two of the three renal corpuscles visible here show the continuity with proximal convoluted tubules. The periodic acid-Schiff (PAS) stain used on this section enhances the staining of the glomerular basement membrane, the basement membrane around the tubules, and the cell coat associated with the brush border of the proximal convoluted tubules. PAS (×335).

TABLE 11-1   Names of the Renal Tubule Segments With Corresponding Nomina Histologica Terminology

Anatomic Terms in Common Use in Renal Literature	Synonyms	Corresponding Nomina Histologica Terminology
Proximal tubule		**Proximal tubule**
Proximal convoluted tubule (Includes S_1 segment and first part of S_2 segment) (PCT)		Proximal convoluted tubule
Proximal straight tubule (Includes latter part of S_2 segment and S_3 segment) (PST)	Thick descending limb of Henle's loop	Proximal straight tubule
Thin limbs of Henle's loop (TL)		**Thin tubules**
Thin descending limb		Thin descending tubule
Thin ascending limb		Thin ascending tubule
Distal tubule		
Thick ascending limb of Henle's loop (MTAL and CTAL)		Distal straight tubule
Distal convoluted tubule (DCT)		Distal convoluted tubule
Connecting segment (CNT)		
Collecting duct		
Initial collecting tubule		Arched collecting tubule
Cortical collecting duct (CCD)		Straight collecting tubule
Outer medullary collecting duct (OMCD)		Straight collecting tubule
Inner medullary collecting duct (IMCD)		
Initial IMCD ($IMCD_1$)		Straight collecting tubule
Terminal IMCD (includes $IMCD_2$ and $IMCD_3$)	Papillary collecting duct	Papillary duct

thus proximal tubule profiles dominate histologic sections of the cortex. The first portion of the proximal tubule is called the **proximal convoluted tubule** (PCT), because it twists and turns in the cortical labyrinth until it enters the medullary ray, where it becomes the **proximal straight tubule** (PST). The PST runs through the medullary ray and extends into the outer stripe of the outer medulla. Proximal tubule segments are also classified as segments S_1, S_2, and S_3, based on differences in the length or abundance of features that are common to all proximal tubule cells.

In general, the apical surface of the proximal tubule is covered by a brush border formed by extensive projections of the apical plasma membrane called microvilli (Figs. 11-13 and 11-14). The lateral borders of the epithelial cells are characterized by elaborate interdigitation of lateral cell processes. In addition, the basal surface of the cells has a remarkably folded membrane with processes from adjacent cells located between the folds. The arrangement of the epithelial cells is like a group of buttressed tree stumps packed closely together with their roots growing beneath one another. The apical brush border and the basolateral plasma membrane infoldings significantly increase the surface area of the cell and thus permit the high rates of transepithelial transport that occur in this segment.

Numerous long mitochondria are interposed among the lateral plasma membrane folds, creating vertical striations that are visible by light microscopy. The close association of the mitochondria with the plasma membrane provides a ready source of energy for adenosine triphosphate (ATP)-dependent transport proteins located in the basolateral plasma membrane.

Near the apical surface, the lateral sides of the cells are joined together by tight junctions (zonulae occludens), zonulae adherens, and desmosomes (maculae adherens). Occasional gap junctions also link the cells. The tight junctions form continuous bands around the cells, but in the proximal tubule the tight junctions are relatively permeable to solutes and water, compared to the tight junctions of distal tubule and collecting duct segments. The single nucleus is spherical and situated in the middle to basal part of the cell. Proximal tubule cells contain an extensive endocytotic apparatus including numerous apical vesicles, endosomes, and lysosomes. Peroxisomes, organelles that contain oxidative enzymes for metabolism of toxic substances, are abundant in the PST. In cats, the PCT cells contain numerous lipid droplets (Fig. 11-15). In dogs, PST cells contain similar lipid droplets and thus the medullary rays appear lighter than the surrounding parenchyma (Fig. 11-16).

Unfortunately, the distinctive structural features of proximal tubules are not evident in many histologic sections because interruption of blood flow to the kidney causes collapse of the tubules, swelling of the epithelial cells, obliteration of the tubule lumens, and disintegration of the brush border. Many of the structural features that exist in the live animal can only be preserved with careful perfusion fixation techniques.

The PST extends into the outer medulla and typically makes an abrupt transition to the simple squamous epithelium of the thin descending limb (Fig. 11-17) at the border between the inner and outer stripes of the outer medulla. In dogs, the change occurs at the corticomedullary junction; therefore, the dog kidney lacks an outer stripe.

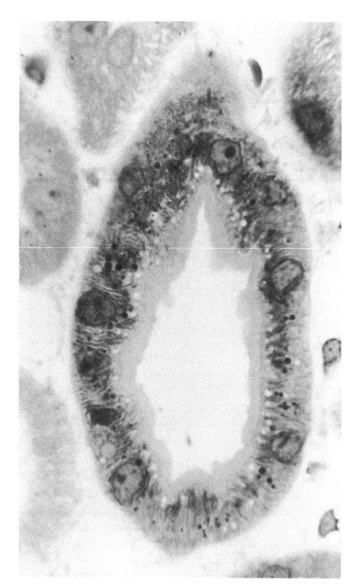

FIGURE 11-13 Proximal convoluted tubule (dog). The brush border composed of microvilli covers the apical surface of the cells. White vacuoles near the lumen and dark, round granules deeper in the cytoplasm are endocytotic vacuoles and lysosomes, respectively. The elongated dark structures oriented perpendicular to the basement membrane are mitochondria. Epon-Araldite. Azure II, methylene blue (×1320).

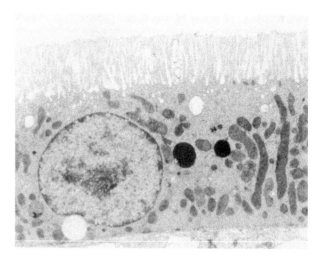

FIGURE 11-14 Transmission electron micrograph of proximal straight tubule (S$_3$) cell (rat). Numerous microvilli cover the apical surface. Small endocytotic vesicles are present in the apical region; large endosomes with unstained contents and densely staining lysosomes are also visible. Numerous mitochondria are present (×8800).

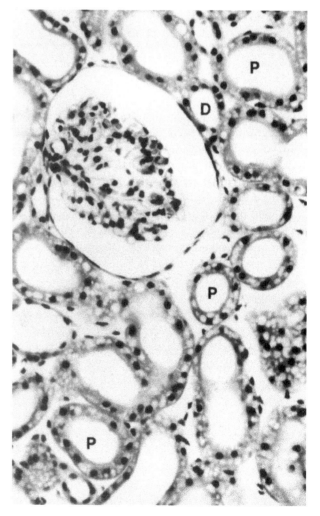

FIGURE 11-15 Cortical labyrinth (cat). In cats, the proximal convoluted tubules (P) contain numerous lipid droplets. Distal convoluted tubule (D) profiles are relatively rare. Hematoxylin and eosin (×335).

The Loop of Henle

The structure known as the loop of Henle includes four tubule segments: the descending thick limb, now more commonly called the **proximal straight tubule**; the **descending thin limb**; the **ascending thin limb**, which is present in long-looped nephrons; and the **thick ascending limb**, which is sometimes called the distal straight tubule.

Thin limbs of the loop of Henle

The thin portion of the loop of Henle (TL) begins at the end of the proximal tubule (Figs. 11-4 and 11-17) and extends a variable

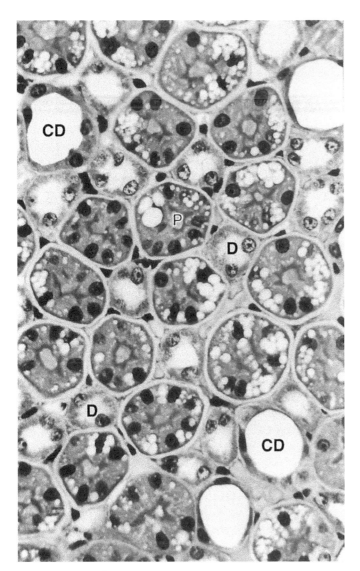

FIGURE 11-16 Medullary ray (dog). The three major components of the medullary ray are the proximal straight tubules (P), distal straight tubules (D), and the collecting ducts (CD). In dogs, the proximal straight tubules contain numerous lipid droplets, which appear as unstained vacuoles in this image. JB-4 plastic. Hematoxylin and eosin and phloxine (×530).

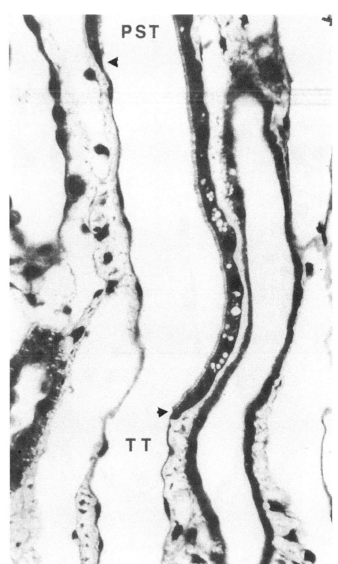

FIGURE 11-17 Proximal straight tubule to thin descending limb of Henle's loop (dog). The cuboidal epithelium with apical brush border of the proximal straight tubule (PST) abruptly changes to the simple squamous epithelium with a smooth apical surface in the thin tubule (TT). Note that the transition occurs at different points (arrows) around the circumference of the tubule. JB-4 plastic. Hematoxylin and eosin and phloxine (×510).

distance in the medulla before making a hairpin turn (Fig. 11-18) and continuing out to the border of the inner and outer medulla. In long-looped nephrons, the thin epithelium extends into the inner medulla. The portion from the PST to the hairpin turn is called the **thin descending limb**; the portion from the hairpin turn out to the inner/outer medulla border is called the **thin ascending limb**. Four distinct parts of the thin tubule have been described, based on ultrastructural differences in the height of the epithelium, the amplification of the apical and basolateral cell membranes, the number of mitochondria, and the complexity of the tight junctions, all of which relate to functional differences along its length. In general, the thin limbs have a simple squamous epithelium, with either abrupt or gradual changes to low cuboidal epithelium at the two ends of the thin segments, depending on the species. The nuclei protrude into the lumen to

a greater degree than do the nuclei of the endothelial cells of adjacent capillaries. In addition, the nuclei are round as viewed from the lumen, whereas endothelial nuclei are elongated in the direction of the longitudinal axis of the vessel.

Thick ascending limb of the loop of Henle

The **thick ascending limb** of the loop of Henle originates at the border of the inner and outer medulla and ascends into the renal cortex in the medullary ray (Fig. 11-19). The medullary thick ascending limb (MTAL) epithelium is taller than the cortical thick ascending limb (CTAL) epithelium. In short-looped nephrons, the thick ascending limb begins at the hairpin turn of Henle's loop at various depths in the outer medulla. In long-looped nephrons, the

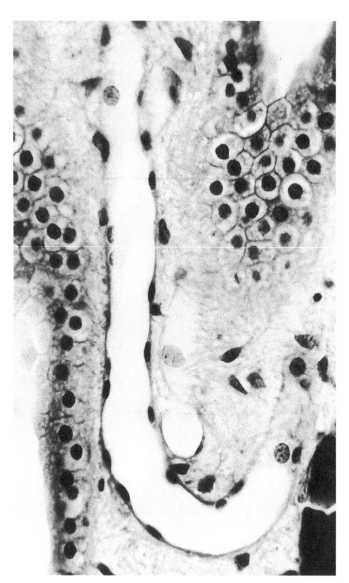

FIGURE 11-18 Hairpin turn of Henle's loop (horse). The thin tubule of long-looped nephrons makes a hairpin turn in the inner medulla. It is not possible to distinguish the thin descending limb from the thin ascending limb in this image. Hematoxylin and eosin (×530).

hairpin turn occurs in the inner medulla and the thin ascending limb extends from the turn to the transition to the thick ascending limb at the border of the inner and outer medulla. The thick ascending limb of each nephron returns to the vascular pole of its own glomerulus. At this site the thick ascending limb contains a specialized cluster of epithelial cells, the macula densa, which is part of the juxtaglomerular apparatus, described below. The transition from the thick ascending limb to the distal convoluted tubule occurs at a variable distance beyond the macula densa.

Cells of the thick ascending limb are cuboidal with short, stubby apical microprojections, undulating cell borders, and a single central cilium on the apical surface. The cells have an impressive array of vertically oriented mitochondria and basolateral plasma membrane infoldings, which are necessary to accomplish the high rate of active transport that occurs in this segment. The mitochondrial density and vertical orientation are so distinctive that they appear as dark vertical striations in the tubule even by light microscopy.

Distal Convoluted Tubule

The **distal convoluted tubule (DCT)** is much shorter than the proximal convoluted tubule; therefore, its profiles are relatively rare in the cortical labyrinth. Distal convoluted tubule cells are taller than cortical thick ascending limb cells and the apical cell borders are simple, not undulating. However, like the thick ascending limb, the apical surface is covered by short microprojections and the cells have a high mitochondrial density. The nucleus is located in the apical region of the cell, and extensive basolateral plasma membrane infoldings with vertically oriented mitochondria arrayed among them fill the entire basal region (Fig. 11-20). Although the distal convoluted tubule is largely composed of a uniform cell population, in some species occasional intercalated cells are present. Intercalated cells are described in detail below.

Connecting Segment

The epithelium of the **connecting segment (CNT)** is approximately the same height as the distal convoluted tubule. However, unlike the distal convoluted tubule, the connecting segment contains a variety of epithelial cell types, which may include distal convoluted tubule cells, connecting segment cells, intercalated cells, and principal cells. The mixture of a variety of cell types with different cell heights, staining density, and shape produces an irregular appearance to the connecting segment profile by light microscopy, compared to the homogeneous appearance and smooth luminal surface of the distal convoluted tubule. Connecting segment cells are similar in morphology to distal convoluted tubule cells, with prominent basolateral plasma membrane infoldings, vertically oriented mitochondria, few short apical plasma membrane microprojections, and an apical nucleus. Differences between the connecting segment cell and the distal convoluted tubule cell are appreciable by electron microscopy; there are usually fewer apical microprojections, a lower mitochondrial density, and a rounder nucleus in the connecting segment cells. However, definitive identification of individual profiles of these two cell types in the connecting segment may require immunocytochemical localization of cell-specific transporters, which highlights the fact that although the structure of the distal convoluted and connecting segment cells may be similar, their functions are quite distinct. Principal cells and intercalated cells are structurally distinct and will be described in the section on collecting ducts.

Collecting Ducts

Several nephrons empty into a single **cortical collecting duct (CCD)**, a straight tubule segment in the medullary ray. The collecting ducts descend through the medulla and repeatedly merge. The terminal inner medullary, or papillary, collecting ducts terminate at the apex of the papilla or along the renal crest and form a perforated area on the surface called the **area cribrosa**, where the tubule fluid, now considered urine, is emitted.

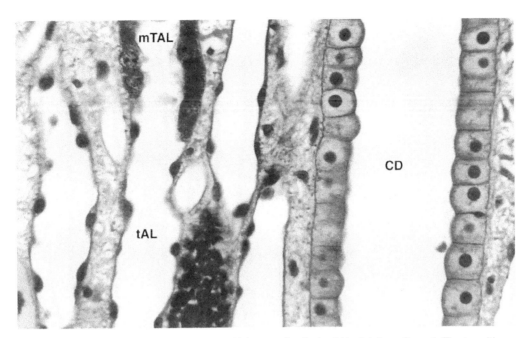

FIGURE 11-19   Thin ascending limb to thick ascending limb of Henle's loop (horse). The transition between the simple squamous epithelium of the thin ascending limb (tAL) and the simple cuboidal epithelium of the medullary thick ascending limb of Henle's loop (mTAL) defines the border between the inner and outer medulla. The inner medullary collecting duct (CD) shown has a tall cuboidal epithelium. JB-4 plastic. Hematoxylin and eosin and phloxine (×530).

The collecting duct is not considered part of the nephron because it has a separate origin during development. In fact, the initial collecting tubule and the collecting duct arise from the ureteric bud, whereas all of the components of the nephron develop from the metanephric blastema. During development, these two components fuse to form a continuous tubule. The term **renal tubule** encompasses both the nephron and the collecting duct. In the past, the collecting duct was thought to be simply a conduit for urine. It is now well known that the collecting duct has major roles in the regulation of salt, water, and acid-base excretion. Thus, the classic definition of the nephron as the "functional unit" of the kidney is somewhat misleading, since the collecting duct, although not part of the nephron, contributes significantly to renal function.

Connecting segments merge with the **initial collecting tubule** in the cortical labyrinth, and these merge with the **cortical collecting duct** in the medullary ray. The initial collecting tubule is made up of **principal cells** and **intercalated cells,** and thus is a heterogeneous epithelium. The height of the initial collecting tubule epithelium is typically intermediate between that of the connecting segment and the cortical collecting duct.

The collecting duct descends through the medullary ray, passes through the outer and inner medulla, and after merging several times with other collecting ducts, opens at the apex of the papilla or the edge of the renal crest. For most of their length, the collecting ducts are lined with simple cuboidal epithelium (Figs. 11-19, 11-21, and 11-22). In carnivores, the epithelium remains low throughout, whereas in ungulates, the epithelium in the medullary portions can be simple columnar or even transitional near the papillary apex.

Cortical and **outer medullary collecting ducts (OMCD)** contain both principal cells and intercalated cells (Fig. 11-22). **Principal cells** account for approximately two thirds of the cells; they are low in profile and have a smooth apical surface, with few short apical microprojections, and a single central cilium. Principal cells contain relatively few organelles and the mitochondria are small and randomly oriented. They have prominent basolateral plasma membrane infoldings and relatively straight, lateral cell membranes. Principal cells are involved in potassium secretion and sodium, chloride, and antidiuretic hormone–regulated water reabsorption. **Intercalated cells** are found throughout most of the collecting duct. In the connecting segment, initial collecting tubule, and cortical collecting duct, there are at least three distinct types of intercalated cells: type A, an acid-secreting cell type; type B, a bicarbonate-secreting cell type; and non-A, non-B intercalated cells, the function of which is not fully characterized. The intercalated cell subtypes are distinguishable both by their ultrastructural characteristics and by the subcellular location of specific transporters involved in acid-base regulation. The locations of specific transporter proteins in intercalated cell subtypes will be described in the section describing structural–functional relationships.

Under basal conditions, type A intercalated cells contain numerous mitochondria, moderate apical plasma membrane microprojections, prominent apical cytoplasmic tubulovesicles, moderate basolateral plasma membrane infolding, and a central nucleus. Type B intercalated cells have a denser cytoplasm and higher mitochondrial density than type A cells, a smooth apical surface, small cytoplasmic vesicles throughout most of the cell with a vesicle-free band of cytoplasm beneath the apical plasma

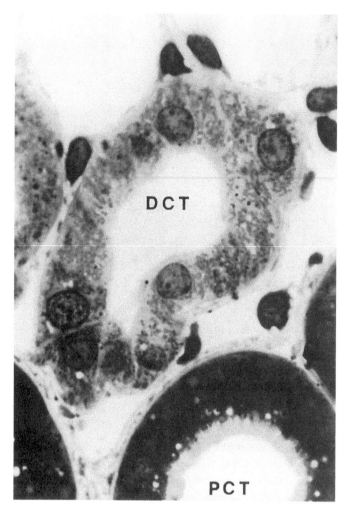

FIGURE 11-20 Distal convoluted tubule (dog). The cells of the distal convoluted tubule (DCT) lack a brush border, contain numerous mitochondria, and have nuclei in the apical region. Note the proximal convoluted tubule (PCT) with its distinct brush border. Epon-Araldite. Azure II, methylene blue (×1320).

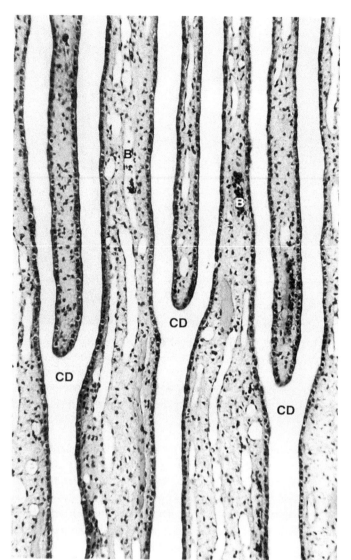

FIGURE 11-21 Confluence of inner medullary collecting ducts (horse). Illustrated are six smaller collecting ducts coalescing to form three larger ones (CD). A few blood vessels (B) and a relatively extensive interstitium are also present. Hematoxylin and eosin (×170).

membrane, prominent basolateral plasma membrane infoldings, and an eccentric nucleus. The non-A, non-B cells are most easily identified in the connecting segment. They have a very high mitochondrial density, prominent apical plasma membrane microprojections that bulge into the tubule lumen, and relatively few cytoplasmic vesicles.

The outer medullary and initial inner medullary collecting duct segments contain principal cells and acid-secreting intercalated cells similar to the type A intercalated cells. The prevalence of intercalated cells gradually diminishes in the distal collecting duct segments, and they are essentially absent in the terminal inner medullary collecting duct.

In the terminal **inner medullary collecting duct (IMCD)**, principal cells also disappear and the predominant cell type, called the inner medullary collecting duct cell, is a taller epithelial cell with short, stubby apical microprojections with a prominent glycocalyx, relatively little basolateral plasma membrane, and few cytoplasmic organelles.

Vasculature of the Kidney

Each kidney is supplied by a single **renal artery** that arises from the abdominal aorta. Branching of the renal artery can occur near the hilus or within the renal sinus. These branches divide into **interlobar arteries,** which ascend in the renal parenchyma to the corticomedullary junction (Fig. 11-23). Here, the interlobar arteries form variably arched vessels called **arcuate arteries.**

The arcuate arteries give off **interlobular arteries,** which course within the cortical labyrinth and give rise to the **afferent arterioles** that supply the glomeruli. The wall of the afferent arteriole is the major location of renin-producing juxtaglomerular cells. The glomerular capillary tufts are drained by **efferent arterioles.** Efferent arterioles from glomeruli located in the superficial or middle cortex distribute to **peritubular capillary**

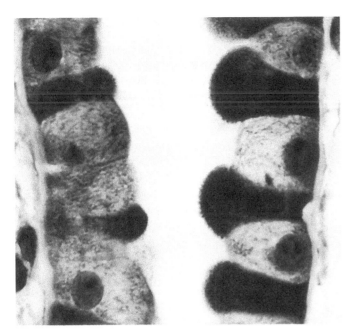

FIGURE 11-22 Collecting duct in medullary ray (horse). This collecting duct is lined by two cell types. The principal cell stains lightly and contains relatively few irregularly shaped mitochondria. The intercalated cells are the dark-staining cells protruding into the lumen. The apical surface of the intercalated cells appears irregular due to numerous apical microprojections. JB-4 plastic. Hematoxylin and eosin and phloxine (×1320).

networks of fenestrated capillaries. Strong evidence suggests that endothelial cells of cortical peritubular capillaries synthesize the hormone erythropoietin, which stimulates the production of red blood cells.

Efferent arterioles from juxtamedullary glomeruli supply blood to the entire medulla. These arterioles divide in the outer stripe of the outer medulla into **descending vasa recta** (straight vessels). The descending vasa recta supply adjacent peritubular capillary networks throughout the medulla. The capillaries drain into **ascending vasa recta**, which ascend in the medulla. The descending vasa recta are arterioles with a continuous endothelium, whereas the ascending vasa recta are venules with a fenestrated endothelium. Many of the descending and ascending vasa recta come together to form vascular bundles that are evenly distributed throughout the medulla (Fig. 11-24).

Veins typically accompany arteries and share the same name. Venous drainage of the medulla is accomplished by the ascending vasa recta that enter the arcuate or occasionally the interlobular veins. Venous drainage of the cortex is primarily from the peritubular capillaries into the **stellate veins, interlobular veins,** or **arcuate veins**. The arcuate veins empty into the **interlobar veins**, which coalesce to form a single renal vein, which exits the hilus and enters the caudal vena cava. In carnivores, a system of superficial and deep cortical veins connects the capillaries in these regions to larger veins. The superficial cortical veins empty into the stellate veins near the cortical surface, whereas the deep cortical veins empty into the arcuate veins. The stellate veins are

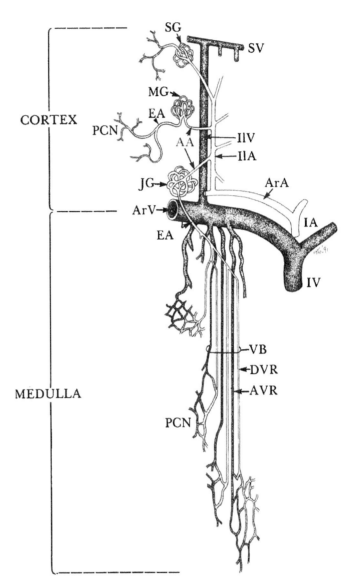

FIGURE 11-23 Schematic drawing of the vasculature of the kidney. Arterial blood flow is through the renal artery, interlobar arteries (IA), arcuate arteries (ArA), interlobular arteries (IIA), afferent arterioles (AA), glomeruli, and efferent arterioles (EA). The efferent arterioles from the superficial glomeruli (SG) and the midcortical glomeruli (MG) supply the peritubular capillary network (PCN) in all parts of the cortex. The efferent arterioles from the juxtamedullary glomeruli (JG) supply the descending vasa recta (DVR) and the peritubular capillary networks (PCN) of the medulla. Venous drainage of the peritubular capillary networks in the cortex involves the stellate veins (SV), the interlobular veins (IIV), and/or the arcuate veins (ArV). Venous drainage of the peritubular capillary networks in the medulla is primarily through the ascending vasa recta (AVR). The interlobular veins of the cortex and the ascending vasa recta of the medulla converge on the arcuate veins at the corticomedullary junction. The arcuate veins are drained by the interlobar veins (IV), which empty into the renal vein. The descending and ascending vasa recta often form vascular bundles (VB). *(Redrawn from Koushanpour E, Kriz W. Renal Physiology. Principles, Structure and Function. New York: Springer-Verlag, 1986.)*

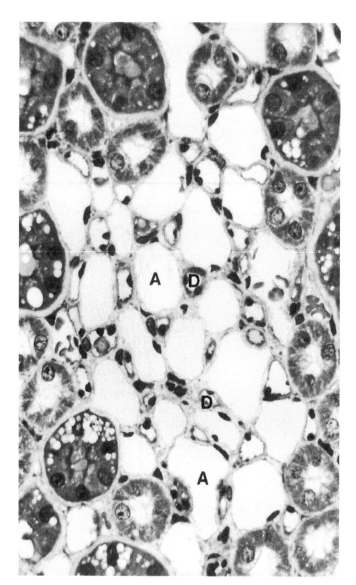

FIGURE 11-24 Vascular bundle in outer medulla (dog). The descending vasa recta (D) are the small, round arterioles in the vascular bundle, and the ascending vasa recta (A) are the large, irregularly shaped, venous capillaries in the bundle. These vessels are the primary supply and drainage of the medulla. JB-4 plastic. Hematoxylin and eosin and phloxine (×530).

large in carnivores. In dogs, they are embedded in the cortical tissue near the surface of the kidney, whereas in cats, they are superficial and are called capsular veins. The stellate veins in most species empty into the interlobular veins, but the capsular veins in cats converge toward the hilus of the kidney to join the renal vein.

The intrarenal arterial system does not provide a good collateral circulatory system. As a result, when a major artery is occluded, death of the tissue supplied by that artery results. For example, when an arcuate artery becomes occluded, a wedge-shaped piece of the kidney, including both cortex and medulla, becomes damaged.

Interstitium, Lymphatics, and Nerves

The interstitium between the renal tubules and the blood vessels is normally sparse, particularly in the cortex, where the tubules and vessels are packed tightly together. More interstitium is present in the medulla, particularly in the inner medulla. The interstitium contains several types of interstitial cells and the extracellular matrix, which is made up of collagen fibrils, glycoproteins, and proteoglycans. Interstitial cells include fibroblasts, bone marrow–derived cells, and a unique lipid-laden interstitial cell that is especially prominent in the inner medulla. The lipid-laden cells are stellate-shaped and produce prostaglandin E_2.

Lymphatics are found in the interstitium surrounding intrarenal arteries; they begin at the vascular pole of the glomerulus or more distally along the afferent arteriole and continue to the renal hilus.

The kidney has efferent innervation to the smooth muscle of arteries, afferent and efferent arterioles, and descending vasa recta; the nerves run in the interstitium surrounding the vessels. Numerous axons and nerve terminals are also present in the area of the juxtaglomerular apparatus and contact the renin-producing juxtaglomerular cells of the afferent arteriole.

Juxtaglomerular Apparatus

The **juxtaglomerular apparatus** is located at the vascular pole of the glomerulus (Figs. 11-6 and 11-25). Its components include the macula densa, the extraglomerular mesangial cells, and the juxtaglomerular cells. The **macula densa** is a patch of specialized epithelial cells in the cortical thick ascending limb where it passes between the afferent and efferent arterioles (Figs. 11-5, 11-6, and 11-25). The cells are tall and narrow compared to typical thick ascending limb cells, and the intercellular spaces between them appear dilated. The basal region of the macula densa is adjacent to the extraglomerular mesangial cells. The **extraglomerular mesangial cells** (Polkissen cells, lacis cells, Goormaghtigh cells) are found between the macula densa and the two arterioles and are continuous with the mesangial cells within the glomerulus. The cells are flattened and arranged into several layers. Gap junctions connect extraglomerular mesangial cells with each other, with intraglomerular mesangial cells, and with juxtaglomerular cells, but not with macula densa cells. **Juxtaglomerular (JG or granular) cells** are primarily found in the afferent arteriole and are derived from smooth muscle (Fig. 11-25). They contain membrane-bounded renin granules of irregular size and shape. Sympathetic nerve endings found near the JG cells are consistent with sympathetic stimulation of renin release.

Structure–Function Relationships in the Kidney

General Function

The kidney excretes metabolic wastes, regulates the volume and composition of body fluids, and regulates systemic blood pressure. Elimination of nitrogenous wastes, such as creatinine, urea, and uric acid, occurs largely by filtration of these substances at

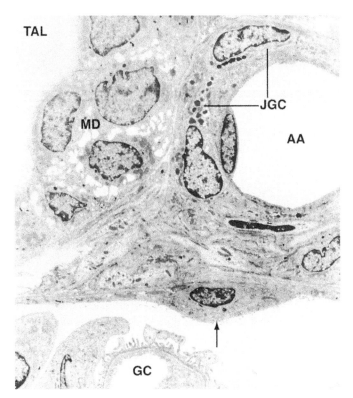

FIGURE 11-25 Transmission electron micrograph of juxta-glomerular apparatus (rat). The macula densa (MD) is located in the thick ascending limb (TAL) where it passes between the afferent and efferent arterioles. Macula densa cells are typically taller and narrower than surrounding thick ascending limb cells and have dilated intercellular spaces. Two juxtaglomerular cells (JGC) with electron-dense granules are present in the wall of the afferent arteriole (AA). Extraglomerular mesangial cells lie between the macula densa and the vascular pole of the glomerulus. A parietal epithelial cell (arrow) and portion of a glomerular capillary (GC) are also visible (×3700).

the glomerulus. Renal regulation of the volume and composition of body fluids is accomplished by changes in both the glomerular filtration rate and the transport processes of the various renal tubule epithelia. The kidney responds to local and systemic factors to maintain fluid, electrolyte, and acid-base homeostasis.

Filtration and Regulation of Blood Pressure

Although the kidneys account for only a small percentage of the body weight of domestic animals, ranging from at most 1% in cats to 0.2% in cattle, they receive a phenomenal 20 to 25% of the cardiac output. Approximately 20% of the volume of blood delivered to the kidney filters across the glomerular capillary wall and forms the glomerular filtrate. However, about 99% of the glomerular filtrate is reabsorbed by the renal tubules, and thus only about 1% of the filtrate volume is excreted as urine. Filtration across the glomerular capillary wall is primarily driven by the hydrostatic pressure of the intracapillary blood; both the systemic blood pressure and the resistance in the afferent and efferent arterioles contribute to the intracapillary hydrostatic pressure.

Filtration is primarily opposed by the osmotic pressure exerted by plasma proteins; the hydrostatic pressure in the urinary space also opposes filtration, but this is negligible under normal circumstances. The filtration barrier created by the glomerular capillary wall is both size and charge selective. Thus, substances over approximately 40,000 kD molecular weight are typically retained within the capillary lumen. Smaller anionic macromolecules are retained more effectively than cationic macromolecules due to the anionic charges of the filtration barrier.

The endothelium blocks filtration of blood cells and platelets. Water and filterable solutes move through the endothelial pores, across the GBM, and through the filtration slits between the podocyte foot processes into the urinary space. The size selectivity of the filtration barrier is primarily created by the tightly knit proteins in the GBM lamina densa. The charge selectivity is created by the anionic molecules coating the endothelial cells and podocytes and in the GBM. These elements repel and block filtration of small anionic plasma proteins, even though neutral or cationic molecules of the same size and shape could be filtered. Normal filtration also requires clearance of macromolecules trapped by the filtration barrier; mesangial cells phagocytose molecules trapped in the GBM and podocytes phagocytose or endocytose molecules trapped at the podocyte surface and slit membrane.

Mesangial cells and podocytes maintain the structural integrity of the capillary tuft. Mesangial cells also contribute to regulation of glomerular capillary perfusion. Largely in response to signals from the macula densa, mesangial cells contract or relax and thus alter resistance within the capillary loops, thereby altering glomerular blood flow. Filtration is also regulated by the resistance in the afferent and efferent arterioles.

Finally, the juxtaglomerular apparatus (Fig. 11-25) not only regulates the rate of flow and perfusion pressure in individual glomeruli, but also contributes to the regulation of systemic blood pressure. Juxtaglomerular cells release **renin** in response to reduced renal perfusion pressure, sympathetic nerve stimulation, or signaling from the macula densa. Renin catalyzes plasma angiotensinogen conversion to angiotensin I, which is converted to **angiotensin II** in many tissues. Angiotensin II increases systemic blood pressure by vasoconstriction and by increasing intravascular volume. Angiotensin II increases intravascular fluid volume by stimulating sodium (and thus water) reabsorption in the proximal tubule and by stimulating adrenal aldosterone secretion, which enhances sodium uptake in the collecting duct.

Tubule Function

The glomerular filtrate traverses the renal tubules where solute and water reabsorption and solute secretion take place. Solute and water reabsorption across the renal tubular epithelium into the peritubular capillaries occurs by transcellular and paracellular pathways.

The **transcellular pathway** uses active and passive processes to move substances through the plasma membranes and cytoplasm. Active transport requires plasma membrane **transport proteins** and energy from ATP to move specific ions across the membrane, often against an electrochemical gradient. Plasma membranes also contain **channel proteins** and **carrier proteins** that do not use ATP; these facilitate ion or water movement across the lipid membranes, often driven by gradients generated by active transporters.

The **paracellular pathway** involves passive movement of water and solute from the tubule lumen to the interstitium through epithelial cell junctions and lateral intercellular spaces. Movement through the paracellular pathway is also driven by gradients produced by active transporters, but is limited by the permeability of the tight junctions joining the cells. Proximal tubules have permeable tight junctions; significant paracellular transport is permitted, but the epithelium cannot maintain large gradients. In the thick ascending limb, distal convoluted tubule, and collecting duct, the tight junctions are relatively impermeable; little paracellular transport occurs, but high salt and water gradients can be sustained.

The structure of renal tubule epithelial cells reflects their function. For example, transmembrane transport depends on plasma membrane surface area and mitochondrial ATP generation. The high capacity for transcellular transport in the proximal tubule is permitted by amplification of both the apical and basolateral plasma membranes and high mitochondrial density. At the other extreme, only limited transcellular transport occurs in the thin limbs of Henle's loop, which have relatively simple plasma membranes and few mitochondria.

Proximal Tubule

The proximal tubule (Figs. 11-13 and 11-14) normally reabsorbs about 85% of the water and salts in the glomerular filtrate and 100% of filtered glucose, amino acids, peptides, and low–molecular-weight proteins. Solute and water uptake are driven by the lumen-to-blood sodium gradient created by active sodium transport across the basolateral plasma membrane. The extensive apical plasma membrane surface area created by the brush border contains numerous specific **transport proteins** that couple sodium uptake with other transport processes, such as bicarbonate and glucose uptake. Water reabsorption follows the chemical gradient created by active sodium reabsorption; water channels (**aquaporins**) allow water to pass through the hydrophobic lipid membrane. The proximal tubule is not a tight epithelium and cannot generate large electrochemical gradients. Thus, although the majority of filtered water and solute is reabsorbed in the proximal tubule, the tubule fluid that enters the thin descending limb is essentially isotonic.

Low–molecular-weight proteins and peptides are filtered but normally are entirely reabsorbed in the proximal tubule. These molecules are taken up from the lumen by receptor-mediated endocytosis into endocytic vesicles and are metabolized in endosomes and lysosomes. A hallmark of glomerular disease is an increase in the amount and size of filtered proteins, with a concurrent increase in the proximal tubule lysosomal system that is visible by light microscopy. When the capacity of the lysosomal system is exceeded, protein appears in the urine; this is often the earliest sign of renal disease.

The proximal tubule also secretes organic ions, which include many drugs and toxins. Uptake of such substances from the blood and secretion into the lumen can concentrate the organic ion in the proximal tubule, sometimes to toxic levels. Proximal tubule damage is often the first sign of toxic injury and may lead to renal failure. An example in clinical settings is renal failure produced by administration of the antibiotic gentamicin, which is secreted by the proximal tubule.

Thin Limbs and Thick Ascending Limb of the Loop of Henle

The physical arrangement and transport characteristics of the thin limbs (Figs. 11-4, 11-17, 11-18, and 11-19) and thick ascending limb of Henle's loop (Fig. 11-19) allow the kidney to produce concentrated urine with minimal energy expenditure. A **countercurrent system** is created by the close apposition of the descending and ascending thin limbs and the opposite direction of tubule fluid flow in these tubules. The descending and ascending vasa recta have a similar countercurrent arrangement. The countercurrent mechanism, along with the active reabsorption of NaCl by the thick ascending limb and the selective permeabilities of the thin limbs to water, salt, and urea, generates and maintains a hypertonic medullary interstitium and permits production of concentrated urine.

The tubule fluid leaves the proximal straight tubule, traverses the thin descending limb through deeper regions of the medulla, makes a hairpin turn, and then ascends through the thin ascending limb and thick ascending limb in long-looped nephrons, or the thick ascending limb in short-looped nephrons. The descending and ascending thin limbs, although structurally similar, have distinct permeabilities that are necessary elements of the countercurrent concentrating mechanism. Also fundamental to this system are the progressively increasing interstitial osmolarity in the medulla and the countercurrent arrangement of the descending and ascending vasa recta. These components function together as follows. The thin descending limb of long-looped nephrons is permeable to water, but impermeable to sodium and urea. Isosmotic tubule fluid enters the thin descending limb and passes through increasing ambient osmolarity in the medulla; water is reabsorbed by passive mechanisms, and by the hairpin turn, luminal fluid tonicity is high. The thin tubule turns and ascends through progressively lower interstitial osmolarity. The thin ascending limb is permeable to sodium, but relatively impermeable to water. Thus, sodium moves down its concentration gradient to the interstitium and is reabsorbed without water; when the tubule fluid reaches the thick ascending limb it is nearly isotonic. These processes occur almost entirely by passive mechanisms. The low level of active transport and the selective permeabilities of the thin limbs correlate with their structure, including uncomplicated plasma membranes, few mitochondria, and complex tight junctions that do not allow leaks.

The vasa recta (Figs. 11-23 and 11-24) are arranged in a similar pattern as the thin limbs, with descending and ascending portions connected by a hairpin turn. The plasma osmolarity entering the descending vasa recta (DVR) is approximately that of the cortical interstitium. The DVR pass through progressively higher interstitial concentrations of NaCl and urea. DVR are not fenestrated, but they permit paracellular diffusion of NaCl and transcellular movement of urea and water into the medullary interstitium via specific proteins. Ascending vasa recta (AVR) are fenestrated and thus are permeable to water, NaCl, and urea, allowing equilibration nearly to isotonicity when the AVR leaves the hypertonic medulla. This system permits adequate blood supply to the inner medulla without degradation of the interstitial hypertonicity.

The thick ascending limb also generates medullary hypertonicity by salt reabsorption without water. The thick ascending limb epithelium has extensive basolateral plasma membrane infoldings that contain abundant **Na$^+$-K$^+$ ATPase** (adenosine triphosphatase), which actively pumps sodium from the cell into the interstitium; the numerous mitochondria interposed among the plasma membrane infoldings produce the necessary energy. The electrochemical gradients created by the basolateral Na$^+$-K$^+$ ATPase drive ion uptake from the lumen via the **NaK2Cl cotransporter** in the apical plasma membrane. This transporter is exclusive to the thick ascending limb; it is inactivated by the drugs furosemide and bumetanide, which are known as "loop diuretics," because they enhance salt and water excretion in Henle's loop. The thick ascending limb is impermeable to water; thus, the avid ion uptake reduces the tubular fluid tonicity and increases the medullary interstitial tonicity.

Distal Convoluted Tubule

In the distal convoluted tubule (DCT) (Fig. 11-20), active transport drives sodium and chloride reabsorption. Because the DCT is impermeable to water, the tubule fluid osmolarity falls to approximately 100 mOsm/kg; thus, the DCT has been called the "diluting segment." Basolateral Na$^+$-K$^+$ ATPase transports sodium to the interstitium; a **NaCl cotransporter** in the apical plasma membrane, the site of action of thiazide diuretics, mediates sodium and chloride uptake from the lumen. The DCT reabsorbs calcium via active transport by basolateral **Ca-ATPase** and secondary active transport through apical calcium channels and a basolateral sodium/calcium exchanger. The complex basolateral plasma membrane infoldings accommodate the many ion transport proteins and the abundant mitochondria produce the energy necessary for high rates of active transport.

Collecting Duct

The collecting duct (Figs. 11-19, 11-21, and 11-22) regulates the final composition of urine and maintains systemic acid-base, sodium, potassium, and water homeostasis. The various epithelial cell types in the collecting duct perform these specific physiologic functions.

Intercalated cells are involved in acid-base regulation. The cortical collecting duct (CCD) can secrete both acid and bicarbonate; this is accomplished by different intercalated cell subtypes. Type A intercalated cells actively secrete acid via apical **H-ATPase** and **H,K-ATPase;** bicarbonate is reabsorbed by the basolateral Cl$^-$/HCO$_3$− **anion exchanger,** AE1. Type B intercalated cells secrete bicarbonate via a distinct apical anion exchanger, pendrin; protons are transported to the interstitium by basolat-

eral proton pumps. The function of non-A, non-B intercalated cells is not clear. They have apical **pendrin,** which suggests they may secrete bicarbonate; they also have apical H-ATPase, which suggests they may secrete protons. Medullary collecting ducts can secrete acid, but not bicarbonate. These segments contain only acid-secreting intercalated cells similar to the type A intercalated cells in the CCD.

Acid-secreting intercalated cells undergo structural changes to enhance acid secretion. The apical cytoplasmic tubulovesicles contain proton pumps. During acidosis, these vesicles fuse with the apical plasma membrane, amplifying the apical plasma membrane and moving proton pumps where they can pump acid into the tubule fluid. Activation of bicarbonate secretion causes similar structural changes in type B intercalated cells; vesicles containing the anion exchanger pendrin are inserted into the apical plasma membrane.

Principal cells and inner medullary collecting duct (IMCD) cells regulate sodium and water excretion. Principal cells reabsorb sodium via Na$^+$-K$^+$ ATPase in the basolateral plasma membrane and sodium channels in the apical plasma membrane. Both of these avenues of sodium uptake are enhanced by the adrenal hormone **aldosterone.**

Principal cells and IMCD cells regulate renal water excretion, but this depends on a hypertonic medullary interstitium and **antidiuretic hormone** (ADH). Principal cells contain apical and basolateral water channels (aquaporins). The apical water channel, **aquaporin 2,** is regulated by ADH. When water must be conserved, ADH released from the pituitary activates the apical water channels. The osmotic gradient between the tubule fluid and the interstitium drives water through the water channels in the plasma membranes to the interstitium. The gradient is sustained despite progressive concentration of the tubule fluid because the medullary interstitium is progressively more hypertonic. When excess water must be excreted, ADH is absent, the apical water channels are not functional, and water stays in the tubule lumen.

In the IMCD, principal cells and IMCD cells also contain urea transporters. Urea transporters in the apical plasma membrane (UT-A1 and UT-A3) facilitate urea uptake. Basolateral facilitated urea transport is also present, but the specific transporters are not yet known. Urea uptake via these transporters is stimulated by ADH and contributes to maintenance of the hypertonic medullary interstitium and thus water conservation.

Both intercalated cells and principal cells participate in regulation of potassium excretion. Principal cells secrete potassium via the basolateral Na$^+$-K$^+$ ATPase and apical potassium channels. Intercalated cells are capable of potassium reabsorption via apical H,K$^+$-ATPase and basolateral potassium channels.

URINARY PASSAGES

The urinary passages include the calyces (large ruminant and pig [Fig. 11-26]), renal pelvis (horse [Fig. 11-27], carnivores, small ruminants and pig), ureters (Fig. 11-28), urinary bladder (Fig. 11-29), and urethra (Fig. 11-30). These structures have a similar

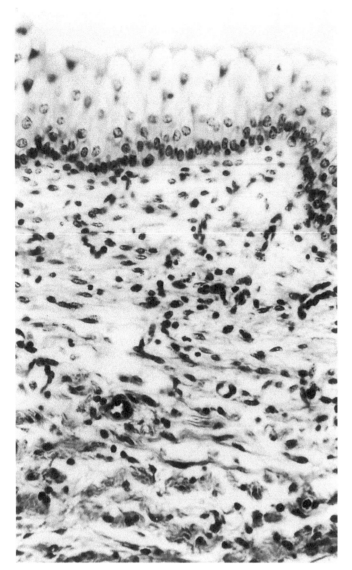

FIGURE 11-26   Calyx (pig). Transitional epithelium lines the inner surface of the calyx. The propria-submucosa is a loose connective-tissue layer with numerous small vessels. A few widely separated smooth muscle fibers form the tunica muscularis. Hematoxylin and eosin (×335).

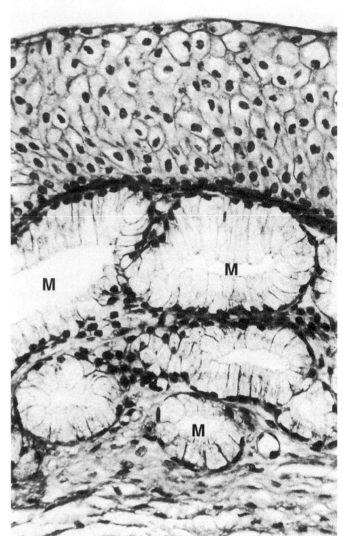

FIGURE 11-27   Renal pelvis (horse). Mucous glands (M) are found in the mucosa just beneath the transitional epithelium of the renal pelvis and the proximal ureter in horses, mules, and donkeys. Ducts, not seen in this section, penetrate the overlaying epithelium and carry the secretion to the lumen. Hematoxylin and eosin (×335).

histologic organization that includes a tunica mucosa of transitional epithelium up to eight cells deep; an underlying loose connective-tissue layer (propria-submucosa); a tunica muscularis of smooth muscle forming inner longitudinal, middle circular, and outer longitudinal layers; and a tunica adventitia of loose connective tissue or a tunica serosa of mesothelium and connective tissue when a visceral peritoneal covering is present. Variations of this general pattern include the following:

1. **Renal pelvis:** In horses, mucous glands (simple branched tubuloalveolar glands) present in the mucosa contribute to the viscous, stringy nature of equine urine (Fig. 11-27). The transitional epithelium is only a few cells deep.
2. **Ureter:** The ureter has a narrow lumen. When the ureter is not distended, the mucosa folds longitudinally, giving the lumen a stellate appearance in cross section. In horses, mucous glands are present in the proximal ureter.
3. **Urinary bladder: Superficial cells** are large transitional epithelial cells that line the lumen. When the urinary bladder is relaxed, the superficial cells contain extensive intracytoplasmic membrane tubulovesicles that are believed to be inserted into the plasma membrane when the bladder is distended. The superficial transitional cells have extensive basolateral plasma membrane infoldings that interdigitate with the plasma membrane of underlying transitional cells. Adjacent transitional cells are connected by numerous desmosomes with long intermediate filaments that extend into the cytoplasm; the desmosomes and intermediate filaments are believed to maintain the epithelial integrity as it stretches and flattens during bladder distention. A lamina muscularis

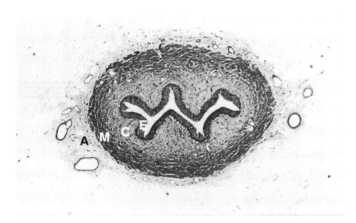

FIGURE 11-28 Ureter (dog). Longitudinal mucosal folds create a stellate-shaped lumen. The epithelial (E), connective tissue (C), muscular (M) and adventitial (A) layers are distinguishable. Hematoxylin and eosin (×50).

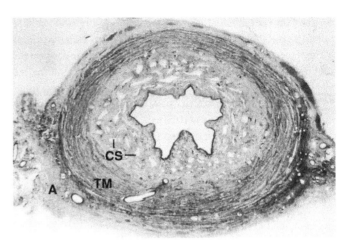

FIGURE 11-30 Urethra (bitch). The mucosa has longitudinal folds. Within the loose connective tissue of the propria-submucosa are numerous irregularly shaped, cavernous blood spaces (CS). The tunica muscularis (TM) is made up primarily of circularly arranged smooth muscle. An adventitia (A) of loose connective tissue surrounds the tunica muscularis. Masson's trichrome (×21).

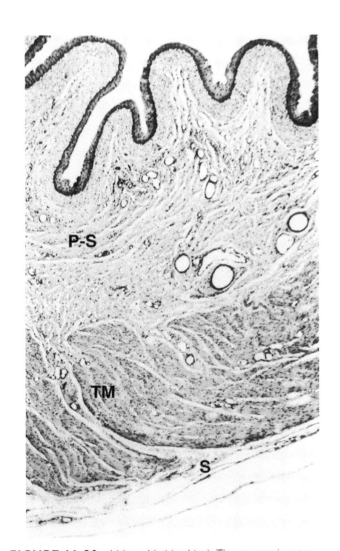

FIGURE 11-29 Urinary bladder (dog). The mucosa is extensively folded and the transitional epithelium and propria-submucosa (P-S) are thick. These are all characteristic features of an empty bladder. The three layers of the tunica muscularis (TM) are not identifiable in this section. A serosa (S) covers the outer surface of the bladder. Hematoxylin and eosin (×50).

of small, isolated bundles of smooth muscle is present in horses, ruminants, dogs, and pigs, but is absent in cats. The lamina muscularis divides the loose connective-tissue layer into an inner lamina propria and an outer submucosa. The smooth muscle of the tunica muscularis, called the detrusor muscle, is composed of three sometimes ill-defined layers of smooth muscle.

4. **Urethra** (female): The epithelium is primarily transitional, but near the external urethral orifice the epithelium changes to stratified squamous. Vessels described as endothelial-lined cavernous spaces are scattered in the connective tissue of the propria-submucosa, giving it the appearance of erectile tissue. The amount and distribution of cavernous tissue in the urethra are species-dependent. A few bundles of longitudinally oriented smooth muscle may form a rudimentary lamina muscularis. The smooth muscle in the tunica muscularis includes irregularly arranged circular and longitudinal components. In the distal urethra, bundles of longitudinally and circularly oriented skeletal muscle are mixed with, or replace, the smooth muscle in the tunica muscularis. A **suburethral diverticulum** lined by transitional epithelium and an underlying loose connective-tissue layer is present ventral to the external urethral orifice in pigs and in ruminants. The male urethra is described in Chapter 12.

These passageways provide a conduit and reservoir for urine plus a mechanism for bladder filling and urine release. Urine is moved from the kidney to the bladder by peristaltic contractions of the smooth muscle of the calices renal pelvis and ureter. The ureters enter the bladder at an acute angle. This angle acts as a valve that prevents reflux of urine back into the ureter. The nervous system controls the muscular components of the bladder and urethra while the bladder fills and is emptied. Bladder filling requires both restriction of outflow and relaxation of the bladder wall. Restriction of outflow results from (a) urethral sphincter constriction via pudendal nerve stimulation of urethral skeletal muscle and (b) sympathetic (hypogastric nerve) stimulation of bladder neck smooth muscle (α-receptors). Bladder relaxation results from (a) inhibition of parasympathetic innervation (pelvic nerve) to the detrusor muscle and (b) inhibition of detrusor muscle contraction by sympathetic nerve stimulation (β-receptors). Voiding of urine is called **micturition**. Voluntary micturition is mediated by the caudal brainstem under cortical and cerebellar control. Normal micturition requires essentially the reverse of bladder filling, that is, relaxation of the urethral sphincter and bladder neck and bladder contraction. Thus, urine outflow is permitted by (a) inhibition of pudendal innervation to urethral skeletal muscle and (b) inhibition of sympathetic innervation to the bladder neck smooth muscle. Bladder contraction results from (a) parasympathetic stimulation of the detrusor muscle and (b) inhibition of sympathetic innervation to the detrusor.

SUGGESTED READINGS

Bulger RE, Cronin RE, Dobyan DC. Survey of the morphology of the dog kidney. Anat Rec 1979;194:41.

Getty R, ed., with editorial coordination and completion by Rosenbaum CE, Ghoshal NG, Hillman D. Sisson and Grossman's Anatomy of the Domestic Animals. 5th Ed. Philadelphia: WB Saunders, 1975.

Kriz W, Kaissling B. Structural organization of the mammalian kidney. In: Seldin DW, Giebisch G, eds. The Kidney: Physiology and Pathophysiology. 3rd Ed. Philadelphia: Lippincott Williams and Wilkins, 2000.

Madsen KM, Brenner BM. Structure and function of the renal tubule and interstitium. In: Tisher CC, Brenner BM, eds. Renal Pathology with Clinical and Functional Correlations. 2nd Ed. Philadelphia: Lippincott, 1994.

Madsen KM, Verlander JW. Renal structure in relation to function. In: Wilcox CS, Tisher CC, eds. Handbook of Nephrology and Hypertension. 5th Ed. Philadelphia: Lippincott Williams and Wilkins, 2004.

Sands JM, Verlander JW. Functional anatomy of the kidney. In: Goldstein RS, ed. Comprehensive Toxicology, Vol. 7, Renal Toxicology. New York: Pergamon Press, 1997.

Tisher CC, Brenner BM. Structure and function of the glomerulus. In: Tisher CC, Brenner BM, eds. Renal Pathology with Clinical and Functional Correlations. 2nd Ed. Philadelphia: Lippincott, 1994.

Tisher CC, Madsen KM. Anatomy of the kidney. In: Brenner BM, ed. The Kidney. 7th Ed. Philadelphia: WB Saunders, 2004.

Verlander JW. Physiology of the kidney. In: Cunningham JG, ed. Textbook of Veterinary Physiology. 3rd Ed. Philadelphia: WB Saunders, 2002.

Verlander JW. Ultrastructural morphology of the urinary tract. Toxicol Pathol 1998;26(1):1–17.

Yadava RP, Calhoun ML. Comparative histology of the kidney of domestic animals. Am J Vet Res 1958;19:958.

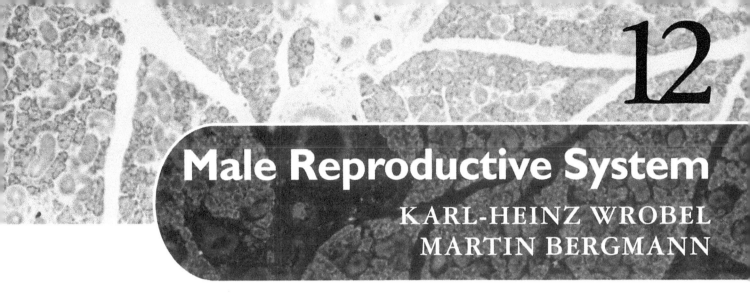

12

Male Reproductive System

KARL-HEINZ WROBEL
MARTIN BERGMANN

Testis
  Stroma and Interstitium
    Tunica vaginalis
    Tunica albuginea
    Septula testis and mediastinum testis
    Interstitial endocrine cells
  Convoluted Seminiferous Tubules
    Lamina propria
    Sustentacular cells
    Spermatogenic cells
    Spermatocytogenesis
    Meiosis
    Spermiogenesis
    Spermatozoon
      Head
      Neck
      Middle piece
      Principal piece
      End piece
    Cyclic events in the seminiferous tubules
  Straight Testicular Tubules

Rete testis
Testicular blood supply and testicular innervation
Epididymis
  Ductuli Efferentes
  Ductus Epididymidis
Ductus Deferens
Accessory Glands
  Vesicular Gland
    Species differences
  Prostate
    Species differences
  Bulbourethral Gland
    Species differences
Urethra
Penis
  Corpora Cavernosa Penis
  Glans Penis
  Species Differences
  Mechanism of Erection
Prepuce

The male reproductive system consists of (a) the testes surrounded by the tunica vaginalis and the testicular tunics, (b) the epididymides, (c) the ductus deferens, (d) the accessory glands (glandular portion of the ductus deferens, vesicular and bulbourethral glands, prostate), (e) the urethra, and (f) the penis surrounded by the prepuce.

TESTIS

Stroma and Interstitium

Tunica Vaginalis

The **tunica vaginalis** consists of mesothelium and a connective-tissue layer that blends with underlying connective tissue of the scrotum (described in Chapter 16) and testis. When the testis is

233

removed from the scrotum, the parietal layer of the tunica vaginalis remains attached to the inner surface of the scrotum, whereas the visceral layer, the peritoneal covering of the testis (and epididymis), remains intimately associated with the underlying capsule (tunica albuginea) of the testis. A space, the vaginal cavity, separates the parietal and visceral layers.

Tunica Albuginea

The **tunica albuginea** (Fig. 12-1) is a solid capsule of dense irregular connective tissue. It consists predominantly of collagen fibers, a few elastic fibers, and myofibroblasts. Intratunical interstitial endocrine cells occur in the cat. Meandering branches of the testicular artery and a network of anastomosing veins constitute the vascular layer (tunica vasculosa) of the tunica albuginea.

Septula Testis and Mediastinum Testis

The tunica albuginea is continuous with connective-tissue trabeculae, the so-called **septula testis,** which converge toward the mediastinum testis. These trabeculae are rather complete septa

in dogs and boars, whereas in the other domestic animals, they are inconspicuous connective-tissue strands surrounding the large intratesticular vessels. The septula testis divide the testicular parenchyma into a varying number of testicular **lobules,** each containing one to four convoluted seminiferous tubules (Fig. 12-2). The septula testis are continuous with the **mediastinum testis** (Fig. 12-3), a connective-tissue area containing the channels of the rete testis and large blood and lymph vessels. The mediastinum testis of stallions and many rodents is relatively small and located in a marginal position, whereas in ruminants, pigs, cats, and dogs, it occupies a central position along the longitudinal axis of the gonad.

Interstitial Endocrine Cells

The intertubular spaces of the testis contain loose connective tissue, blood and lymph vessels, fibrocytes, free mononuclear cells, and interstitial endocrine (Leydig) cells (Fig. 12-4). **Interstitial endocrine cells** constitute approximately 1% of the entire testicular volume in adult rams, approximately 5% in bulls, and 20 to 30% in boars. In seasonally breeding males (e.g., camel), interstitial endocrine cell volume and number may change during the year. The interstitial endocrine cell is a large polymorphous cell with a spherical nucleus. The cell occurs in cords or clusters, and not every interstitial endocrine cell is in close contact with a capillary. Smooth endoplasmic reticulum (sER) (in bulls, a granular endoplasmic reticulum) is the dominating organelle in interstitial endocrine cells. sER membranes incorporate most of the enzymes necessary for steroid biosynthesis. Mitochondria of the interstitial endocrine cell have tubular cristae and are involved in the first step of steroid hormone production (e.g., transformation

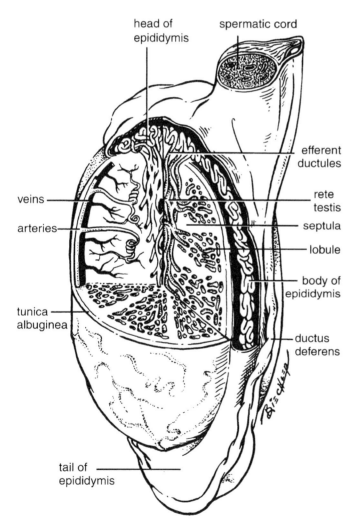

FIGURE 12-1 Schematic drawing of a bovine testis, epididymis, ductus deferens, and spermatic cord. The testicular lobules contain seminiferous tubules. Branches of the arteries and veins in the vascular layer supply and drain the testicular parenchyma and stroma.

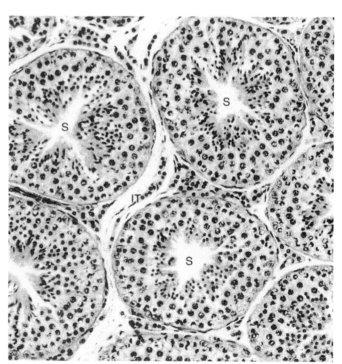

FIGURE 12-2 Seminiferous tubules (S) and intertubular tissues (IT) of the canine testis. Hematoxylin and eosin (×140).

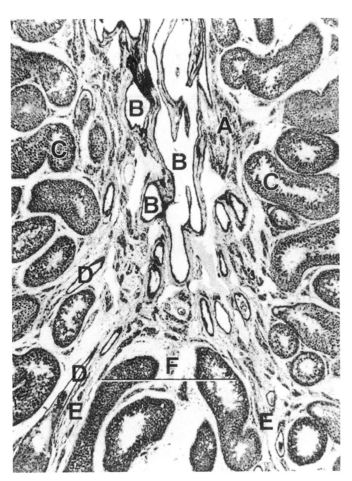

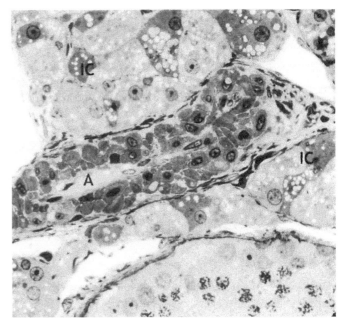

FIGURE 12-4 Intertubular region of the cat testis. The interstitial endocrine cells (IC) have round nuclei and many lipid inclusions. The small artery (A) with loosely arranged muscle cells represents the type with dual innervation by noradrenergic and cholinergic fibers. Semithin section (×450).

FIGURE 12-3 The mediastinum testis (A) of the cat is a connective-tissue area in the central longitudinal axis of the gonad and contains the anastomosing channels of the rete testis (B). Convoluted seminiferous tubules (C) empty into straight testicular tubules (D), which connect with the rete. The septula testis (E) are located between testicular lobules (F). Masson-Goldner (×35).

of cholesterol to pregnenolone). The relatively small Golgi complex does not participate in secretion of androgen. Release of androgen from interstitial endocrine cells is morphologically inconspicuous. Lipid inclusions are found in all species, but are particularly abundant in cats (Fig. 12-4). Between adjacent cells are intercellular canaliculi and gap junctions.

Two generations of interstitial endocrine cells, fetal and pubertal, develop from mesenchymelike precursors. In some species (e.g., bovine and porcine), a third generation of interstitial endocrine cells (early postnatal) is encountered.

Interstitial endocrine cells produce testicular androgens (testosterone) and, in boars, large amounts of estrogen as well. More than 90% of all androgens in the organism are produced by the testis. Among the main functions of testosterone (in some tissues, to be effective, testosterone must be converted by the enzyme 5-α reductase to dihydrotestosterone) are (a) promotion of normal sexual behavior (libido); (b) triggering of the growth and maintenance of the function of the penis, male accessory glands, and secondary sex characteristics; (c) control of spermatogenesis (together with follicle-stimulating hormone [FSH]); (d) negative

feedback action on the hypophysis and hypothalamus; (e) general anabolic effects; and (f) the prenatal maintenance of the mesonephric (wolffian) duct and its differentiation into the epididymis and ductus deferens.

Convoluted Seminiferous Tubules

The **convoluted seminiferous tubules** (tubuli seminiferi convoluti) in most mammals are tortuous two-ended loops with a diameter between 150 and 300 µm (Fig. 12-3). They are lined by the stratified **spermatogenic epithelium** (germinal epithelium), surrounded by a lamina propria, and connected at both ends to straight testicular tubules by a specialized terminal segment (see Fig. 12-12). The length of all seminiferous tubules in the testis of the adult bovine amounts to approximately 5000 m. Histologically, the seminiferous tubules have three components: lamina propria, sustentacular cells (somatic, supporting, or Sertoli cells), and spermatogenic cells.

Lamina Propria

The lamina propria surrounds the seminiferous tubule. Its innermost layer is a basement membrane, often with club-shaped projections that extend into basal infoldings of sustentacular cells and spermatogonia. Collagen and elastic fibers connect the basement membrane to the flat **peritubular cells**, which form a stratum of one to five layers, depending on the species. At birth, these peritubular cells resemble mesenchymal cells, which gradually differentiate into contractile cells postnatally. In some species (e.g., boars), the cells acquire all features of typical smooth muscle cells; in other species (e.g., bulls), they represent myofibroblasts.

The peritubular cells contain actin filament bundles that are arranged in both circular and longitudinal directions and are responsible for tubular contractions. Thus, the peritubular cells participate in transport of tubular content and in **spermiation**, that is, the release of spermatozoa into the tubular lumen. The outermost layer of the tubular lamina propria consists of fibrocytes and collagen fibrils. Lymphocytes and monocytes invade the lamina propria but never the intact tubular epithelium.

Sustentacular Cells

Sustentacular (Sertoli) cells are derived from undifferentiated supporting cells of the prepubertal gonad. The undifferentiated cells are mitotically active, contain large amounts of rough endoplasmic reticulum (rER), and produce **antiparamesonephric hormone**, a glycoprotein that suppresses development of uterine tubes, uterus, and vagina in the male. During puberty, sustentacular cell differentiation is accompanied by a morphologic transformation and loss of mitotic capability.

The adult sustentacular cells are irregularly outlined, elongated cells (Fig. 12-5). Their broad base rests on the basement membrane, and the remaining cytoplasm extends upward to the tubular lumen. They are rather evenly spaced; approximately 20 sustentacular cells are seen in a cross section of an adult seminiferous tubule. Lateral and apical cytoplasmic processes of the sustentacular cells fill all the spaces between adjacent spermatogenic cells. The oval or pear-shaped nucleus is generally located in the broad basal portion of the cell, is often deeply infolded, and contains a large nucleolus. The basal portion and the central trunk region of the sustentacular cell contain mitochondria, an inconspicuous Golgi complex, abundant sER, little rER, free ribosomes, microtubules, actin and vimentin filaments, lysosomes, and lipid inclusions. Only a few organelles are found in the lateral and apical sustentacular cell processes.

The shape of the cell, the surface area, volume percentages of the nucleus and organelles (sER, lysosomes, lipid inclusions), and the amount, and organization of the cytoskeleton change in accordance with spermatogenic events (**sustentacular cell cycle**) (Fig. 12-6). Sustentacular cells form hemidesmosomes with the basement membrane. Temporary junctions with adjacent germ cells play a part in vertical displacement and release (spermiation) of the germ cells into the lumen of the tubule. Adjacent sustentacular cells are joined by tight junctions associated with actin filaments and subsurface cisternae of the ER. These junctions separate a **basal compartment** from an **adluminal (apical) compartment**, and constitute a diffusion barrier, also referred to as the **blood-testis barrier**. Renewal of spermatogenic stem cells and multiplication of spermatogonia take place in the basal compartment, to which intertubular tissue fluid has relatively free access. The blood-testis barrier selectively prevents many substances from entering the adluminal compartment, where the vital processes of meiosis and spermiogenesis take place in a controlled microenvironment. Another function of the blood-testis barrier is to prevent autoimmune reactions against postspermatogonial germ cells. Early spermatocytes must pass through these specialized intercellular junctions

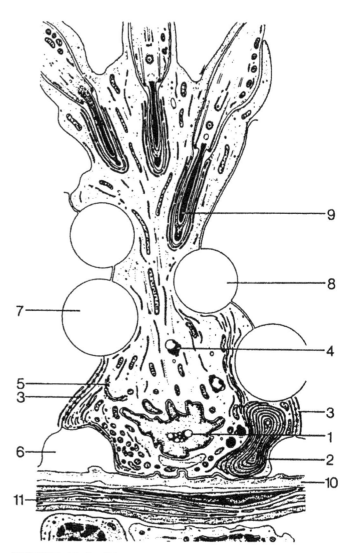

FIGURE 12-5 Diagrammatic representation of sustentacular cell–germ cell interrelationships in the bull. **1.** Sustentacular cell nucleus. **2.** Smooth endoplasmic reticulum. **3.** Tight junctions between adjacent sustentacular cells constituting the morphologic equivalent of the blood-testis barrier. **4.** Phagolysosomes. **5.** Golgi complex. **6.** Space occupied by a spermatogonium. **7.** Space occupied by a primary spermatocyte. **8.** Space occupied by a spherical spermatid. **9.** Elongated spermatid within apical recess of sustentacular cell. **10.** Basement membrane. **11.** Peritubular cell (myofibroblast). *(With permission from Mosimann M, Kohler T. Zytologie, Histologie und mikroskopische Anatomie der Haussäugetiere. Hamburg: Paul Parey, 1990.)*

joining sustentacular cells without interrupting the physiologic blood-testis barrier. Such passage is probably accomplished by a zipperlike opening of these junctions, which closes again below the spermatocytes before they reach the adluminal compartment.

Sustentacular cells have nutritive, protective, and supportive functions for the spermatogenic cells. In addition, they phagocytize degenerating spermatogenic cells and detached residual bodies of spermatids. Sustentacular cells release the spermatozoa into the lumen of the seminiferous tubules (spermiation). They mediate the action of FSH and testosterone on the germ cells,

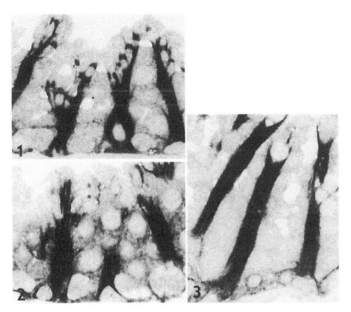

FIGURE 12-6 Shape and size of the sustentacular cells (ovine; dark cells) vary characteristically in accordance with the stages of the seminiferous epithelial cycle. **1.** Stage 2. **2.** Stage 4. **3.** Stage 8. Alpha-tubulin reaction (×560).

participate in the synchronization of spermatogenic events, and secrete constituents of the intratubular fluid such as transferrin, androgen-binding protein, and inhibin. **Inhibin** is reabsorbed from the lumen of the efferent ductules and the initial segment of ductus epididymidis; it then reaches the bloodstream and exerts negative feedback on hypophyseal FSH secretion. Paracrine signals from sustentacular cells modulate the activity of nearby interstitial endocrine cells. Although normal sustentacular cells have minimally proven steroidogenic function, sustentacular cell tumors may produce large amounts of estrogen, leading to feminization of the animal.

Spermatogenic Cells

Various **spermatogenic cells,** representing different phases in the development and differentiation of the spermatozoon, are located between the sustentacular cells. The sequence of events in the development of spermatozoa from spermatogonia is referred to as **spermatogenesis** and is subdivided into three phases: (a) **spermatocytogenesis,** the process during which spermatogonia divide mitotically several times and finally develop into primary spermatocytes; (b) **meiosis,** the maturation division of spermatocytes that results in spermatids with a reduced (haploid) number of chromosomes; and (c) **spermiogenesis,** the process of transformation of spermatids into spermatozoa. The duration of spermatogenesis is approximately 39 days in boars; 50 days in bulls, rams, and stallions; and 55 days in dogs.

Germ cell loss by apoptosis or degeneration is low during spermatocytogenesis, but affects between 6% and 18% of the cells during the two meiotic divisions in the ruminant spermatogenic epithelium. The main reason for this numerical decrease is an escape of cells into the tubular lumen during the second meiotic division. As a consequence, exfoliated germ cells are regu-

larly observed within the lumen of the testicular excurrent duct system (see Fig. 12-15).

In addition to the cell population involved in spermatogenesis (cycling population), the spermatogenic epithelium contains a separate spermatogonia stem and precursor cell line, which guarantees uninterrupted spermatogenesis and can adapt to changing demands. Spermatogonia stem and precursor cells are morphologically similar to cycling spermatogonia and are also located in the basal tubular compartment.

Spermatocytogenesis

During **spermatocytogenesis,** spermatogonia multiply mitotically, resulting in A-, I- (intermediate), and B-spermatogonia and finally in preleptotene primary spermatocytes (Figs. 12-7 and 12-8). Primary spermatocytes no longer divide mitotically, but instead undergo two meiotic divisions, which result in a fourfold increase in the number of germ cells. Therefore, the number of spermatozoa that originate from one A-spermatogonium is decisively influenced by spermatogonial proliferation during spermatocytogenesis. In most mammals, a variable number of generations of A-spermatogonia are followed by one generation each of I- (intermediate) and B-spermatogonia, respectively. In a given tubular segment, the few A-spermatogonia are irregularly distributed. Daughter cells of A- and I-mitoses drift apart to achieve an even distribution. **A-spermatogonia** are the largest spermatogonia and share an extensive contact area with the tubular basement membrane. They possess prominent nucleoli and nuclei with a pale or cloudy appearance. The small **B-spermatogonia** have spherical nuclei containing numerous chromatin particles and less prominent nucleoli. Most spermatogonia of a given tubular segment are interconnected by cytoplasmic processes and form a network composed of individual cells (Fig. 12-7). The mitotic division of B-spermatogonia results in the formation of **preleptotene primary spermatocytes.** These cells and their descendents are interconnected by true cytoplasmic bridges and form a syncytium until shortly before spermiation. Preleptotene primary spermatocytes gradually lose contact with the basement membrane and are passively translocated into the adluminal tubular compartment across the intercellular junctions between the sustentacular cells. In preleptotene primary spermatocytes, the nuclear deoxyribonucleic acid (DNA) is replicated and all chromosomes consist of two sister chromatids.

Meiosis

During **meiosis,** two successive nuclear divisions occur, resulting in the formation of four haploid spermatids from one primary spermatocyte. **Primary spermatocytes** are the largest spermatogenic cells in the tubular epithelium and are located in the intermediate position between spermatogonia and spermatids. Because the prophase of the first maturation division is extremely prolonged, two generations of primary spermatocytes are present in many tubular sections (Fig. 12-8; see also Fig. 12-11). The prophase of the **first maturation division** is subdivided into the leptotene, zygotene, pachytene, diplotene, and diakinesis stages according to characteristic changes in nuclear chromatin. During

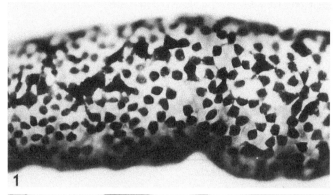

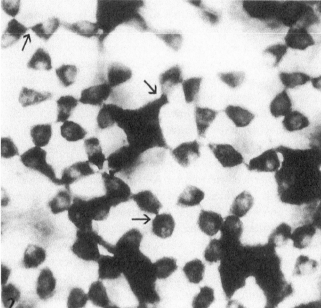

FIGURE 12-7 **1.** Surface of a tubular whole mount (bovine) showing evenly distributed small B-spermatogonia and irregularly spaced larger A-spermatogonia. Protein gene product 9.5 reaction (×225). **2.** Surface of tubular whole mount at higher magnification (×560). The small B-spermatogonia and the large future A-spermatogonia for the next round of spermatocytogenesis are both members of a common cellular network and are interconnected by narrow mutual processes (arrows) but remain individual cells. On the contrary, postspermatogonial germ cells undergo incomplete cell divisions and form true syncytia.

the **leptotene stage,** the chromosomes become arranged in thin threadlike strands. In the **zygotene stage,** homologous chromosomes begin to pair and tetrads of four chromatids emerge. Visible evidence of pairing is the synaptic complexes seen under the electron microscope. Completion of pairing initiates the **pachytene phase,** during which crossing over occurs between the nonsister chromatids of the paired chromosomes. In microscopic preparations, primary spermatocytes are best identified when they are in this phase of meiosis (Fig. 12-8; see also Fig.12-11). During the **diplotene phase,** the paired chromosomes pull away from each other, but sister chromatids remain attached through chiasmata (i.e., sites where crossing over has occurred). During the prophase of the first meiotic division, the cells grow consider-

ably. For instance, between preleptotene and diplotene, ovine primary spermatocytes increase in volume 4.8 times and their nuclei increase in volume 3.3 times. During **diakinesis,** the chromosomes shorten and broaden and the four separate chromatids are clearly evident. At the end of prophase, the nuclear membrane disappears.

The metaphase, anaphase, and telophase of the first maturation division occur rapidly. During these phases, the paired chromosomes are first arranged at the equatorial plate. Subsequently, homologous chromosomes move to opposite poles of the cell to be distributed to the secondary spermatocytes, which have only half the number of chromosomes, but two chromatids each (dyads). **Secondary spermatocytes** are short-lived (a few hours), intermediate in size between diplotene primary spermatocytes and spherical spermatids, and occur exclusively in phase 4 of the seminiferous epithelial cycle (Fig. 12-8).

After a short period of interphase, during which no duplication of genetic material occurs, the secondary spermatocytes undergo the **second maturation division,** with a short prophase followed by metaphase, anaphase, and telophase, which are essentially similar to those of mitotic divisions. During this division, the centromeres divide and the sister chromatids of the secondary spermatocytes separate and are distributed to each of the spermatids resulting from that division. Thus, these cells possess a haploid set of chromosomes with 1N DNA each.

Spermiogenesis

The process by which interconnected clones of newly formed spermatids differentiate into individual testicular spermatozoa is referred to as **spermiogenesis.** The most important morphologic changes during spermiogenesis are formation of the acrosome, condensation of the nuclear chromatin, outgrowth of a motile tail, and loss of excess spermatid material (cytoplasm, water, organelles) not necessary for the later spermatozoon.

Spermiogenesis is divided into the Golgi phase, cap phase, acrosomal phase, and maturation phase (Fig. 12-9). In histologic sections, the Golgi and cap phases are characterized by spherical nuclei, whereas the acrosomal and maturation phases have elongated nuclei (Fig. 12-8; see also Fig. 12-11).

During the **Golgi phase,** proacrosomal granules appear in Golgi vesicles and eventually fuse to form a single acrosomal granule within a single acrosomal vesicle. Both structures make contact with an indentation of the nucleus, thus marking the anterior pole of the future sperm head.

During the **cap phase,** the acrosomal vesicle grows and forms the head cap that covers the anterior two thirds of the nucleus. In the late cap phase, the still spherical spermatid becomes polarized, and the nucleus and head cap are shifted to an eccentric position. The two centrioles assemble at the posterior pole of the nucleus, and the distal centriole gives rise to the outgrowing flagellum.

In the early **acrosomal phase,** the nucleus and cell body start to elongate in a craniocaudal direction. At the same time, the spermatids rotate so that the nucleus is directed toward the periphery of the tubule and the developing tail is directed toward the lumen. The spermatids, formerly separated by lateral susten-

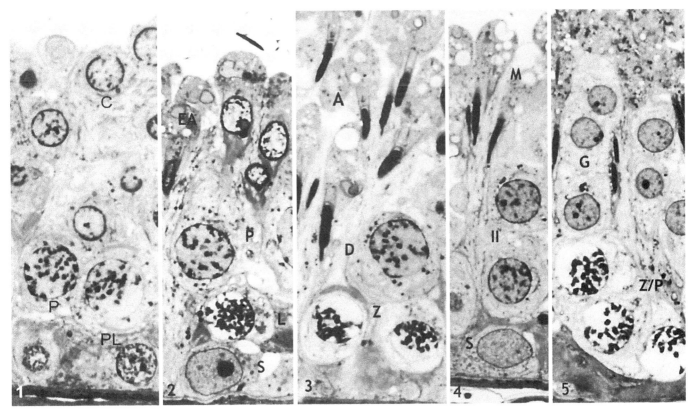

FIGURE 12-8 Typical morphology of the various cells in the spermatogenic epithelium (water buffalo). The numbers on the images correspond to the stages of the epithelial cycle (compare to Figure 12-11). Spermatogonia (S); preleptotene primary spermatocytes (PL); leptotene primary spermatocytes (L); zygotene primary spermatocytes (Z); zygotenes entering pachytene (Z/P); pachytene primary spermatocytes (P); diplotene primary spermatocytes (D); secondary spermatocytes (II); Golgi-phase spermatids (G); cap-phase spermatids (C); early acrosome–phase spermatids (EA); acrosome-phase spermatids (A); maturation-phase spermatids (M). Semithin sections (×1560).

tacular cell processes, are now embedded in apical recesses of these cells. As the nucleus begins to elongate, nuclear histones, which are responsible for the normal spatial nucleosomal arrangement of nuclear DNA, are gradually replaced by basic proteins (protamines), which allow dense packing of the chromatin. After this condensation, the DNA is transcriptionally inactive and resistant to noxious influences. During fertilization, protamines must be replaced by histones before decondensation of the chromatin. These histones are provided by the oocyte.

During the **maturation phase,** nuclear condensation is completed. In the region of the future middle piece of the spermatozoon, most of the mitochondria gather around the axoneme in a helicoidal manner. The system of the outer fibers and the fibrous sheath of the future principal piece develop. The volume of a spermatid in the late maturation phase amounts to only 20 to 30% of that of a cap-phase spermatid. Autolytic processes are generally responsible for this reduction. In the bovine, sustentacular cell processes contacting the spermatids participate in absorption of spermatid material. Before spermiation, the cytoplasmic bridges between maturation-phase spermatids are disconnected and excess cytoplasm is detached as residual body. Residual bodies have different fates; they may be phagocytosed by sustentacular cells, lost into the tubular lumen, or subjected to rapid autolysis when attached to the apical border of the tubular epithelium. A small remaining portion of spermatid cyto-

plasm, the cytoplasmic droplet of young spermatozoa, is lost during epididymal passage.

Spermatozoon

Spermatozoa vary in length from approximately 60 µm (boars, stallions) to 75 µm (ruminants). Under the light microscope, the spermatozoon consists of two portions: the head and the tail. With the electron microscope, the tail is subdivided further into the neck, middle piece, principal piece, and end piece (Fig. 12-10).

Head

The shape of the nucleus and acrosome determines the shape of the **head** of the spermatozoon, which is species-dependent and subject to great variations. The anterior pole of the nucleus is covered by the **acrosomal cap,** with an outer and an inner acrosomal membrane that fuse at the caudal end. The acrosomal cap contains several hydrolytic and proteolytic enzymes (e.g., acrosin), which are set free during the **acrosome reaction** of capacitated spermatozoa in the uterine tube. Acrosomal enzymes are needed for the penetration of the zona pellucida during fertilization. The posterior region of the acrosome is characterized by a narrowing of the cap and condensation of its contents. This area is the equatorial segment of the acrosome. The base of the nucleus is surrounded by the postacrosomal sheath, which consists of fibrous

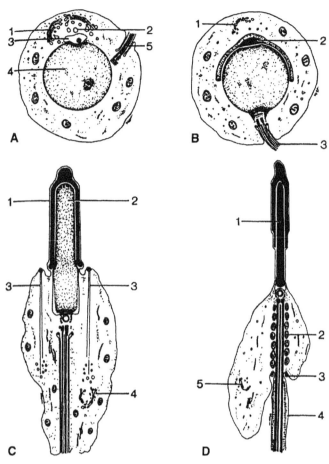

FIGURE 12-9 Spermiogenesis (bull). **A.** Spherical spermatid, Golgi phase. 1. Golgi complex; 2. Golgi vesicle; 3. acrosomal vesicle containing acrosomal granule; 4. nucleus; 5. developing tail. **B.** Spherical spermatid, cap phase. 1. Golgi complex; 2. head cap containing acrosome; 3. developing tail. **C.** Elongated spermatid, acrosomal phase. 1. acrosomal cap containing acrosome; 2. nucleus; 3. manchette; 4. Golgi complex. **D.** Elongated spermatid, maturation phase. 1. nucleus (condensation completed); 2. middle piece with mitochondrial sheath; 3. annulus; 4. principal piece; 5. Golgi complex. *(With permission from Mosimann W, Kohler T. Zytologie, Histologie und mikroskopische Anatomie der Haussäugetiere. Hamburg: Paul Parey, 1990.)*

proteins rich in sulfur. In dead spermatozoa, the sheath stains intensely with certain dyes, such as eosin or bromophenol blue. This reaction is used to evaluate the quality of an ejaculate. The plasma membrane of the postacrosomal head region contains receptor molecules necessary for the recognition of a homologous oocyte. At the posterior surface of the sperm head, the nuclear envelope lines an implantation groove where the tail is inserted in a jointlike manner.

Neck

The **neck** is a relatively short and narrow structure between the head and middle piece. It consists of a centrally located centriole and nine peripheral, longitudinally oriented coarse fibers (connecting piece) continuous with the outer dense fibers of the middle piece.

Middle piece

The core of the **middle piece** has the characteristic structure of a flagellum: two central microtubules and nine peripheral doublets (microtubules) making up the axial filament complex. They are surrounded by nine longitudinally oriented, tapered outer fibers that are connected to the fibers of the connecting piece in the neck. These, in turn, are surrounded by the mitochondria in a helicoid arrangement. In ruminants, the mitochondrial helix consists of approximately 40 turns. A ring-shaped thickening of the plasma membrane (annulus) of the middle piece marks the limit between the middle piece and the principal piece.

Principal piece

The **principal piece** is the longest portion of the spermatozoon. The axial filament complex has a structure identical to that of the middle piece and is surrounded by the continuing outer fibers of the middle piece. The fibers are subject to variations in size and shape and gradually taper toward the end of the principal piece. Semicircular ribs of structural proteins in a helicoid arrangement fuse to two of the outer fibers to form the characteristic peripheral fibrous sheath of the principal piece.

End piece

The termination of the fibrous sheath marks the beginning of the **end piece,** which contains only the axial filament complex. Proximally, in the end piece, this complex has its characteristic nine peripheral doublets; distally, these doublets gradually become reduced to singlets and terminate at various levels.

Cyclic Events in the Seminiferous Tubules

Before one spermatogenic series is completed, several (generally four) new spermatogenic series are initiated at the same level within the seminiferous tubule. As all the descendents of each B-spermatogonium develop synchronously, successive cell generations follow each other with cyclic regularity, from the periphery toward the center of the seminiferous tubule (seminiferous epithelial cycle).

Changes in the shape and staining of the nuclei during cell division and release of spermatozoa into the tubular lumen provide a basis for dividing the spermatogenic cycle into stages. In testes of bulls, rams, and boars, eight stages can be identified (Fig. 12-11):

Stage 1. After spermiation, spherical spermatids lie nearest to the lumen, followed basally by two generations of primary spermatocytes, that is, old pachytenes and young preleptotenes/leptotenes (Fig. 12-11-1).

Stage 2. The spermatids and their dark-stained nuclei are elongated. The two generations of primary spermatocytes are old pachytenes and young leptotenes/zygotenes (Fig. 12-11-2).

Stage 3. Elongated spermatids are arranged in bundles and lie in deep apical recesses of the sustentacular cells (Fig. 12-11-3). The pachytenes of stage 2 have reached diplotene. A second generation of primary spermatocytes in zygotene is present in the basal region.

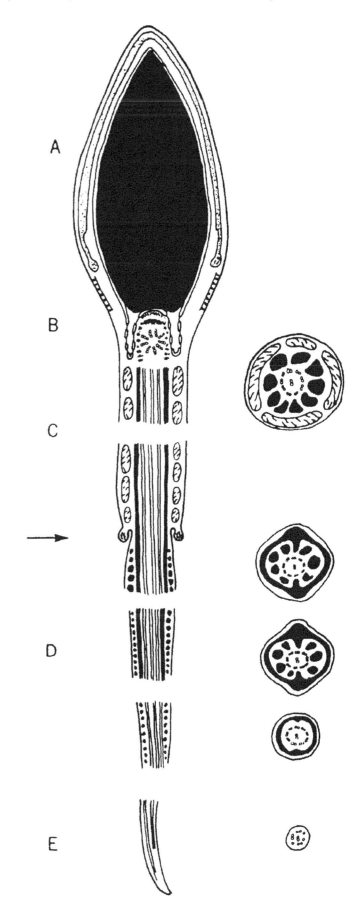

FIGURE 12-10 Schematic drawing of a spermatozoon. **Left,** Longitudinal section. **Right,** Cross sections located at the levels from which they are taken. **A.** Head containing the nucleus covered by the acrosome. Note the equatorial segment of the acrosome and postacrosomal sheath. **B.** Neck. **C.** Middle piece with central axial filament complex, nine outer dense fibers, and the surrounding mitochondria. The middle piece terminates at the annulus (arrow). **D.** Principal piece in which the outer dense fibers are surrounded by the fibrous sheath; they terminate before the end of the principal piece. **E.** In the end piece, the microtubules of the axial filament complex terminate at various levels.

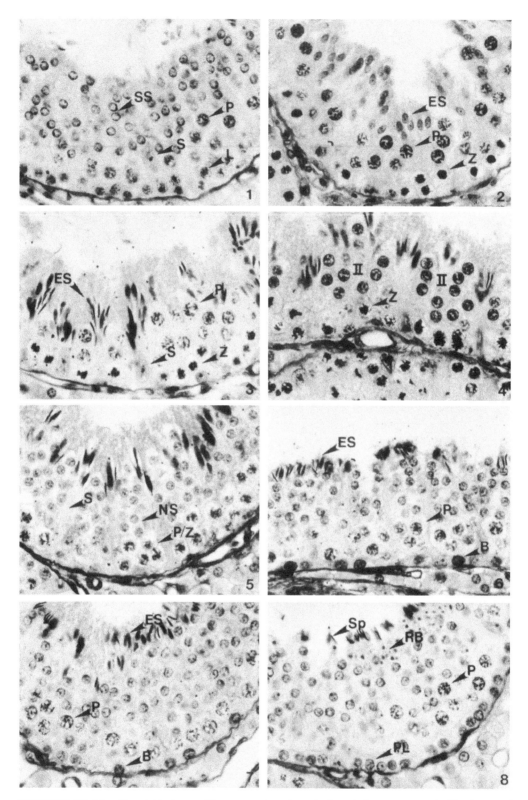

FIGURE 12-11   The eight stages of the spermatogenic cycle (boar). B spermatogonia (B); elongated spermatids (ES); leptotene primary spermatocytes (L); newly formed spermatids (NS); pachytene primary spermatocytes (P); preleptotene primary spermatocytes (PL); primary spermatocytes leaving zygotene and entering pachytene (P/Z); zygotene (Z); residual bodies (RB); sustentacular cell (S); spermatozoa in spermiation (Sp); spherical spermatids (SS); secondary spermatocytes (II). Periodic acid-Schiff (×500).

Stage 4. The first and second maturation divisions take place. In addition to bundles of maturing spermatids and zygotene primary spermatocytes, either diplotenes, secondary spermatocytes, or spherical spermatids are seen (Fig. 12-11-4).

Stage 5. Two generations of spermatids are present: older elongated spermatids and newly formed spherical spermatids. The zygotenes of stage 4 enter the pachytene stage and are displaced in the direction of the tubular lumen (Fig. 12-11-5).

Stage 6. The bundles of older spermatids have moved away from the vicinity of the sustentacular cell nuclei. In addition to spherical spermatids, pachytenes and numerous spermatogonia (I- or B-) are present (Fig. 12-11-6).

Stage 7. The maturation-phase spermatids achieve a position close to the tubular lumen. All other cells are as in stage 6 (Fig. 12-11-7).

Stage 8. Spermatozoa leave the tubular epithelium (spermiation) after separation from their residual bodies. Remaining within the epithelium are spherical spermatids and two generations of primary spermatocytes (older pachytenes and young preleptotenes) (Fig. 12-11-8).

In all domestic animals, not only are the descendents of one spermatogonium all more or less at the same stage of development, but identical cellular associations are found over a certain distance in cross and longitudinal sections of seminiferous tubules. These **spermatogenic segments** (portions with synchronized development of germ cells) are usually arranged so that one specific segment is located between the preceding and following stages of the spermatogenic cycle. If stages 1 through 8 succeed each other along the length of the seminiferous tubule, the sequence is referred to as a regular **spermatogenic wave**, which is approximately 10 mm long in bulls. Variations, such as repetition of wave fragments (1-2-3-4-1-2-3-4) or inversions (1-2-3-4-5-4-3-2), seem to occur more frequently, however. Exactly what determines the spermatogenic cycles, segments, and waves is not known at this time.

Straight Testicular Tubules

In all domestic mammals, most of the convoluted seminiferous tubules terminate into the **straight testicular tubules** (tubuli recti), which are connected to the rete testis (Fig. 12-1). Straight testicular tubules are generally short and have a straight course. In stallions and boars, some of the convoluted seminiferous tubules terminate at the periphery of the testis and join the rete testis by long, straight testicular tubules situated within the septula testis. The terminal segment of the convoluted seminiferous tubule is composed of modified sustentacular cells that occlude the tubular lumen and project their apices into the cup-shaped initial portion of the straight testicular tubule (Fig. 12-12). All spermatozoa must pass through the narrow intercellular slits between adjacent modified sustentacular cells on their way to the straight tubule. The terminal segment may further function as a valve that prevents reflux of rete testis fluid into the seminiferous tubules.

The straight testicular tubules are lined with a simple squamous to columnar epithelium. In bulls, a simple cuboidal epithe-

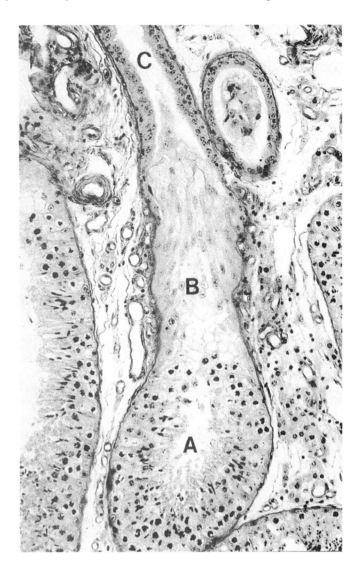

FIGURE 12-12 Convoluted seminiferous tubule (A), terminal segment (B) surrounded by a vascular plexus, and straight testicular tubule (C) in the bovine testis. Iron hematoxylin (×140).

lium lines the proximal portion of the straight tubules, and a simple columnar epithelium lines the distal portion (Fig. 12-13). This epithelium contains numerous macrophages and lymphocytes and is able to phagocytize spermatozoa.

Rete Testis

Irregularly anastomosing channels, surrounded by loose connective tissue, form the **rete testis** (Figs. 12-1 and 12-14). Most of the rete is situated within the mediastinum testis, but smaller intratunical and extratesticular portions are generally also present. The rete testis is lined by a simple squamous to columnar epithelium. Elastic fibers and contractile cells are present under the epithelium. Most of the testicular fluid, which is reabsorbed in the head of the epididymis, is produced in the rete testis (in the ram, approximately 40 mL/day). Rete testis fluid differs in composition from seminiferous tubular fluid, testicular lymph, and blood plasma.

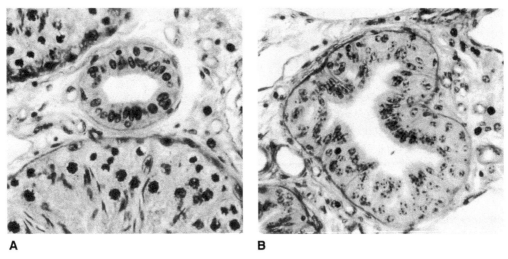

FIGURE 12-13   Proximal (**A**) and distal (**B**) portions of the straight testicular tubules in the bovine testis. Note the differences in tubule diameter and the lining epithelium. Masson-Goldner (×350).

Testicular Blood Supply and Testicular Innervation

The testicular artery has a straight abdominal portion and becomes highly coiled after reaching the spermatic cord. Small nutritive twigs and larger epididymal arteries branch from the coiled portion. As the artery reaches the testis, it courses parallel to the epididymis and is embedded in the tunica albuginea. The testicular artery divides at the caudal testicular pole to form the arterial contributions to the vascular layer of the tunica albuginea. Within the septula testis, centripetal septal arteries course to the mediastinum testis, where they form very convoluted coils in ruminants. From

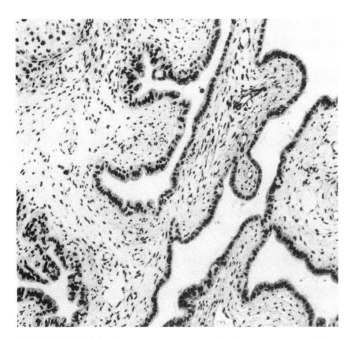

FIGURE 12-14   Bovine rete testis lined with simple cuboidal epithelium and surrounded by a relatively large amount of connective tissue. Masson-Goldner (×140).

these convolutes or from the septal arteries, smaller arterial vessels deviate to supply the testicular parenchyma (Fig. 12-1). Most of the testicular veins empty into superficial veins situated in the vascular layer of the tunica albuginea. The albugineal veins converge at the base of the spermatic cord to form the pampiniform plexus, which completely surrounds the windings of the testicular artery. This remarkable vascular topography in the mammalian spermatic cord is believed to allow venous–arterial steroid hormone transfer and cooling of the arterial blood entering the testis. Thus, testicular androgen levels are increased and testicular temperature is lowered; these are two important requirements for spermatogenesis. Valves are present in the veins of the spermatic cord of all domestic species and in the septal veins of the porcine testis.

The senses of pain and touch in the scrotal area involve primarily the testicular coverings, which are innervated by myelinated and nonmyelinated branches of the lumbosacral plexus. The intrinsic nerves to the testis itself are nonmyelinated, mainly vasomotor fibers that reach the gonad by three access routes: (a) with the spermatic cord to its cranial extremity; (b) via the ligamentous bridge (proper ligament of the testis) between the epididymal tail and testis to its caudal extremity; and (c) through the mesorchium to the epididymal border of the testis. Considerable species-specific differences in the testicular innervation pattern have been recorded. Whereas in the cat many nerves are present in tunica albuginea, septula, mediastinum, and lobuli testis, the large testis of the adult boar is not innervated at all. Also, in the testis of the bull and donkey, large areas of the testicular interior are devoid of nerve fibers. The majority of the intrinsic testicular nerve fibers contain dopamine-β-hydroxylase and neuropeptide Y and thus represent postganglionic sympathetic fibers. Only in the cat, medium-sized arterioles within the mediastinum, septula, and testicular lobules receive a dual innervation by noradrenergic and cholinergic axons (Fig. 12-4). Besides vasomotor fibers, the testis of most species also contains a varying number of calcitonin gene–related peptide (CGRP)–positive axons, which run independently from blood vessels in the connective tissue and seem to be the most important sensory nerves in the male gonad. The autonomous innervation of testicular interstitial endocrine cells and the functional correlations between neural and endocrine regulations in the testis are still a matter of debate. In the camel testis, which displays distinct volume changes over the year, an inverse relation between neural and endocrine activities has been reported as follows: the greatest volume and highest 3-β-hydroxysteroid-dehydrogenase (3-β-HStDH) content of the interstitial endocrine cell compartment seen in the winter is paralleled by a regression of testicular innervation. A weak or absent 3-β-HStDH activity and a decreasing volume of the interstitial endocrine cells in summer is accompanied by an increase in intertubular nerve fibers.

EPIDIDYMIS

The mammalian **epididymis** is a dynamic accessory sex organ that is dependent on testicular androgens for the maintenance of a differentiated state of its epithelium. It comprises several (8 to 25) ductuli efferentes and a long, coiled ductus epididymidis (Fig. 12-1). Macroscopically, the epididymis is divided into a head, body, and tail. It is surrounded by a thick tunica albuginea of dense irregular connective tissue covered by the visceral layer of the tunica vaginalis. In stallions, the tunica albuginea has a few smooth muscle cells scattered throughout the dense connective tissue.

Ductuli Efferentes

Between 8 and 25 **ductuli efferentes** with regionally varying diameters connect the rete testis to the ductus epididymidis (Figs. 12-1 and 12-15-1). The ductules are gathered in small lobules (coni vasculosi) with distinct boundaries of connective tissue. There is generally an abrupt border between the epithelia of rete testis and efferent ductules (Fig. 12-15-2). The epithelium of the efferent ductules is simple columnar and consists of ciliated and nonciliated principal cells (Fig. 12-16-1). Scattered free mononuclear cells that have invaded the basal epithelial area have been misinterpreted as a third genuine cell type. The ciliated cells (apical row of nuclei) help to move the spermatozoa toward the ductus epididymidis. The nonciliated principal cells (basal row of nuclei) display a brush border of microvilli and morphologic characteristics of fluid-phase endocytosis with membrane recycling, such as coated pinocytotic invaginations, coated and transport vesicles, and endosomes. Besides generating an osmotically driven water flow by transcellular transport of ions, most of the nonciliated principal cells are involved in resorptive processes and, after resorption and digestion of ductular fluid and macromolecules, may contain globular periodic acid-Schiff (PAS)–positive residual bodies (Fig. 12-16-2); others may have a secretory activity. Intermediate forms between ciliated and nonciliated epithelial cells are occasionally observed. The ratio between ciliated and nonciliated principal cells varies along the ductule, but ciliated cells increase in number toward the epididymal duct. The ductular epithelium is surrounded by three to six loosely arranged lay-

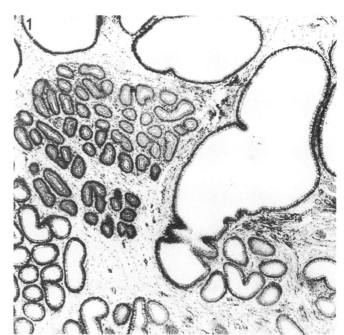

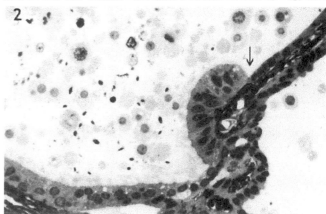

FIGURE 12-15 1. Ductuli efferentes of the cat. The lumen decreases from the initial portion toward the epididymidis. A segment of the ductus epididymidis is seen at the upper left (tubular profiles with thick walls and small lumina). Masson-Goldner (×55). **2.** Transition (arrow) of the simple cuboidal epithelium of the rete testis into the columnar epithelium of the ductuli efferentes (cat). In addition to spermatozoa (small, dark cells), the lumen of the testicular excurrent duct system contains many exfoliated spermatocytes and spermatids. Semithin section (×350).

ers of myofibroblasts and connective tissue. The ductuli efferentes and the initial portions of the ductus epididymidis constitute the head of the epididymis.

Ductus Epididymidis

The **ductus epididymidis** is extremely tortuous and coiled. The length of the duct varies considerably among species and has been estimated to be 40 m in bulls and boars and 70 m in stallions. Despite these differences, transport of sperm through the epididymis seems to require 10 to 15 days in most mammalian species.

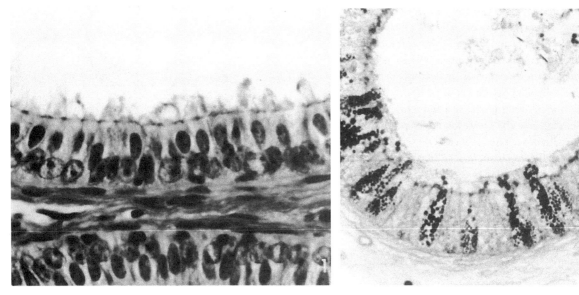

FIGURE 12-16   1. The simple columnar epithelium of the efferent ductules consists of secretory and resorptive cells (light spherical nuclei) and ciliated cells (dense ovoid nuclei). Masson-Goldner (×560). **2.** Selective staining of nonciliated cells. Periodic acid-Schiff reaction after digestion by diastase (×350).

The ductus epididymidis is lined by a pseudostratified columnar epithelium, surrounded by a small amount of loose connective tissue and circular smooth muscle fibers, the number of which increases significantly toward the tail of the epididymis (Fig. 12-17). In seasonal breeders such as the camel, the height of the epididymal epithelium and the innervation density of the muscular layer display characteristic changes over the year. Two cell types are invariably present in the epididymal epithelium of all domestic mammals: columnar principal cells and small, polygonal basal cells. In many species, additional cell types, such as apical cells and clear cells, are present. Macrophages and lymphocytes also occur within the epithelium.

The **principal cells** are generally taller in the head of the epididymis than in the remainder of the organ. The apical surfaces of these columnar cells bear long and sometimes branching microvilli (stereocilia) that become gradually shorter toward the tail. The occurrence of pinocytotic invaginations at the base of the microvilli and the presence of coated vesicles and multivesicular bod-

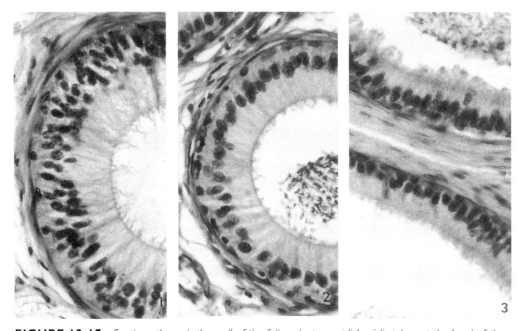

FIGURE 12-17   Sections through the wall of the feline ductus epididymidis taken at the level of the head (**1**), body (**2**), and tail (**3**) of the epididymis. Note the variations in the position of the nuclei, height of the pseudostratified columnar epithelium, length of the microvilli, and thickness of the muscular coat. Hematoxylin and eosin (×435).

ies in the apical cytoplasm indicate that the epididymal epithelium has a high resorptive capacity. Most of the fluid (more than 90%) that leaves the testis is reabsorbed in the ductuli efferentes and the proximal part of the epididymal duct. Androgen-binding protein and inhibin produced by the sustentacular cells of the seminiferous tubules are also reabsorbed in the initial segment of the ductus epididymidis. The secretion of various substances, such as glycerophosphoryl choline, and glycoproteins, such as phosphatase and glycosidase, is also well established.

On the basis of histologic, histochemical, and ultrastructural criteria, the ductus epididymidis may be subdivided into several segments, the distribution and number of which (six in bulls) are characteristic for each species. Generally, the proximal parts of the duct (head and body) are involved in the maturation process of spermatozoa. The tail of the epididymis serves as their main storage place (e.g., 45% of bovine epididymal spermatozoa are stored here). Spermatozoa leaving the testis are both immotile and infertile, whereas spermatozoa leaving the epididymis have gained motility and fertility. During their passage through the ductus epididymidis, spermatozoa undergo a series of morphologic and functional changes that lead to the acquisition of full fertilizing capacity by the time they reach the tail. The change in the functional status of the spermatozoa is reflected in (a) development of progressive motility, (b) modification of their metabolism, (c) alteration of the plasma membrane surface characteristics (activation of membrane-bound molecules necessary for recognition processes during fertilization), (d) stabilization of plasma membrane by oxidation of incorporated sulfhydryl groups, and (e) caudad movement and eventual loss of the cytoplasmic droplet, a remnant of the spermatid cytoplasm. Spermatozoa with persisting droplets are probably infertile. Once fully mature, spermatozoa can be stored in the tail of the epididymis for a remarkably long period; much longer than if they were maintained at a similar temperature in vitro. Epididymal spermatozoa can carry a wide range of potent antigens and easily trigger an autoimmune response by antisperm antibodies. This is generally prevented by an effective blood-epididymal barrier whose morphologic equivalent is represented by the apical epithelial junctional complex containing one of the best developed tight junctions anywhere.

DUCTUS DEFERENS

The ductus epididymidis, after a sharp bend at the end of the tail, gradually straightens and acquires the histologic characteristics of the **ductus deferens**. In stallions and ruminants, the ductus deferens unites with the excretory duct of the vesicular gland to form a short ejaculatory duct, which opens at the colliculus seminalis into the urethra. The pseudostratified lining epithelium of the bovine ejaculatory duct contains engulfed spermatozoa. In boars, the ductus deferens and the excretory duct open separately into the urethra. In carnivores, the ductus deferens joins the urethra alone because the vesicular gland is absent.

The mucosa of the ductus deferens is lined by a pseudostratified columnar epithelium (Fig. 12-18) similar to that of the ductus epididymidis, but with a higher amount of basal cells; toward the end of the duct, it may become a simple columnar epithelium. In the proximity of the epididymis, the columnar cells possess short, branched microvilli. In bulls, small lipid droplets are present in the basal cells. The loose connective tissue of the propria-submucosa is highly vascularized, is rich in fibroblasts and elastic fibers, and contains a network of cholinergic nerves, whereas the tunica muscularis is densely innervated by postganglionic sympathetic fibers. In stallions, bulls, and boars, the tunica muscularis consists of intermingled circular, longitudinal, and oblique layers; in small ruminants and carnivores (Fig. 12-18-1), an inner circular layer and an outer longitudinal layer are present. A tunica serosa with its usual components covers the organ.

The terminal portion of the ductus deferens is one of the male accessory glands, regardless of whether it forms an ampulla (stallions, ruminants, dogs) (Fig. 12-19-1) or does not (boars, cats); it contains simple branched tubuloalveolar glands in the propria-

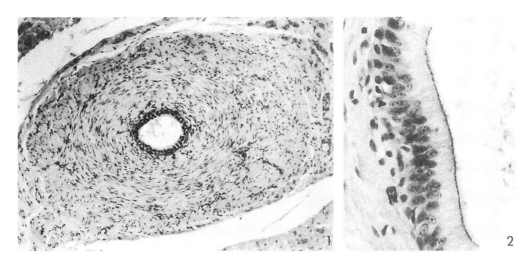

FIGURE 12-18 **1.** Cross section through the intraabdominal portion of the feline ductus deferens. Hematoxylin and eosin (×130). **2.** Pseudostratified columnar epithelium of the canine ductus deferens taken at the same level. Hematoxylin and eosin (×435).

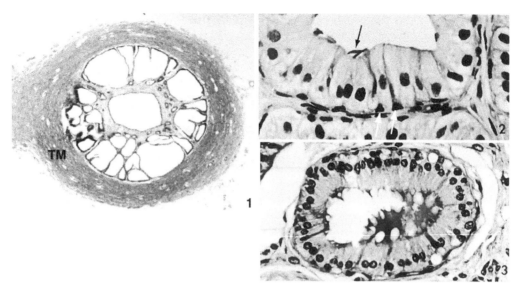

FIGURE 12-19 1. Cross section through the glandular portion of the canine ductus deferens. The tunica muscularis (TM) is relatively thin. Hematoxylin and eosin (×38). **2.** Part of a secretory alveolus of the glandular portion of the ductus deferens of a buck. Basal (white arrows) and columnar cells are present and heads of spermatozoa (black arrow) are seen in the lumen. Weigert's hematoxylin (×560). **3.** In this secretory alveolus of the glandular portion of the ductus deferens of a bull, some of the basal cells contain a huge lipid droplet (vacuole). Weigert's hematoxylin (×350).

submucosa. In stallions, bulls, and rams, these glands occupy practically the entire propria-submucosa, which is rich in smooth muscle cells. In dogs and bucks, the glands are surrounded by periglandular connective tissue devoid of smooth muscle cells. The glands are lined by cells that vary from tall columnar cells with ovoid nuclei to cuboidal cells with spherical nuclei (Figs. 12-19-2 and 12-19-3). Apical, bleblike protrusions suggestive of secretory activity are often observed. Spherical or polyhedral basal cells are distributed irregularly between the columnar cells (Fig. 12-19-2). In ruminants, the glandular epithelium is rich in glycogen and the basal cells contain lipid droplets of variable size. Lipid droplets are also present in the columnar cells of bulls. The lipids in bovine basal cells may coalesce, thereby giving these cells the appearance of fat cells (Fig. 12-19-3). The tunica muscularis of the terminal portion of the ductus deferens consists of variably arranged smooth muscle bundles surrounded by the highly vascularized loose connective tissue of the tunica adventitia.

The lumen of the glandular portion of the ductus deferens and the wide openings of the glands into the lumen contain a considerable number of spermatozoa in all domestic animals. In the bull, the number is sufficient for at least one normal ejaculate after recent castration or vasectomy.

ACCESSORY GLANDS

The ejaculate consists of spermatozoa and seminal plasma, which is composed of secretions from the epididymis and male accessory glands. These glands are (a) the glandular portion of the ductus deferens, which has been described together with the ductus deferens; (b) the vesicular gland; (c) the prostate; and (d) the bulbourethral gland. All accessory glands are present in stallions, rumi-

nants, and boars; the vesicular glands are absent in carnivores, and the bulbourethral gland is absent in dogs.

Vesicular Gland

The paired **vesicular glands** are compound tubular or tubuloalveolar. The glandular epithelium is pseudostratified with tall columnar cells and often sparse, small, spherical, basal cells (Fig. 12-20-1). The intralobular and main excretory ducts are lined by a simple cuboidal epithelium, or by a stratified columnar epithelium in horses.

The highly vascularized loose connective tissue of the propria-submucosa is continuous with the denser connective tissue of the trabeculae, which may subdivide the organ into lobes and lobules. A tunica muscularis of varying width and arrangement surrounds the organ, covered by a tunica serosa or a tunica adventitia.

Species Differences

In stallions, the vesicular glands are true vesicles, with short, branched tubuloalveolar glands that open into wide central lumina (ducts), separated by relatively thin connective-tissue trabeculae with irregularly arranged smooth muscle cells.

In boars, the two vesicular glands possess a common connective-tissue capsule; the tunica muscularis is thin. The interlobular septa consist predominantly of connective tissue and a few smooth muscle cells. The tubular lumina are wide and the secretory epithelium is folded (Fig. 12-21).

In bulls, the vesicular gland is a compact, lobulated organ. Intralobular secretory ducts drain the slightly coiled tubular portions of the tubuloalveolar gland and, in turn, are drained by the main excretory duct. The secretory columnar cells have small lipid droplets and glycogen (Figs. 12-20-2 and 12-20-3) and

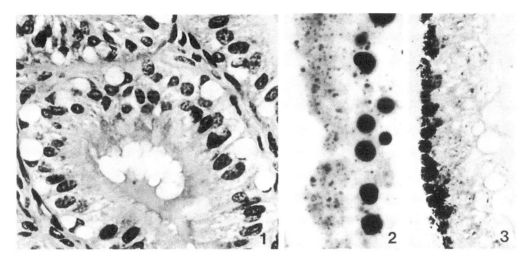

FIGURE 12-20 Vesicular gland (bull). **1.** The basal cells in the pseudostratified columnar epithelial lining of the alveoli are characterized by large vacuoles containing lipid in vivo. Masson-Goldner (×560). **2.** Lipids were specifically stained with Sudan black B. Note the large lipid droplets in the basal cells and small lipid droplets in the secretory columnar cells (×560). **3.** The apices of the secretory columnar cells contain large amounts of glycogen. Periodic acid-Schiff (×560).

react positively for alkaline phosphatase. Some of the columnar cells possess light, bleblike apical projections. The basal cells are characterized by large lipid droplets (Fig. 12-20-1). Approximately 50% of the lipid material in the bovine vesicular gland is cholesterol and its esters, approximately 25% is triglycerides, and approximately 10% is phospholipids. The interlobular septa are predominantly muscular, derived from the thick tunica muscularis, which is surrounded by a capsule of dense irregular connective tissue with a few smooth muscle cells.

The vesicular gland of rams and bucks is similar to that of bulls. Lipid droplets in the basal cells are absent in rams but may be present in bucks. The epithelium of the vesicular gland of bucks is considerably higher during the breeding season than during the nonbreeding season. The gelatinous, white, or yellowish-white secretory product of the vesicular gland amounts to approximately 25 to 30% of the total ejaculate in bulls, 10 to 30% in boars, and 7 to 8% in rams and bucks. It is rich in fructose, which serves as an energy source for ejaculated spermatozoa.

Prostate

The **prostate** consists of a varying number of individual tubuloalveolar glands (Fig. 12-22) derived from the epithelium of the pelvic urethra. Two portions may be distinguished, according more to topographic than to histologic features: the **body** (corpus

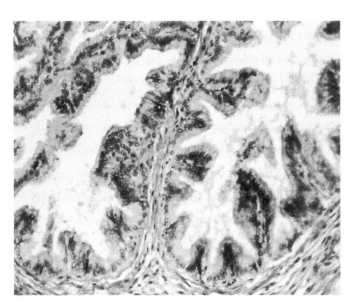

FIGURE 12-21 Vesicular gland (boar). Epithelial folds project into the secretory alveoli. Hematoxylin and eosin (×130).

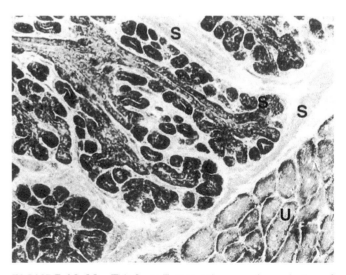

FIGURE 12-22 This figure illustrates the general organization of the porcine disseminate prostate; smooth muscle fibers (light gray; S) are present in the capsule and the septa. The striated urethralis muscle (U) is visible in the lower right corner. β-D-galactosidase reaction (×100).

prostatae) and the **disseminate** part (pars disseminata prostatae). The body either entirely surrounds the pelvic urethra at the level of the colliculus seminalis or covers part of its dorsal aspect. The disseminate part is located in the propria-submucosa of the pelvic urethra.

The secretory tubules, alveoli, and intraglandular ducts of the prostate are lined by a simple cuboidal or columnar epithelium, with occasional basal cells (Fig. 12-23). The simple epithelium changes to stratified columnar or transitional epithelium toward the terminal portions of the ducts. Some of the epithelial cells give a positive mucous reaction; most contain proteinaceous secretory granules. The tall columnar cells possess microvilli and sometimes bleblike apical protrusions. Occasionally, concentrically laminated concretions of secretory material (corpora amylacea) are found in the tubules and alveoli. The duct system of the prostate possesses saccular dilations in which secretory material may be stored.

The prostate is surrounded by a capsule of dense irregular connective tissue that contains many smooth muscle cells around the disseminate part, which is also surrounded by the striated urethral muscle (Figs. 12-22 and 12-24). Large trabeculae originate from the capsule and separate the body and the disseminate part into individual lobules. They are predominantly muscular in the body of the gland.

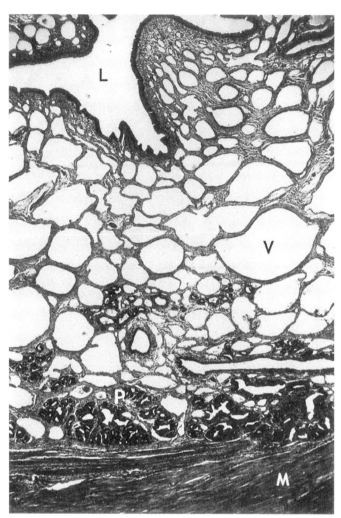

FIGURE 12-24 In this cross section through part of the bovine prostatic urethra, note the large veins (V) of the spongiose stratum and the disseminate prostate (P) in the propria-submucosa, surrounded by the urethral muscle (M). Lumen (L). Hematoxylin and eosin (×35).

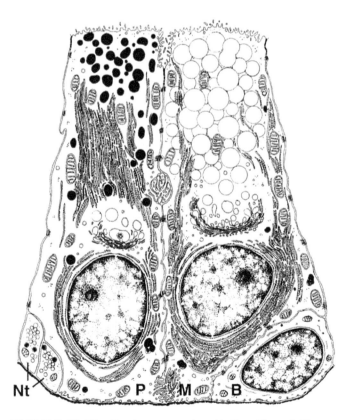

FIGURE 12-23 Ruminant prostatic epithelium. The cell (P) on the left side is a specific secretory cell containing proteinaceous granules. The cell (M) on the right secretes mucus. Basal cell (B); intraepithelial autonomic nerve terminals (Nt).

Secretory portions and ducts of the prostate are surrounded by loose connective tissue containing smooth muscle cells, which are particularly abundant in the body of the gland.

Species Differences

In carnivores, the body of the prostate is particularly well developed and separated into two distinct bilateral lobes. In dogs, these lobes completely surround the proximal portion of the pelvic urethra. In cats, they are located on the lateral and dorsal aspects of the urethra. The disseminate part in dogs consists of a few glandular lobules. In cats, individual lobules of the disseminate part are found scattered between the colliculus seminalis and the bulbourethral glands. Lamellar corpuscles may be observed in the interstitium.

In stallions, only the body of the prostate is present and consists of right and left lobes, both connected by a narrow dorsal isthmus. The individual lobes empty through 15 to 30 ducts into the pelvic urethra. The capsule, trabeculae, and interstitial connective tissue are rich in smooth muscle.

The body of the prostate gland of the bull is relatively inconspicuous; it is absent in small ruminants. The disseminate portion (Fig. 12-24) encircles the urethra in bulls and bucks; in rams, it is U-shaped, and the midline of the ventral aspect of the urethra is free of glandular tissue.

In boars, the body of the prostate is a platelike organ; the disseminate part is well developed and completely encircles the pelvic urethra.

The contribution of the prostatic secretions to the total volume of the ejaculate varies with the species. In ruminants, it is 4 to 6%; in stallions, 25 to 30%; and in boars, 35 to 60%. One of the functions of the prostate is to neutralize the seminal plasma, made acidic by accumulation of metabolic carbon dioxide and lactate, and to initiate active movements of the ejaculated spermatozoa.

Bulbourethral Gland

The paired **bulbourethral glands** are located dorsolateral to the penile portion of the urethra, at the bulb of the penis. The gland is compound tubular (boars, cats, bucks) or tubuloalveolar (stallions, bulls, rams) (Fig. 12-25); it is absent in dogs.

The secretory portions of the bulbourethral gland are lined with a tall simple columnar epithelium and occasional basal cells (Fig. 12-25-1). They open into collecting ducts either directly or through connecting pieces lined by simple cuboidal epithelial cells with dark cytoplasm. The collecting ducts, lined by a simple cuboidal or columnar epithelium, unite to form larger intraglandular ducts lined by a pseudostratified columnar epithelium. These, in turn, open into a single (or multiple) bulbourethral duct with a lining of transitional epithelium.

The gland is sheathed by a fibroelastic capsule containing a variable amount of striated muscle. Trabeculae, extending from the capsule, consist of dense irregular connective tissue and some smooth and striated muscle fibers. The interstitium consists of loose connective tissue and a few smooth muscle fibers.

Species Differences

In cats, the gland consists of spacious, sinuslike intraglandular ducts and short, narrow, mostly unbranched tubular end pieces. The secretory surface of the cells is increased by a well-developed system of intercellular canaliculi.

In stallions, the bulbourethral gland is completely surrounded by the bulboglandularis muscle. Three to four individual bulbourethral ducts are present.

The exceptionally large bulbourethral gland of boars is also surrounded by the bulboglandularis muscle. Only a few smooth muscle cells are present in the interstitium. The collecting ducts are lined by simple columnar epithelium.

In ruminants, the gland is surrounded by the bulbospongiosus muscle. In bulls and rams, short connecting pieces link the secretory portions to the collecting ducts, lined by a simple cuboidal epithelium that is sometimes also secretory. In bucks, the secretory portions empty directly into these ducts. Smooth muscle cells are particularly abundant within the interstitium.

The mucous and proteinaceous secretory product of the bulbourethral gland is discharged before ejaculation in ruminants (Fig. 12-25-2), where it apparently serves to neutralize the urethral environment and to lubricate both the urethra and the vagina. In boars, the exclusively mucous, sialic acid-rich secretory product is part of the ejaculate (15 to 30%). The secretion is possibly involved in the occlusion of the cervix to prevent loss of sperm following insemination. In cats, the secretory product is mucus and also contains glycogen. In the absence of a vesicular gland, this bulbourethral glycogen may be the source of feline seminal fructose, providing energy for the metabolism of the spermatozoa.

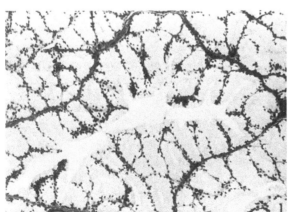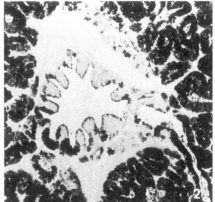

FIGURE 12-25 Bulbourethral gland (bull). **1.** The light tall columnar secretory epithelial cells are almost entirely filled with mucous secretory product; the heterochromatic nuclei are located in the cell base. Masson-Goldner (×100). **2.** Positive periodic acid-Schiff mucin reaction in the parenchyma and some of the lining cells of the central duct (×100).

URETHRA

The male **urethra** is divided into the prostatic, pelvic, and penile portions. The prostatic portion extends from the urinary bladder to the caudal edge of the body of the prostate. The pelvic portion begins here and terminates where the urethra enters the bulb of the penis, from which level the penile portion continues to the external urethral opening.

The entire urethral mucosa is thrown into longitudinal folds that flatten or disappear during erection and micturition. In the prostatic urethra, a prominent, permanent dorsomedian fold, the urethral crest, is present. It terminates as a slight enlargement, the **colliculus seminalis.** There, the following ducts open into the urethra: the ejaculatory ducts in ruminants and stallions, the ductus deferentes and the excretory ducts of the vesicular glands in boars, and the deferent ducts in carnivores. Between these ducts, vestiges of the fused paramesonephric ducts, the uterus masculinus, may be found as either a solid epithelial cord or a short canal.

The predominant lining of the urethra is a transitional epithelium with variably sized patches of simple columnar epithelium or stratified cuboidal or columnar epithelium. The propria-submucosa consists of a loose connective tissue with many elastic fibers and smooth muscle cells and frequent diffuse lymphatic tissue or lymphatic nodules (dog). In stallions and cats, simple tubular mucous (urethral) glands are present. Regulatory peptide-containing cells of the diffuse neuroendocrine system are regularly found in the epithelia of the urethra and the glands derived from the urogenital sinus (i.e., prostate and bulbourethral).

Throughout the entire length of the urethra, the propria-submucosa possesses erectile properties by virtue of endothelium-lined caverns of variable size that constitute the so-called **vascular stratum** in the prostatic (Fig. 12-24) and pelvic urethra. Around the penile urethra, the quantity and size of the cavernous spaces are greatly increased (Fig. 12-26); here, the vascular stratum is referred to as the **corpus spongiosum,** which begins at the ischiadic arch with a bilobed expansion, the bulb of the penis.

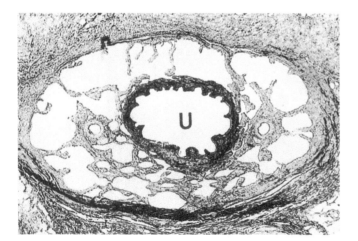

FIGURE 12-26 Penile urethra (cat). The urethra (U) is surrounded by the cavernous spaces of the corpus spongiosum. Hematoxylin and eosin (×35).

The tunica muscularis of the pelvic part of the urethra consists of smooth muscle in the vicinity of the bladder or striated muscle in the remainder of the urethra. It is surrounded by a tunica adventitia of loose or dense irregular connective tissue.

In ruminants and stallions, the terminal portion of the urethra protrudes incompletely (bulls) or completely (stallions, rams, and bucks) above the glans penis to form the urethral process. The transitional or stratified squamous epithelial lining is surrounded by a corpus spongiosum containing many cavernous spaces in stallions, and fewer, smaller spaces in ruminants. Two longitudinal fibrocartilaginous cords flank the urethra in bucks and rams. The urethral process is covered by a cutaneous mucous membrane.

PENIS

The penis consists essentially of (a) the corpora cavernosa penis, (b) the corpus spongiosum penis surrounding the penile urethra, and (c) the glans penis.

Corpora Cavernosa Penis

The paired **corpora cavernosa penis** arise from the ischiadic tuberosities and merge with the corpus spongiosum to form the body of the penis. They are surrounded by the tunica albuginea, a thick layer of dense irregular connective tissue containing variable numbers of elastic fibers and smooth muscle cells. A connective-tissue septum completely (dogs) or partially divides the corpora cavernosa penis.

The spaces between the tunica albuginea and the trabecular network arising from the tunica albuginea are filled with erectile tissue. In stallions (Fig. 12-27-1) and carnivores (Fig. 12-27-2), this tissue consists of caverns lined by endothelium and surrounded by connective tissue, the appearance of which varies between loose and dense irregular, and by smooth muscle cells (Fig. 12-27-1). In stallions, these muscle bundles are oriented with the longitudinal axis of the penis, often causing a virtually complete obturation of the lumina of the cavernous spaces. Relaxation of these muscle cells causes the penis to elongate and emerge from the prepuce, which usually happens during micturition. In boars (Fig. 12-27-3) and ruminants (Fig. 12-27-4), the connective tissue surrounding the caverns contains few, if any, smooth muscle cells.

The cavernous spaces receive their main blood supply from arteries with a helical arrangement that are referred to as **helicine arteries** (arteriae helicinae). Characteristically, they have epithelioid smooth muscle cells in the tunica intima that protrude into the lumina of these vessels as ridges or pads, causing partial obliteration. As the smooth muscle cells relax, the blood flow into the caverns increases considerably and causes erection. The cavernous spaces are drained by venules, several of which give origin to thick-walled veins.

The penis of stallions is classified as a vascular penis because of the predominance of caverns in the corpus cavernosum. In ruminants and boars, the caverns are less extensive and connective tissue prevails, thus the designation of the penis as fibroelastic. The penis of dogs and cats is best classified as an intermediate type.

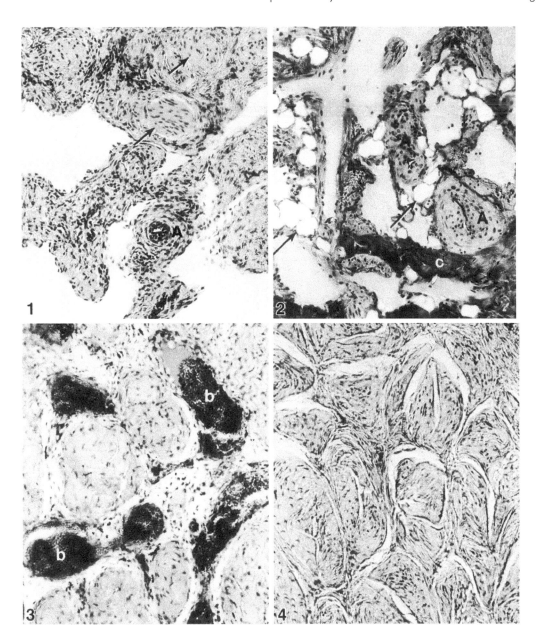

FIGURE 12-27 **1.** Corpus cavernosum (stallion). Bundles of smooth muscle (arrows) and a helicine artery (A) are present within the connective-tissue trabeculae between the cavernous spaces. **2.** Corpus cavernosum (cat). Connective-tissue trabecula (c) between cavernous spaces, adipose cells (arrows), and numerous helicine arteries (A). **3.** Corpus cavernosum (boar). Cavernous spaces contain coagulated blood (b) between abundant connective-tissue trabeculae. **4.** Corpus cavernosum (bull). Note the slitlike, empty cavernous spaces and abundant connective-tissue trabeculae. Masson-Goldner (×140).

Glans Penis

A well-developed **glans penis** is present only in stallions and dogs. The glans is surrounded by a tunica albuginea rich in elastic fibers. The tunica albuginea continues into trabeculae that delineate spaces containing erectile tissue similar to that of the corpus spongiosum penis (stallions) or a plexus of large caverns (dogs) (Fig. 12-28). The glans penis is covered by the prepuce (see section later in this chapter).

Species Differences

The corpora cavernosa penis of dogs are completely separated by a connective-tissue septum and are continued cranially by the **os penis,** which terminates in a fibrocartilaginous tip. The glans penis consists of the bulbus glandis and the pars longa glandis. Both almost completely surround the os penis and the distal portion of the penile urethra and its associated corpus spongiosum. The **bulbus glandis** consists of large venous caverns separated

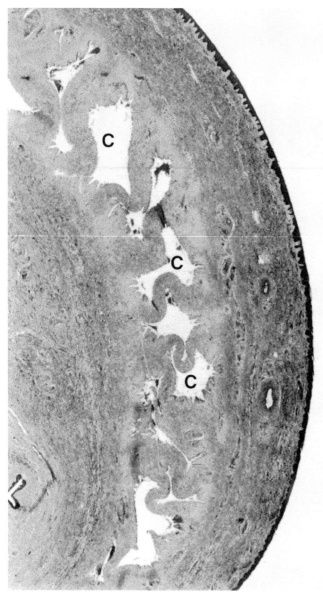

FIGURE 12-28 Glans penis, pars longa (dog). Note the large cavernous spaces (C) in the erectile tissue. Hematoxylin and eosin (×11).

by connective-tissue trabeculae rich in elastic fibers. The **pars longa glandis** forms the cranial portion of the glans penis; its structure is identical to that of the bulbus.

In cats, many adipose cells are present between the caverns of the corpus cavernosum penis. They increase in number toward the tip of the corpus cavernosum, which contains little erectile tissue. A small os penis surrounded by the corpus spongiosum of the glans is present.

The connective tissue of the corpus cavernosum of stallions contains many elastic fibers and smooth muscle cells. The glans covers the corpus cavernosum penis cranially and possesses a long, caudally directed, **dorsal process** and an enlargement, the corona glandis, the epithelial covering of which bears cylindric papillae. An indentation of the glans, the fossa glandis, contains the slightly protruding end of the urethra (urethral process). At

the level of the glans, the bulbospongiosus muscle bundles are interrupted by the retractor penis muscle.

A corkscrewlike, left spiral characterizes approximately the cranial third of the penis of the boar. The structure of the rest of the porcine penis is similar to that of the penis of the bull.

The corpus cavernosum penis of bulls contains a central connective-tissue strand formed by the converging trabeculae. The tip of the penis (glans) consists of mucous (gelatinous) connective tissue, adipose cells, and large intercellular spaces (Fig. 12-29). An extensive, erectile venous plexus is present. The penis of bucks and rams is similar to that of bulls. The glans is a large cap-like enlargement that is similar to that of bulls. The urethra projects from the glans as a twisted urethral process.

Mechanism of Erection

In animals with either a vascular- or an intermediate-type penis, erection causes an increase in size and a stiffening of the organ. Relaxation of the smooth muscle cells in the helicine arteries results in increased blood flow into the spaces of the corpora cavernosa. The increased blood volume compresses the veins and subsequently decreases the outflow, eventually filling the erectile tissue spaces in the corpora cavernosa and spongiosa penis and in the glans penis.

Detumescence is initiated by contraction of the musculature of the helicine arteries and thus by a decrease in arterial inflow. The contraction of the smooth muscle cells of the tunica albuginea, the trabeculae, and the erectile tissue causes the penis to return to the flaccid state.

In animals with a fibroelastic penis, erection results essentially in an increase in the length of the penis that emerges from the prepuce. In ruminants and boars, the retractor penis muscle plays an essential role during detumescence in retracting the penis into the prepuce.

During copulation, the constrictor vestibuli muscle of bitches constricts the veins that drain the entire glans and especially the

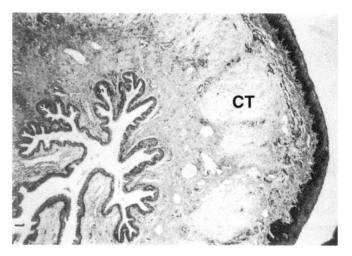

FIGURE 12-29 In the bovine glans penis, the urethra is surrounded by relatively little subepithelial erectile tissue and a thick connective-tissue layer (CT). Hematoxylin and eosin (×40).

bulbus glandis. This constriction causes the bulbus to enlarge to such a degree that immediate withdrawal of the penis from the vagina is impossible; consequently, coitus is prolonged.

PREPUCE

The cranial portion of the body of the penis and the glans penis are located in a tubelike reflection of the skin, the **prepuce,** composed of an external and an internal layer. The external layer re-

flects inward at the preputial opening to form the internal layer of the prepuce. It reflects on the cranial portion of the penis and is securely attached cranially to the glans penis.

The external layer is typical skin. Numerous sebaceous glands, not always related to hairs, are present at the preputial opening. In addition, long, bristlelike hairs are found in ruminants and boars. In stallions, ruminants, boars, and dogs, fine hairs and sebaceous and sweat glands are located over a variable distance in the internal layer. In stallions, occasional hairs occur in the penile skin, which is also rich in sebaceous and sweat glands (Fig. 12-30). In dogs and ruminants, both the internal layer of the prepuce and the skin covering the penis contain solitary lymphatic nodules; in boars, they are present only in the internal layer. In cats, the mucosa covering the glans has numerous keratinized papillae.

In boars, a dorsal evagination of the internal layer of the prepuce is referred to as the preputial diverticulum. It is incompletely separated into two lateral portions by a median septum. Frequently, the keratinized cutaneous mucous membrane is folded. A mixture of desquamated epithelial cells and urine forms smegma, which collects in the diverticulum and is odiferous.

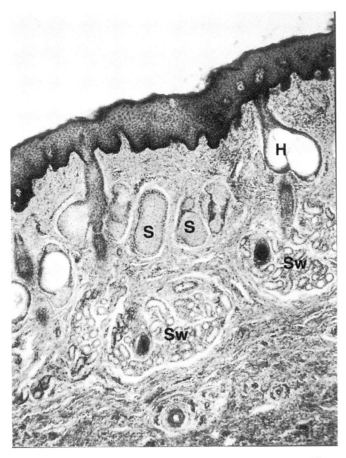

FIGURE 12-30 Skin with hair follicles (H) and sebaceous (S) and sweat (Sw) glands covering the corpus penis (stallion). Hematoxylin and eosin (×40).

SUGGESTED READINGS

Aumüller G. Prostate gland and seminal vesicles. In: Handbuch der mikroskopischen Anatomie des Menschen. Berlin: Springer-Verlag, 1979;7(6).

Cole HH, Cupps PT. Reproduction in Domestic Animals. 3rd Ed. New York: Academic Press, 1977.

Fawcett DW, Bedford JM, eds. The Spermatozoon. Maturation, Motility, Surface Properties and Comparative Aspects. Baltimore: Urban and Schwarzenberg, 1979.

Guraya SS. Biology of Spermatogenesis and Spermatozoa in Mammals. New York: Springer-Verlag, 1987.

Knobil E, Neill JD, eds. The Physiology of Reproduction. New York: Raven Press, 1988.

Russell LD, Griswold MD, eds. The Sertoli Cell. Clearwater, FL: Cache River Press, 1993.

Setchell BP. The Mammalian Testis. London: Paul Elek, 1978.

Steinberger A, Steinberger E. Testicular Development, Structure and Function. New York: Raven Press, 1980.

Van Blerkom J, Motta P, eds. Ultrastructure of Reproduction. Boston: M. Nijhoff, 1984.

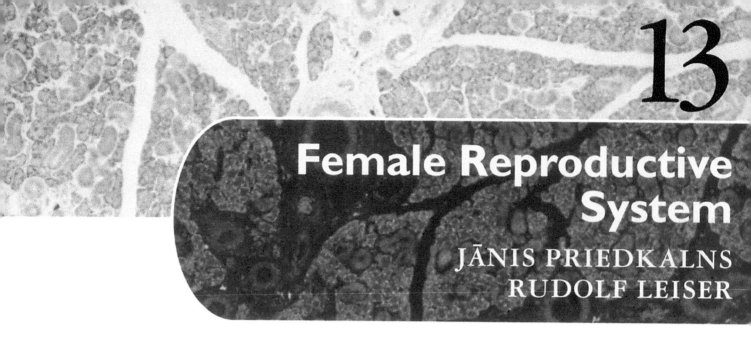

13

Female Reproductive System

JĀNIS PRIEDKALNS
RUDOLF LEISER

Ovary
 Cortex
  Follicular development
  Ovulation
  Follicular atresia and interstitial endocrine cells
  Corpus luteum
 Medulla
 Blood Vessels, Lymphatics, and Nerves
Uterine Tube (Oviduct)
 Histologic Structure
 Blood Vessels, Lymphatics, and Nerves
 Histophysiology
Uterus
 Histologic Structure
  Endometrium
  Myometrium
  Perimetrium
 Blood Vessels, Lymphatics, and Nerves
Cervix
 Histologic Structure
Vagina
 Histologic Structure

Vestibule, Clitoris, and Vulva
The Estrous Cycle
 Hormones of the Ovary
 Phases of the Estrous Cycle
 Cyclic Changes of the Endometrium
  Cow
  Bitch
  Primates
 Cyclic Changes of the Vaginal Epithelium
  Cow
  Bitch
Avian Female Reproductive System
 Ovary
 Oviduct
  Infundibulum
  Magnum
  Isthmus
  Uterus
  Vagina
 Cloaca

The female reproductive system consists of bilateral ovaries and uterine tubes (oviducts), a usually bicornuate uterus, cervix, vagina, vestibule, vulva, and associated glands. It is concerned with the production and transport of ova, the transport of spermatozoa, fertilization, and the accommodation of the conceptus until birth.

OVARY

The ovary is a combined exocrine and endocrine gland; that is, it produces both ova (exocrine "secretion") and ovarian hormones, chiefly estrogens and progesterone (endocrine secretion). The structure of the normal ovary varies greatly with the species, age, and phase of the sexual cycle. It is an ovoid structure divided into an outer cortex and an inner medulla (Fig. 13-1). In the mature mare, these areas become reversed, and the cortical tissue remains on the surface only in the ovulation fossa, which is the site of all ovulations.

Cortex

The cortex is a broad peripheral zone containing **follicles** in various stages of development and **corpora lutea** embedded in a loose connective tissue stroma (Fig. 13-1). It is covered by a low cuboidal **surface epithelium**. A thick connective tissue layer, the **tunica albuginea**, lies immediately beneath the surface epithelium. It is disrupted by the growth of ovarian follicles and corpora lutea and may be inconspicuous during increased ovarian activity. In the ovary of rodents, bitches, and queens, the cortical stroma contains cords of polyhedral **interstitial endocrine cells**. In the ovary of bitches, **cortical tubules** are also prominent; these are narrow channels lined by a cuboidal epithelium that, in some sites, are continuous with the surface epithelium.

Follicular Development

An **ovarian follicle** is a structure composed of an oocyte surrounded by specialized epithelial cells; during follicular development, the epithelial cells become surrounded by specialized stroma cells and a fluid-filled cavity develops among the epithelial cells.

Primordial (unilaminar, preantral, resting) follicles are composed of a **primary oocyte** surrounded by a simple squamous epithelium of **follicular cells** (Figs. 13-1 and 13-2). Primordial follicles arise prenatally by mitotic proliferation of **internal epithelial cell masses** in the ovarian cortex. In some species (e.g., bitches), they may arise also postnatally. The internal epithelial cell masses are believed to arise after interaction of cortical stroma, ovarian surface epithelium, or irregular epithelioid cell cords or channels, termed **rete ovarii**, with **primordial germ cells (PGCs)**; the PGCs arrive in the gonadal ridge from the wall of the yolk sac. During proliferation, the internal epithelial cell masses become separated into cell clusters. The central cell of a cluster becomes the **oogonium**. The oogonia enlarge, enter the prophase of the first meiotic division, and are then termed **primary oocytes**, approximately 20 μm in diameter in most species. The primary oocytes then go through the leptotene, zygotene, pachytene, and diplotene stages and then remain in the dictyotene stage. As the primary oocyte forms, the surrounding cells form a single layer of flat follicular cells resting on a basal lamina. Together, these components constitute the primordial follicle, approximately 40 μm in diameter. Primordial follicles are located mainly in the outer cortex. They are evenly distributed in ruminants and the sow and occur in clusters in carnivores.

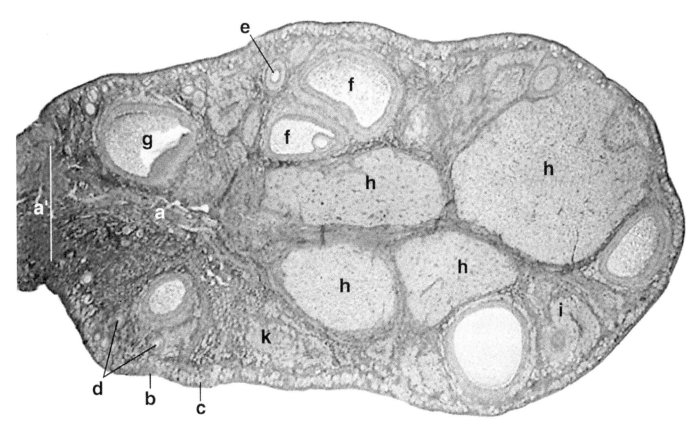

FIGURE 13-1 Ovary of queen showing the development and the regression of follicles and corpora lutea in the ovarian cortex. The ovarian medulla contains blood vessels (a) that enter the ovary at the hilus from the mesovarium (a′). Surface epithelium with adjacent tunica albuginea (b); subtunical layer with primordial follicles (c); primary follicles (d); secondary follicle (e); tertiary follicles, in one case containing an oocyte within the cumulus oophorus (f); early atretic follicle (g); corpora lutea (h); corpus regressivum (i); interstitial endocrine cells (k) (×56).

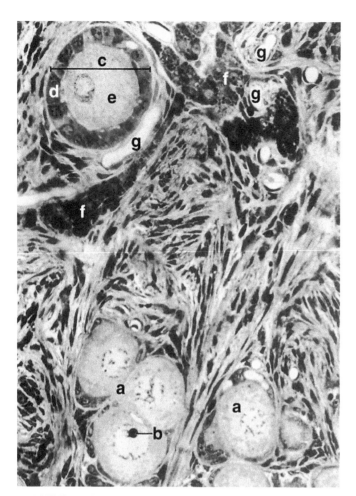

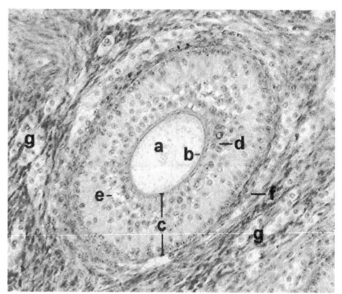

FIGURE 13-3 Ovary of queen showing a secondary follicle, in which the primary oocyte (a) is surrounded by a thin (initially) zona pellucida (b) and a stratified epithelium of polyhedral cells (c), of which the inner cell layer forms the corona radiata (d). Call-Exner bodies (e) are present in some cells. The connective tissue cells that surround the follicle will form the theca interna (f). Interstitial endocrine cells (g) are located in the connective tissue outside the follicle (×175).

FIGURE 13-2 Ovary of queen showing primordial follicles (a), which consist of primary oocytes surrounded by a simple squamous epithelium. Nucleus with nucleolus (b). Primary follicle (c), in which a cuboidal epithelium (d) encloses an enlarged primary oocyte (e). Interstitial endocrine cells containing granules (f) are seen near capillaries (g) (×300).

Primary (unilaminar, preantral, growing) follicles are composed of a **primary oocyte** surrounded by a simple cuboidal epithelium of follicular cells (Figs. 13-1 and 13-2). The primary oocytes begin the first meiotic division before birth, but the completion of prophase does not occur until the time of ovulation. The primary oocytes thus remain in suspended prophase (dictyotene stage) until after puberty. Several hundred thousand to 1 million potential oocytes may be present at birth in a single ovary in various species. Most of these regress before or after birth, and only several hundred ovulate during a normal lifetime. The processes involved in the selection of follicles for growth from a pool of nonproliferating primordial follicles are poorly understood.

Secondary (multilaminar, preantral, growing) follicles are composed of a primary oocyte surrounded by a stratified epithelium of polyhedral follicular cells, termed **granulosa cells** (Figs. 13-1 and 13-3). The multilaminar stratum of granulosa cells arises from proliferating follicular cells of the primary follicle. In carnivores, sows, and ewes, polyovular follicles, which contain several oocytes, may develop. In cows, the late secondary

follicle is approximately 120 μm in diameter and contains an oocyte approximately 80 μm in diameter. Secondary follicles are marked by the development of a 3- to 5-μm-thick glycoprotein layer, the **zona pellucida,** around the plasma membrane of the oocyte (Fig. 13-3). The zona pellucida is secreted by the granulosa cells immediately surrounding the oocyte and, in part, by the oocyte itself. There is partial penetration of this zone by the oocyte microvilli. Cytoplasmic extensions of the granulosa cells situated around the oocyte penetrate the zona pellucida and associate closely with these microvilli. As follicular development continues, small fluid-filled clefts are formed among the granulosa cells. A vascularized multilaminar layer of spindle-shaped stroma cells, termed **theca cells,** begins to form around the granulosa cell layer in late secondary follicles.

Tertiary (multilaminar, antral, growing) follicles, also termed **vesicular** or **Graafian follicles,** are composed of a **primary oocyte** (or, immediately before ovulation, a **secondary oocyte** in most species) surrounded by a stratified epithelium of granulosa cells; the granulosa cells are surrounded by a multilaminar layer of specialized stromal cells, termed the **theca,** and a fluid-filled cavity, the **antrum,** develops among the granulosa cells (Figs. 13-1, 13-4, and 13-5). The antrum, which characterizes tertiary follicles, is formed when the small, fluid-filled clefts among the granulosa cells of secondary follicles coalesce to form a single large cavity containing **liquor folliculi.** Late tertiary follicles, just before ovulation, are termed **mature follicles** (Fig. 13-6). In mature follicles, just before or just after ovulation, depending on the

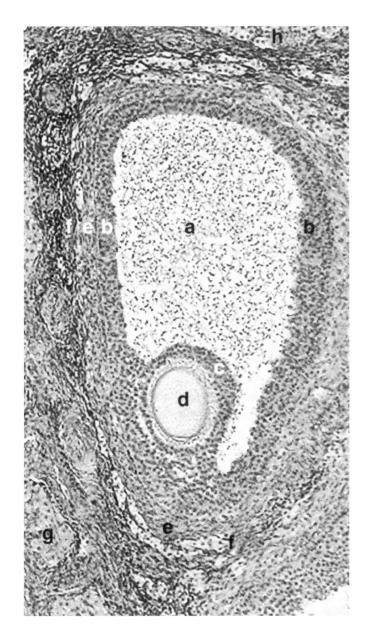

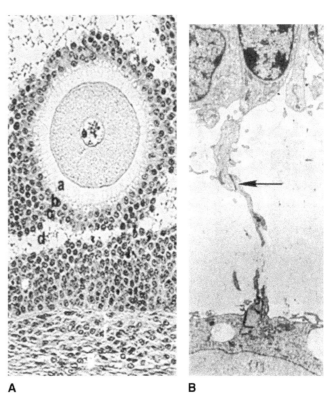

A   **B**

FIGURE 13-5 **A.** A bovine oocyte, surrounded by the zona pellucida (a), the corona radiata (b), and cells of the cumulus oophorus (c), is separated from the stratum granulosum of the follicular wall (e) by a gap (d) that developed during oocyte detachment from the follicle wall during the beginning stages of ovulation. Basal lamina of stratum granulosum (f); theca interna (g) (×220). **B.** An electron micrograph from the bovine ovary showing projections of a corona radiata cell (top) and of an oocyte (bottom), traversing a homogeneous zona pellucida, being in gap-junctional contact (arrow) with each other (×9000). *(Courtesy of P. Hyttel. From Leiser R. Weibliche Geschlechtsorgane. In: Mosimann W, Kohler T, eds. Zytologie, Histologie und mikroskopische Anatomie der Haussäugetiere. Berlin: Verlag Paul Parey, 1990:232.)*

FIGURE 13-4 Ovary of queen showing a tertiary follicle, which contains an antrum (a) and a multilayered epithelium, the stratum granulosum (b); a cumulus oophorus (c) enclosing the primary oocyte (d) forms in the stratum granulosum. The antrum contains a flocculent liquor folliculi. A connective tissue layer, the theca, which surrounds the stratum granulosum, can be divided into an inner theca interna, with light voluminous cells (e), and an outer theca externa, with dark fibrocytes (f). Marginal cells of the corpus luteum (g) have features of interstitial endocrine cells (h) (×110).

species, the primary oocyte completes the first meiotic division, thereby giving rise to a secondary oocyte and the **first polar body.**

The primary oocyte in tertiary follicles measures 150 to 300 μm in diameter, depending on the species. It has a spherical, centrally located nucleus with a sparse chromatin network and a prominent nucleolus. The Golgi complex, initially dispersed in the cytoplasm, becomes concentrated near the plasma membrane. Lipid granules and lipochrome pigment occur in the cytoplasm. As the antrum enlarges through the accumulation of liquor folli-

culi, the oocyte is displaced eccentrically, usually in a part of the follicle nearest to the center of the ovary (Fig. 13-1). The oocyte then lies in an accumulation of granulosa cells, the **cumulus oophorus** (Fig. 13-4). In large tertiary follicles, the granulosa cells immediately surrounding the oocyte become columnar and radially disposed; they are termed the **corona radiata** (Fig. 13-5A). The corona radiata cells are believed to provide nutrient support for the oocyte. They are lost at the time of ovulation in ruminants but generally persist until just before fertilization in other species.

In tertiary follicles, the granulosa cells form a parietal follicular lining, the **stratum granulosum** (Figs. 13-4 and 13-5A). Most of the parietal granulosa cells are polyhedral, but the basal layer may be columnar. Some of the granulosa cells in secondary and tertiary follicles may contain large periodic acid-Schiff (PAS) positive inclusions, the **Call-Exner bodies,** which represent intracellular precursors of liquor folliculi (Fig. 13-3). In the large tertiary follicle, the granulosa cells have the fine structural characteristics of protein-secreting cells, notably an extensive granu-

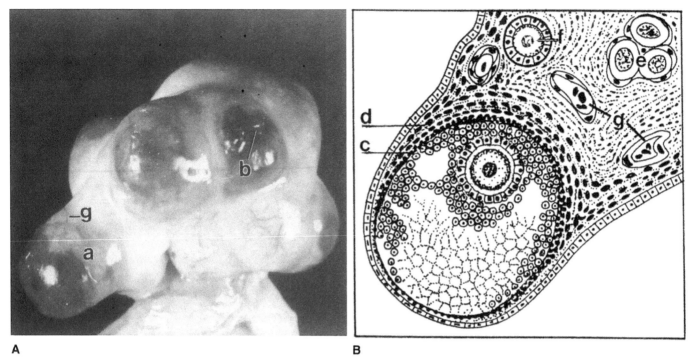

A   **B**

FIGURE 13-6   A. Ovary of sow with mature tertiary follicles immediately before ovulation (a) and one just ovulated as indicated by the stigma (b). A subepithelial vein (g) (×2.7). **B.** A schematic drawing of the follicle in **A** (left) shows the oocyte ready to disengage itself from the stratum granulosum at a site opposite the thinned, protruding follicular wall at the ovulation site, the stigma. Note the theca interna (c), theca externa (d), primordial follicles (e), primary follicle (f), and blood vessels (g).

lar endoplasmic reticulum (ER). Before ovulation, the granulosa cells of the mature follicle assume the characteristics of steroid-secreting cells, especially an agranular ER and mitochondria with tubular cristae.

The stratum granulosum is surrounded by the theca, which in tertiary follicles differentiates into two layers: an inner vascular **theca interna** and an outer supportive **theca externa** (Fig. 13-6). The **theca interna** cells are spindle-shaped in early tertiary follicles and located in a delicate reticular fiber network. An extensive blood and lymph capillary network is present in the theca interna, but it does not penetrate the stratum granulosum. Sympathetic nerve endings are present around the larger follicles. In mature follicles, many of the spindle-shaped theca interna cells adjacent to the stratum granulosum increase in size and become polyhedral and epithelioid. The nuclei of the epithelioid cells have a lighter chromatin pattern and more distinct nucleoli than those of the spindle-shaped cells. Cytoplasmic organelles in the epithelioid cells become typical of steroid-secreting cells: the mitochondria with tubular cristae, agranular tubular ER, and lipid inclusions are present. The epithelioid cells are abundant in mature follicles during proestrus and estrus and during their early regression.

The **theca externa** consists of a thin layer of loose connective tissue with fibrocytes arranged concentrically around the theca interna. Blood vessels of the theca externa supply capillaries to the theca interna.

One or more **mature follicles** reach maximal development near the time of ovulation. The **primary oocyte** (containing a diploid number of chromosomes) in these follicles completes the first meiotic division to become a **secondary oocyte** (containing a haploid number of chromosomes). During the first meiotic division, chromosome pairs are established and a mixture of parental genetic material occurs. Separation of the pairs and the production of the secondary oocyte and the first polar body (also containing a haploid number of chromosomes but little cytoplasm) follow as the division is completed. In domestic animals, the first meiotic division is completed shortly before ovulation, except in the bitch and the mare, in which it is completed shortly after ovulation (i.e., a primary oocyte is ovulated in the bitch and the mare). The **second meiotic division** begins immediately after the first meiotic division is completed but is arrested in metaphase; it is not completed unless fertilization occurs. At fertilization, the second meiotic division is completed, the secondary oocyte becomes an **ovum,** and a **second polar body** (also with little cytoplasm) is given off. The ovum becomes a **zygote** when the male and female chromosomes come together, establishing a diploid number of chromosomes.

Ovulation

When the follicle is fully developed, it protrudes from the surface of the ovary. Abundant blood and lymph vessel networks surround the follicle and an increased rate of secretion of a thin liquor folliculi occurs. The increased secretion rate is facilitated by increases in the follicular blood capillary pressure and permeability during proestrus and estrus. The increased accumulation of liquor folliculi causes the follicles to swell, but intrafollicular pressure does not significantly increase. Small hemorrhages occur in the follicular wall. The follicular wall becomes thin and transparent at the future site of follicular rupture, the **stigma.** The mature ovulatory follicles attain a size of 15 to 20 mm in cows; 50 to 70 mm in mares; approximately 10 mm in ewes, goats, and sows (Fig. 13-6A); and approximately 2 mm in bitches and queens.

Changes in the wall of the follicle preceding rupture are caused by the release of collagenases. Luteinizing hormone (LH) stimulates the production of prostaglandins (PG) F_2 and E_2. PGF_2 is believed to release collagenases from follicular cells, causing digestion of the follicular wall and its distension at the stigma. The process of digestion also releases proteins that provoke an inflammatory response with leukocytic infiltration and the release of histamine. All of these processes degrade the connective tissue of the follicular wall and the ground substance of the cumulus oophorus, so that the follicle ultimately ruptures at the stigma and the oocyte is released. The oocyte, usually surrounded by the corona radiata, escapes into the peritoneal cavity, from which it is swept directly into the infundibulum of the uterine tube. On rare occasions, an oocyte may fail to enter the uterine tube and, if fertilized, may establish ectopic pregnancy. In most species, the corona radiata cells disperse in the uterine tube in the presence of spermatozoa; in ruminants, they already are lost at the time of ovulation. The oocyte generally remains fertilizable for less than 1 day; when not fertilized, it degenerates and is resorbed. Most domestic animals ovulate spontaneously, but ovulation in queens is induced by a copulatory stimulus.

Follicular Atresia and Interstitial Endocrine Cells

Most follicles regress at some time during their development, and only a small percentage of all potential oocytes is ovulated from the ovary. This regression is called **atresia;** many more follicles become atretic than ever attain maturity. Prominent signs of atresia in follicular wall cells are nuclear pyknosis and chromatolysis. During atresia, the basal lamina of the granulosa layer may fold, thicken, and hyalinize; it is then called the **glassy membrane** (Fig. 13-7A). Eventually, atretic follicles are resorbed, except that small fibrous tissue scars may remain after atresia of large follicles.

In cows, in atresia of primary and secondary follicles, the oocyte commonly degenerates before the follicular wall, whereas in tertiary follicles, the reverse is true. Atretic changes in bovine tertiary follicles may result in the formation of two different morphologic types of atretic follicles: obliterative and cystic. In **obliterative atresia,** the granulosa and theca layers both infold, hypertrophy, and extend inward to occupy the antrum. In **cystic atresia,** both the granulosa and theca layers may atrophy, or only the granulosa layer may atrophy and the theca layer may luteinize, become fibrotic, or hyalinize around the antrum (Fig. 13-7B). In cystic atretic follicles, the theca interna cells containing LH receptors may continue to synthesize androgens after the regression of the granulosa cells, which converted the androgens to estrogens.

In the ovaries of the bitch, the queen, and rodents, **interstitial endocrine cells** are prominent; they arise chiefly from the epithelioid theca interna cells of atretic antral follicles or from hypertrophied granulosa cells of atretic preantral follicles (Fig. 13-8). They are usually absent from the ovaries of other adult domestic animals. The interstitial endocrine cells are polyhedral and ep-

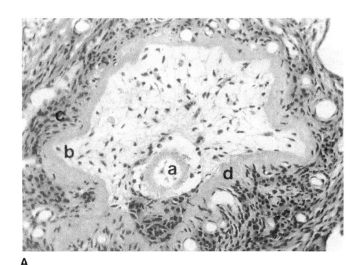

A

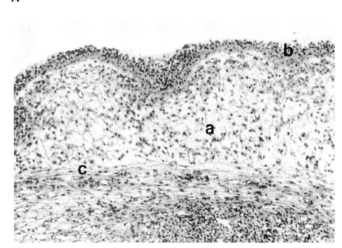

B

FIGURE 13-7 A. Atretic tertiary follicle (mature bitch). The oocyte (a) and granulosa layer (b) have degenerated, and the theca layer (c) has fibrosed. "Glassy membrane" (d) (×170). (With permission from Adam WS, Calhoun ML, Smith EM, et al. Microscopic Anatomy of the Dog: A Photographic Atlas. Springfield, IL: Charles C. Thomas, 1970.) **B.** Atresia of a large tertiary ovarian follicle (cow). Extensive hyalinization of theca interna (a) and loss or pyknosis of granulosa cells (b). Theca externa (c) (×100). *(From Priedkalns J. Effect of melengestrol acetate on the bovine ovary. Z Zellforsch 1971;122:85.)*

ithelioid and contain lipid droplets. In species such as rabbits and hares, they show an abundance of steroid-synthesizing organelles.

Corpus Luteum

At ovulation, the follicle ruptures, collapses, and shrinks as the liquor pressure is reduced. Folding of the follicular wall is extensive. The ruptured follicle is referred to as a **corpus hemorrhagicum** because of the blood that may fill the antrum. Bleeding after rupture of the follicle in mares, cows, and sows is greater than that in carnivores and small ruminants. Immediately before ovulation, some cells of the stratum granulosum exhibit signs of pyknosis. After ovulation, the stratum becomes vascularized by

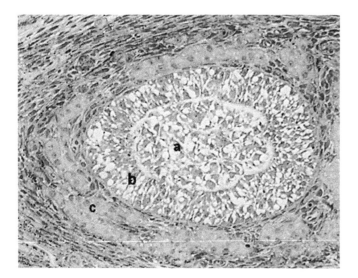

FIGURE 13-8 Atretic tertiary follicle (queen). The former antrum (a) and the stratum granulosum (b) have fibrosed, and the theca (c) has been replaced by epithelioid interstitial endocrine cells (×230).

an extensive capillary network originating from blood vessels in the theca interna. The granulosa cells enlarge, luteinize, and contribute to the **large luteal (lutein) cell** population of the corpus luteum. Simultaneously, folding of the follicular wall results in the incorporation of the theca interna into the corpus luteum, and, in most species, the theca interna cells contribute initially to the **small luteal (lutein) cell** population of the corpus luteum.

Luteinization is the process by which the granulosa and theca cells transform into luteal cells. It includes hypertrophy and hyperplasia of both cell types. A yellow pigment, lutein, appears in the luteal cells in cows, mares, and carnivores; it is absent in ewes, goats, and sows. A black pigment has been observed in the luteal cells of mares. In cows, postovulatory mitosis lasts for approximately 40 hours in the granulosa luteal cells and for approximately 80 hours in the theca luteal cells. The increase in size of the corpus luteum, after the period of mitotic activity, results mainly from hypertrophy of the large luteal cells. The small luteal cells make up a minor part of the corpus luteum and occupy mainly trabecular and peripheral areas.

The large luteal cells are polygonal, measure approximately 40 μm in diameter, and have a large spherical vesicular nucleus. They contain numerous metabolic lipid inclusions (Fig. 13-9). During metestrus and diestrus, the cells contain organelles characteristic of steroid-synthesizing cells, such as mitochondria with tubular cristae and abundant tubular agranular ER (Fig. 13-9C). The small luteal cells have more lipids but fewer steroid-synthesizing types of organelles than do the large luteal cells (Fig. 13-9A and B). The two luteal cell types eventually become mixed in the corpus luteum and are then difficult to distinguish. They both produce progesterone. Progesterone receptor expression and associated messenger ribonucleic acid (mRNA) activity are evident in luteal cells, especially during metestrus and diestrus and in pregnancy, suggesting that luteal autoregulatory mecha-

nisms have a role in progesterone production. In cows, the corpus luteum is fully developed and vascularized 9 days after ovulation but continues to grow until day 12, when it attains a diameter of approximately 25 mm.

The first sign of luteal regression is seen in late diestrus and involves the condensation of lutein pigment, which then appears reddish, followed by fibrosis and resorption of most of the corpus luteum. In cows, these signs are first observed 15 days after ovulation; further shrinkage of the corpus luteum occurs rapidly after day 18, and regression is complete 1 to 2 days after estrus. Large lipid droplets and crystalloid inclusions are typical of regressing luteal cells (Figs. 13-10 and 13-11). The vascular connective tissues of the corpus luteum become conspicuous in regression, with muscle cells in the walls of luteal arteries transformed by cellular hypertrophy and sclerosis. The connective tissue scar remaining after luteal regression is called the **corpus albicans**. In older ovaries, there is an abundance of such scars.

Medulla

The medulla is the inner area of the ovary containing nerves, many large and coiled blood vessels, and lymph vessels (Fig. 13-1). It consists of loose connective tissue and strands of smooth muscle continuous with those in the mesovarium. Retia ovarii are located in the medulla; they are solid cellular cords or networks of irregular channels lined by a cuboidal epithelium. They are prominent in carnivores and ruminants. It is claimed that the cells of the rete may differentiate into follicular cells when in juxtaposition to an oocyte.

Blood Vessels, Lymphatics, and Nerves

Arteries enter the ovary at the hilus. In the medulla, they form plexuses and give off branches to the follicular thecae, corpora lutea, and stroma. Around the larger follicles, arterial branches form a capillary wreath. During cyclic regression of the corpora lutea and the follicles, muscle hypertrophy and sclerosis occur in the walls of the arteries supplying these structures. The venous return is parallel to the arterial supply. Lymph capillaries accompany blood vessels in the follicular thecae and in the corpus luteum.

The nerves that supply the ovary are generally nonmyelinated. They are vasomotor in nature but include some sensory fibers. The nerves follow blood vessels and terminate in the walls of the vessels and around the follicles, in the corpora lutea, and in the tunica albuginea. They are derived mainly from the sympathetic system through renal and aortic plexuses, but vagal supply of the ovary also has been claimed.

UTERINE TUBE (OVIDUCT)

The uterine tubes are bilateral, tortuous structures that extend from the region of the ovary to the uterine horns and convey ova, spermatozoa, and zygotes. Three segments of the uterine tube can be distinguished: (a) the **infundibulum**, a large funnel-shaped portion (Fig. 13-12); (b) the **ampulla**, a thin-walled

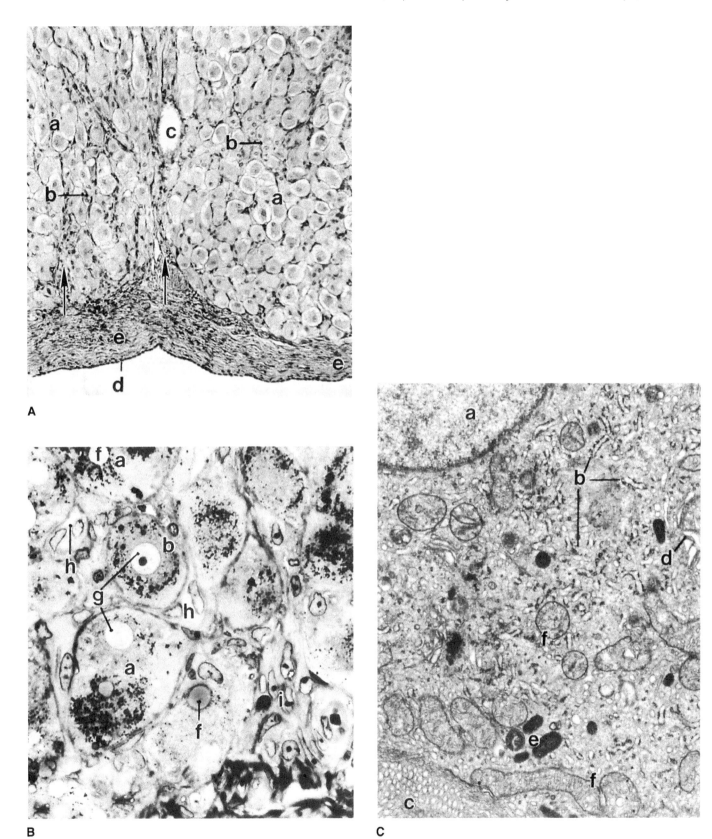

A

B

C

FIGURE 13-9 **A.** Part of a mature corpus luteum (sow). The corpus luteum consists of large luteal cells (a) intermingling with groups of small luteal cells (b). The corpus luteum is supplied with blood vessels (c) entering from the periphery by the trabeculae (arrows). Ovarian surface epithelium (d); adjacent tunica albuginea (e) (×120). **B.** Enlarged segment of **A** showing large (a) and small (b) luteal cells containing fine granular inclusions and lipid droplets (f). Nuclei (g); capillaries (h); strand of connective tissue (i) (×830). **C.** Large luteal cell from a corpus luteum from the same ovary of the sow as in **A** and **B.** Nucleus (a); granular endoplasmic reticulum (b); tubular and smooth endoplasmic reticulum (c); Golgi complex (d); secretory granules (e); mitochondria with tubular cristae (f) (×15,700).

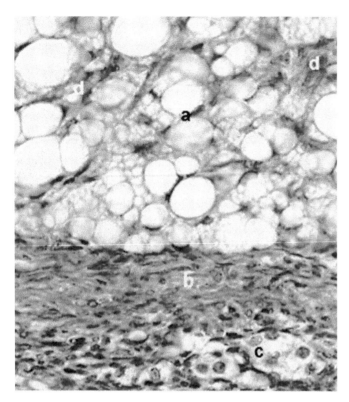

FIGURE 13-10 Corpus luteum (queen) in regression (corpus regressivum) (a) with adjacent connective tissue of theca origin (b) and ovarian interstitial endocrine cells (c). Lipid droplets of varying sizes are typical of regressing luteal cells. Connective tissue in the corpus regressivum (d) (×420).

section extending caudally from the infundibulum (Fig. 13-13A); and (c) the **isthmus**, a narrow muscular segment joining the uterus (Fig. 13-13B).

Histologic Structure

The epithelium is simple columnar or pseudostratified columnar with motile cilia on most cells (Fig. 13-12). Both ciliated and nonciliated cell types possess microvilli. Morphologic signs of secretory activity are evident only in the nonciliated cells. During the luteal phase, the secretory cells become taller than the ciliated cells. Their secretion provides the ovum and zygote with the necessary nutrients.

The mucosa is continuous with the submucosa in the female reproductive tract because the thin lamina muscularis (which separates these tunics in other tubular structures) is absent. In the uterine tube, the propria-submucosa consists of loose connective tissue with many plasma cells, mast cells, and eosinophils. The tunica mucosa-submucosa of the ampulla is highly folded, especially in sows and mares. In cows, approximately 40 primary longitudinal folds are present in the ampulla, each with secondary and tertiary folds (Fig. 13-13A). In the isthmus, with increasing distance from the ampulla, secondary and tertiary folds gradually disappear, and at the isthmus—uterus junction, where the isthmus is embedded in the uterine wall, only four to eight primary folds and no secondary or tertiary folds are present.

The tunica muscularis consists chiefly of circular smooth muscle bundles, but isolated longitudinal and oblique bundles also

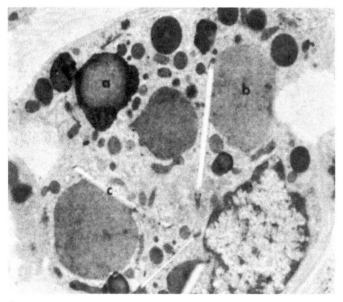

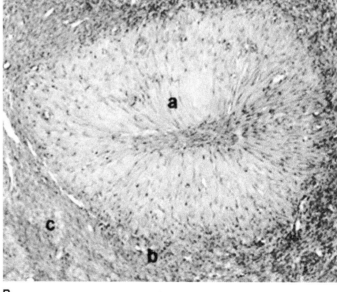

A   **B**

FIGURE 13-11 A. Electron micrograph of a regressed luteal cell, ovary (cow). Note the characteristic large remnant lipid droplets (a), granular bodies (b), and crystalloid inclusions (c) (×8725). (From Priedkalns J, Weber AF. Ultrastructural studies of the bovine Graafian follicle and corpus luteum. Z Zellforsch 1968;91:554.) **B.** Corpus luteum (cow) in regression (corpus regressivum) (a) with adjacent connective tissue of theca origin (b) and interstitial endocrine cells (c) (×100).

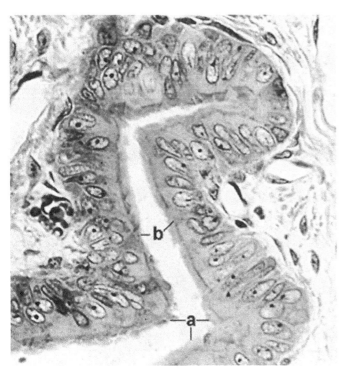

FIGURE 13-12 Columnar epithelium of the infundibulum of the uterine tube (queen) in estrus. Ciliated cells (a) are more numerous than dark-stained nonciliated cells (b) (×470).

The caudal ampulla is the site of fertilization. In the ampulla, ciliary activity is the primary force propelling the oocyte or zygote toward the isthmus, but in some species, muscle contractility is also involved. In the isthmus, muscle contractility is the primary force propelling the zygote toward the uterus, with ciliary activity involved in some species. The directionality of isthmus contractions varies according to the phase of the estrous cycle. In the follicular phase, antiperistaltic contractions of the isthmus tend to move the luminal contents toward the ampulla, whereas in the luteal phase, segmental contractions gradually propel the zygote toward the uterus. Zygotes require 4 to 5 days to traverse the isthmus. This length of time is independent of the isthmus length or of the gestation time in various species.

The passage of spermatozoa to the ampulla is accounted for by muscular contractions of the uterine and tubal walls. Inert particles and nonmotile spermatozoa can ascend the uterine tube at the same speed as motile spermatozoa, suggesting that the ascent of spermatozoa is not primarily the result of their innate motility. In cows, spermatozoa can reach the ampulla within 5 minutes after mating. Ascent at this rate is too fast to be accounted for by the motility of spermatozoa and/or by the ciliary movement of tubal cells.

Although spermatozoa develop in the male reproductive tract, their ability to fertilize is attained in domestic animals only after **capacitation** in the uterine tube.

UTERUS

The uterus is the site of attachment of the conceptus. It undergoes a definite sequence of changes during the estrous cycle and pregnancy. In most species, it consists of bilateral horns (cornua) connected to the uterine tubes and an unpaired body (corpus) and a neck (cervix), which joins the vagina. The cervix is considered separately in this chapter. In primates, the entire uterus is a single tube, called the uterus simplex.

Histologic Structure

The uterine wall consists of three layers (Figs. 13-14 and 13-15): (a) the mucosa-submucosa or **endometrium,** (b) the muscularis or **myometrium,** and (c) the serosa or **perimetrium.** The perimetrium, the longitudinal layer of the myometrium, and the vascular layer of the myometrium are all continuous with corresponding structures in the broad ligament of the uterus (Fig. 13-14A).

Endometrium

The endometrium is composed of two zones that differ in structure and function. The superficial layer, called the **functional zone,** degenerates partially or fully after pregnancy or after estrus. A thin deep layer, the **basal zone,** persists after these events, and the functional zone is restored from this layer.

The surface epithelium of the functional zone is simple columnar in the mare, the bitch, and the queen. It is pseudostratified columnar and/or simple columnar in sows and ruminants. In iso-

occur. The muscle layer gives off radial strands into the mucosa-submucosa. In the infundibulum and ampulla, the tunica muscularis is thin (Fig. 13-13A). In the isthmus, the inner muscle layer is prominent and blends with the uterine circular muscle (Fig. 13-13B).

A tunica serosa is present and contains many blood vessels and nerves.

Blood Vessels, Lymphatics, and Nerves

The blood vessels form subepithelial vascular plexuses and proliferate during pregnancy. Lymph vessels have capillary networks in the mucosal and serosal layers and drain into the lumbar lymph nodes.

Both myelinated and nonmyelinated nerve fibers with many subepithelial branches are present. They are derived mainly from the sympathetic system.

Histophysiology

The infundibulum secures oocytes extruded from the ovary. It is enclosed in the ovarian bursa or, in species without a definite ovarian bursa (e.g., the mare), it is applied partly around the ovary at estrus. It has fingerlike projections called **fimbriae.** At the time of ovulation in most species, blood vessels in the fimbriae become engorged. The turgid fimbriae move over the surface of the ovary due to rhythmic smooth muscle contractions. At the same time, cilia of the infundibular epithelial cells, mostly beating toward the uterus, transport the oocyte into the ampulla.

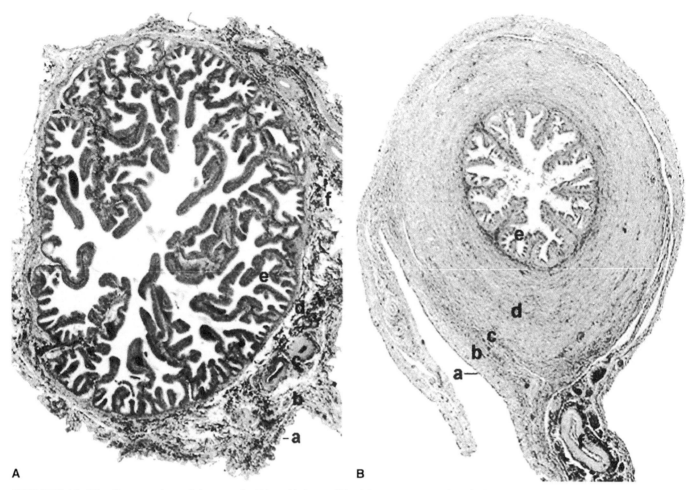

A

B

FIGURE 13-13 Cross sections of the ampulla (**A**) and isthmus (**B**) of the uterine tube (cow). Tunica serosa (a); longitudinal muscle layer (b); stratum vasculare (c); circular muscle layer (d); mucosal-submucosal folds (e); mesosalpinx with blood vessels (f) (×25).

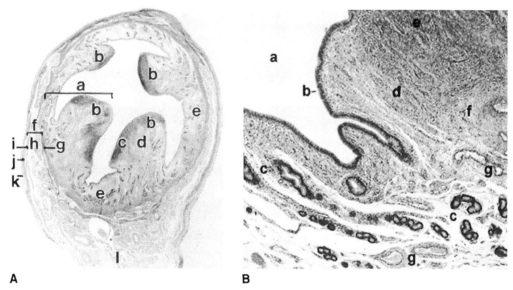

A

B

FIGURE 13-14 **A.** Cross section of the uterine horn (cow). Endometrium (a) forms four caruncles (b) with a distinct (dark) stratum cellulare (c) and a (clear) stratum reticulare (d). Glands (e) are present between the caruncles. Myometrium (f) consists of an inner muscle layer (g), a stratum vasculare (h), and an outer muscle layer (i). Perimetrium or serosa (j); mesothelium (k); mesometrium (l) (×6). (From Leiser R. Weibliche Geschlechtsorgane. In: Mosimann W, Kohler T, eds. Zytologie, Histologie und mikroskopische Anatomie der Haussäugetiere. Berlin: Verlag Paul Parey, 1990:232.) **B.** Endometrium, cow, 10 days postestrum. Uterine lumen (a); pseudostratified columnar epithelium (b); tubular uterine glands (c); caruncle (d) with a stratum cellulare (e) and a stratum reticulare (f); blood vessels (g) (×44).

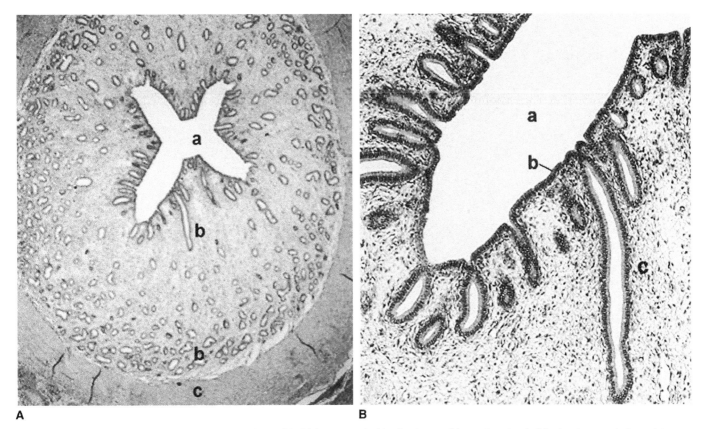

A   **B**

FIGURE 13-15 Sections through the uterine horn (bitch) in estrus. **A.** Uterine lumen (a); uterine glands (b); circular muscle layer (c) (×22). **B.** Magnification of **A** with uterine lumen (a), endometrial epithelium (b), and tubular glands (c) (×90).

lated areas, the epithelium may be simple cuboidal. The height and structure of the epithelial cells are related to the secretion of ovarian hormones throughout the cycle. The subepithelial, superficial part of the functional zone consists of a richly vascular, loose connective tissue with many fibrocytes, macrophages, and mast cells. Neutrophils, eosinophils, lymphocytes, and plasma cells are also present; melanophores are present in sheep. The deep part of the functional zone consists of loose connective tissue that is less cellular than that of the superficial part. In ruminants, during estrus, large irregular fluid-filled tissue spaces are present in the functional zone; this is termed **endometrial edema.**

Simple coiled, branched tubular glands are present throughout the endometrium in most species (Fig. 13-15). The glands are absent from the caruncles of ruminants (Fig. 13-14). The simple columnar glandular epithelium includes secretory and nonsecretory ciliated cells (Fig. 13-16). Rising estrogen levels stimulate the growth and branching of the glands, but coiling and a copious secretion from the glands generally do not occur until progesterone stimulation occurs. The branching and coiling of the glands are extensive in mares, whereas less branching is seen in carnivores (Fig. 13-15B). **Endometrial cups** occur in mares in early pregnancy after endometrial invasion by fetal cells (see Chapter 14).

In ruminants, circumscribed thickenings of the endometrium, known as **caruncles,** are present (Fig. 13-14). They are rich in fibrocytes and have an extensive blood supply. Approximately

15 caruncles in each of four rows are present in each uterine horn in ruminants. They are dome-shaped in cows and cup-shaped (i.e., a dome with a central depression) in ewes. Caruncles are the endometrial structures providing attachment of the maternal placenta to the corresponding structures of the fetal placenta, the cotyledons (see Chapter 14).

Myometrium

The myometrium consists of a thick inner layer, which is mostly circular, and an outer longitudinal layer of smooth muscle cells that increase in number and size during pregnancy. Between the two layers, or within the inner layer, is a vascular layer (stratum vasculare).

Perimetrium

The perimetrium consists of loose connective tissue covered by the peritoneal mesothelium. Smooth muscle cells occur in the perimetrium. Numerous lymph and blood vessels and nerve fibers are present in this layer.

Blood Vessels, Lymphatics, and Nerves

Between the inner and outer layers of the myometrium, or deep in the inner layer, is a vascular layer consisting of large arteries, veins, and lymph vessels that supply the endometrium (Fig. 13-14).

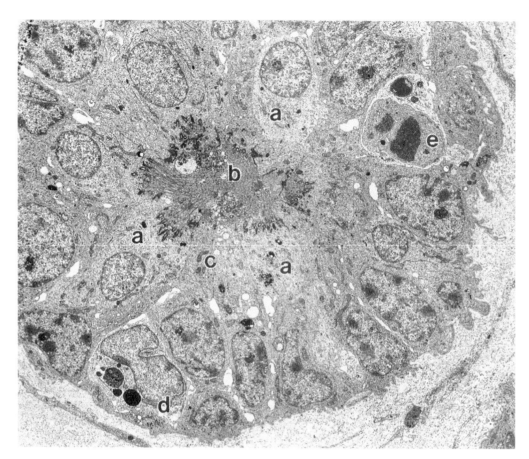

FIGURE 13-16 Electron micrograph of a section through a uterine gland (sow) in estrus. Columnar cells (pale appearance) (a) are ciliated with the cilia filling the gland lumen (b). Dark cells with microvilli and containing secretory granules (c); macrophage (d); and mitotic cell (e) (×2700).

They are especially large in the caruncular regions in ruminants. Numerous lymph and blood vessels and nerve fibers are present in the perimetrium.

The nerves are derived mainly from the sympathetic system through the uterine and pelvic plexuses. They branch in all of the tunics. Parasympathetic supply from the sacral spinal cord segments reaches the uterus through the pelvic plexus.

CERVIX

The cervix or the neck of the uterus is thick-walled, muscular, and rich in elastic fibers. The mucosa-submucosa forms high primary folds with secondary and tertiary folds. In cows, four large circular and 15 to 25 longitudinal primary folds, each with many secondary and tertiary folds, are present (Fig. 13-17A). The folding may give a false impression of glandular structure. The glandular elements present in the cervix are mostly mucigenous (Fig. 13-17B). Uterine glands do not extend into the cervix.

Histologic Structure

In most species, the epithelium is of the simple columnar type with many mucigenous cells, including goblet cells. Increasing quantities of mucus are secreted during estrus, and much of the mucus passes to the vagina. In pregnancy, the mucus thickens to form the cervical seal. A small proportion of the epithelial cells is ciliated in some species. Intraepithelial and simple tubular glands may be present in ruminants. In sows, more than 90% of the cervix may have a vaginal type of mucosa with stratified squamous epithelium that undergoes cyclic alterations as in the vagina. These features and alterations have relevance for the porcine copulatory mechanism.

The propria-submucosa consists of dense irregular connective tissue, which becomes edematous and assumes a loose areolar structure during estrus. In mares and bitches, venous plexuses are present in the deep part of the propria-submucosa.

The tunica muscularis consists of inner circular and outer longitudinal smooth muscle layers. Elastic fibers are prominent in the circular layer. Both muscle and elastic fibers are important in reestablishing cervical structure after parturition. The muscle layers of the cervix are continuous with those of the body of the uterus and the vagina. The cervical circular muscle layer is variously modified in different species. Thickening and infolding of the circular layer occurs in the region of the circular folds or prominences in the small ruminants and sows. In mares and cows, the thickened circular layer forms the body of the vaginal portion of the cervix. The orifice (external uterine ostium) of the

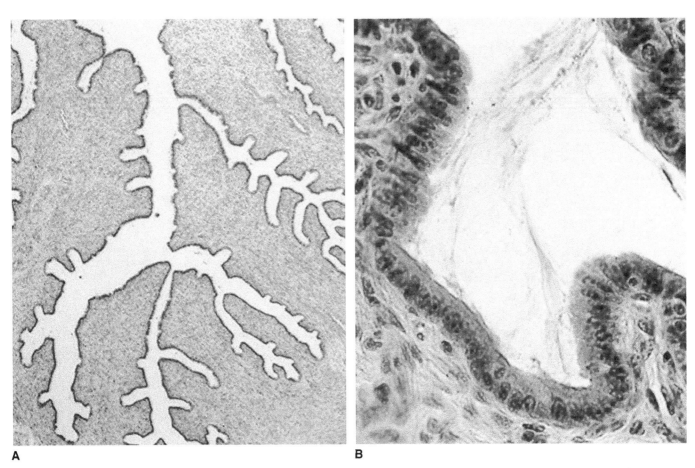

A   B

FIGURE 13-17   Cervix uteri (cow). **A.** Section of a large primary mucosal-submucosal fold with small secondary and tertiary folds projecting into the cervical lumen (×46). **B.** Note the mucous secretory activity of the epithelial cells as evidenced by the coagulated mucus in the cervical lumen (×430).

vaginal portion of the cervix in bitches is surrounded by a loop of the vaginal muscle.

The tunica serosa of the cervix consists of loose connective tissue covered by mesothelium. A longitudinal duct of the epoophoron (Gärtner's duct) may be present in this layer on one or both sides.

VAGINA

The vagina is a muscular tube extending from the cervix to the vestibule. Flat longitudinal mucosal-submucosal folds extend throughout the length of the vagina. In cows, prominent circular folds are also present in the cranial portion of the vagina. Cyclic variations occur in epithelial height and structure. Intraepithelial glands are present in some species. The increased amounts of vaginal mucus during estrus originate mainly in the cervix.

Histologic Structure

The vaginal mucosa is lined mostly by a stratified squamous epithelium that increases in thickness during proestrus and estrus (Fig. 13-18). In the cranial part of the bovine vagina, a surface layer of columnar and goblet cells containing PAS-positive mucosubstances is present on the stratified squamous epithelium. In mares, the epithelial cells are generally polyhedral, with a few

layers of flattened cells on the surface. The propria-submucosa consists of loose or dense irregular connective tissue, containing lymphatic nodules in the caudal part of the vagina.

The tunica muscularis consists of two or three layers. A thick inner circular smooth muscle layer is separated into bundles by connective tissue and is surrounded by a thin outer longitudinal smooth muscle layer. In sows and bitches, and to a small extent in queens, an additional thin layer of longitudinal smooth muscle is present inside the circular layer.

Cranially, the vagina is covered by a typical tunica serosa (loose connective tissue covered by mesothelium), while caudally, a tunica adventitia, consisting of loose connective tissue, is present. Both the serosa and adventitia contain large blood vessels and extensive venous and lymph plexuses. Numerous nerve bundles and ganglia occur in the tunica serosa and adventitia. The innervation is primarily sympathetic, derived from the pelvic plexus.

VESTIBULE, CLITORIS, AND VULVA

The wall of the **vestibule** is similar to that of the caudal portion of the vagina, except for the presence of more subepithelial lymphatic nodules, especially in the region of the clitoris. Blood ves-

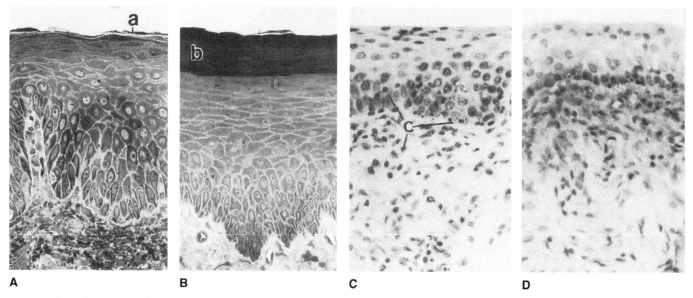

FIGURE 13-18 Stratified squamous epithelium of the vagina in the bitch. Proestrus (**A**): the epithelium has a thin layer of keratinized cells (a). Early estrus (**B**): a thick layer of keratinized cells (b) is present. Metestrus (**C**): the epithelium is nonkeratinized and leukocytes (c) are present within the relatively thin epithelium. Diestrus/anestrus (**D**): the epithelium comprises only a few layers of epithelial cells (×240).

sels, erectile cavernous tissue, venous plexuses, and small lymph vessels are abundant in the vestibular wall. They become congested during estrus. A discrete mass of erectile tissue, called the **bulbus vestibuli**, is present on each side beneath the vestibular mucosa in the mare and the bitch. It resembles the corpus spongiosum penis.

Major vestibular glands are bilateral compound tubuloacinar mucous glands located in the deep part of the propria-submucosa. They occur in cows, sheep, and queens. The terminal secretory acini contain large mucigenous cells. The small ducts draining the acini are lined by columnar mucous cells, with isolated areas of goblet cells. The large ducts leading to the vestibule are lined by a thick stratified squamous epithelium. Individual or aggregated lymphatic nodules may surround the large ducts. The glands provide mucous lubrication of the vestibule. They may be compressed during coitus and secrete mucus, thereby providing mucous lubrication also of the caudal vagina. They are homologous with the male bulbourethral glands.

Minor vestibular glands are bilateral small, branched, tubular mucous glands scattered in the vestibular mucosa in most domestic animals. They are homologous with the male urethral glands.

The **clitoris** consists of paired, joined erectile corpora cavernosa clitoridis, a rudimentary glans clitoridis, and a preputium clitoridis. The corpus cavernosum clitoridis, homologue of the corpus cavernosum penis, is well developed in mares. The glans clitoridis, homolog of the glans penis, is functionally erectile only in mares. A nonerectile fibroelastic tissue cover replaces the glans clitoridis in queens, sows, and ewes; in ewes, the cover contains a venous plexus. The clitoris contains many lymphatic nodules and is richly supplied with sensory and autonomic nerve endings.

The **vulva** is formed by the labia vulvae, which are covered by skin that is richly supplied with apocrine and sebaceous glands.

Striated muscle fibers of the constrictor vulvae are found in the hypodermis. The labia are well supplied with small blood and lymph vessels, which become congested during estrus, especially in sows and bitches.

THE ESTROUS CYCLE

Hormones of the Ovary

The ovary has important endocrine functions. It secretes the female sex hormones, mainly estrogens and progesterone. **Estrogens** are produced primarily during estrus by the granulosa cells, which convert androgens, secreted by the theca interna cells, to estrogens. **Progesterone** is produced primarily by the large luteal cells during metestrus, diestrus, and pregnancy and by the placenta. In certain species, the interstitial endocrine cells secrete large amounts of steroid sex hormones. Estrogen induces the growth and development of the female reproductive tract and estrous behavior. Progesterone stimulates the development of uterine glands, induces them to secrete, and renders the endometrium receptive to the implantation of the blastocyst. It also prevents follicular maturation and estrus and promotes behavior appropriate to pregnancy. Estrogens and progesterone promote the development of the mammary gland.

The growth and maturation of ovarian follicles and their estrogen secretion are controlled by pituitary **gonadotropins**. Both the granulosa and theca cells of late secondary or early tertiary follicles become responsive to gonadotropic hormones. The granulosa cells develop follicle-stimulating hormone (FSH) receptors, and the theca cells develop LH receptors. In mature tertiary follicles, the granulosa cells are induced by FSH also to develop LH receptors.

In tertiary follicles, LH interacts with receptors on the theca interna cells to stimulate the production of androgens and small amounts of estradiol. The androgens either are secreted into capillaries or traverse the basal lamina to reach the granulosa cell layer. Receptors on the granulosa cells interact with FSH to activate the aromatase enzyme system, which converts the thecal androgens (testosterone, androstenedione) to estrogens (estradiol-17, estrone). Granulosa cells themselves are unable to produce the androgens. The estrogens are secreted into the follicular fluid and also enter capillaries. The antral concentration of estradiol-17 is some 1,000 times greater than that of the bloodstream. The high local concentration of estrogens maintains a favorable environment for follicular maturation. The action of FSH, as well as of LH, on follicular cells is mediated by an increased production of cyclic adenosine-3′,5′-monophosphate (cAMP), which acts as an intracellular "second messenger."

Immediately before ovulation, the ovulatory surge of LH interacts with the LH receptors on the granulosa cells to induce events leading to ovulation. In addition, the LH surge seems to inhibit the aromatase activity of granulosa cells and thus to diminish estrogen secretion. In the mature preovulatory follicle, LH is involved also in the induction of oocyte maturation (i.e., the completion of the first meiotic division). Several other physiologically active substances accumulate in the fluid of the mature preovulatory follicle, including inhibin, a large protein that selectively suppresses pituitary FSH secretion.

Ovarian secretion of estrogens triggers the release of an ovulatory surge of LH, usually on the day of estrus, thereby inducing the processes leading to ovulation. The peak level of FSH occurs on the day before estrus; the peak level of LH, like that of estrogens, occurs on the day of estrus. Pituitary LH also initiates the formation of the corpus luteum. LH interacts with receptors on the cells of the ruptured follicular wall to initiate luteinization and progesterone secretion. In some species, such as rats and mice, luteotropic hormone (LTH) is needed to maintain the corpus luteum and its progesterone secretion. The expression of progesterone receptors in and on luteal cells in metestrus, diestrus, and pregnancy suggests that local luteal autoregulatory mechanisms may also control progesterone production.

Luteal cells produce progesterone during late metestrus and most of diestrus. Secretion peaks in late diestrus shortly before luteal regression sets in. Luteal cells also secrete estrogens and relaxin. In cells of the developing and the mature corpus luteum, the lipids are mostly phospholipids with traces of triglycerides and cholesterol and its esters. During regression, cholesterol accumulates in the luteal cells, suggesting decreased cholesterol utilization for steroid hormone synthesis. In active luteal cells, the lipid droplets are small and even in size and distribution, whereas during regression, they are large and unevenly distributed. With the light microscope, they appear as large vacuoles (Fig. 13-10). Regression of the corpus luteum is triggered by a uterine luteolytic factor reaching the ovary by local blood supply in the ewe, the cow, and the sow. The main luteolytic factor is $PGF_{2\alpha}$. If pregnancy occurs, the corpus luteum persists as the corpus luteum of pregnancy for different periods of time in various species. In cows and does, progesterone production by the corpus luteum continues through-

out gestation. The corpus luteum of pregnancy is supported by luteotropic hormones from the pituitary as well as from the placenta and by local luteal autoregulatory mechanisms. The embryo in ewes provides, in addition to luteotropic hormones, an antiluteolytic factor that overcomes the luteolytic effect of the uterus. In later stages of pregnancy in most species, the corpus luteum is not important because the placenta secretes the progesterone required for the successful maintenance of pregnancy. Ovarian and placental steroid hormones in turn influence pituitary gonadotropin secretion by a feedback effect on the hypothalamus, regulating mainly the release of the hypothalamic gonadotropin-releasing hormones. Other diencephalic structures, such as the pineal gland, also influence gonadotropic functions.

Phases of the Estrous Cycle

The estrous cycle is regulated by an intrinsic hypothalamo–hypophysial–ovarian rhythm that is modulated by environmental and internal neuroendocrine factors. In domestic animals, the estrous cycle is generally divided into the following sequential phases.

1. **Proestrus** is the phase of follicular maturation and endometrial proliferation following regression of the corpus luteum of the previous cycle. During this phase, the progesterone level falls, thus allowing release of FSH. Rising estrogen levels lead to estrus.
2. **Estrus** is the phase of sexual receptiveness, during which ovulation occurs in most species. Ovulation is preceded by a surge of LH. At the end of estrus, estrogen levels decline.
3. **Metestrus** is the phase of corpus luteum development and initial progesterone secretion.
4. **Diestrus** is the phase of the active corpus luteum in which the influence of luteal progesterone on accessory sex structures predominates. Endometrial glandular hyperplasia and secretion are maximal during diestrus. Toward the end of diestrus, however, the corpus luteum regresses and endometrial involution, including glandular regression, sets in. Diestrus can be prolonged into pseudopregnancy or gestational and lactational diestrus.
5. **Anestrus** is the prolonged period of sexual inactivity.

The average duration (in days) of the phases of the estrous cycle in cows and sows, respectively, is as follows: proestrus—3, 3; estrus—1, 2; metestrus—3, 3; and diestrus—14, 12. Thus, during proestrus and estrus, large ovarian follicles produce estrogens, whereas during metestrus and diestrus, the corpus luteum produces mainly progesterone.

Cyclic Changes of the Endometrium

The cyclic changes in the endometrium (Fig. 13-19 and 13-20) are, to a large extent, caused by the ovarian hormones estrogens and progesterone. During pregnancy, these hormones are produced chiefly by the placenta.

Some animals (e.g., bitches) are **monestrous** and have one or two estrous cycles per year, followed by a long anestrous period.

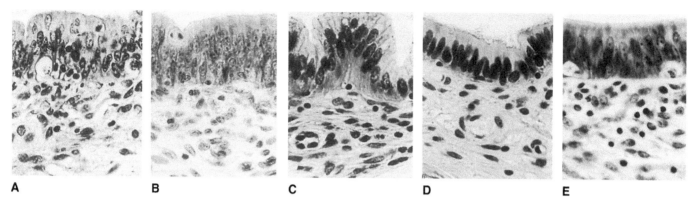

A   B   C   D   E

FIGURE 13-19 Endometrial epithelium through the estrous cycle (sow). Estrus (**A**); metestrus (**B**); early diestrus (**C**); late diestrus (**D**); proestrus (**E**) (×250).

Continuously cycling animals, without an anestrous period (e.g., cows and sows), or seasonally cycling animals (e.g., queens, mares, ewes, and goats) are **polyestrous.** The endometrium of monestrous animals degenerates and regenerates to a much greater extent than that of polyestrous animals. The immediate factor precipitating uterine degenerative changes is probably local ischemia. Uterine regenerative changes are induced by estradiol and continued by progesterone, which induces glandular secretory activity and causes the endometrium to produce a maternal placenta when stimulated by the presence of the blastocyst. A detailed description of the cyclic changes in the cow and the bitch follows.

Cow

In the cow, the estrous cycle lasts 21 days (Fig. 13-20). Ovulation occurs on the day after estrus, or approximately 30 hours after the onset of estrus. The day of estrus may be called "day 0" or "day 21" of the cycle, and the last day of proestrus may be referred to as "day 20." During the last 3 to 4 days of **diestrus,** the endometrial stroma shrinks and the epithelium becomes lower. The glands become shorter, their epithelium becomes lower, and their secretions cease. During **proestrus,** under the influence of estrogens, the endometrium is restored; the mucosa becomes thickened, congested, and edematous with a predominance of mucin-filled epithelial cells. Glandular proliferation, however, is limited to straight lumen growth without significant branching or coiling. During **estrus,** endometrial edema and hyperemia are maximal. During **metestrus,** the edema lessens, and a breakdown occurs in some of the congested endometrial blood vessels. With the onset of **diestrus,** under the influence of progesterone, the endometrium transforms from a proliferative to a secretory type, with glandular epithelial growth and glandular branching, coiling, and secretion. During the first 11 days of diestrus, endometrial glandular secretion is greatest. If pregnancy does not occur, the glands again regress along with the corpus luteum during the last 3 days of diestrus.

Mitotic activity begins in the surface and glandular epithelia and in the interstitial elements during estrus and continues for approximately 6 days after estrus. Neutrophils invade the lamina propria, epithelia, and uterine lumen from late proestrus to approximately day 3 or 4 after estrus. An invasion of agranulocytes, mainly lymphocytes, occurs from day 3 to 5 after estrus. These cells are especially abundant in the basal zone of the endometrium. An eosinophilic invasion may occur from estrus to midcycle. Mast cells increase in number at the time of maximal edema, especially in the caruncular areas. **Metrorrhagia** refers to the microscopic hemorrhages in the functional zone of the endometrium that begin shortly before the time of ovulation in the cow. At ovulation, metrorrhagia becomes widespread and is prominent in the pitted central areas of the caruncles. Metrorrhagia is greatest immediately after maximal endometrial edema. Capillaries rupture in the mucosa and blood accumulates in "blisters" beneath the surface epithelium. The blisters rupture, and blood and shreds of mucosa are liberated into the uterine lumen. Blood in the caruncular areas is mainly phagocytized and resorbed and generally does not reach the uterine lumen. Tissue fluid, as well as blood, may be lost at points of rupture in the intercaruncular areas. Metrorrhagia ends abruptly near the end of day 2 after estrus. A bloody vulvar discharge occurs at this time.

Bitch

Proestrus and estrus each lasts approximately 1 to 2 weeks in the bitch. If pregnancy does not follow estrus, pseudopregnancy and anestrus ensue. Endometrial edema, congestion, and hemorrhages occur during proestrus. Ovulation occurs soon after the onset of estrus. On approximately day 6 of estrus, corpora lutea become functional, and uterine glands and interstitial elements begin to proliferate. The glandular epithelium becomes high columnar, and the glands become coiled. In the nonpregnant state, involution of the endometrial glands and stroma begins approximately 20 to 30 days after the onset of estrus. During anestrus, the endometrium is thin and regressed, and the epithelium is mainly cuboidal. A prolonged and incomplete endometrial regression may occasionally result in pyometra.

Primates

Menstruation in primates is an entirely different phenomenon from the uterine bleeding seen in the bovine and the canine species. The uterine hemorrhages in the cow and the bitch occur during a **regenerative phase** of the endometrium near estrus.

Menstruation, on the other hand, occurs during a **degenerative phase** of the endometrium, precipitated by the withdrawal

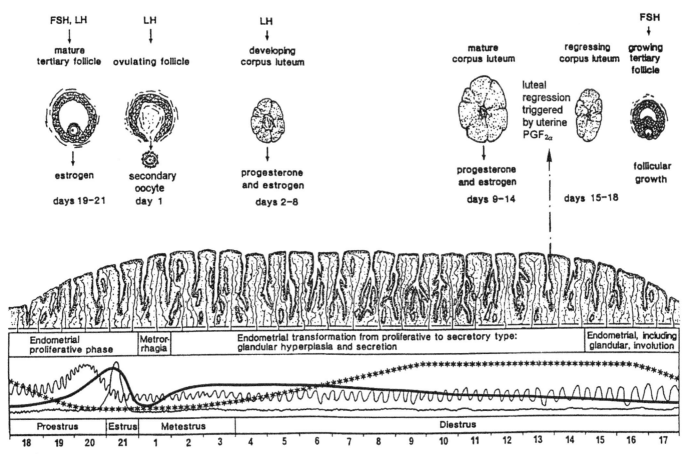

FIGURE 13-20 The ovarian and uterine changes during the estrous cycle in the cow are shown schematically. The ovarian follicular (days 15–21) and luteal (days 1–14) phases; the endometrial proliferative and secretory stages, with maximal glandular branching and activity on days 8–12; and endometrial involution (triggered by local prostaglandin $F_{2\alpha}$) are indicated. The relative blood levels of the following hormones are shown:

********** *progesterone*
_____ *estrogens*
〜〜〜 *follicle-stimulationg hormone (FSH)*
_____ *luteinizing hormone (LH)*
The scale indicates days 1–21 of the estrous cycle.

of estrogens and, more importantly, of progesterone after the involution of the corpus luteum. The occurrence of hemorrhage in primates has been related to special coiled arteries in the endometrial functional zone that periodically constrict and dilate as the support of progesterone and estrogens wanes. The arterial constriction causes ischemia and necrosis of tissue, and the dilation that follows leads to the rupture of the blood vessels, hemorrhage, and loss of tissues of the functional zone.

In certain animal species, the period most analogous to the period of human menstrual regression is the termination of pseudopregnancy. In bitches, pseudopregnancy invariably follows estrus and spontaneous ovulation if the animal has not become pregnant. In other animals, pseudopregnancy follows estrus and ovulation only if a mating stimulus resulting in a corpus luteum of pseudopregnancy has occurred (i.e., a corpus luteum of prolonged and sometimes greater activity than that of the corpus luteum of diestrus). Regression of the corpus luteum results in decreased progesterone and estrogen supply, and consequent regression of the endometrium and the termination of pseudopregnancy. Although

no external bleeding occurs in bitches at this time, microscopic hemorrhages of the endometrium have been observed.

Cyclic Changes of the Vaginal Epithelium

Cow

The epithelium varies with the site and hormonal status of the animal. Under the influence of **progesterone,** the epithelium in the cranial part of the vagina consists of approximately three layers of cells and increases to approximately 10 layers in the caudal part.

Under the influence of **estrogens,** the rate of epithelial cell proliferation is increased throughout the vagina and the epithelium thickens. In early estrus, the superficial layer of columnar and goblet cells in the cranial part of the vagina attains maximal height as a result of stored mucus. The epithelium of the caudal part is at maximal height from 2 days after estrus until midcycle, during which period the surface cells are more squamous than at other times and desquamation occurs. True keratinization (cornification) of the superficial epithelial cells is not observed, however.

Neutrophils invade the vaginal epithelium from estrus until 2 days after estrus. Lymphocytes and plasma cells are more common under the influence of progesterone. (Attempts to identify the stage of the estrous cycle by the vaginal smear method are not as successful as in the bitch.)

Bitch

Cyclic cellular changes that occur in the vaginal epithelium of the bitch are clinically useful and important for estimating the times of estrus and breeding (Fig. 13-21). The assessment of cellular changes by the vaginal smear method is widely used. After staining, vaginal smears appear as follows:

1. **Proestrus** (approximately 9 days in duration). Numerous erythrocytes (of uterine origin) and many large flat keratinized cells are present.
2. **Estrus** (approximately 9 days in duration). Some erythrocytes and numerous keratinized cells are present. As estrus

progresses, the keratinized cells become wrinkled and distorted and are frequently invaded by bacteria.
3. **Metestrus-diestrus** (approximately 3 months in duration). Epithelial cells are less keratinized and appear more like unstained living cells. Neutrophils are numerous on day 3 of metestrus and gradually disappear until day 10 to 20 of metestrus.
4. **Anestrus** (approximately 2 months in duration). Numerous unstained nonkeratinized epithelial cells, a few large stained cells with pyknotic nuclei, and a few neutrophils and lymphocytes are present.

The cyclic histologic changes in the vaginal epithelium in the bitch are shown in Figure 13-18. Although the epithelial lining of the vagina is thin in anestrus, with only approximately two to three layers of cells, it proliferates during proestrus and may be 12 to 20 cells thick at the beginning of estrus, with keratinization of the surface layers (Fig. 13-22). By late estrus, desquamation of the

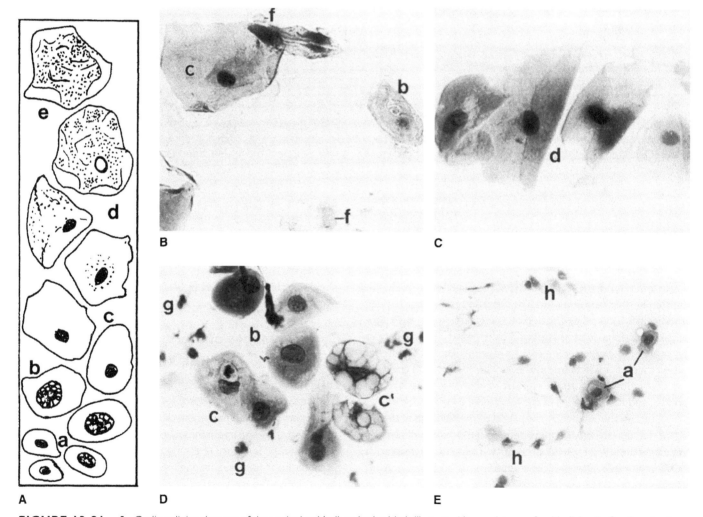

FIGURE 13-21 **A.** Cyclic cellular changes of the vaginal epithelium in the bitch illustrated by a scheme of epithelial cells. Parabasal cells (a); small intermediate cells (b); large intermediate cells (c); superficial cells (d); keratinized cells (e, without nuclei). Vaginal smears (epithelial and blood cells): **B.** Proestrus; note small intermediate cells (b), large intermediate cells (c, centrally keratinized), and erythrocytes (f). **C.** Estrus; note superficial cells (d, keratinized, pyknotic nuclei). **D.** Metestrus, note small intermediate cells (b), large intermediate cells (c) undergoing disintegration (c′), and granulocytes (g). **E.** Anestrus, note parabasal cells (a), and cell debris (h) (×680).

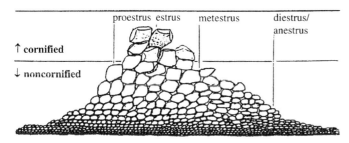

FIGURE 13-22 Schematic drawing of the cyclic changes of the vaginal epithelium in the bitch. (Modified from Tammer I, Blendinger K, Sobiraj A, et al. Über den Einsatz der exfoliativen Vaginalzytologie im Rahmen der gynœkologischen Befunderhebung bei der Hündin. Tierärztl Praxis 1994;22:199.)

keratinized layers begins (Fig. 13-23). Intraepithelial glands are common during estrus.

AVIAN FEMALE REPRODUCTIVE SYSTEM

Ovary

In adult birds, only the left ovary is present. The ovarian cortex and medulla are distorted by the presence of large "follicles" in various stages of development or atresia. Each is attached to the ovary by a peduncle. True follicles are not present in the avian ovary because a fluid-filled follicular antrum does not develop. In the follicle, the oocyte is surrounded by one or several layers of granulosa cells. The granulosa cells are surrounded by cells of the theca interna and theca externa. The granulosa cells are shed with the oocyte at ovulation, whereas the theca cells remain to

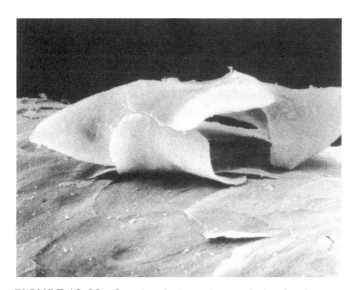

FIGURE 13-23 Scanning electron micrograph showing the desquamation of keratinized superficial cells from the vaginal epithelium in the bitch in estrus (×650).

form a transient corpus luteum. Interstitial endocrine cells are found at the periphery of the ovary.

Formation of follicles usually begins in the posthatching period, during which time the oogonia enlarge and become primary oocytes surrounded by follicular cells. The primary oocytes then enter the first meiotic division. At the time of sexual maturity (5 to 6 months in hens), secondary oocytes are ovulated. The second meiotic division is completed at fertilization, and an ovum, then a zygote, results. While the primary oocyte is primarily protoplasmic, the secondary oocyte contains mainly yolk. Abundant yolk is accumulated at one end of the cell; the nucleus is at the other end. The secondary oocyte and ovum are thus termed **macrolecithal, telolecithal cells.** The yolk contains lipids, such as lecithin, cholesterol, and carotene, arranged in concentric layers. The oocyte is surrounded by a plasma membrane, termed the **vitelline membrane.** After ovulation, other layers are added to the outside of the oocyte during passage through the female reproductive tract.

Oviduct

The term **oviduct** in the bird is used to describe the entire reproductive duct. It is present in the adult only on the left side. The left oviduct consists of the **infundibulum, magnum, isthmus, uterus,** and **vagina** (Fig. 13-24). Although each of these divisions has special structural and functional features, they all have two morphologic elements essential for egg formation: (a) a muscle layer, which supports the oviduct and propels the egg, and (b) a glandular epithelial lining, which secretes all the parts of the egg outside the yolk-filled oocyte/zygote. Moreover, the mucous membrane produces a slimy secretion that forms a soft resilient cushion for the egg as it passes through the oviduct.

The following secretions of the oviduct are added onto the oocyte/zygote:

1. Four layers of albumen are added in the magnum (the cranial part of the oviduct).
2. A shell membrane, consisting of a thin inner and a thick outer layer of protein (mainly keratin) filaments, is added in the isthmus; the two layers become separated in the air chamber at the blunt end of the egg.
3. A porous shell is formed in the uterus. This shell consists of an inner layer of conical calcareous masses, surrounded by a spongy organic layer, and an outer shell cuticle. An organic pigment layer may be added externally in some breeds.

Infundibulum

The cranial extremity of the infundibulum is dilated and has long fimbriae that grasp the secondary oocyte as it is released from the ovary. The infundibulum is the usual site of **fertilization.** The mucosa-submucosa is thrown into low longitudinal ridges or primary folds; in addition, secondary mucosal-submucosal folds are present in the caudal infundibulum. The egg remains in the infundibulum for approximately 25 minutes.

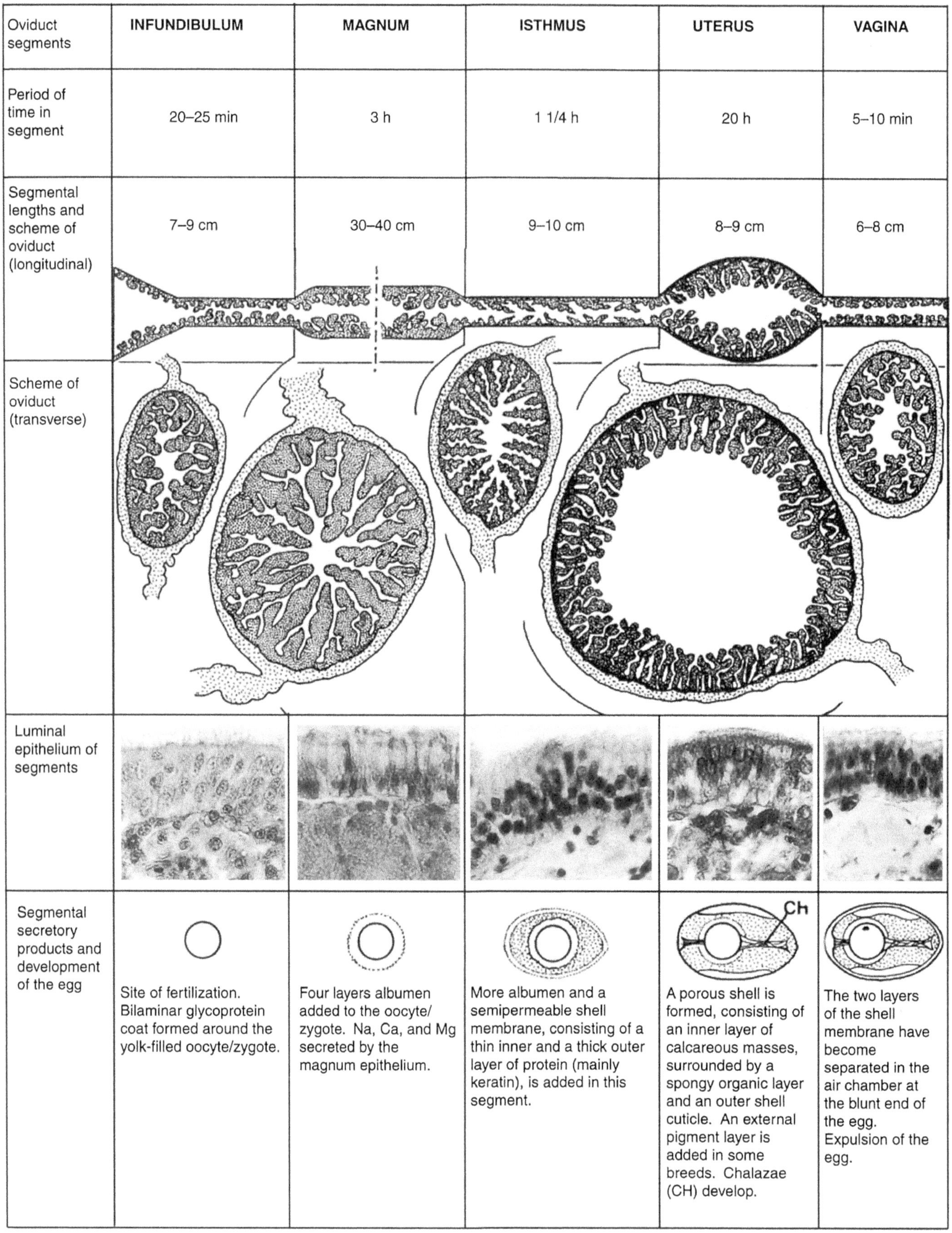

Oviduct segments	INFUNDIBULUM	MAGNUM	ISTHMUS	UTERUS	VAGINA
Period of time in segment	20–25 min	3 h	1 1/4 h	20 h	5–10 min
Segmental lengths and scheme of oviduct (longitudinal)	7–9 cm	30–40 cm	9–10 cm	8–9 cm	6–8 cm
Scheme of oviduct (transverse)					
Luminal epithelium of segments					
Segmental secretory products and development of the egg	Site of fertilization. Bilaminar glycoprotein coat formed around the yolk-filled oocyte/zygote.	Four layers albumen added to the oocyte/zygote. Na, Ca, and Mg secreted by the magnum epithelium.	More albumen and a semipermeable shell membrane, consisting of a thin inner and a thick outer layer of protein (mainly keratin), is added in this segment.	A porous shell is formed, consisting of an inner layer of calcareous masses, surrounded by a spongy organic layer and an outer shell cuticle. An external pigment layer is added in some breeds. Chalazae (CH) develop.	The two layers of the shell membrane have become separated in the air chamber at the blunt end of the egg. Expulsion of the egg.

FIGURE 13-24 Egg development in the laying domestic hen: structural changes of the egg in the various segments of the oviduct. Luminal epithelium of oviduct segments (×510). (Modified from Salomon F-V. Lehrbuch der Geflügelanatomie. Stuttgart: Gustav Fischer Verlag Jena, 1993).

The epithelium is ciliated pseudostratified columnar. It contains occasional goblet cells, except at the bottom of the folds, where the epithelium is nonciliated simple columnar. Toward the caudal portion of the infundibulum, glandular cells increase in number and become aggregated in **glandular grooves** that resemble the tubular glands of the magnum.

The propria-submucosa consists of loose connective tissue containing many lymphocytes and plasma cells. The tunica muscularis is composed of scattered bundles of longitudinal smooth muscle. The tunica serosa consists of loose connective tissue and mesothelium.

Magnum

The magnum has a thick wall and tall thick longitudinal primary and secondary mucosal-submucosal folds. **Albumen** is added to the egg in the magnum. The egg remains in the magnum for approximately 3 hours.

The epithelium of the magnum is simple columnar with close to equal numbers of ciliated cells and goblet cells. The loose connective tissue of the propria-submucosa is packed with many long, branched, coiled tubular glands. The cells are pyramidal and contain coarse basophilic granules. An inner circular and an outer longitudinal smooth muscle layer are present. A thin tunica serosa consists of loose connective tissue and mesothelium. The magnum is sharply divided from the next portion of the oviduct, the isthmus, by a 1- to 3-mm segment devoid of glands.

Isthmus

The isthmus has pronounced longitudinal ridges. The egg remains in the isthmus for approximately 1.25 hour. The bilaminar **shell membrane** is formed in this region.

The epithelium is simple columnar with close to equal numbers of ciliated and goblet cells.

The propria-submucosa is filled with distended branched tubular glands. The glands are lined by pyramidal cells with cytoplasm that contains many acidophilic secretory granules. The tunica muscularis consists of circular and longitudinal smooth muscle layers. The tunica serosa consists of loose connective tissue and mesothelium.

Uterus

The uterus, or **shell gland,** is thick-walled, saclike, and distensible. Primary and secondary longitudinal folds are obscured by a series of primary and secondary circular folds. Rotation of the egg, associated with twisting of the chalazae, occurs here. The egg remains in the uterus for approximately 20 hours. Shell components, such as organic matrix, shell cuticle, and inorganic material, are formed here.

The epithelium is ciliated pseudostratified columnar. The propria-submucosa contains branched, coiled tubular glands. The cells of these glands are pyramidal and have a diffusely granular and vacuolated cytoplasm. Loose connective tissue is sparse between the glands. The tunica muscularis consists of two layers of smooth muscle. The inner circular layer is thick and forms a sphincter at the boundary with the vagina. The tunica serosa consists of loose connective tissue and mesothelium.

Vagina

The vaginal wall is thick and has low primary and secondary longitudinal folds. The egg remains in the vagina for a short time, and the vagina does not participate in the formation of the egg. It is glandless, except for the so-called **sperm-host glands** at the uterovaginal junction that are used for the storage of spermatozoa.

The epithelium is ciliated pseudostratified columnar with few goblet cells. The propria-submucosa is loose connective tissue, frequently containing lymphocytes, plasma cells, and granulocytes. The tunica muscularis is functional in expelling the egg and consists of a thick inner circular layer and an outer longitudinal layer. The tunica serosa consists of loose connective tissue and mesothelium.

Cloaca

The vagina, colon, and ureters open into the cloaca. The epithelium of the cloaca is simple columnar and contains many goblet cells.

SUGGESTED READINGS

Baird DT. The ovary. In: Austin CR, Short RV, eds. Reproduction in Mammals, Vol. 3. 2nd Ed. Cambridge: Cambridge University Press, 1984:91.

Byskov AGS. Primordial germ cells and regulation of meiosis. In: Austin CR, Short RV, eds. Reproduction in Mammals, Vol. 1. 2nd Ed. Cambridge: Cambridge University Press, 1982:1.

Goodman RL, Karsch FJ. The hypothalamic pulse generator: a key determinant of reproductive cycles in sheep. In: Follett BK, Follett DE, eds. Biological Clocks and Seasonal Reproductive Cycles. Colston Papers No. 32. Bristol: John Wright, 1981:223.

Juengel JL, Niswender GD. Molecular regulation of luteal progesterone synthesis in domestic ruminants. J Reprod 1999;Suppl 54:193.

Leiser R. Weibliche Geschlechtsorgane. In: Mosimann W, Kohler T, eds. Zytologie, Histologie und mikroskopische Anatomie der Haussäugetiere. Berlin: Verlag Paul Parey, 1990:232.

Liebig H-G. Funktionelle Histologie der Haussäugetiere. Stuttgart: Schattauer, 1990:255.

Liggins GC. The fetus and birth. In: Austin CR, Short RV, eds. Reproduction in Mammals, Vol. 2. 2nd Ed. Cambridge: Cambridge University Press, 1983:114.

Knobil E, Neill JD. The Physiology of Reproduction. 2nd Ed. New York: Raven Press, 1994:II.

McDonald LE. Veterinary Endocrinology and Reproduction. 3rd Ed. Philadelphia: Lea & Febiger, 1982.

Milvae RA, Hinckley ST, Carlson JC. Luteotropic and luteolytic mechanisms in the bovine corpus luteum. Theriogenology 1996;45:1327.

Moore RM, Seamark RF. Cell signaling, permeability and microvascularity changes during antral follicle development in mammals. J Dairy Sci 1986;69:927.

Priedkalns J. Pregnancy and the central nervous system. In: Steven DH, ed. Comparative Placentation: Essays in Structure and Function. London: Academic Press, 1975:189.

Priedkalns J, Weber AF, Zemjanis R. Qualitative and quantitative morphological studies of the cells of the membrana granulosa, theca interna, and corpus luteum of the bovine ovary. Z Zellforsch 1968; 85:501.

Rajakoski E. The ovarian follicular system in sexually mature heifers with special reference to seasonal, cyclical and left-right variations. Acta Endocrinol (Kbh.) 1960;34(Suppl 52):1.

Salomon F-V. Weibliches Geschlechtssystem. In: Lehrbuch der Geflügel-anatomie. Stuttgart: Gustav Fischer Verlag Jena, 1993:197.

Sjöberg N-O, Hamberger L, Janson PO, et al., eds. Local Regulation of Ovarian Function. Carnforth, UK: Parthenon, 1992.

Van Blerkom J, Bell H, Weipz D. Cellular and developmental biological aspects of bovine meiotic maturation, fertilization and pre-implantation embryogenesis in vitro. J Electron Microsc Tech 1990; 16:298.

Wrobel K-H, Laun G, Hees H, et al. Histologische und ultrastruk-turelle Untersuchungen am Vaginalepithel des Rindes. Anat Histol Embryol 1986;15:303.

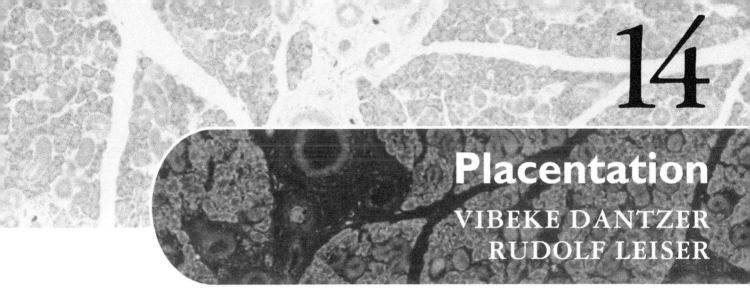

14

Placentation
VIBEKE DANTZER
RUDOLF LEISER

Embryology

Classification

    Fetal Extraembryonic Membrane Contributions

        Choriovitelline placenta

        Chorioallantoic placenta

    Macroscopic Structure of the Placenta

    Three-Dimensional Structure of the Interface Between
        Maternal and Fetal Tissues

    Tissue Layers of the Fetal–Maternal Interhemal Barrier

    Fetal–Maternal Anchoring and Fate of
        Maternal Tissues at Birth

Nourishment of the Embryo

Placental Vascularity and Circulation

Specialized Cells of the Placenta

Changes During Placentation

Function–Structure Relationships

Species Differences

    Sow

    Mare

    Cow

    Ewe and Goat

    Bitch, Queen, and Mink

EMBRYOLOGY

The fusion of a female and male gamete results in a **zygote**. After repeated cleavage during the transport through the uterine tube to the uterine cavity in higher mammals (Eutheria), the zygote develops into a fluid-filled vesicle, the **blastocyst,** with a wall of simple epithelium, the **trophoblast.** An eccentrically located **inner cell mass** extends from the wall into the blastocyst cavity. The free-floating blastocyst is nourished by secretions from the endometrium. Because the increasing demand from the growing embryo necessitates a more efficient nutritive arrangement (i.e., a vascular transport system), the embryo produces membranes that, in a process called **implantation,** gradually attach to the endometrium. A close relationship is established between fetal and maternal circulatory systems for physiologic exchange. As a result, a combined organ, the **placenta,** is formed. A **fetal part** (pars fetalis) and a **maternal part** (pars uterina) are recognized. The fetus and fetal membranes, including the fetal part of the placenta, are known as the **conceptus.** The manner of attachment and subsequent formation of the placenta is termed **placentation.**

The first events in placentation occur in the blastocyst stage. The trophoblast is essential for the transfer of nourishment to the offspring during intrauterine life but has no function after birth of the young and is expelled with the afterbirth (secundinae). The inner cell mass differentiates into three germ layers in two stages, initially forming **ectoderm** and **endoderm** and then **mesoderm** between the two original layers. These three germ layers form the embryo, but they also participate in the formation of the fetal membranes. The ectoderm contributes to a vesicle enclosing the embryo, the **amnion;** it provides buoyancy and protected space for development for the embryo. The amnion contains antiangiogenic factors and is used for eye surgery to prevent unwanted vascularization. The endoderm contributes to the **yolk sac,** communicating with the midgut, and to the **allantois,** a diverticulum from the hindgut (Fig. 14-1).

The further development of the fetal membranes is directed by the mesoderm. Lateral mesoderm splits into a somatic and a splanchnic layer. The resulting intramesodermal cleft gives rise to the body cavity (intraembryonic coelom), which, at this stage, extends to form an extraembryonic cavity called the **exocoelom.** Somatic mesoderm combines with the trophoblast layer to form

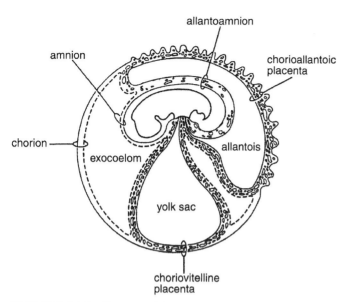

FIGURE 14-1 Diagram of fetal membranes. The arrangement is subject to wide variation in different species. The amnion encloses the amniotic cavity and embryo. Ectoderm and somatic mesoderm (somatopleure) form the amnion and chorion, while the yolk sac and allantois consist of endoderm and splanchnic mesoderm (splanchnopleure). *(From Dellmann H-D, Carithers JR. Cytology and Microscopic Anatomy. Philadelphia: Williams & Wilkins, 1996.)*

the **chorion** or with the ectoderm of the amnion. These membranes constitute the extraembryonic **somatopleure**. Splanchnic mesoderm fuses with the endoderm of the yolk sac and the allantois, and together these layers form the extraembryonic **splanchnopleure**.

Somatic mesoderm, and hence the chorion, is initially avascular. Blood islands and vessels first arise in the splanchnic mesoderm of the yolk sac and later in the splanchnic mesoderm of the allantois. Eventually, the avascular mesoderm of the chorion fuses with the mesoderm of the allantois, forming the **allantochorion**, which then becomes vascularized and filled with allantoic fluid. At birth, the **allantoamnion,** a fusion of the allantois and amnion, protrudes through the ruptured allantochorion and assists in dilation of the cervix at parturition. The placental vessels, together with the vitelline and allantoic ducts, are contained in the **body stalk** and later develop into the **umbilical cord** (see Fig. 14-10A).

Secretions from the fetal membranes play an important role in the maternal recognition of pregnancy and its continuation. The secretions result in an alteration of the endometrial signal to the ovary, leading to the preservation of the corpus luteum. In the pig, estrogen secreted by the blastocyst is antiluteolytic, while in ruminants, interferon τ (IFNτ) exerts a similar effect.

CLASSIFICATION

The placenta is subject to great variation in structure, which is species-dependent. The variation has given rise to many different systems of classification, based on five main criteria: (a) fetal extraembryonic membrane contributions, (b) macroscopic structure of the placenta, (c) three-dimensional structure of the maternal–fetal interface, (d) tissue layers of the fetal–maternal interhemal barrier, and (e) degree of fetal–maternal anchoring and fate of maternal tissues at birth.

Fetal Extraembryonic Membrane Contributions

Two types of placentae occur in domestic mammals: the choriovitelline placenta (omphaloid or yolk sac placenta) and the chorioallantoic placenta. The yolk sac, and hence the choriovitelline placenta, develops before the allantois and subsequent chorioallantoic placenta. Early during gestation, the choriovitelline and chorioallantoic placentae coexist temporarily, and then the choriovitelline placenta regresses.

Choriovitelline Placenta

The **choriovitelline** or **yolk sac placenta** is formed when the yolk sac wall (splanchnopleure) combines with the chorion and then contacts the endometrium (Figs. 14-1 and 14-16). It may be fully or partially vascularized by the vitelline plexus, which connects with the omphalomesenteric vein leading to the developing heart. Blood returns from the embryo to the vitelline circulation in the yolk sac via the omphalomesenteric artery, which branches from the dorsal aorta.

In sows and ruminants, the yolk sac wall is simply apposed to the uterine epithelium, and the yolk sac begins its involution 3 to 4 weeks after conception. However, in carnivores and mares, the yolk sac is well developed early in gestation and persists throughout gestation. In carnivores, a temporary lamellar choriovitelline placenta develops (see Fig. 14-16). In all domestic mammals, the choriovitelline placenta is of minor importance in physiologic fetal–maternal exchange.

In the **inverted yolk sac placenta,** the endoderm of the yolk sac is directly exposed to the uterine luminal content. It occurs in mice, rats, rabbits, and guinea pigs and participates in selective absorption and transmission of maternal immunoglobulins for fetal immunoprotection.

Chorioallantoic Placenta

When the allantois fuses with the chorion, an **allantochorion** is formed. The allantochorion contacts the endometrium, resulting in a **chorioallantoic placenta** (Fig. 14-1). This organ is the most efficient for mediating physiologic exchange between mother and offspring. It is very well vascularized by umbilical arteries and vein.

The principle of providing a vast area of fetal–maternal interchange determines the placental structure at the gross and microscopic anatomic levels. The structural variations of the placenta are numerous. Intermediate forms exist, and the placenta also changes its internal structure during the period of gestation.

Macroscopic Structure of the Placenta

The region of the chorion where folds, lamellae, or villi increase the surface area is called the **frondose chorion** (chorion frondosum); the region without projections is the **smooth chorion** (chorion laeve). Considering the frondose chorion region and its uterine counterpart, four types of placentae are recognized macroscopically. In domestic mammals, diffuse, cotyledonary, and zonary placentae are present (Fig. 14-2), whereas in humans and some other species, the discoid type develops.

In the **diffuse placenta** (placenta diffusa), most of the chorionic sac forms a frondose chorion attached to the endometrial

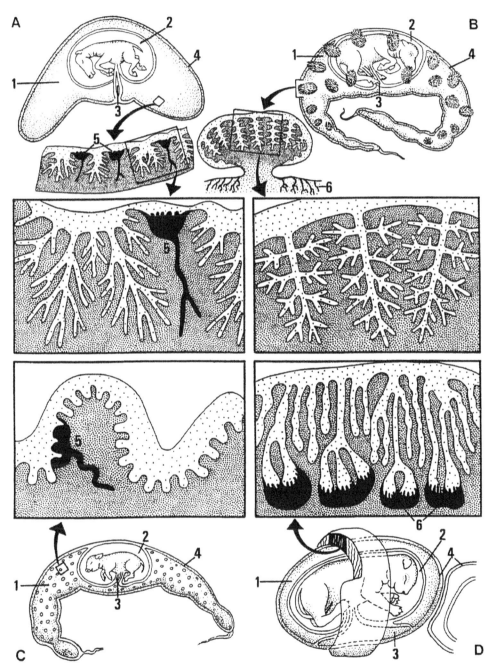

FIGURE 14-2 Schematic drawings of the fetus in the fetal membranes to show differences in placental shape and internal structure among species. Horse with a diffuse villous (microcotyledonary) placenta (**A**); ruminants (cow), with a cotyledonary villous placenta (**B**); pig with a diffuse folded placenta provided with macroscopically visible areolae (**C**); carnivores (here, cat) with a zonary (girdle) lamellar or tightly folded placenta (**D**). Allantoic cavity (1); amnionic cavity (2); yolk sac (3); allantochorion (4). In the higher magnification views, the maternal side is dark, the fetal side is bright, and the areola–gland complex (5) in horse and pig and the endometrial glands (6) in bovine and cat are black.

epithelium (sows, mares, camels) (Figs. 14-2A and C; see also Figs. 14-5 and 14-11A).

In the **cotyledonary placenta** (placenta multiplex), tufts of chorionic protrusions (**cotyledons**) attach to preformed endometrial prominences (**caruncles**) (Fig. 14-2B). Cotyledons and caruncles combine to form **placentomes**. In the intercaruncular area, a smooth chorion is apposed to the endometrial epithelium (ruminants) (see Fig. 14-13).

In the **zonary placenta** (placenta zonaria), the frondose chorion forms a band or girdle around the equator of the chorionic sac (Fig. 14-2D; see also Fig. 14-17). Outside the girdle, the smooth chorion apposes to the endometrial epithelium (carnivores and minks) (see Fig. 14-17).

In the **discoid placenta** (placenta discoidalis), the frondose chorion forms a disc-shaped area of fusion with the endometrium (e.g., humans, apes, mice, rats, rabbits, guinea pigs).

Three-Dimensional Structure of the Interface Between Maternal and Fetal Tissues

The capacity for exchange between maternal and fetal tissues is enhanced by the increased surface area of a folded, villous, or lamellar interface (Fig. 14-2). This vast fetal–maternal contact area is further increased by an irregular cell surface or microvilli on both cells of the trophoblast and endometrial epithelial cells (see Figs. 14-8, 14-9, and 14-12B).

In the **folded placenta**, the fetal–maternal contact surface is increased by the presence of vascularized macroscopic folds (**plicae**) of varying magnitude and microscopic ridges (**rugae**) of varying height (sows) (see Figs. 14-5 through 14-7).

In the **villous placenta**, the allantochorion forms cotyledons (i.e., arborizing chorionic villi with vascular mesenchymal cores that fit into corresponding **caruncular crypts**). Together, the villi and crypts form macroscopic (ruminants) or microscopic placentomes (mares) (see Figs. 14-11 through 14-13), or independently, the villous tree extends into the maternal intervillous blood space (humans).

In **lamellar placentation**, the trophoblast of the allantochorion forms an intercommunicating network that envelopes the endothelium of maternal blood vessels (carnivores) (see Fig. 14-18), or it is in direct contact with maternal blood in trophoblast-lined vascular channels (rats, mice, rabbits).

Tissue Layers of the Fetal–Maternal Interhemal Barrier

The fetal and maternal placental circulations are separated by tissue layers that form the placental or fetal–maternal interhemal barrier. The barrier is a highly selective transport avenue in fetal–maternal exchange (Fig. 14-3). The fetal component of the barrier is chorionic tissue that is vascularized by allantoic vessels; it consists of three tissue layers: endothelium, mesenchyme, and trophoblast. The maternal counterpart consists basically of three corresponding layers in reverse order:

endometrial surface epithelium, connective tissue, and endothelium.

Although the number of tissue layers of the fetal component is constant, the number of maternal layers varies with the species. Therefore, placentae are further classified on the basis of the number of uterine tissue layers.

In the **epitheliochorial placenta** (placenta epitheliochorialis), all three layers of the maternal component are present. This type of placenta occurs in sows, mares, and ruminants (see Figs. 14-8, 14-12A, and 14-15). In ruminants, however, binucleated trophoblast cells migrate and fuse with the endometrial surface epithelium, and the placenta is designated as **synepitheliochorial**.

In the **endotheliochorial placenta** (placenta endotheliochorialis), the endometrial surface epithelium and the underlying maternal connective tissue are absent, and endothelium alone separates the maternal blood from the trophoblast. This type of placenta is primarily present in carnivores and minks (see Fig. 14-18B).

In the **hemochorial placenta** (placenta hemochorialis), all three maternal layers are absent, rendering the trophoblast freely exposed to maternal blood. Up to three layers of trophoblast may be present (hemotrichorial), of which at least one is composed of **syncytiotrophoblast** (fusion of trophoblast cells into a symplasm). This type of placenta is present in humans, rats, mice, rabbits, and guinea pigs.

Fetal–Maternal Anchoring and Fate of Maternal Tissues at Birth

The degree to which the endometrium is changed and the fetal membranes are anchored into the maternal tissue determines the amount of uterine tissue lost at parturition. On this basis, two types of chorioallantoic placentation, nondeciduate and deciduate, are recognized (Fig. 14-3).

In the **nondeciduate placenta**, the fetal components interlock with relatively intact uterine tissue, from which they separate without much loss of endometrium. Epitheliochorial placentation (ungulates) is an example of nondeciduate placentation.

In **deciduate placentae**, the transformed part of the endometrial stroma, the **decidua**, is shed with the fetal membranes after parturition.

NOURISHMENT OF THE EMBRYO

The main physiologic principle of the chorioallantoic placenta is the substantial exchange between maternal and fetal blood. The substance that nourishes the developing offspring is termed **embryotroph**. The portion of embryotroph contributed from maternal blood is **hemotroph**, while the uterine glandular secretions and cell fragments form **histotroph**. Nutrients from both the hemotroph and histotroph are taken up by the trophoblast.

Histotroph nourishes the offspring before implantation. During gestation, histotroph is present in **areolae**, which are indentations of the chorion opposite the openings of endometrial glands. The areolae are scattered in the diffuse placenta of pigs and

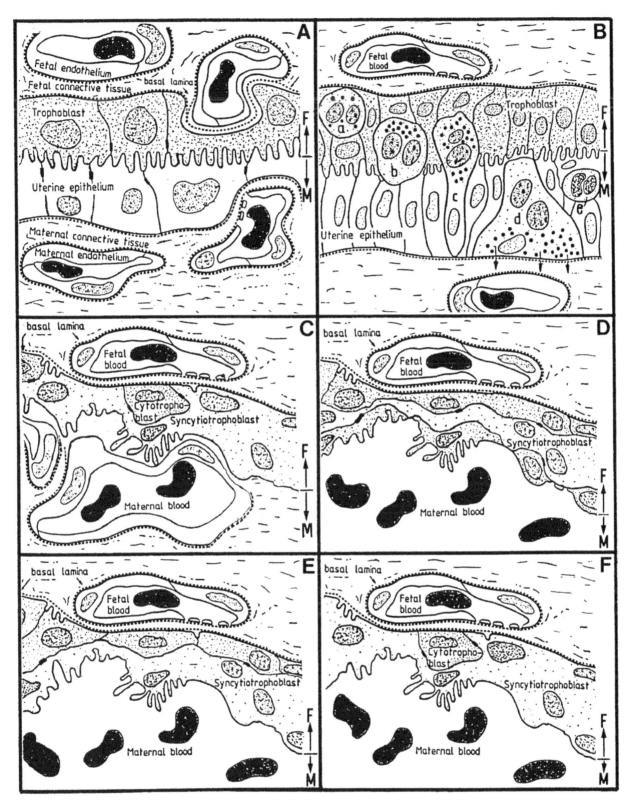

FIGURE 14-3 Schematic drawings of the tissue layers of the fetal–maternal interhemal barrier of placenta, including fetal components of the allantochorion (F) and maternal components (M). Dependent on species a reduction of the maternal components takes place, illustrated here by steps (**A–F**) until the trophoblast of the chorion comes into direct contact with maternal blood. Species differences in the trophoblast are also shown. The different placental types and corresponding species are: **A.** Epitheliochorial—sow, mare. **B.** Synepitheliochorial—ruminants (a–e show migration of binucleate trophoblast cells [a,b], fusion of binucleate cell with uterine epithelial cell [c], maternal–fetal hybrid cell [d], which secretes granular content [arrows] into maternal stroma, and degenerating hybrid cell [e]). **C.** Endotheliochorial—carnivores (bitch, queen). **D.** Hemotrichorial—rat, mouse. **E.** Hemodichorial—rabbit. **F.** Hemomonochorial—human, guinea pig. (Modified from Leiser R, Kaufmann P. Placental structure: in a comparative aspect. Exp Clin Endocrinol 1994;102:122–134.)

mares, or they are located in the smooth chorion of the ruminant placentae. In the carnivore placenta, histotroph is found in the junctional zone; it is typically seen in the areola–gland complex in the diffuse placenta, as well as in relation to the smooth chorion in the cotyledonary placenta (Fig. 14-2).

After successful implantation, the embryo is nourished by hemotroph, metabolites that cross the placental barrier from maternal circulation.

PLACENTAL VASCULARITY AND CIRCULATION

The two blood circulatory systems of the epitheliochorial and endotheliochorial placentae always remain morphologically separated by a species-dependent number of tissue layers (see Tissue Layers of the Fetal–Maternal Interhemal Barrier above). In hemochorial placentae, the uterine vessels are absent from the placental barrier, and the blood flows through trophoblastic tubules or intervillous spaces (lacunae). Regardless of the type of chorioallantoic placentation, trophoblast and fetal endothelium are always present in the placental interhemal barrier (Fig. 14-3).

In the maternal part of the placenta, circulating blood is either contained in vessels or bathes the trophoblast directly. Uterine vessels also form **placental hematomas,** due to local degeneration of endometrial tissue. The hematomas are deposits of stagnant maternal blood between endometrial epithelium and the trophoblast in carnivores and ruminants (see Fig. 14-17).

The fetal placental capillaries have smaller lumina than the maternal capillaries (see Fig. 14-8); both are partially fenestrated and surrounded by basal laminae (Fig. 14-3; see also Fig. 14-18B).

The supply of oxygenated blood to the maternal part of the placenta is derived from the uterine artery and anastomoses from the ovarian and vaginal arteries. The arteries are enlarged during pregnancy, and their placental capillaries develop into a species-specific architecture reflecting the internal three-dimensional structure of the placenta (Fig. 14-4; see also Fig. 14-11B). The maternal part of the placenta is drained by uterine veins.

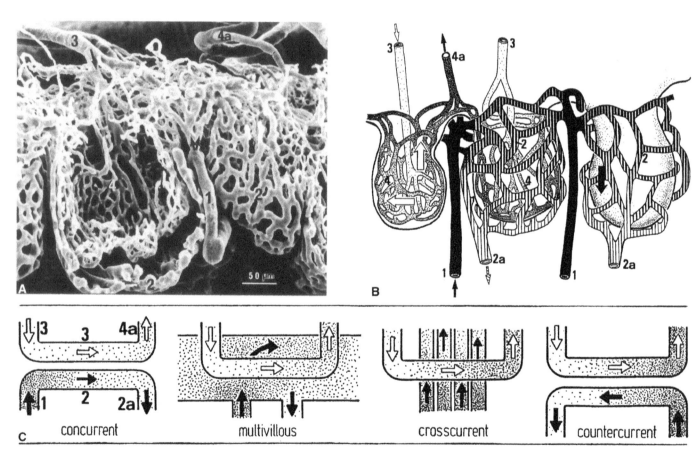

FIGURE 14-4 Combined maternal and fetal vascular cast (**A**), corresponding schematic of blood vessels from the placenta of the pig at day 99 of pregnancy (**B**), and idealized patterns of placental blood flow (**C**). The maternal arterioles (1) run to the top of maternal ridges, where they branch into the maternal capillary networks (2), which are drained by venules (2a). The fetal arterioles (3) can be followed into the fetal capillary networks (4), which have outlets through the fetal venules (4a). The large arrows in **B** demonstrate a mixture of crosscurrent (black/vertical versus white/horizontal arrows) and countercurrent (black/vertical versus white/vertical arrows) maternal–fetal blood flow interrelationship in the pig. The schematic **C** demonstrates, from left to right, blood flow of four different placental exchange types linked to typical species, including concurrent (theoretical), multivillous (human), crosscurrent (queen), and countercurrent (guinea pig). The density of dots in the fetal venules (4a) illustrates the efficiency of the various exchangers in diffusional exchange (e.g., oxygen). **A:** ×260. (**C:** *From Dantzer V, Leiser R, Kaufmann P, et al. Comparative morphological aspects of placental vascularization. Trophoblast Res 1988;3:235.*)

Fetal placental vessels take up oxygen and nutrients from maternal circulation and deliver waste products. To facilitate exchange, the different placental circulatory systems have multivillous, crosscurrent, or countercurrent flows between allantoic and uterine vessels; although the least efficient, the concurrent exchange system is only theoretical (Fig. 14-4). It is also noteworthy that the fetal veins leave the placenta apposed to the origin of uterine arterioles, thus enhancing the capability of exchange. The capillaries underlying maternal epithelium and the trophoblast bend and dilate. The bending of the vessels provides a flow stress that enhances vascular growth through interaction with hormones and cytokines. Dilation of blood vessels slows blood flow, enhancing the possibility for the active exchange of nutrients.

The yolk sac placenta, when present, receives deoxygenated blood from the omphalomesenteric arteries, which arise from the abdominal aorta. Oxygenated blood is then returned to the heart by the omphalomesenteric veins.

The fetal part of the chorioallantoic placenta receives deoxygenated blood from the paired umbilical arteries, which originate from the caudal aorta, and returns oxygenated blood through the umbilical veins. The left umbilical vein carries blood to the heart via the liver and the caudal vena cava, whereas the right vein undergoes involution in the fetus.

SPECIALIZED CELLS OF THE PLACENTA

Decidual cells are specialized cells derived from fibroblasts in the endometrium. They may develop in the endotheliochorial placenta of carnivores (see Fig. 14-18A) and are always present in hemochorial placentae. Decidual cells are enlarged and rounded or polyhedral; they are subject to considerable species variations in size, contents (lipid, glycogen, hormones, and growth factors), and structure.

The trophoblast (simple epithelium that forms the wall of the blastocyst) performs many different functions including absorption, exchange of metabolites, and synthesis of hormones and other signal transmitter substances. This diversity is reflected in the complex structure of individual cells and the cell types developed by differentiation (see Sow Placenta below, as a species example). The discrete cell of the trophoblast is termed a **cytotrophoblast** (Fig. 14-3). Another form of differentiation is the **binucleate trophoblast cell**, or giant cell, found in ruminants and mares (see Figs. 14-14 and 14-15). If multiple trophoblast cells fuse, they form a **syncytiotrophoblast** (Fig. 14-3; see also Fig. 14-18). When both cytotrophoblasts and syncytiotrophoblasts are present (carnivores), the cellular form is primitive, whereas the syncytial form is more differentiated with respect to the development of organelles. The presence of binuclear or multinuclear trophoblast cells corresponds to increasing invasion of the endometrium. In ruminants and mares, a relatively low degree of invasion occurs in the presence of binucleate cells, compared to the extensive endometrial invasion of multinucleated syncytiotrophoblasts in carnivores, rodents, and primates.

CHANGES DURING PLACENTATION

The placenta continuously changes in size, shape, and internal structure throughout gestation. After implantation, it grows at a rapid, although gradually decreasing, rate and may be subject to minor involution before term. Rearrangements at the cellular level are reflected in apoptosis (regulated cell death) and mitotic activity. In addition, the physical barrier between the maternal and fetal circulatory systems progressively attenuates with time (for details see Function–Structure Relationships below).

FUNCTION–STRUCTURE RELATIONSHIPS

Structural differences in the various placental types do not necessarily indicate differences in function. The transfer mechanism of the respiratory gases (i.e., oxygen and carbon dioxide under gradient pressure) is essentially simple diffusion. Therefore, the diffusion distance across the interhemal barrier is of major importance. Capillaries from both fetal and uterine sides of the placenta approach and indent the respective epithelia during gestation (Fig. 14-3; see also Fig.14-8). Consequently, despite a varying number of layers in the interhemal barrier, the diffusion barrier thins to 2 μm, which is similar for most species.

The plasma membrane, with its variety of receptors, is an important structure in cellular transport. The membrane regulates cellular uptake and transfer of nutrients as well as export of unusable metabolic components. As parts of the placental barrier, the plasma membranes are present only in epithelium and endothelium. To traverse a cell (or syncytium), a substance must pass both the apical and basal plasma membrane. Therefore, placental selective barrier and transport functions are critically dependent on the number and activity of plasma membranes to be traversed.

A directional preference from mother to fetus generally exists for important inorganic elements (e.g., calcium, phosphorus, iodine, and iron). This characteristic is especially true of iron, as no retrograde transfer of iron from fetus to mother occurs. In different species, however, the iron transfer takes place by different mechanisms. In carnivores, and to a lesser extent in ruminants, iron is absorbed from blood hemoglobin in maternal hemorrhages. In the sow and mare, and also to some extent in ruminants, the source of iron is a glycoprotein complex secreted by the endometrial glands. The trophoblast takes up iron from circulating maternal transferrin in hemochorial placentation. Calcium is transferred in different regions of the fetal membranes, depending on the species. In sows, the transfer occurs across the folded interhemal barrier of the interareolar region, whereas in cows, it occurs at the intercotyledonary region, and in the mare, across the areolar-gland complexes by a different mechanism than for iron.

The hemoglobin of the growing offspring contains different types of polypeptide chains during different phases of development. The earliest (nucleated) erythrocytes from the yolk sac mesoderm contain embryonic hemoglobin. Later in intrauterine life, hepatic and splenic erythrocytes carry fetal hemoglobin, and near the time of birth, a gradual change to bone marrow cells with adult hemoglobin takes place. Embryonic and fetal hemoglobins have a higher affinity for oxygen than adult hemoglobin, and thus, they are able to more efficiently extract oxygen, which diffuses across the placental barrier. This difference is an adaptation for intrauterine life with low oxygen pressure.

Maternal proteins of high molecular weight, such as immunoglobulin G, which protects newborns against infectious diseases, sufficiently bypass some placental barriers. Proteins cross over in endotheliochorial placentae with hematomas and hemochorial placentae, but they do not cross in epitheliochorial placentae, although some proteins may be transferred at hematomas in ruminants. Therefore, neonates of species with epitheliochorial placentae are totally dependent on the immunoglobulins in the colostrum ingested immediately after parturition when the epithelium in the intestinal tract is temporarily permeable for these large molecules.

Placental tissues show a very high degree of expression of various genes. The placental trophoblast secretes hormones, for example, chorionic gonadotropin (mares), placental lactogen (ruminants), estrogens, and progesterone. During pregnancy, the placenta also produces a wide spectrum of other factors for the regulation of metabolic activity, growth, and structural changes (paracrine factors). These factors are used or promoted differently among species to regulate gestation and complete successful placentation.

SPECIES DIFFERENCES

The beginning of placentation and length of gestation vary considerably in different species (Table 14-1).

Sow

In early stages, the yolk sac is unusually large and well vascularized; its maximal development occurs at approximately day 20. A choriovitelline placenta of insignificant extent is formed, but disappears as the yolk sac rapidly decreases in size.

The chorioallantoic placenta is diffuse, folded, epitheliochorial, and nondeciduate (Fig. 14-5). The fusiform chorionic sac adheres to the endometrium over its entire area, except at the

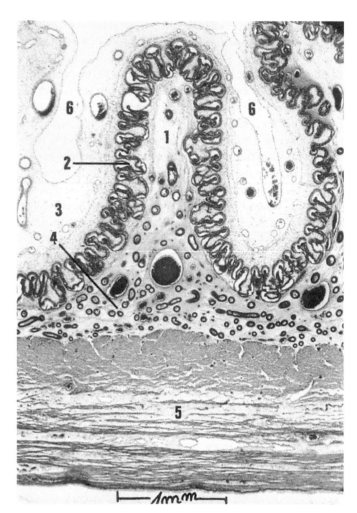

FIGURE 14-5 Longitudinal section of uterine horn with placenta (sow), late midpregnancy. Primary fold (plica) of endometrium (1); rugae (2); plica of allantochorion (3); endometrium with glands (4); myometrium (5); allantoic cavity (6) (×20). *(Courtesy of A. Hansen.)*

avascular extremities and over the uterine gland openings, where **areola–gland complexes** are formed (Figs. 14-2, 14-6, and 14-7).

The blastocyst undergoes extremely rapid elongation from day 10 to day 12. It changes from a sphere of approximately 2 mm in diameter to a membranous hollow "thread" approximately 100 cm in length. At days 12 to 14, the migration of multiple blastocysts is fulfilled and they are evenly distributed in both uterine horns along the mesometrial side. Placentation begins close to the embryo, where the endometrium forms epithelial proliferations covered with corresponding caplike formations of the chorion at days 13 to 14, thus giving an anchoring effect until interdigitating microvilli begin to develop between the uterine epithelium and the trophoblast at day 15.

The chorionic–endometrial contact area is increased approximately three times by macroscopic primary and split circular folds (plicae). The folds are stable on the maternal side but unstable on the fetal side as they passively follow the existing endometrial folds (Figs. 14-2C and 14-5). When the whole chorionic

TABLE 14-1 Implantation and Gestation in Domestic Animals

	Beginning of Implantation (day)	Gestation Time (days)
Bitch	17–18	58–63
Queen	12.5–14	63–65
Mare	35–40	329–345
Sow	13–14	112–115
Cow	16–18	279–285
Ewe	15–20	144–152

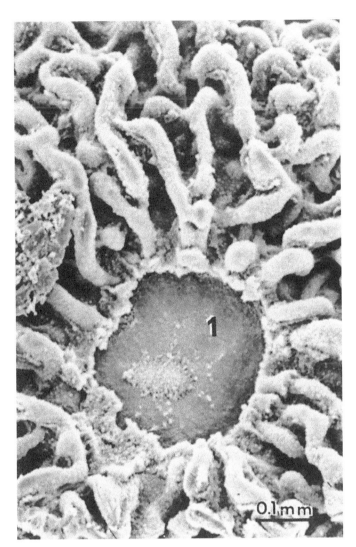

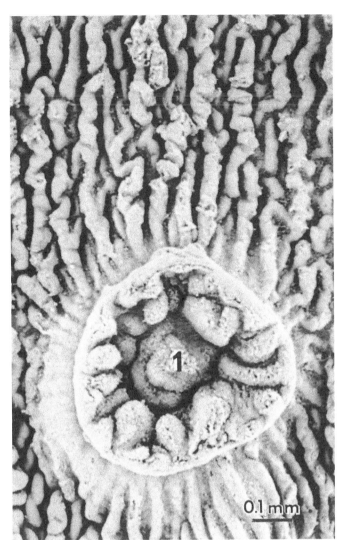

FIGURE 14-6 Maternal part of porcine placenta from midgestation after separation from the fetal side to illustrate the maternal side of an areola (1) with some accumulation of uterine milk covering the opening of the uterine gland. The maternal rugae radiate around the areola and the parallel arrangement can be discerned at the top of the picture. These rugae are complementary to the fetal fossae between the fetal rugae (see Fig. 14-7) (×90). *(From Dantzer V. Scanning electron microscopy of exposed surfaces of the porcine placenta. Acta Anat 1984;118:96.)*

FIGURE 14-7 Complementary surface to Figure 14-6 of the porcine allantochorion from midgestation with a medium-sized fetal areola (1) with villi. The chorionic rugae radiating from its periphery fuse with parallel chorionic rugae after a short distance (×50). *(From Dantzer V. Scanning electron microscopy of exposed surfaces of the porcine placenta. Acta Anat 1984;118:96.)*

sac is spread out, it measures approximately three times the length of the corresponding permanently folded endometrium. The microscopic folds form rugae separated by fossae that are permanent on both maternal and fetal sides. They are irregular at first and later develop into more regular circular rugae (Figs. 14-5, 14-6, and 14-7). In late gestation, the circular rugae become further subdivided, thereby changing into bulbous protrusions. The microscopic foldings increase the exchange area approximately four times. The trophoblastic and uterine epithelial cells have interdigitating microvilli, which further increase the exchange area by a factor of approximately 10 (see Fig. 14-9). Overall, with folding and surface modifications, the total surface area is increased approximately 120 times.

The uterine epithelial cells differentiate as the trophoblast lining the chorionic fossae forms arcades of high columnar epithelium apposed to the low columnar epithelium on the summit of the endometrial rugae. The remaining chorionic and uterine epithelial cells are cuboidal or flattened (Fig. 14-8).

As gestation proceeds, allantoic and uterine capillaries indent those parts of the respective rugae where the trophoblast and endometrial epithelium are low. Thus, the connective tissue interposed between the capillaries and epithelia is reduced to basal laminae (Figs. 14-3A and 14-9). In advanced stages, the thickness of the interhemal membrane can be less than 2 μm, consisting of six layers, four of which are cellular (Fig. 14-8).

The uterine epithelial cells contain spherical nuclei with small nucleoli. Rough endoplasmic reticulum (rER) predominates, the Golgi complex is extensive, and small mitochondria are scattered

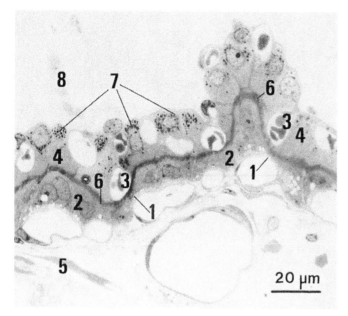

FIGURE 14-8 Detail of placental fold (sow) day 99 of pregnancy; perfusion fixation from maternal side. The distance of the placental barrier is shortened by endometrial capillaries (1) indenting the uterine epithelium (2) and fetal capillaries (3) indenting the trophoblast (4). Uterine connective tissue (5); border of interdigitating microvilli (6); characteristic dense bodies in trophoblast cells (7); fetal mesenchyme (8). Epon section, perfusion-fixed from the maternal side (×660).

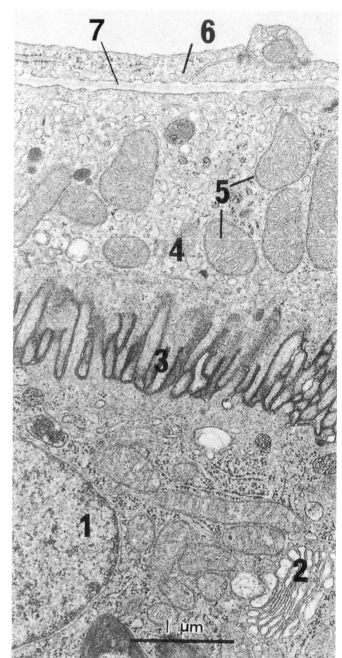

FIGURE 14-9 Transmission electron micrograph from the placenta of the sow illustrates the interdigitating microvilli between the maternal epithelium and the trophoblast, as well as the accumulation of mitochondria in the trophoblast close to the apical exchange area. Nucleus of a maternal epithelial cell (1); Golgi complex (2); interdigitating microvilli (3); trophoblast (4); mitochondria (5); endothelium of fetal capillary (6); basal laminae (7) (×21,000).

in the cytoplasm (Fig. 14-9). Numerous lysosomes are characteristic in the maternal epithelial cells.

The cells of the trophoblast have rounded nuclei with distinct nucleoli. The rER occurs mainly in the basal part of the cells intermingled with electron-dense, periodic acid-Schiff (PAS)–positive bodies and lysosomes, indicating high metabolic and secretory activities. Soon after day 80 of gestation, aggregations of smooth endoplasmic reticulum (sER) are also seen basally and laterally in the cells; their occurrence is correlated with high estrogen synthesis. Evidence of high endocytic activity is indicated by apical mitochondria located among coated pits and vesicles, tubular endosomes, and multivesicular bodies (Fig. 14-9).

The areola–gland complex is macroscopically visible as small opalescent vesicles, the areolae, which contain histotroph (Figs. 14-2C, 14-6, and 14-7). The maternal areolae are smooth-surfaced shallow cups surrounding the openings of uterine glands (Fig. 14-6). The fetal areolae are rosettelike structures composed of villi (Fig. 14-7). Histotroph, composed of secretory products and degenerating cell material, accumulates in the areolae between the uterine and fetal epithelia in the intermicrovillous space. The main transfer of iron from mother to fetus takes place via the areola–gland complex. The uterine glands of the complex secrete an iron-containing glycoprotein, **uteroferrin,** which is subsequently taken up by the areolar trophoblast and transferred to the underlying fetal capillary network. The areola–gland complexes also participate in the transfer of vitamin A (retinoids).

The blood flow relationship between maternal and fetal circulation in the sow is a mixture of crosscurrent and countercurrent (Fig. 14-4). Exchange across the porcine placental barrier is midrange in efficiency compared to other species described in this text.

Mare

A large yolk sac is present in the mare 3 weeks after insemination and becomes an important fetal–maternal interchange medium. The temporary placenta is composed of an avascular portion of the yolk sac wall and, in the marginal zone, a choriovitelline placenta. About the end of week 6, the change from vitelline to allantoic circulation is effected in the placenta, and the yolk sac, although persisting until term, undergoes gradual involution (Fig. 14-10A).

The chorioallantoic placenta of the mare is diffuse, villous, epitheliochorial, and nondeciduate. The embryo emerges from the zona pellucida at days 8 to 9 and then becomes completely encapsulated in an acellular glycoprotein capsule, which persists until at least day 21.

Although the equine blastocyst becomes fixed in position in the uterus at approximately day 16, the allantochorionic villi are not aggregated into tufts, called **microcotyledons,** until approximately day 60. The conceptus thus remains spherical and lies unattached in the uterine lumen, held in place merely by a pronounced increase in uterine tone until day 50.

At the junction of the developing allantochorion and the regressing yolk sac, the chorion forms an annulate **chorionic girdle** consisting of projections of the rapidly proliferating trophoblast. Between days 36 and 38, the trophoblast cells of the girdle become binucleate and begin to invade the endometrium by ameboid movements. They destroy the uterine epithelium almost completely and implant themselves in the endometrial stroma, where they form **endometrial cups** (Fig. 14-10). The cups measure a few millimeters to approximately 5 cm in diameter. Endometrial epithelium regenerates quickly, and the underlying cup cells become densely packed among uterine glands, supplied by the relatively sparse endometrial vasculature. The cup cells grow to large polyhedral cells with two nuclei and predominant rER. Cup cells act as an endocrine gland and elaborate equine chorionic gonadotropin (eCG), which helps to stabilize the hormonal function of the corpora lutea and can be used in diagnosis of pregnancy.

The endometrial cups eventually become surrounded by leukocytes, which invade and destroy the cup cells as they begin to degenerate after approximately 80 days of gestation. From days 120 to 150, the cellular remnants are rejected. This process coincides with regression of the primary and secondary corpora lutea (formed concurrently with the cup formation), after which the placenta takes over the production of progesterone at a reduced level. After detachment from the uterine wall, the cups are encapsulated by chorionic folds and form allantochorionic pouches. Also, flattened oval bodies of disputed origin, **hippomanes,** float freely in the allantoic fluid.

Fetal allantochorionic tufts (microcotyledons) and complementary maternal endometrial crypts begin to develop after the initiation of endometrial cups (days 38 to 40), and at approximately day 150, the typical microcotyledonary placenta has been formed over the entire surface of the endometrium (Fig. 14-2A). The fetal tufts, with a dense capillary system (Fig. 14-11B), and corresponding crypts form placental units known as **micropla-** centomes (Fig. 14-11A). The areola–gland complexes are located between these microplacentomes, with the areolae surrounding the base of the fetal portion of the microplacentomes. Uterine glandular secretory products are released into the areolar cavity between endometrial epithelium and trophoblast cells covering the areolar villi; consequently, these epithelia are not in close contact (Fig. 14-11A). Transfer of iron and calcium from mother to fetus takes place in the areolar–gland complexes.

In the microcotyledons, the fetal villi consist of vascular mesenchyme covered with trophoblast (Fig. 14-12A). The villi fit into crypts lined with simple columnar uterine epithelium of varying height. The crypts are separated by septa consisting of vascular uterine connective tissue. Indentations of capillaries into the trophoblast and maternal epithelium are seen in later pregnancy.

Uterine epithelial cells are light staining (Fig. 14-12A). The trophoblast cells are slightly darker and have a more compact rER. The sER is well developed in the cells of both epithelia, but most prominent in the trophoblast, reflecting the high synthesis of steroids, especially estrogens and progesterone. The apical surface of the trophoblast and uterine epithelial cells bear microvilli that interdigitate and form a dark border as seen with light and electron microscopy (Fig. 14-12). In the later stages of gestation before placental detachment after delivery, local apoptosis of the trophoblast and cryptal epithelium is indicated by dark-staining epithelial cytoplasm and the presence of cellular debris.

Cow

Initially, the yolk sac has a rather large vascular area and forms a functional choriovitelline placenta. The yolk sac is rapidly outgrown by the allantois, and after 3 weeks, it begins to degenerate.

The chorioallantoic placenta is cotyledonary, villous, epitheliochorial of the subtype synepitheliochorial, and nondeciduate. The elongated blastocyst implants close to the embryo at days 18 to 19 and gradually proceeds peripherally. In the intercotyledonary areas, the trophoblast layer develops papillae that extend into the uterine gland openings, possibly functioning as an anchor. The attachment by papillae occurs until day 21. At day 22, the blastocyst extends equally into both uterine horns, and by day 27, an overall intimate contact between trophoblast cells and maternal epithelium by interdigitating microvilli is established. A firm fetal–maternal connection is initiated at days 32 to 34. Simple villi develop from areas of the chorionic sac in contact with elevated, convex structures of the maternal endometrium (**caruncles**). The simple chorionic villi ramify to form branching **cotyledons** (Fig. 14-13B), which project into crypts of the caruncle (Fig. 14-13A). The anchoring stalk of the caruncle contains maternal blood vessels. No uterine glands open at the caruncle. Together, the fetal cotyledon and maternal caruncle form the collective structure, the **placentome** (Fig. 14-13A). During gestation, the placentomes grow approximately 5,000-fold, but undergo a slight involution toward term.

The chorionic villi of the cotyledon consist of vascular mesenchyme covered with a simple layer of trophoblast cells. The trophoblast includes columnar or irregularly shaped mononuclear

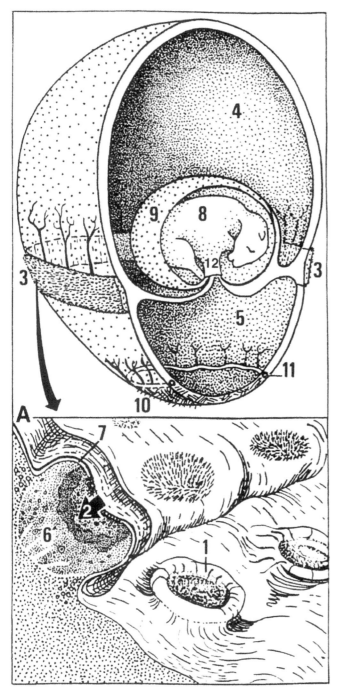

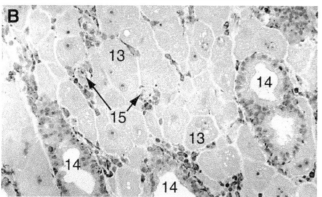

FIGURE 14-10   Endometrial cups (mare) 47 days of pregnancy. **A.** Schematic overview drawings of conceptus with its chorionic girdle (top) and detail with the chorion partly separated from the endometrium (bottom). Formation of endometrial cups (1) is due to trophoblast cell migration (2) from the chorionic girdle (3)—located between allantois (4) and yolk sac (5)—into the endometrial stroma (6). Uterine lumen (7); young fetus (8); allantoamnion (9); choriovitelline placenta (10) bordered by sinus terminalis (11); umbilical cord (12). **B.** Histologic section from a later stage of the endometrial cup showing the large endometrial cup cells (13), uterine glands (14), and few maternal vessels (15) (×330). *(Courtesy of A. C. Enders.)*

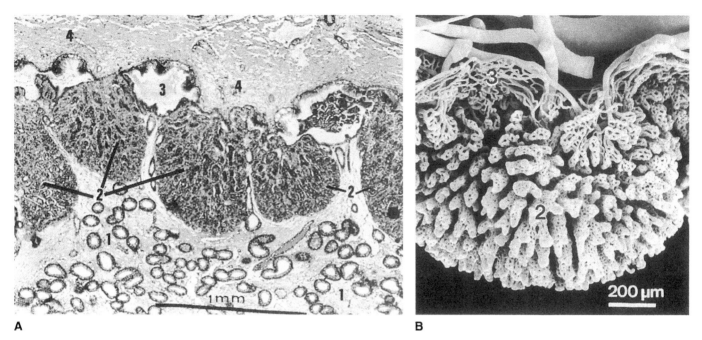

FIGURE 14-11 Histologic cross section of mare placenta (**A**) and scanning electron microscopy of corresponding vascular cast showing the fetal capillary network of a microcotyledon (**B**). **A.** Endometrium with uterine glands (1); microplacentomes (2); areola (3); chorionic mesenchyme (4). **B.** The fine capillary network of the fetal villi of a microcotyledon (2) and the more loose network at the fetal areola (3). **A:** ×40; **B:** ×60. (**A:** *From Björkman N. An Atlas of Placental Fine Structure. Baltimore: Williams and Wilkins, 1970.* **B:** *From Dantzer V, Leiser R. Areola-gland subunits in the epitheliochorial types of placentae from horse and pig. Micron Microscopa Acta 1992;23:79–80.*)

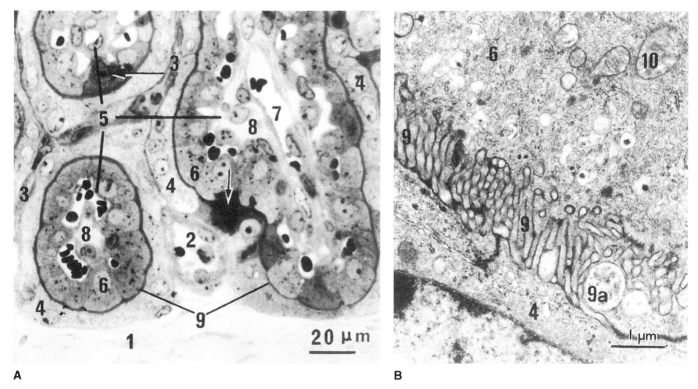

FIGURE 14-12 Light microscopy of epon section of microplacentome (**A**) and transmission electron microscopy (**B**) of interhemal barrier (mare). **A.** Endometrial connective tissue (1); maternal capillary (2); maternal septum (3); uterine epithelium (4); chorionic villi (5); trophoblast (6); fetal capillary (7); fetal mesenchyme (8); border of microvilli (9). The dark parts of trophoblast and uterine epithelium (arrows) are apparently undergoing apoptosis. **B.** Detail of the uterine epithelium (4) and trophoblast (6) showing the complementary interdigitating microvilli (9) closely associated to a multivesicular body (9a); in the trophoblast, many signs of high endocytic activity, including coated pits, endosomes, multivesicular bodies and mitochondria (10), are present. **A:** ×630; **B:** ×15,000.

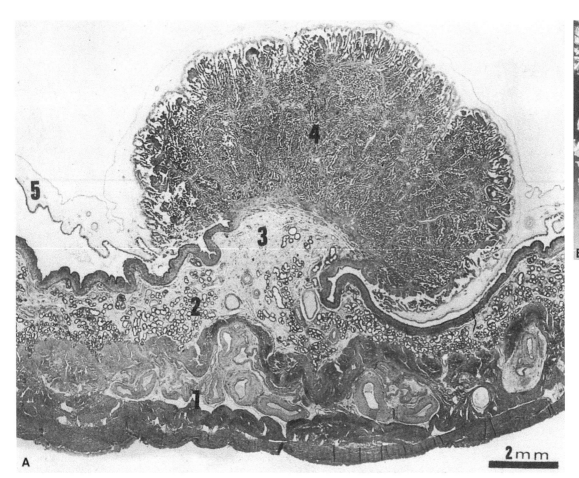
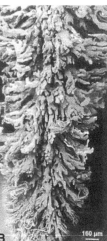

FIGURE 14-13   A. Cross section of a placentome (cow) midpregnancy. Myometrium separated into two layers by uterine vessels (1); endometrium with glands (2); stalk of placentome (3); placentome (4); chorion laeve (5) (×8). (Courtesy of A. Hansen.) **B.** Vascular cast of a villus from a fetal cotyledon, day 220 of pregnancy. Note the rich branching (×50). *(Leiser R, Krebs C, Klisch K, et al. Fetal villosity and microvasculature of the bovine placentome in the second half of gestation. J Anat 1997;191:517–527.)*

cells, and large binucleate cells (Fig. 14-14). The **mononuclear cells** have spherical or irregularly shaped nuclei with large nucleoli. In addition, the cells have sparse rER and relatively numerous apical mitochondria. **Binucleate cells** (trophoblast giant cells) have spherical, separated nuclei with conspicuous nucleoli, and the cytoplasm is voluminous. At the ultrastructural level, the cell surface lacks microvilli. The cytoplasm contains a great diversity of organelles and inclusions. The Golgi complex is well developed and mitochondria are numerous but moderate in size. The cells synthesize progesterone, prostaglandin, and placental lactogen. In contrast to the mononuclear cells, giant cells show no morphologic evidence of absorption. Furthermore, the giant cells lack desmosomes and are mobile within the chorionic epithelium. They migrate into the cryptal epithelium, where they fuse with uterine epithelial cells to form tri- or multinucleate hybrid cells, thus transferring hormone-containing granules from the fetal to the maternal compartment (Figs. 14-3B and 14-14).

The maternal uterine epithelium of the caruncle is cuboidal or flattened (Fig. 14-14). The cells have spherical nuclei with distinct nucleoli. Among them are cryptal giant cells with three or more nuclei, generated by hybridization with trophoblast binu-

cleate cells. Most uterine epithelial cells also contain lipid inclusions in the infranuclear region.

The apical borders of both the trophoblast and the cryptal epithelial cells have interdigitating microvilli that are more irregular in cows than in mares or sows. The narrow space between the microvilli contains dense granular material.

Regressive changes occur frequently in the placentome. Both trophoblast cells and cryptal epithelial hybrid cells undergo apoptosis. In the latter case, functionally insignificant, small areas of temporary syndesmochorial placenta are formed.

Hematomas develop at the convex side of the placentome between the fetal side of the caruncular crypt walls and the base of the chorionic villi. They are formed in the later part of gestation. Blood collects in the fetal tissues surrounding leaky vessels. Erythrocytes are phagocytized by the trophoblast and broken down by lysosomes. Hemoglobin from the erythrocytes is digested and iron is released. These areas may be subject to bacterial infections during pregnancy.

After parturition, the chorionic villi are released from the crypts. Normally, the separation occurs between the interdigitating microvilli and the crypt, and the trophoblast layer and cryptal

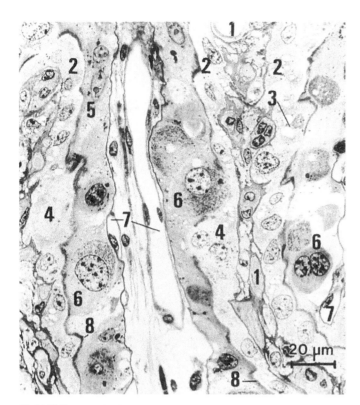

FIGURE 14-14 Detail of placentome (cow) midpregnancy (compare to Fig. 14-3B). Maternal septal stroma with capillaries (1); uterine epithelial cells (2); lipid droplets (3); trophoblast–uterine epithelial hybrid cells (4); mononuclear trophoblast cells (5); binuclear trophoblast giant cells with granules (6); fetal capillaries (7); maternal–fetal contact line (8) (×560).

epithelium remain intact. A common complication of parturition in cattle, however, is **retained afterbirth** (retentio secundinarum), in which the villi are trapped in the crypts and the adhesiveness between the fetal and maternal tissues remains high.

In the intercotyledonary area, a smooth chorion adheres to the endometrium, except over the glandular openings, where areolae are formed. The simple columnar cells of the trophoblast and the uterine epithelium both have interlocking brush borders (microvilli). Interdigitations are tight during early pregnancy and become less pronounced as pregnancy advances. In the intercotyledonary area, binucleate trophoblast cells are also frequent.

Amniotic plaques are yellow irregular elevations of stratified ectodermal epithelium on the inner surface of the amnion. They measure from a fraction of a millimeter to a few millimeters in diameter and contain large quantities of glycogen.

The interrelationship of the maternal and fetal capillary system is predominantly countercurrent with some crosscurrent flow, making it the most efficient system of the species described in this text.

In vitro fertilization may often lead to large offspring syndrome in cattle and sheep. This condition is due to in vitro handling and also the composition of growth media, both of which give a slight imbalance in the timing of gene activation. There is also a high degree of polyploidy in the trophoblast giant cells

as well as changes in placental development and activity. In cloned embryos, this condition is even more pronounced and often leads to an overproduction of fetal fluid, hydrallantois. Insulin-like growth factor (IGF) is one of the supposed key factors involved in this condition.

Ewe and Goat

The placentae of ewes and goats are similar to bovine placentae but differ in some respects. Implantation, occurring as in cows, begins at days 14 to 15, with development of interdigitating microvilli between trophoblast cells and maternal epithelium at days 16 to 18. Chorionic villi are seen from day 13 to day 20. Grossly, the placentome has a concave surface. The placentome of goats is flatter than that of ewes but has a similar internal structure.

Microscopically, the chorionic villi are more irregular than those of the bovine placenta (Fig. 14-15). The cryptal lining consists mainly of multinucleated cell masses arranged as a symplasm or syncytium, which was generated by fusion of binucleate trophoblast cells (hybridization) (Fig. 14-3B), after migration across the fetal–maternal microvillous junction. In contrast to the bovine, the hybridization in the ewe and goat is much more active. The trophoblast layer also has mononuclear cells, which gives rise to the typical ovoid binucleate cells (Fig. 14-15).

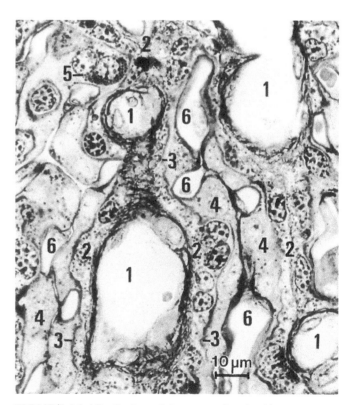

FIGURE 14-15 Section of placentome (ewe) midpregnancy. Maternal capillaries (1); maternal syncytium of trophoblast–uterine epithelial hybrid cells (2); maternal–fetal contact border of microvilli (3); trophoblast (4) with a binucleate cell with typical granules (5); fetal capillaries, which often deeply indent the trophoblast (6). Silver staining (×810).

Hematomas are more pronounced and are located in the central concave area of the placentome; they occur earlier than in cows. Amniotic plaques are also present in ewes.

Bitch, Queen, and Mink

The yolk sac forms a choriovitelline placenta, with trophoblastic villi invading eroded uterine mucosa. This transient lamellar placenta is originally extensive (Fig. 14-16), but eventually disappears. The yolk sac, however, persists until term.

The chorioallantoic placenta is zonary, lamellar, endotheliochorial, and deciduate. Implantation occurs at day 17 in bitches, whereas it is delayed in minks. In queens, implantation begins at day 13 with the formation of gap junctions between the trophoblast and maternal epithelium. At day 14, the trophoblast cells of the girdle area have intruded into the endometrium, thereby forming an endotheliochorial placenta with cytotrophoblast and syncytiotrophoblast. Here, the frondose chorion and uterine capillaries form tightly arranged **lamellae** (Figs. 14-2D, 14-17A, and 14-18A), which are localized in a girdle around the equator of the chorionic sac. In the girdle, a **junctional zone** containing termi-

nal parts of placental lamellae, maternal vessels, cell debris, and glandular secretions is located beneath the lamellar zone. The junctional zone is specifically enlarged in bitches and located adjacent to the dense connective tissue of the **supraglandular zone** (Fig. 14-17A). The **glandular zone,** which is formed by the dilated lower parts of the uterine glands, lies just above the myometrium (Fig. 14-17A). In the late stages of gestation, the invasion into the glandular zone progresses almost to the deep part of the glands where histotroph and cell debris accumulate (Fig. 14-2D). Remnants of the glandular zone are left at parturition. Outside the girdle, a chorion laeve is apposed to the uterine surface epithelium, and here the glandular development is restricted.

Hemorrhage of uterine blood within and outside the placental girdle gives rise to hematomas. In bitches, distinct **marginal hematomas** with large blood compartments are formed (Fig. 14-17A). In queens, smaller hemorrhages occur in irregular positions in the placental girdle and between the smooth chorion and the endometrium along the girdle. In minks, the hematoma is located centrally and antimesometrially. The columnar trophoblast cells lining the compartments of the hematoma have phagocytic characteristics and are believed to be involved in

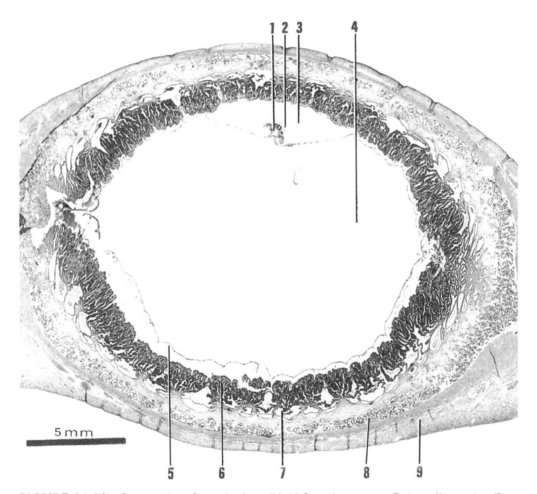

5 mm

FIGURE 14-16   Cross section of a uterine horn (bitch) 3 weeks pregnant. Embryo (1); amnion (2); exocoelom (3); yolk sac cavity (4); yolk sac wall (splanchnopleure) (5); hypertrophied epithelial surface of the endometrium containing chorionic villi (choriovitelline placenta) (6); junctional zone (7); glandular zone (8); myometrium (9) (×5). *(Courtesy of A. Hansen.)*

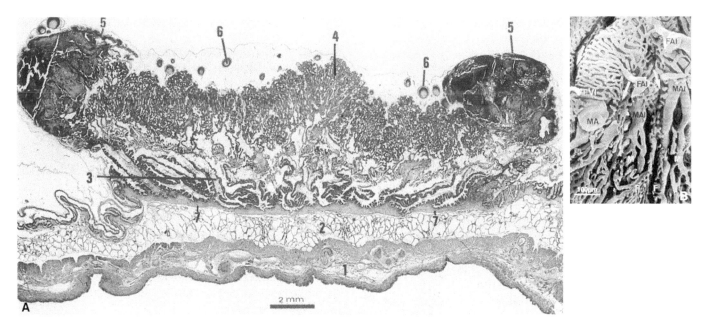

FIGURE 14-17 **A.** Cross section of placental girdle (bitch) midpregnancy. Myometrium (1); glandular zone (2); junctional zone (3); placental lamellae/labyrinth (4); marginal hematomas (5); fetal vessels in mesenchyme (6); the supraglandular layer (7), above which the placenta is separated from the endometrium at parturition (×2.7). (Courtesy of A. Hansen.) **B.** Double cast from cat placenta late gestation. Maternal arterioles (MAI) branch into maternal capillaries (M); fetal arterioles (FAI) branch into fetal capillaries (F). Note that maternal capillaries are wider than the fetal capillaries. Maternal stem artery (MA); fetal vein (FVI).

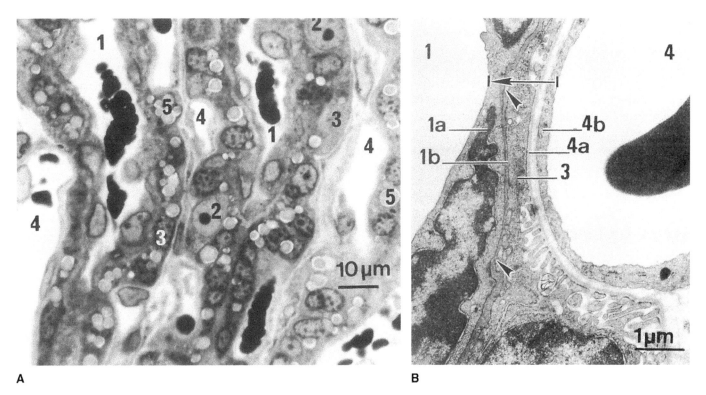

FIGURE 14-18 Histology of placental lamellae (**A**) and transmission electron microscopy of interhemal barrier (**B**) (queen) late pregnancy. Maternal capillaries (1); maternal endothelium (1a); maternal interstitial layer (1b); decidual cells (2); syncytiotrophoblast (3); fetal capillaries (4); fetal basal lamina (4a); fetal endothelium (4b); lipid droplets (5); endotheliochorial contact (arrowheads); minimal interhemal distance of about 1.5 μm (arrow). No distinct cytotrophoblasts are seen due to the late stage of gestation. **A:** ×1,000; **B:** ×12,500. *(B: From Leiser R, Koob B. Development and characteristics of placentation in a carnivore, the domestic cat. J Exp Zool 1993;266:642–656.)*

the absorption of large molecules and iron from destroyed maternal erythrocytes. After breakdown of the blood, the hematomas become brown (in queens) or green (uteroverdin in bitches) because of degradation of the hemoglobin.

The fetal part of the placenta is composed of trophoblast-covered mesenchymal lamellae, which contain small thin-walled capillaries (Fig. 14-17B). In bitches, the lamellae are branched, whereas in queens, the lamellae are more regularly stacked (Figs. 14-17A and 14-18), and in minks, they are rigorously twisted villi giving a labyrinthine appearance. Relatively wide and thick-walled maternal capillaries are enclosed by trophoblast and surrounded by a mesh of fetal capillaries (Fig. 14-18A), which gives a labyrinthine appearance in histologic sections. The maternal capillaries are surrounded by a thick, basal laminalike amorphous layer, the **interstitial layer,** which is especially irregular in queens (Figs. 14-3C and 14-18B). Giant decidual cells occur in queens (Fig. 14-18A) and, less frequently, in bitches. In minks, the maternal stem arteries lack smooth muscle cells, but some periendothelial cells do show intense staining for actin, thus providing some contractility for blood flow regulation.

The trophoblast layer originally consists of discrete cells. A syncytium is formed by the coalescence of some cells. Thus, the trophoblast includes cytotrophoblast (discrete cells) and syncytiotrophoblast (fused cells). The syncytium constitutes the major part of the lamellae and forms a continuous interhemal barrier. The cytotrophoblast is discontinuous, and the cells occur mainly along the mesenchymal parts of the lamellae (Figs. 14-3C). The discrete cells contain free ribosomes and a poorly developed ER. The syncytium possesses a conspicuous ER, numerous mitochondria, and dense bodies, which appear to be lysosomes. In queens, the syncytium contains numerous lipid droplets (Fig. 14-18A).

In queens, in the placental girdle, the maternal and fetal capillary systems meet in a simple crosscurrent blood flow interrelation. Therefore, transplacental diffusion in the queen is of low efficiency when compared to other species.

At parturition, the placenta separates from the endometrium through the junctional zone above the supraglandular layer (Fig. 14-17A).

SUGGESTED READINGS

Abd-Elnaeim M, Pfarrer C, Saber AS, et al. Feto-maternal attachment in the early diffuse epitheliochorial placenta of the camel (Camelus dromerarius). Light, transmission, and scanning electron microscopy study. Cells Tissues Organs 1999;164:141–154.

Allen WR. Immunological aspects of the endometrial cup reaction and the effect of xenogeneic pregnancy in horses and donkeys. J Reprod Fertil 1982;31(Suppl):57.

Amoroso EC. The mammalian placenta. In: Parkes AS, ed. Marshall's Physiology of Reproduction. 3rd Ed. London: Longmans, Green and Co., 1952;II:138.

Anderson JW. Ultrastructure of the placenta and fetal membranes of the dog. 1. The placental labyrinth. Anat Rec 1969;165:15.

Bertolini M, Anderson GB. The placenta as a contributor to production of large calves. Theriogenology 2002;57:181–187.

Björkman N. An Atlas of Placental Fine Structure. Baltimore: Williams and Wilkins, 1970.

Björkman N, Dantzer V, Leiser R. Comparative placentation in laboratory animals. A review. Scand J Lab Anim Sci 1989;16:129.

Burton GJ. Review article. Placental uptake of maternal erythrocytes: a comparative study. Placenta 1982;3:407.

Dantzer V. An extensive lysosomal system in the maternal epithelium of the porcine placenta. Placenta 1984;5:117.

Dantzer V. Electron microscopy of the initial stages of placentation in the pig. Anat Embryol 1985;172:281.

Dantzer V. Endometrium of epitheliochorial and endotheliochorial placentae. In: Glasser SR, Aplin JD, Guidance LC, et al., eds. The Endometrium. London, New York: Taylor and Francis, 2002; 25:352–364.

Dantzer V. Endotheliochorial placentation. In: Knobil E, Neill JD, eds. Encyclopedia of Reproduction. San Diego: Academic Press, 1998;1:1078–1084.

Dantzer V. Epitheliochorial placentation. In: Knobil E, Neill JD, eds. In Encyclopedia of Reproduction. San Diego: Academic Press, 1998;2:18–28.

Dantzer V, Leiser R, Kaufmann P, et al. Comparative morphological aspects of placental vascularization. Trophoblast Res 1988;3:235.

Dantzer V, Svenstrup B. Relationship between ultrastructure and oestrogen levels in the porcine placenta. Anim Reprod Sci 1986;11:139.

Dantzer V, Winther H. Histological and immunohistochemical events during placentation in pigs. Reproduction 2001;58(Suppl): 209–222.

Dellmann H-D, Carithers JR. Cytology and Microscopic Anatomy. Media, PA: Williams & Wilkins, 1996.

Enders AC, Lantz KC, Schlafke S, et al. New cells and old vessels: the remodeling of endometrial cups. Biol Reprod 1995;(Suppl 1): 181–190.

Enders AC, Liu IKM. Trophoblast-uterine interactions during equine chorionic girdle cell maturation, migration and transformation. Am J Anat 1991;192:366.

Engelhardt H, King GJ. Uterine natural killer cells in species with epitheliochorial placentation. Nat Immun 1997;15:53–69.

Friess AE, Sinowatz F, Skolek-Winnisch R, et al. The placenta of the pig. Anat Embryol 1980;158:179.

Friess AE, Sinowatz F, Skolek-Winnisch R, et al. The placenta of the pig. II. The ultrastructure of the areolae. Anat Embryol 1981;163:43.

Guillomot M, Fléchon J-E, Wintenberger-Torres S. Conceptus attachment in the ewe: an ultrastructural study. Placenta 1981;2:169.

Guillomot M, Guay P. Ultrastructural features of the cell surfaces of uterine and trophoblastic epithelia during embryo attachment in the cow. Anat Rec 1982;204:315.

Johansson S, Denker L, Dantzer V. Immunohistochemical localization of retinoid binding proteins at the materno-fetal interphase of the porcine epitheliochorial placenta. Biol Reprod 2001;64:60–68.

King BF, Enders AC. Comparative development of mammalian yolk sac. In: Nogales FF, ed. The Human Yolk Sac and Yolk Sac Tumors. Heidelberg: Springer-Verlag, 1993:1.

King GJ, Atkinson BA, Robertson HA. Implantation and early placentation in domestic ungulates. J Reprod Fertil 1982;31(Suppl):17.

Klisch K, Hecht C, Pfarrer C, et al. DNA content and ploidy level of bovine placentomal trophoblast giant cells. Placenta 1999;20: 451–458.

Krebs C, Winther H, Dantzer V, et al. Vascular interrelationship of near term mink placenta: light microscopy combined with scanning electron microscopy of corrosion casts. Microsc Res Tech 1997; 38:76–87.

Leiser R, Dantzer V. Structural and functional aspects of porcine placental microvasculature. Anat Embryol 1988;177:409.

Leiser R, Kaufmann P. Placental structure: in a comparative aspect. Exp Clin Endocrinol 1994;102:122.

Leiser R, Koob B. Development and characteristics of placentation in a carnivore, the domestic cat. J Exp Zool 1993;266:642.

Leiser R, Koob B. Structural and functional aspects of placental microvasculature studies from corrosion casts. In: Motta PM, Murakami T, Fujita H, eds. Scanning Electron Microscopy of Vascular Casts: Methods and Applications. Boston: Kluwer Academic Publishers, 1992:261.

Leiser R, Krebs C, Klisch K, et al. Fetal villosity and microvasculature of the bovine placentome in the second half of gestation. J Anat 1997;191:517–527.

Leiser R, Pfarrer C, Abd-Elnaeim M, et al. Feto-maternal anchorage in epitheliochorial and endotheliochorial placenta types studied by histology and microvascular corrosion casts. Trophoblast Research 1998;12:21–39.

Lennard SN, Stewart F, Allen WR, et al. Growth factor production in pregnant equine uterus. Biol Reprod Mono 1995;1:161.

Morgan G, Whyte A, Wooding FBP. Characterization of the synthetic capacities of isolated placental binucleate cells from sheep and goats. Anat Rec 1990;226:27.

Morgan G, Wooding FBP, Care AD, et al. Genetic regulation of placental function: a quantitative in situ hybridization study of calcium binding protein (Calbindin-D_{9k}) and calcium ATPase mRNA in sheep placenta. Placenta 1997;18:211.

Mossman HW. Vertebrate Fetal Membranes: Comparative Ontogeny and Morphology, Evolution, Phylogenetic Significance, Basic Functions, Research Opportunities. New York: Macmillan Press, 1987.

Pfarrer C, Winther H, Leiser R, et al. The development of the endotheliochorial mink placenta: Light microscopical and scanning electron microscopical morphometry of maternal vascular casts. Anat Embryol 1999;199:63–74.

Ramsey EM. The Placenta. Human and Animal. New York: Praeger Publishers, 1982.

Reimers TJ, Ullmann MB, Hansel W. Progesterone and prostanoid production by bovine binucleate trophoblastic cells. Biol Reprod 1985; 33:1227.

Steven DH. Comparative Placentation. New York: Academic Press, 1975.

Stewart F. Roles of mesenchymal-epithelial interactions and hepatocyte growth factor-scatter factor (HGF-SF) in placental development. Rev Reprod 1996;1:144.

Stroband HWJ, Van der Lende T. Embryonic and uterine development during early pregnancy in pigs. J Reprod Fertil 1990; 40(Suppl):261.

Winther H, Dantzer V. Co-localization of vascular endothelial growth factor and its two receptors Flt-1 and KDR in the mink placenta. Placenta 2001;22:457–465.

Winther H, Leiser R, Pfarrer C, et al. Localization of micro and intermediate filaments in non-pregnant uterus and placenta of the mink suggests involvement of maternal endothelial cells and periendothelial cells in blood flow regulation. Anat Embryol 1999; 200:253.

Wooding FBP. Frequency and localization of binucleate cells in placentomes of ruminants. Placenta 1983;4:527.

Wooding FBP. The synepitheliochorial placenta of ruminants: binucleate cell fusions and hormone production. Placenta 1992;13:101.

Wooding FBP, Flint APF. Placentation. In: Lamming GE, ed. Marshall's Physiology of Reproduction. 4th Ed. London: Chapman and Hall, 1994;II:233.

Wooding FDB, Morgan G, Fowden AL, et al. Separate sites and mechanisms for placental transport of calcium, iron and glucoses in the equine placenta. Placenta 2000;21:635–645.

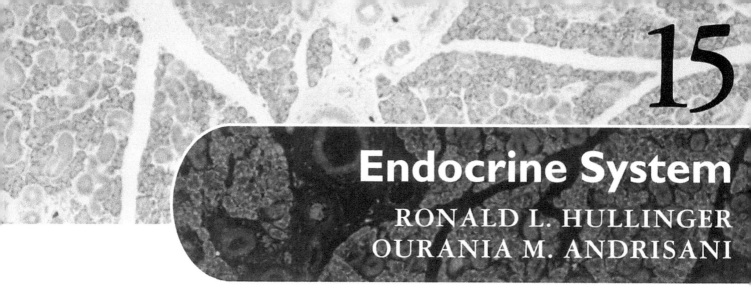

15

Endocrine System

RONALD L. HULLINGER
OURANIA M. ANDRISANI

Endocrine Organs
  Hypothalamus
  Hypophysis Cerebri (Pituitary Gland)
    Adenohypophysis
      Pars distalis
        Acidophils
        Basophils
        Chromophobes
      Pars intermedia
      Pars tuberalis
    Neurohypophysis
      Hypothalamo-neurohypophyseal tract
      Hypothalamo-adenohypophyseal axis
  Epiphysis Cerebri (Pineal Gland)
  Thyroid Gland

Parathyroid Gland
Adrenal Gland
  Adrenal cortex
  Adrenal medulla
Endocrine Tissues and Cells
  Pancreatic Islets
  Paraganglia
  Diffuse Neuroendocrine System Cells
  Other Endocrine Cells
    Adipocytes
    Endocrine cells of the heart
    Juxtaglomerular cells of the kidney
    Endocrine cells of the ovary
    Endocrine cells of the placenta
    Endocrine cells of the testis

The **endocrine system** is the *ductless* gland system (Greek *endo,* meaning "within"; Greek *krino,* meaning "to separate"), that is, the glands of *internal secretion.* Endocrine secretions are released into the intercellular compartment rather than onto a surface or into a duct leading to a surface (as is the case with exocrine glands). Most organs and tissues of the endocrine system are characterized by a dense epithelioid parenchyma and a sparse, delicate, interstitial stroma. The reticular fiber stroma supports individual parenchymal cells and conveys blood and lymph capillaries and the distal arborizations of neurons. Endocrine cells are typically nonpolar, releasing their secretory products, **hormones,** into the interstitial space from the entire cell surface. Hormones may diffuse locally in the interstitial fluid, binding to their specific cellular receptors, signaling adjacent cells in an **autocrine** or **paracrine** mode. Alternatively, they may enter the blood or lymph capillaries, signaling **target cells** located at a greater distance. Circulating hormones are diluted by interstitial fluid and plasma to relatively low concentrations (10^{-9} to 10^{-11}M) and bind to their receptors with high affinity. The endocrine system plays a major role in the maintenance of **homeostasis,** the dynamic steady state of the body, ensuring minimum variability of the organism's internal environment. Hormones modulate target cell function by up-regulating (stimulating) or down-regulating (inhibiting) processes in a dynamic fashion. Functions of the endocrine system are integrated and regulated by complex neural, endocrine, and immune molecular signaling and feedback mechanisms.

The endocrine system is composed of endocrine organs, as well as tissues and cells found in small numbers in nonendocrine organs. Classically, the **endocrine organs** include the hypophysis cerebri (pituitary gland), epiphysis cerebri (pineal gland), thyroid gland(s), parathyroid glands, and adrenal glands. **Endocrine tissues** typically have well-differentiated epithelial/epithelioid cells. The organelles and inclusions are indicative of secretory activity, and the cells have an intimate association with large, highly permeable blood capillaries (sinusoids) as well as lymphatics. In addition to dense vascularity, other characteristics of endocrine tissue include sparse stroma, high metabolic activity of the parenchyma, and a potent ability to stimulate angiogenesis. Interestingly, endocrine tissues are found in organs having additional, nonendocrine functions, for example, neurosecretory neurons of the hypothalamus; pancreatic islet cells; adipocytes; cardiac myocytes; juxtaglomerular cells of the kidney; internal theca cells, follicular epitheliocytes, interstitial cells, and corpus luteum cells of the ovary; hormone-producing cells of the placenta; interstitial and sustentacular cells of the testis; and paraganglia associated with blood vessels. Relatively isolated **endocrine cells** are dispersed in the epithelium of the digestive, urinary, reproductive, and respiratory systems; together these cells constitute the **diffuse neuroendocrine system.**

All embryonic germ layers contribute parenchyma to endocrine organs and tissues. For example, ectoderm gives rise to hypothalamic nuclei, the hypophysis cerebri, the epiphysis cerebri, and the neural crest, the latter providing precursor cells to multiple endocrine cells and tissues; differentiation of mesoderm forms the adrenal cortex and endocrine tissues of the ovary and testis; and endoderm contributes the parenchyma of the thyroid and parathyroid.

ENDOCRINE ORGANS

Hypothalamus

The hypothalamus is the most ventral part of the diencephalon and forms a significant portion of the expansive circumventricular region (Fig. 15-1). The hypothalamus contains neurons that integrate and regulate vital body functions (e.g., temperature, blood volume, blood osmolarity, and food intake). Clusters of neurons of the hypothalamus are referred to as **nuclei,** including the paired supraoptic, paraventricular, and arcuate nuclei. Afferent neural input to the hypothalamic neurons comes from many regions of the brain, spinal cord, and special senses. The hypothalamic neurons receive signals that reflect the status of the internal and external environments of the body, and respond with signals to the endocrine system and the autonomic portion of the nervous system. In the circumventricular region, the blood-brain barrier is reduced or absent, allowing hypothalamic neurons to easily respond to ionic and molecular signals (importantly, hormonal signals) in the blood. This combined input from the nervous system and the vascular system provides the basis for both a **hormonal feedback system** and **neuroendocrine integration.**

Peptidergic neurons of the hypothalamus (e.g., neurons of the supraoptic, suprachiasmatic, paraventricular, or arcuate nu-

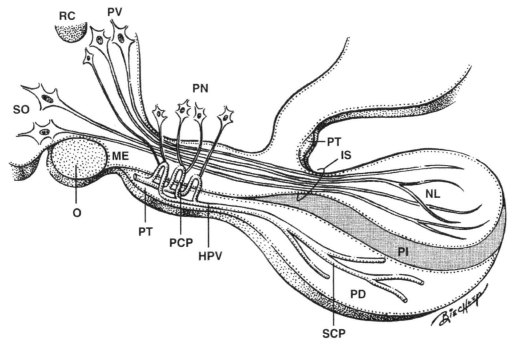

FIGURE 15-1 Schematic drawing of the hypothalamo-adenohypophysial and the hypothalmo-neurohypophysial systems. Optic chiasm (O); rostral commissure (RC). Axons from the parvicellular neurons (PN) of the hypothalamus terminate in contact with a primary capillary plexus (PCP) of the hypophysial portal system in the external zone of the median eminence, into which they secrete releasing hormones; in the case of prolactin, dopamine-producing neurons of the hypothalamus inhibit its release from the lactotrophs. These hormones are conveyed to the pars distalis (PD) through the hypophysial portal venules (HPV) and gain access to the cells of the pars distalis via a secondary capillary plexus (SCP). Pars intermedia (PI); pars tuberalis (PT). Axons originating from the magnocellular hypothalamic supraoptic (SO) and paraventricular (PV) nuclei course through the median eminence (ME) and the infundibular stalk (IS) to terminate in the neural lobe (NL), where oxytocin and vasopressin are stored and released.

clei, which have peptides as neurotransmitters) contribute axons to the neurohypophysis and secrete **releasing hormones** (releasing factors) to the adenohypophysis (Table 15-1). These axons projecting from the hypothalamus constitute the hypothalmoneurohypophyseal tract described below. Releasing hormones are distributed to the hypophysis cerebri through a blood circulation system (hypothalamo-hypophyseal portal system) described below.

Hypophysis Cerebri (Pituitary Gland)

Adenohypophysis

The hypophysis cerebri is composed of the **adenohypophysis** and **neurohypophysis** (in humans, the anterior lobe and posterior lobe, respectively). During development, the adenohypophysis forms from a midline epithelial evagination (Rathke's pouch) of the roof of the stomodeum, eventually losing the stomodeal connection. Simultaneously, the neurohypophysis forms as a midline evagination of neural tissue from the floor of the hypothalamus (diencephalon). As the oral epithelial pouch advances, it surrounds the neural evagination, and forms a double-layered envelope. Together these primordia form the hypophysis cerebri, with the neurohypophysis remaining attached to the developing hypothalamus (Fig. 15-2A). This organogenesis brings the adenohypophysis near the hypothalamus, creating a structural proximity that is important for the hypothalamic regulation of hypophyseal function.

The adenohypophyseal (Latin *adeno,* meaning "gland"; Greek *hypo,* meaning "beneath"; Greek *physis,* meaning "growth") parenchyma differentiates, forming three parts: **pars distalis, pars intermedia,** and **pars tuberalis.** The relative size and orientation of each part depends upon the species (Fig. 15-3). As the pouch contacts and envelops all but the distal aspect of the developing neurohypophysis, those cells contacting the neural tissue form the pars intermedia (Fig. 15-2B and D). The pars distalis forms the most diverse cell population and largest part of the adenohypophysis (Fig. 15-2B and E), and constitutes the majority of the outer envelope formed by the embryonic stomodeal pouch. The pars tuberalis is the portion of the pouch that contacts the base of the brain (median eminence/tuber cinereum), forming a collarlike

TABLE 15-1 Relationship of Hypothalamic Releasing Hormones, Hormones Released From Adenohypophysis, and Hormones Released by Target Cells

Hypothalamus Secretion	Cell of Origin in Hypothalamus	Hormone From Adenohypophysis, Pars Distalis	Cell of Origin in Adenohypophysis	Chief Target Cell	Hormone Released by Target Cell
Growth hormone–releasing hormone (GHRH)	Hypothalamic neuron	Growth hormone (GH)	Somatotroph	All cells	—
				Hepatocyte	Insulinlike growth factor I (IGF-I)
Prolactin-releasing factor (PRF)	Hypothalamic neuron	Prolactin (PRL)	Lactotroph	Mammary ductal/alveolar epitheliocyte	—
Thyrotropin-releasing hormone (TRH)	Hypothalamic neuron	Thyroid-stimulating hormone (TSH)	Thyrotroph	Thyroid follicular epitheliocyte	Triiodothyronine (T_3) and tetraiodothyronine (T_4)
Gonadotropin-releasing hormone (GnRH)	Hypothalamic neuron	Follicle-stimulating hormone* (FSH)	Gonadotroph*	Ovarian follicular epitheliocyte	Estrogen, inhibin, activin
				Testicular sustentacular cell	Estrogen, inhibin, activin
		Luteinizing hormone (LH)*	Gonadotroph*	Corpus luteum epitheliocyte	Progesterone
				Ovarian internal thecal cell	Testosterone
				Testicular interstitial cell	Testosterone
Corticotropin-releasing hormone (CRH)	Hypothalamic neuron	Adrenocorticotropin (ACTH)	Corticotroph	Zona glomerulosa epitheliocyte**	Mineralocorticoid
				Zona fasciculata epitheliocyte	Glucocorticoid
				Zona reticulans epitheliocyte	Androgen

*FSH and LH are coexpressed by the same gonadotroph.
**Cells of the zona glomerulosa are 10-fold less responsive than those of the zona fasciculata.

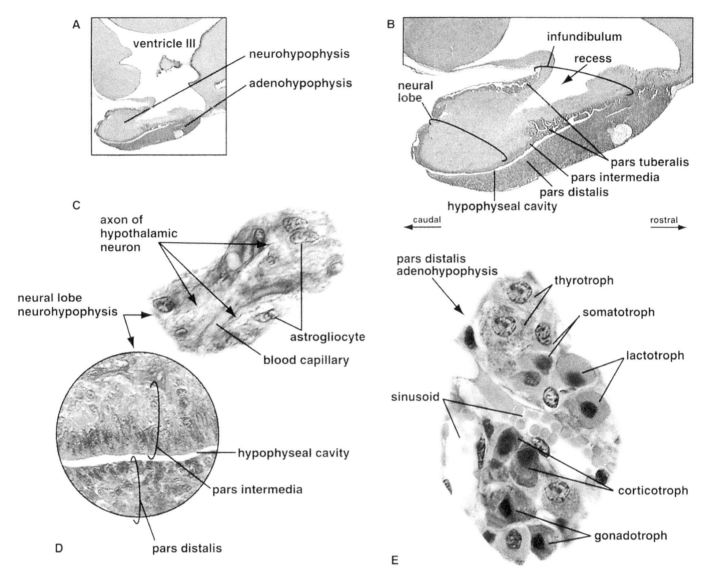

FIGURE 15-2 **A.** Midsagittal (median) section of the hypophysis cerebri, hypothalamus, and thalamus of a puppy (×2). **B.** Blood arrives in sinusoids of pars distalis only after perfusing the hypothalamus; a large cyst is present in the pars distalis (×4.5). **C.** Portion of the hypothalamo-neurohypophyseal tract (×100). **D.** Adenohypophysis contacting neural lobe (×40). **E.** Parenchyma of the adenohypophysis (×100). Hematoxylin and eosin.

investment of the stalk of the neurohypophysis (Fig. 15-2B), and links the pars distalis and pars intermedia proximally. The lumen of the pouch may remain in some species/individuals as the **hypophyseal cavity** between the pars intermedia and the pars distalis (Fig. 15-2B and D).

As an extension of the ventral aspect of the hypothalamus, the neurohypophysis is a continuation of the median eminence. Proximally, the third ventricle extends as a recess into the neurohypophysis (Fig. 15-2A and B). The proximal segment of the neurohypophysis is a funnel-shaped stalk, the **infundibulum,** which attaches to the **median eminence.** The infundibulum is continued distally as the **neural lobe** (pars nervosa) (Fig. 15-2B).

The hypophysis is oriented ventrocaudally from the hypothalamus, straddling the midline (Fig. 15-2B). Like the brain, the hypophysis is invested by the pia-arachnoid; distally, these leptomeninges are fused with the periosteum in a depression of the

basisphenoid bone, the sella turcica (Latin *sella,* meaning "saddle"; Latin *turcica,* meaning "Turkish"). In species in which this depression is deep, the meninges, including the dura mater, extend as a diaphragm (the diaphragma sellae) from the lateral margins of the saddle at the level of the infundibular stalk. Due to its cryptic location, the common surgical approach to the hypophysis is transpharyngeal. At necropsy, meningeal adhesions with the periosteum (and the diaphragm in some species) make it difficult to remove the hypophysis intact and still attached to the brain.

Pars Distalis

The **pars distalis** comprises parenchymal cell clusters perfused with sinusoidal capillaries (Fig. 15-2E). The sinusoidal capillaries of the pars distalis form the **secondary capillary plexus** of the hypothalamo-hypophyseal portal system. Based on routine staining of their stored secretions, the cells of the pars distalis have

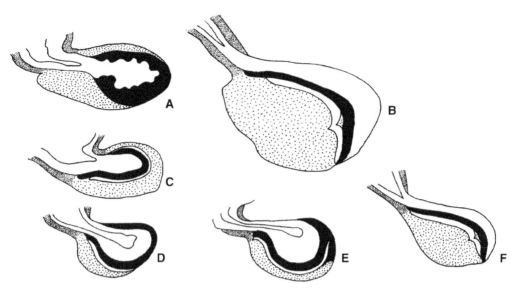

FIGURE 15-3 Schematic drawings of midsagittal sections of the hypophysis cerebri. **A.** Horse. **B.** Cow. **C.** Dog. **D.** Pig. **E.** Cat. **F.** Sheep. White: neurohypophysis with infundibular recess; small dots: pars tuberalis adenohypophysis; large dots: pars distalis adenohypophysis; black: pars intermedia adenohypophysis. *(From Dellmann H-D. Veterinary Histology: An Outline Text–Atlas. Philadelphia: Lea & Febiger, 1971.)*

been classified as **acidophils, basophils,** or **chromophobes.** These cell types vary in size, shape, number, and position depending on species, gender, age, and physiologic status (e.g., during pregnancy and lactation or after gonad removal). Five subtypes of cells have been further identified with immunohistochemistry. Each cell type (called a "-troph") expresses a peptide, protein, or glycoprotein hormone (called a **tropin** [Greek *troph,* meaning "food"]) (Fig. 15-2E) and represents a definitive and terminal differentiation. Secretory vesicles store the secretions in the cytoplasm prior to signals for their exocytosis (Fig. 15-4). Secretions include somatotropin hormone (growth hormone); lactotropin (mammotropin, prolactin); thyrotropin (thyroid-stimulating hormone); two gonadotropins (follicle-stimulating hormone and luteinizing hormone); and corticotropin (adrenocorticotropic hormone) (see Table 15-1).

Acidophils. Specifically, **somatotrophs** that synthesize and secrete **growth hormone (GH)** are concentrated laterally in the pars distalis; their abundant acidophilic secretory granules stain with orange G dye and are approximately 300 to 400 nm in diameter. **Lactotrophs,** which produce **prolactin (PRL),** stain lightly with erythrosin and carmine dyes. Lactotroph cell size and dye affinity increase during pregnancy and lactation. The acidophilic secretory granules of lactotrophs may be as large as approximately 800 nm in diameter.

Basophils. **Thyrotrophs** produce **thyroid-stimulating hormone (TSH),** are more numerous midventrally, and may be detected with aldehyde-fuchsin dye; their basophilic secretory granules measure approximately 150 nm in diameter. **Gonadotrophs** coexpress **follicle-stimulating hormone (FSH)** and **luteinizing hormone (LH),** are relatively small, and stain with aldehyde-thionine dyes; their stored basophilic secretory granules are approximately 200 nm in diameter. **Corticotrophs** pro-

duce **adrenocorticotropic hormone (ACTH)** and are uniformly dispersed in the pars distalis. These cells are less conspicuous within the parenchymal cell clusters and are difficult to identify with the light microscope. Corticotrophs may be spherical, ovoid, or stellate, depending on the species. Their basophilic granules measure approximately 150 to 200 nm in diameter and stain with antibody for both ACTH and **β-lipotropin** hormone (β-LPH). These peptide hormones are derived from the posttranslational processing of **proopiomelanocortin** (POMC). All three basophilic cell types stain with periodic acid-Schiff (PAS) and Alcian blue dyes.

Chromophobes. **Chromophobes** stain poorly with dyes used to identify acidophils and basophils. Some are considered postsecretory acidophils and basophils. Other chromophobes occasionally form the simple epithelium that lines cysts of unknown significance. Still other stellate-shaped chromophobes are interspersed between the other cells of the pars distalis, and it has been suggested that they may represent an undifferentiated stem cell of the adenohypophyseal parenchyma.

Pars Intermedia

In some species, the parenchyma of the **pars intermedia** is arranged as a simple columnar epithelium; in others, it is a pseudostratified columnar epithelium that invades the neural lobe; while in others (e.g., horse), the parenchyma is extensively developed. **Melanotrophs** are the most abundant parenchymal cell of the pars intermedia, secreting **α-melanocyte-stimulating hormone** (α-MSH) and β-LPH. These peptide hormones are processed products of POMC expressed by the melanotrophs. Other parenchymal cells include those lining cysts, corticotrophs, stellate cells, and simple epithelium lining the hypophyseal cavity. Blood capillaries are not as extensive as in the pars distalis. Hypothalamic axons terminate in the pars intermedia and include dopaminergic,

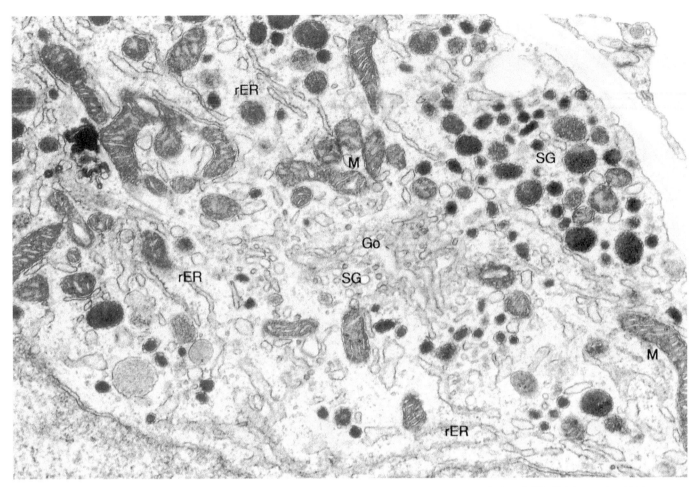

FIGURE 15-4 Organelles typical of an adenohypophyseal cell: granular (rough) endoplasmic reticulum (rER); Golgi complex (Go); mitochondria (M); secretory granules (SG) of varying maturational stages (×28,000).

serotoninergic, adrenergic, and GABAergic (γ-aminobutyric acid) axons that modulate the activity of the parenchyma.

Pars Tuberalis

The **pars tuberalis** is composed of cell clusters that form a folded tissue with occasional small cysts (Figs. 15-2B and 15-5). This region of the pituitary is traversed by hypophyseal portal venules that carry blood from the primary capillary plexus in the median eminence to the secondary capillary plexus in the pars distalis. The parenchymal cells of the pars tuberalis have melatonin receptors and are believed to regulate the seasonal reproductive cycle of some domesticated mammals (see Epiphysis Cerebri below). Other cells include those lining cysts, as well as a few gonadotrophs and thyrotrophs.

Neurohypophysis

Hypothalamo-Neurohypophyseal Tract

Large (magnocellular) neurons clustered in the hypothalamus make up the majority of the **supraoptic** and **paraventricular nuclei.** These neurons receive afferent synaptic input that signals the exocytosis of secretory vesicles from their axons. Bundles of these axons and their supporting astroglial cells constitute the median

eminence, infundibulum, and neural lobe of the **neurohypophysis** (Fig. 15-2B), together forming a major portion of a tractlike extension of the hypothalamus known as the **hypothalamo-neurohypophyseal tract.** The neurohypophysis contains the axons of hypothalamic neurons and **central gliocytes** ("pituicytes"), but no neuron cell bodies. The neuron cell bodies in the hypothalamus and secretory granules in their axons stain positively with antibody to **oxytocin** (OT) and **antidiuretic hormone** (ADH) (Figs. 15-6 and 15-7), also called arginine vasopressin (AVP). In the pig, lysine is substituted for arginine, producing lysine vasopressin (LVP). ADH-producing neurons and OT-producing neurons are present in both the supraoptic nuclei and the paraventricular nuclei. Secretory vesicles containing the hormone are transported along microtubules to axon terminals near blood capillaries in the neural lobe. Along the course of the axon, secretory vesicles form focal accumulations (Herring bodies); when stained with aldehyde-fuchsin, these can be resolved by light microscopy (Fig. 15-8).

In the hypothalamic nuclei, neurons synthesize preprooxytocin, which is processed to oxytocin and neurophysin and packaged in secretory granules. Exocytosis of the secretory granules is via a calcium-mediated mechanism, initiated by a neural synapse from sensory networks in the brainstem (e.g., sensory input from

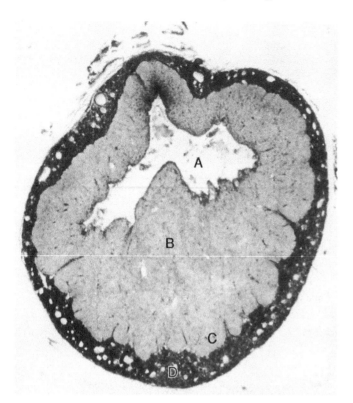

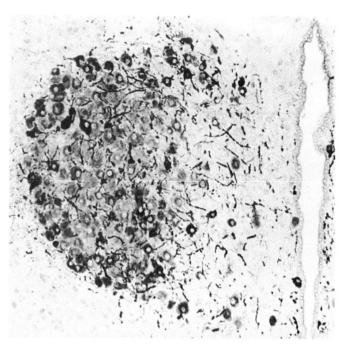

FIGURE 15-5 Section in the dorsal plane through the median eminence (large ruminant). Infundibular recess (A); internal zone (B); external zone (C); pars tuberalis of the adenohypophysis with numerous portal venules (D). Masson's trichrome (×2).

FIGURE 15-6 Neurosecretory neurons of hypothalamic paraventricular nucleus labeled with antibodies directed against antidiuretic hormone. Transverse section (×20).

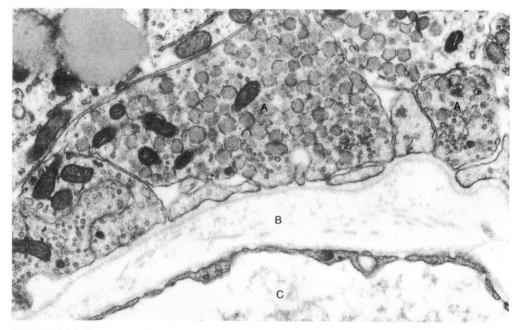

FIGURE 15-7 Axons of neurosecretory neurons (A) adjacent to a basal lamina, interstitial connective tissue (B), and a fenestrated capillary (C) in the neural lobe of neurohypophysis. Axon terminals have large electron-dense, hormone-containing secretory vesicles; upon depolarization of the neuron, the contents of the vesicles are released by exocytosis (×31,500).

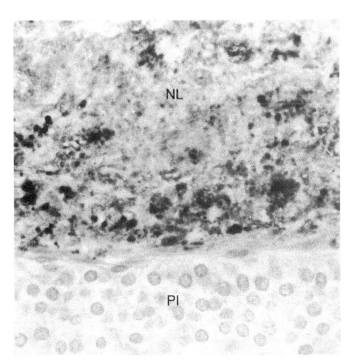

FIGURE 15-8 Hypophysis cerebri of cat. Dark staining within the neural lobe (NL) marks accumulations of neurosecretory granules (Herring bodies). Pars intermedia of the adenohypophysis (PI). Aldehyde-fuchsin (×40).

washing the cow's udder in the milking parlor or sounds from the sow's litter). When released, oxytocin binds to its receptor on myoepithelial cells of the mammary alveoli and ducts, causing myofilament-driven cell contraction, thereby resulting in "milk letdown." In addition, oxytocin binds to its receptor on smooth myocytes of the myometrium, causing uterine contraction and parturition, and to its receptor in the brain, initiating species-specific maternal behaviors (e.g., sheep).

Other neurons in the hypothalamus synthesize preprovasopressin, which is processed to ADH and neurophysin. Secretory granules for ADH are stored and released similar to oxytocin granules. The release is signaled by sensory synapses from neurons monitoring properties of the internal environment, for example, increased plasma osmolality or decreased blood volume (hypovolemia). ADH acts on the kidney by binding to the V2 receptor and activating water channels (aquaporin 2) in the apical membrane of the collecting tubule cells, decreasing water loss through the urine (an antidiuretic effect). ADH also binds to its V1 receptor on vascular smooth muscle, causing increased myocyte tone, vascular constriction, and elevated blood pressure. In addition, binding of ADH to the V3 receptor on hypophyseal corticotrophs causes release of ACTH and a rise in aldosterone secretion. Insufficient production of ADH results in diabetes insipidus, characterized by an increased volume of dilute urine.

Hypothalamo-Adenohypophyseal Axis

Neurons of the hypothalamus also regulate the neuroendocrine and autonomic nervous systems. Within the hypothalamus, a generally diffuse population of small (parvicellular) neurons syn-

thesizes hormones, which target the cells of the pars distalis. These hormones are termed **releasing hormones** (factors); they effect the release, by exocytosis, of the specific hormones expressed and synthesized in the pars distalis. In contrast, functions of the pars intermedia are regulated by innervation, whereas regulation of cells in the pars tuberalis remains unclear.

The releasing hormones from the hypothalamus are transported within axons of hypothalamic neurons to the periphery of the median eminence, where they are released near the **primary capillary plexus** of the hypothalamo-hypophyseal portal system (Greek *portal,* meaning "gateway"). The capillaries are drained by **hypophyseal venules** that flow through the pars tuberalis to the **secondary capillary plexus** in the pars distalis. This portal vascular system establishes the anatomic basis of a functional **hypothalamo-adenohypophyseal axis.**

In the pars distalis, the hypothalamic neurosecretions leave the secondary capillary (sinusoidal) plexus and bind specific receptors on their respective adenohypophyseal target cells. Hormones are then released from the target cells and affect other target cells in the periphery. In turn, peripheral target cells synthesize and release hormones into the circulation that mediate either **negative feedback** in other target cells or **positive feedback** to the hypothalamic neurons and cells of the pars distalis.

Growth hormone–releasing hormone (GHRH) (somatotropin-releasing hormone [SRH]) is released from neurons of the arcuate nucleus in response to neural stimulation (e.g., during sleep and exercise). It binds to its receptor on the somatotrophs of the pars distalis. The GHRH receptor is a **G protein–coupled receptor** (GPCR) that, when activated, elevates intracellular concentration of 3′, 5′-cyclic adenosine monophosphate (cAMP), triggering calcium-mediated exocytosis of secretory vesicles containing growth hormone. **Growth hormone (GH)** is a 22 Kda protein. The GH receptor is a tyrosine kinase (cytokine receptor family) that, upon binding GH, forms a dimer, leading to tyrosine phosphorylation of downstream signaling molecules (transcription factors). GH targets all cells, but especially hepatocytes, skeletal myocytes, adipocytes, and growth plate chondrocytes. GH induces an anabolic effect in muscle; in liver and cartilage, GH induces synthesis and release of insulinlike growth factor I (IGF-I; somatomedin). IGF-I mediates additional GH effects by acting on chondroblasts, promoting their proliferation and thus causing growth of the skeleton. GH causes its own downregulation (negative feedback) by stimulating somatostatin-producing neurons in the hypothalamus. Somatostatin binds to its GPCR on the GH-producing somatotrophs, uncoupling cAMP production and suppressing release of GH.

Prolactin-releasing factor (PRF) remains poorly understood. **Prolactin (PRL)** is principally regulated by tonic inhibition provided by dopamine from the hypothalamus. Dopamine binds to its D2 membrane receptor on lactotrophs of the pars distalis, uncoupling cAMP, lowering intracellular calcium, and inhibiting release of prolactin. Several stimuli result in PRL release from the lactotrophs (e.g., TRH, OT, ADH, angiotensin II). Neurogenic stress and sensory stimuli of suckling can override the dopamine inhibition. PRL is a 23 Kda protein; the PRL receptor is a tyrosine kinase. PRL targets its receptor on epithelial cells of the mammary gland, causing tyrosine phosphorylation of signaling molecules that stimulate proliferation and differentiation of the epitheliocytes as milk-synthesizing cells. Further, PRL binds to its receptor on dopaminergic neurons of the hypothalamus, increasing dopamine synthesis and release, thus causing inhibition of PRL release in the pars distalis. Together with GH, PRL also stimulates the immune system, specifically the proliferation and differentiation of lymphocytes.

Thyrotropin-releasing hormone (TRH) is released from small neurons in the paraventricular nucleus and binds to its GPCR on thyrotrophs (see Fig. 15-13). The binding results in the activation of phospholipase C and PI3-kinase and the elevation of intracellular calcium concentration, which is involved in exocytosis of **thyroid-stimulating hormone** (TSH; thyrotropin). TSH is a glycoprotein that is transported in the blood to the thyroid epithelial cells where it binds to its GPCR, stimulating the synthesis and storage of thyroglobulin and the release of thyroid hormones, **triiodothyronine** (T_3) or **tetraiodothyronine** (T_4). In turn, negative feedback of T_3 or T_4 to the hypothalamus and the pars distalis regulates the production of TRH and TSH, respectively.

Gonadotropin-releasing hormone (GnRH) is a protein hormone released from neurons diffusely scattered in the hypothalamus; it binds to its GPCR on the gonadotroph, elevating the intracellular concentration of calcium and activating protein kinase C. Protein kinase C signals the coexpression, synthesis, and release of the glycoprotein hormones **follicle-stimulating hormone** (FSH) and **luteinizing hormone** (LH). In the female, FSH binds to its GPCR on the **follicular epithelial cells**; in the male, FSH binds to its GPCR on **sustentacular cells** (Sertoli cells) of the testis. In both sexes, production of **estrogen** is signaled by FSH. In the female, LH binds to its GPCR on **internal thecal cells**, signaling the production of **testosterone**, and on follicular and thecal cells of the postovulatory follicle, signaling production of **progesterone**. Cells of the ovarian interstitial stroma in the pig, dog, cat, rabbit, and human also produce testosterone. In the male, LH (also called interstitial cell–stimulating hormone [ICSH]) binds to its GPCR on the **interstitial cells** (Leydig cells) and signals production of testosterone. In addition to effects on other target cells, these gonadal steroids bind to cells of the hypothalamus and the pars distalis, negatively regulating production of GnRH and gonadotropins. FSH also stimulates follicular cells, corpus luteal cells, and sustentacular cells to synthesize **inhibin** and **activin**. As members of the TGF-β superfamily of growth factors, inhibin and activin either inhibit or activate, respectively, production of FSH from the hypophysis.

Corticotropin-releasing hormone (CRH) is a protein hormone released from small neurons in the paraventricular nucleus in response to neural signaling (see Fig. 15-20). CRH binds to its GPCR on the corticotrophs, elevating intracellular concentration of cAMP and triggering calcium-mediated exocytosis of secretory vesicles containing **adrenocorticotropic hormone** (ACTH). ADH potentiates the release of ACTH from corticotrophs; ADH and CRH are coexpressed in neurons of the paraventricular nucleus that terminate in the median eminence, near the primary capillary plexus of the portal system. IL-1β, IL-6, and TNF-α act

in the hypothalamus to enhance CRH production. ACTH is one of the posttranslational cleavage products of the prohormone POMC, processed in corticotrophs to form ACTH, α-MSH, and β-LPH. ACTH binds to its GPCR on adrenal cortical parenchymal cells and, via adenylate cyclase and cAMP, activates proteins that increase transcription of the enzymes involved in steroid hormone biosynthesis (e.g., glucocorticoids). Glucocorticoids negatively regulate CRH production in the hypothalamus and negatively regulate POMC synthesis and ACTH release in the pars distalis. In response to stress, signals creating increased neurogenic input to the hypothalamus overcome this inhibition of ACTH by glucocorticoid.

Epiphysis Cerebri (Pineal Gland)

The pineal gland is a midline evagination of the dorsocaudal aspect of the epithalamus of the diencephalon, to which it remains attached by a stalk that contains a small recess of ventricle III (Fig. 15-9A). The pineal (Latin *pinus*, meaning "pine, pine cone") is enveloped by pia-arachnoid from which the blood supply to the gland originates. As a derivative of neural epithelium, the parenchyma is composed of **pinealocytes** and astrocytelike, **central gliocytes**; the processes of both cell types form the **neuropil** between the cells (Fig. 15-9B). The blood-brain barrier is not functional in this circumventricular organ and pinealocyte secretions have easy access to blood capillaries; pineal secretions also appear in the cerebrospinal fluid. In old animals, calcified protein deposits (concretions) termed **corpora arenacea** (brain sand) may be present. The deposits are easily resolvable in the intercellular neuropil, but are of no known functional significance.

Pinealocytes share gap junctions and extend axons to multiple sites, including other pinealocytes, adjacent capillaries (Fig. 15-9C), and the base of the ependymal lining of the ventricular recess. The pinealocyte receives synaptic input from sympathetic axons coursing in the adventitia of arterioles supplying the pineal. Sympathetic neurons from which these axons arise are in the cranial cervical ganglia. These neurons receive input from preganglionic neurons in the intermediate gray matter of the first thoracic segment of the spinal cord. The thoracic neurons are linked to optic input via a reticulospinal tract to the trigeminal reticular nucleus and, in turn, axonal projections from the suprachiasmatic nucleus of the hypothalamus. The optic nerve sends projections to synapses in the suprachiasmic nucleus.

Pineal function is linked to visual signals relaying information about environmental light. Most understanding of the mechanism of pineal function is based on data from the rat, sheep, and horse. A biorhythm, also known as circadian rhythm, has been linked to the intensity of yellow-green light in the environment and characterizes the secretory activity of the pinealocyte. The primary signal to the pinealocyte is norepinephrine, released from the sympathetic axon, which binds to its β-adrenergic receptor. Light received by an intact visual system inhibits this adrenergic stimulation, and the pinealocyte releases **serotonin**. In the dark phase, the adrenergic stimulation is operational, resulting in activation of the β-adrenergic GPCR on the pinealocyte. The resulting elevation of cAMP induces the expression of *N*-acetyltransferase,

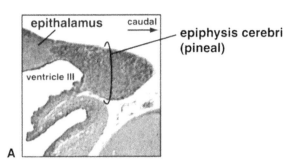

A

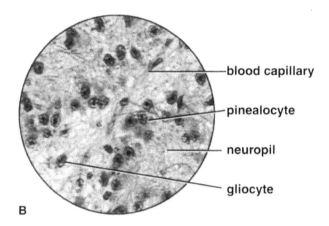

B

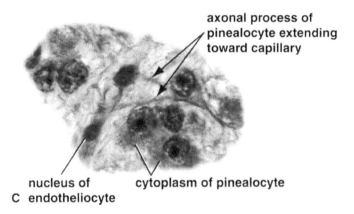

C

Adrenergic stimulation of pinealocyte
results in serotonin conversion to melatonin;
melatonin is released near capillaries.

FIGURE 15-9 Midsagittal section, pineal and epithalamus of puppy. **A:** ×2; **B:** ×40; **C:** ×100. Saffron-modified Masson's trichrome.

which converts serotonin to **melatonin**. Melatonin is released as it is synthesized, rather than stored. Melatonin, released from axons terminating near capillaries, circulates via the blood. At the target cells, melatonin binds to its GPCR, inhibiting neurons in the suprachiasmatic nucleus; it also inhibits gonadotropin release from the pars distalis by an unknown mechanism. In domesticated animals that are seasonally polyestrous, pineal activity resulting in melatonin synthesis is linked to species-dependent, seasonal (circannual) variation in ambient photoperiod, blocking release of gonadotropins and having an "antigonadotrophic effect."

Thyroid Gland

The thyroid (Greek *thyreos,* meaning "oblong shield"; Greek *eidos,* meaning "form") parenchyma is derived from the pharyngeal endoderm as a ventral, tubular extension caudally along the midline, beginning at the root of the tongue. Initially the thyroid develops as an exocrine gland; however, the duct is lost, and the parenchyma develops as many follicles supported by a delicate interstitial stroma (mesodermal) of reticular or loose collagenous connecting tissue (Fig.15-10B). The stroma bears a profuse plexus

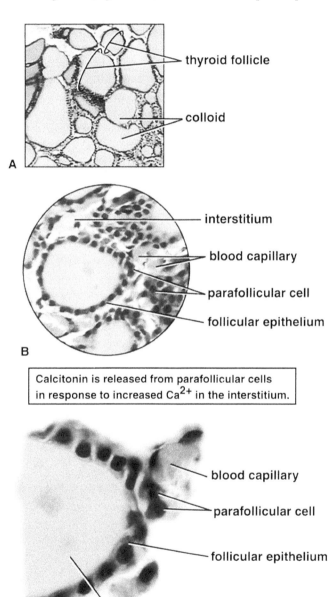

Calcitonin is released from parafollicular cells
in response to increased Ca^{2+} in the interstitium.

T_3 and T_4 are stored within thyroglobulin of the follicle;
proteolysis releases T_3 and T_4 from the epitheliocyte;
T_3 and T_4 enter target cells; T_3 binds to its nuclear receptor.

FIGURE 15-10 Random sectional plane, thyroid of dog. **A:** ×4.5; **B:** ×40; **C:** ×100. Hematoxylin and eosin.

of blood sinusoids, lymph capillaries, and adrenergic axons. A later migration of cells from pharyngeal pouch IV forms the ultimobranchial body. As this body advances to fuse with the developing thyroid, it is colonized by migrating neural crest cells. These neural crest cells differentiate in the thyroid as parafollicular (calcitonin-producing, "C") cells (Fig. 15-10B and C).

The **thyroid follicle** is delineated by a simple epithelium, the cells of which are joined by junctional complexes near the lumen. The size of follicles varies from a few to several hundred micrometers in diameter (Fig. 15-10A). Interestingly, in contrast to other endocrine tissues, the follicular epithelium displays polarity. The polarized **follicular epithelial cells** (Figs. 15-10C and 15-11) vary in height (columnar, cuboidal, squamous), depending upon their synthetic activity. Columnar cells indicate highly secretory follicles, whereas squamous cells are linked to follicles in a resting state. Follicular cells display an elaborate granular endoplasmic reticulum, Golgi complex, and secretory vesicles, characteristic of cells active in the synthesis of protein. **Thyroglobulin,** a glycoprotein, is exocytosed at the apical surface of the follicular epithelial cell; this iodinated glycoprotein, accumulating in the follicular lumen, is also called **colloid.** Furthermore, these follicular epithelial cells are simultaneously active in the endocytosis of the colloid from the follicular lumen via apical cell processes and the proteolysis of thyroglobulin, as evidenced also by the presence of lysosomes and phagolysosomes (secondary lysosomes).

Both TSH and adrenergic input stimulate GPCRs, leading to elevation of intracellular cAMP, which mediates both the synthesis of thyroglobulin and the release of thyroid hormone. Thyroglobulin is a glycosylated dimer containing tyrosyl sites capable of being iodinated. The enzymes participating in the iodination of thyroglobulin include the iodide symporter and thyroid peroxidase (Fig. 15-12). At its basolateral membrane, the epithelial cell expresses an integral membrane protein, the **sodium iodide symporter,** that actively imports sodium and iodide and effectively concentrates iodide in the epitheliocyte. **Thyroid peroxidase** is also expressed and incorporated in the apical membrane. In the presence of hydrogen peroxide, iodide is converted to iodine and one or two ions are incorporated into each tyrosyl residue, forming **mono-** or **diiodotyrosine** (T_1 or T_2). The peroxidase catalyzes the coupling of iodotyrosyl residues within the thyroglobulin dimer, forming **tri-** or **tetraiodothyronine** (T_3 or T_4). T_4 is commonly called **thyroxin.** Should production of thyroid hormones decline, stored thyroglobulin can provide required hormone for many days.

The release of stored thyroglobulin is effected by endocytosis of colloid via the extension of microvilli and lamellipodia of the follicular cells. Endocytotic vesicles containing colloid fuse with lysosomes, and proteolysis of the thyroglobulin releases T_1, T_2, T_3, or T_4. Only T_3 and T_4 are released into the blood from the basolateral cell surface, by diffusion through the membrane.

The synthesis, iodination, and proteolysis of thyroglobulin occur simultaneously in the same cell, and are regulated by TSH (Fig. 15-13). Gap junctions provide for a synchronized activity of all cells lining a given follicle.

T_3 and T_4 are soluble in the membrane of target cells. T_3 is the active form of the hormone; T_4, which enters the cytoplasm of a target cell, is deiodinated to form T_3. T_3 target cells express the T_3 receptor, a member of the steroid nuclear receptor family. T_3 acts in target cells by entering the nucleus and binding to its receptor. In the absence of T_3, the receptor is already in the nucleus, bound to the hormone response element (HRE) of the DNA, and acting as a repressor of transcription. Binding of the T_3 ligand to

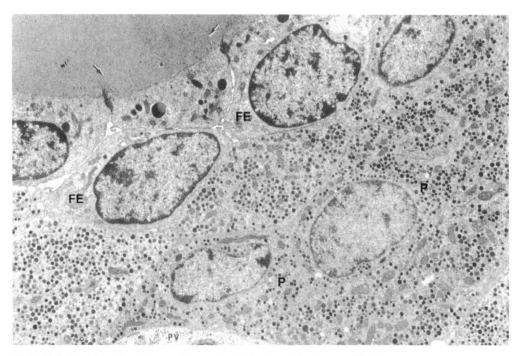

FIGURE 15-11 Thyroid parenchyma, dog. Follicular epitheliocytes (FE) form lining of follicle. Microvilli (arrows) project into colloid; calcitonin-producing, parafollicular cells (P) lie near a pericapillary space (PV) (×7,900). *(Courtesy of K. R. Moore and S. L. Teitelbaum.)*

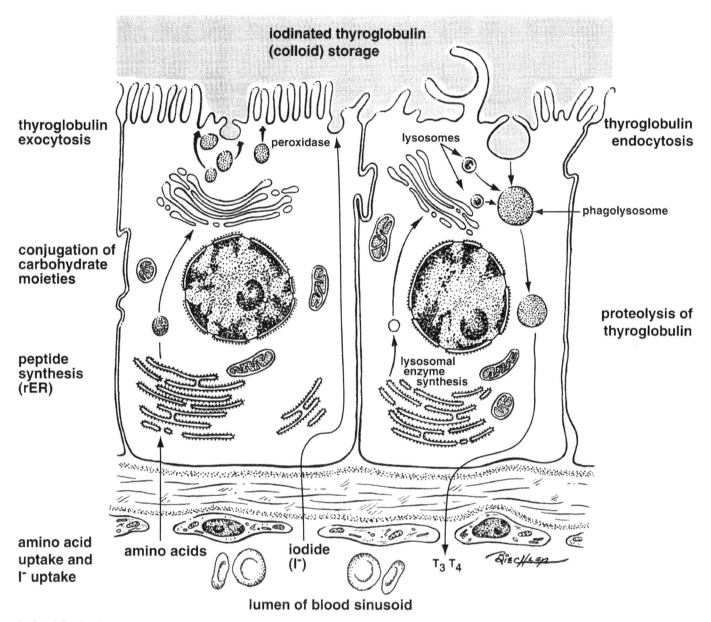

iodinated thyroglobulin (colloid) storage

thyroglobulin exocytosis

thyroglobulin endocytosis

peroxidase

lysosomes

phagolysosome

conjugation of carbohydrate moieties

proteolysis of thyroglobulin

peptide synthesis (rER)

lysosomal enzyme synthesis

amino acid uptake and I⁻ uptake

amino acids

iodide (I⁻)

T_3 T_4

lumen of blood sinusoid

FIGURE 15-12 Schematic drawing of the biosynthesis of thyroglobulin (left) and its resorption and proteolysis (right). For didactic purposes, events are depicted in two cells but they occur simultaneously in the same cell. Rough endoplasmic reticulum (rER).

its nuclear hormone receptor displaces transcriptional corepressor complexes and allows the T_3-bound receptor to activate transcription. Thus, the T_3 receptor is a ligand-induced transactivator; genes transcribed affect basal metabolic rate, thermogenesis, and gluconeogenesis. In the median eminence and pars distalis, T_3 acts to negatively regulate the release of TRH and TSH, respectively.

The **parafollicular cells** often are positioned in the basolateral compartment between follicular epithelial cells and within the basal lamina, while others form clusters between the follicles (Figs. 15-10B and C). These large epithelioid cells (prominent in the dog) synthesize **calcitonin** and are APUD (amine precursor uptake and decarboxylation) cells (see Diffuse Neuroendocrine System Cells below). Synthesis and release of calcitonin is regulated, not by the pars distalis, but by the concentration of calcium in the intercellular fluid. When the intercellular calcium concentration rises, the

calcium-sensing GPCRs on the parafollicular cell detect the calcium increase and trigger calcitonin release. Gastrin also promotes calcitonin release (see Enteroendocrine Cells). Calcitonin binds to its GPCR on osteoclasts and kidney epithelium, lowering calcium concentration in blood and interstitial fluid by inhibiting osteoclast activity and lowering tubular resorption of calcium, respectively.

Parathyroid Gland

Parathyroid glands are derived from endoderm of pharyngeal pouches III and IV. As the thyroid primordium is displaced caudoventrally from the root of the tongue into the neck, clusters of endodermal cells from the pouches join the thyroid tissue to form the parathyroids. The cranial external parathyroid (Fig. 15-14A) forms from pouch III, while the caudal internal parathyroid

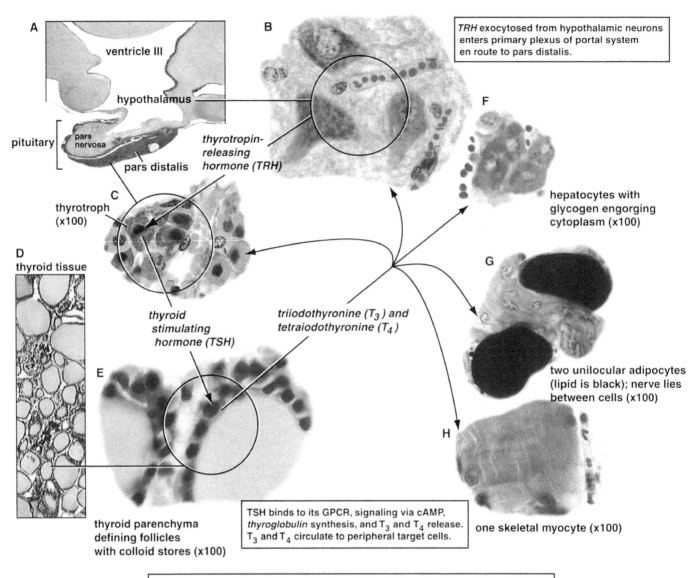

FIGURE 15-13   Cartoon summarizing molecular, cellular, and tissue biology of thyroid. **A.,** Hypothalamus and hypophysis cerebri. Hematoxylin and eosin (×2). **B.,** Parenchyma of hypothalamus. Saffron-modified Masson's trichrome (×100). **C.,** Parenchyma of pars distalis. Hematoxylin and eosin (×100). **D.,** Thyroid tissue. Hematoxylin and eosin (×4.5). **E.,** Parenchyma of thyroid. Hematoxylin and eosin (×100). **F.,** Parenchyma of liver. Periodic acid-Schiff (×100). **G.,** Interstitial unilocular adipocytes. Sudan black B (×100). **H.,** Skeletal muscle. Saffron-modified Masson's trichrome (×100).

forms from pouch IV. Each gland is separated from the thyroid by a stroma forming a capsule (Fig. 15-14B); the parenchyma is supported by a delicate interstitium that bears an extensive capillary plexus (Fig. 15-14D). The parenchyma is arranged as a large, uniform, and tightly packed cluster of small **principal cells** (chief cells) (Fig. 15-14C and D). Slight variations in the staining affinity of the principal cells are thought to merely reflect differences in the secretory cycle. The parathyroid glands of the horse, cow, and human have a few scattered, large **oxyphilic cells** (acidophils) of unknown function.

The principal cell synthesizes **parathyroid hormone (PTH)**, which elevates and maintains normal calcium concentration in

blood and interstitial fluid. PTH synthesis and release is regulated by calcium concentration in the intercellular fluid. The principal cell has calcium-sensing GPCRs that monitor decreased extracellular calcium concentration. When stimulated, the receptor activates phospholipase C and PI3-kinase, leading to a rise in concentration of intracellular calcium. The increased calcium concentration effects an opening of plasma membrane calcium channels, increased intracellular calcium, and exocytosis of PTH. PTH binds to its GPCR on target cells, elevating the concentration of cAMP and enhancing the activity of enzymes in osteocytes and osteoclasts, kidney epithelium, and intestinal epithelium. PTH enhances the resorption of calcium from bones (activation

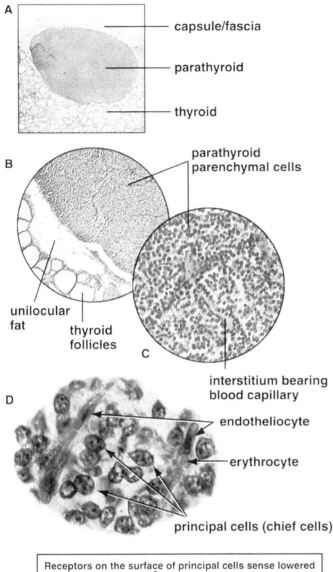

A

capsule/fascia

parathyroid

thyroid

B

parathyroid
parenchymal cells

unilocular
fat

thyroid
follicles

C

interstitium bearing
blood capillary

endotheliocyte

erythrocyte

D

principal cells (chief cells)

Receptors on the surface of principal cells sense lowered
levels of interstitial (Ca^{2+}), signaling exocytosis of
parathyroid hormone; parathyroid hormone affects target
tissue to increase (Ca^{2+}).

FIGURE 15-14 Random sectional plane parathyroid of dog. **A.** Parathyroid with thyroid (×4.5). **B.** ×10. **C.** Parenchyma and vascular stroma (×40). **D.** Parenchyma and blood capillaries (×100). Hematoxylin and eosin.

of osteoclasts) and the absorption of calcium across kidney and intestinal epithelia.

Adrenal Gland

The adrenal (Latin *ad*, meaning "near"; Latin *rene*, meaning "kidney") glands are composed of an outer cortex, derived from intermediate mesoderm, and an inner medulla, derived from neural crest ectoderm. The differentiation of the medullary cells results from signals available along the migratory path during development and is maintained by exposure to glucocorticoids leaving the cortex through the medulla. A robust capsule of dense irregular collagenous connective tissue envelops the cortex, and a del-

icate connective tissue envelope separates the cortex and medulla. The stroma is sparse in both the cortex and medulla, with a few trabeculae extending from the capsule to the medulla bearing arterioles and preganglionic sympathetic axons. The dual blood supply of the cortex and medulla is from an arteriolar plexus in the capsule that supplies the fenestrated sinusoids of the cortex, as well as arterioles passing directly to the medulla. These circulations merge in the medulla, forming medullary sinusoids, venous sinuses, and eventually the medullary vein.

Adrenal Cortex

The tissue architecture and staining affinities of the adrenal cortical parenchyma give rise to a pattern of zonation (from the outermost to innermost): zona glomerulosa (arcuata), zona fasciculata, and zona reticularis (Fig. 15-15A and B). The zona glomerulosa (arcuata) constitutes the **outer cortex**; the zonae fasciculata and reticularis form the **inner cortex**. At the interface of the outer and inner cortices, there is a narrow band, the **zona intermedia,** of small, undifferentiated cells that make up the blastemic stem cells, which generate replacement parenchyma for both the inner and outer cortex (Fig. 15-15D).

Arranged as tufts of epithelial cells (**zona glomerulosa** in ruminants and humans) (Fig. 15-16A) or as arches of columnar cells (**zona arcuata** in horses, pigs, and carnivores) (Figs. 15-15B and 15-16B), the outer cortex is the source of **mineralocorticoids (aldosterone and corticosterone).** This zone develops in the perinatal period as the last of the cortical zones to appear. The organelles and inclusions of the outer cortical parenchyma are those of steroidogenesis, but, unlike the rounded mitochondria in the inner cortex, the mitochondria are elongated with lamellar cristae. When present, columnar cells are bipolar with lipid droplets at both poles (Fig. 15-15C). Arising from the zona intermedia, cells of the zona glomerulosa (outer cortex) differentiate and, in turn, undergo apoptosis in this zone.

The **zona fasciculata** is composed of radiating columns (cords) of spherical cells, separated by sinusoids and bundled as fascicles; these cells produce **glucocorticoids (cortisol and cortisone)** (Figs. 15-15E and 15-17). The **zona reticularis** is formed by polyhedral cells, arranged as a network of anastomosing cords and plates, separated by large sinusoids (Figs. 15-15F and 15-18). These cells synthesize small amounts of **androgens.** Cells of the zona reticularis are the oldest of the inner cortex, and apoptotic cells are frequently observed. Cells of the inner cortex migrate from the zona intermedia, in turn forming the zona fasciculata and then the zona reticularis. As they migrate, the cells differentiate, initially expressing the enzymes of glucocorticoid synthesis, and later, those of sex steroid synthesis. The organelles and inclusions of the inner cortical parenchyma are those of most steroidogenesis, namely, profuse smooth endoplasmic reticulum, large and rounded mitochondria with tubulovesicular cristae, and numerous lipid droplets. Regarding lipid storage, pigs are an exception in that they do not store lipid in their cortical parenchymal cells. Cells in the reticularis often have lipofuscin granules and the pyknotic nuclei indicative of apoptosis.

Aldosterone is released from cells in the outer adrenal cortex as a consequence of angiotensin II signaling. Angiotensin II

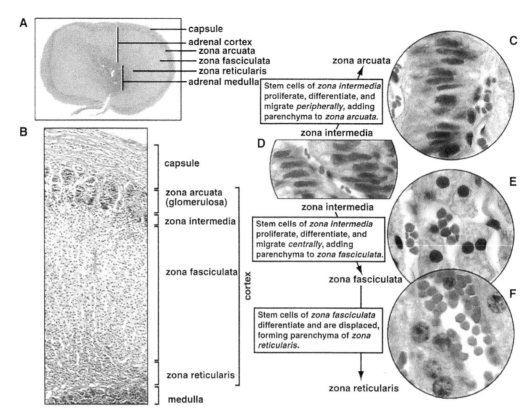

FIGURE 15-15 Adrenal gland of dog. **A.** (×1). **B.** Parenchyma and stroma, adrenal cortex (×10). **C.** Parenchyma zona arcuata (×100). **D.** Parenchyma, zona intermedia (×100). **E.** Parenchyma, zona fasciculata (×100). **F.** Parenchyma, zona reticularis (×100). Hematoxylin and eosin.

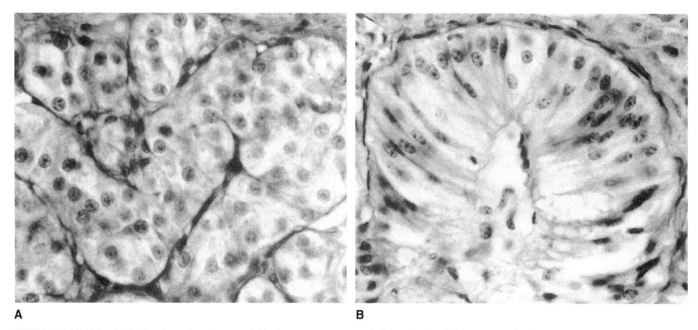

FIGURE 15-16 In the bovine adrenal cortex (**A**), the outermost zone is formed of cell clusters or tufts (glomeruli), whereas in the donkey (**B**), the cells are arranged in arcs. Hematoxylin and eosin (×20). *(From Dellmann H-D. Veterinary Histology: An Outline Text–Atlas. Philadelphia: Lea & Febiger, 1971.)*

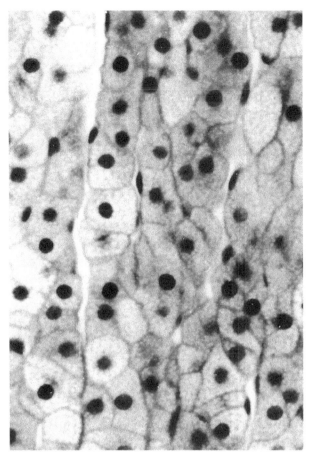

FIGURE 15-17 Cells in the zona fasciculata are arranged as radiating, anastomosing columns separated by sinusoids. The cells appear vesiculated due to extraction of lipid droplets during processing. Hematoxylin and eosin (×40).

synthesis involves the enzyme renin. **Renin** is synthesized in juxtaglomerular cells (modified smooth muscle cells, see Juxtaglomerular Cells of the Kidney below), especially prominent in the tunica media of afferent arterioles of the renal glomerulus; renin release is triggered by lowered blood perfusion pressure (pressoreceptor signal) in the arteriole. The substrate for renin is a plasma protein, **angiotensinogen,** that is converted to **angiotensin I,** which then is converted enzymatically to **angiotensin II.** Cells of the zona glomerulosa express the angiotensin (AT1) receptor. The AT1 is a GPCR that, when ligated, activates phospholipase C and PI3-kinase, resulting in increased intracellular calcium concentration, transcription of the aldosterone synthase gene, and synthesis of aldosterone. Essentially, within these steroidogenic cells, cholesterol is converted by a series of the cytochrome P450 family of enzymes to the mineralocorticoid **corticosterone,** which is then converted by aldosterone synthase to aldosterone. The cells of the zona glomerulosa have extensive smooth endoplasmic reticulum and mitochondria that harbor the dehydrogenases and hydroxylases of this synthetic sequence. (The outer zone does not express a 17α-hydroxylase and therefore cannot synthesize glucocorticoids.) Although the principal signal is angiotensin II, the outer zone is also signaled to synthesize and release mineralocorticoids (aldosterone or corticosterone) in response to elevated potassium (a chemoreceptor signal) and ACTH. The release of the steroid hormone from the parenchymal cell is by diffusion through the cell membrane. Chronic stimulation of the zona glomerulosa (e.g., kidney disease) leads to cell proliferation within the zona intermedia, growth of the zona glomerulosa, invasion of parenchyma into and through the capsule, and formation of accessory nodules of the parenchyma (Fig. 15-19).

At its target tissues, aldosterone diffuses through the cell membrane into epithelial cells of the distal convoluted and col-

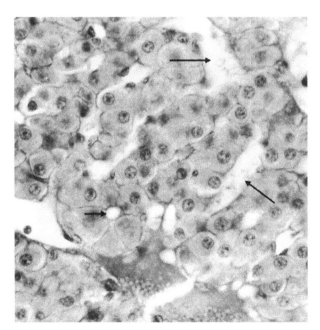

FIGURE 15-18 Cells of zona reticularis appear as irregular plates ("cords") of polyhedral cells separated by sinusoidal capillaries (arrows). Hematoxylin and eosin (×40). *(From Dellmann H-D. Veterinary Histology: An Outline Text–Atlas. Philadelphia: Lea & Febiger, 1971.)*

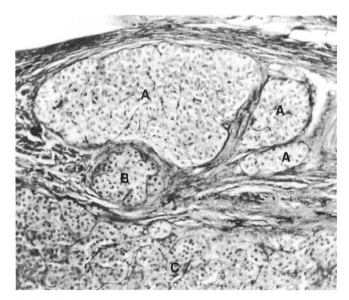

FIGURE 15-19 Adrenal gland of cow. Clusters of parenchymal cells within a hyperplastic nodule in the capsule (A). Note that cells in the small cluster (B) resemble those of the zona glomerulosa (C). Hematoxylin and eosin (×10). *(From Dellmann H-D. Veterinary Histology: An Outline Text–Atlas. Philadelphia: Lea & Febiger, 1971.)*

lecting tubules of the kidney and epithelial cells of the colon. The hormone binds to its cytosolic receptor and is transported into the nucleus to its specific hormone response elements on target genes. The increased expression of these genes in the distal convoluted and collecting tubule cells produces more Na^+-K^+ ATPase (adenosine triphosphatase) transporters in the basolateral cell membrane and more sodium channels in the apical membrane. These membrane changes cause increased release of potassium in the urine and increased sodium retention, resulting in increased blood volume. Negative feedback, due to the increased fluid volume and reduction of potassium concentration, suppresses renin and aldosterone release. (Glucocorticoids are also able to bind the same cytosolic receptor, potentially exacerbating the mineralocorticoid response. However, specificity of action for mineralocorticoids is accomplished by the epithelial target cells in the distal nephron and collecting tubule through their expressing a glucocorticoid-degrading enzyme, hydroxysteroid dehydrogenase.)

In the zona fasciculata, synthesis of glucocorticoids is promoted by ACTH. ACTH is released from the corticotrophs in response to "stress signals" affecting the hypothalamus. ACTH binds to its GPCR and, via adenylate cyclase and elevated concentrations of cAMP, activates proteins that increase transcription of the enzymes of steroid hormone synthesis. Synthesis proceeds as in the zona glomerulosa, except that the parenchymal cells also express 17α-hydroxylase. Progesterone is modified by a series of hydroxylations that form cortisol, the principal glucocorticoid.

Cortisol is bound to a carrier protein as it circulates in the plasma. When freed from the carrier, cortisol diffuses into the target cell and binds to its cytoplasmic steroid receptor. A dimer of the ligand-bound receptor enters the nucleus and binds to its hormone response elements on target genes, activating gene transcription. The effects are marked in hepatocytes, skeletal myocytes, and adipocytes (Fig. 15-20). In hepatocytes, glucocorticoids act to favor glycogen storage and gluconeogenesis, whereas in myocytes,

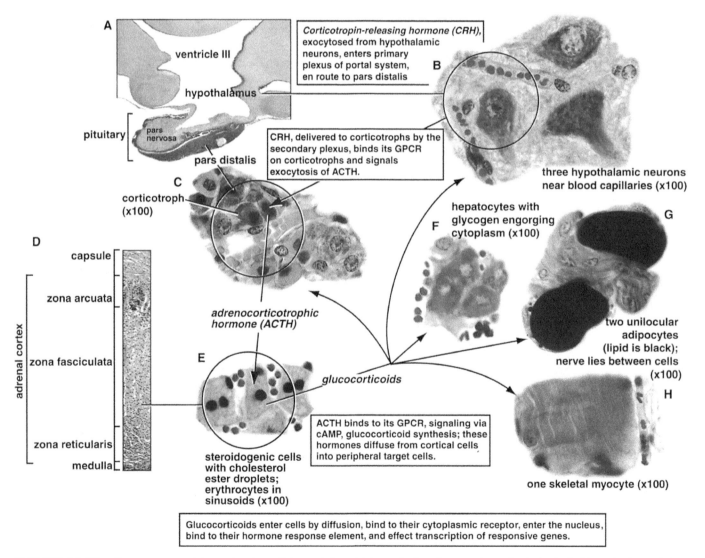

FIGURE 15-20 Cartoon summarizing molecular, cellular, and tissue biology of adrenal cortex (zona fasciculata). **A.** Hypophysis cerebri. Hematoxylin and eosin (×2). **B.** Parenchyma, hypothalamus. Saffron-modified Masson's trichrome (×100). **C.** Parenchyma, pars distalis. Hematoxylin and eosin (×100). **D.** Adrenal cortex. Hematoxylin and eosin (×4.5). **E.** Parenchyma, zona fasciculata. Hematoxylin and eosin (×100). **F.** Parenchyma, liver. Periodic acid-Schiff (×100). **G.** Unilocular adipocytes. Sudan black (×100). **H.** Skeletal muscle. Saffron-modified Masson's trichrome (×100).

they inhibit glucose uptake; in adipocytes, they inhibit glucose uptake, stimulate lipolysis and fatty acid release, and stimulate adipogenesis (by stimulating proliferation and differentiation of adipocytes). Catabolic effects of glucocorticoids result in skeletal muscle breakdown and atrophy and a generalized wasting of connective tissues, including bone. Glucocorticoids also exert anti-inflammatory effects by stimulating apoptosis of lymphocytes and inhibiting cytokine synthesis. In addition, glucocorticoids exert negative feedback to the pars distalis and inhibit POMC synthesis. In the hypothalamus, they inhibit CRH and ADH synthesis. Hyperactivity of the adrenal cortex is clinically recognized as Cushing's disease; hypoactivity (insufficiency) is termed Addison's disease.

In the zona reticularis, ACTH stimulates androgen synthesis, depending on the relative activities of cytochrome P450 family enzymes, forming androgen. Androgens of the adrenal cortex are relatively more important in the female than the male.

Adrenal Medulla

The adrenal medullary parenchymal cells are modified sympathetic neurons, essentially constituting a large sympathetic gan-glion. They synthesize **epinephrine** and **norepinephrine**, and store these neurotransmitters as secretory granules. When exposed to chromium salts, the cells containing the granules stain boldly brown; accordingly, these and other similarly staining cells are referred to as **chromaffin cells**. The epithelioid cells form clusters separated by sinusoids (Fig. 15-21A and B); although they represent modified neurons, the medullary endocrine cells do not extend axonal projections. Occasionally sympathetic neurons are found among the endocrine cells (Fig. 15-21C). At the periphery of the medulla and adjacent to medullary sinusoids, columnar cells (in horses, ruminants, and pigs) produce epinephrine; rounded, epithelioid cells of the medulla produce norepinephrine. Epinephrine is formed by the columnar cells from norepinephrine by the action of a methyltransferase; the cytodifferentiation of the columnar cell and synthesis of this enzyme is induced by glucocorticoids flowing into the medulla from the cortex.

Connective tissue trabeculae extend from the capsule, bearing arterioles and preganglionic, sympathetic axons that synapse with multiple medullary cells. The release of epinephrine and norepinephrine occurs in response to acetylcholine that binds to its postsynaptic receptor. The activated acetylcholine receptor

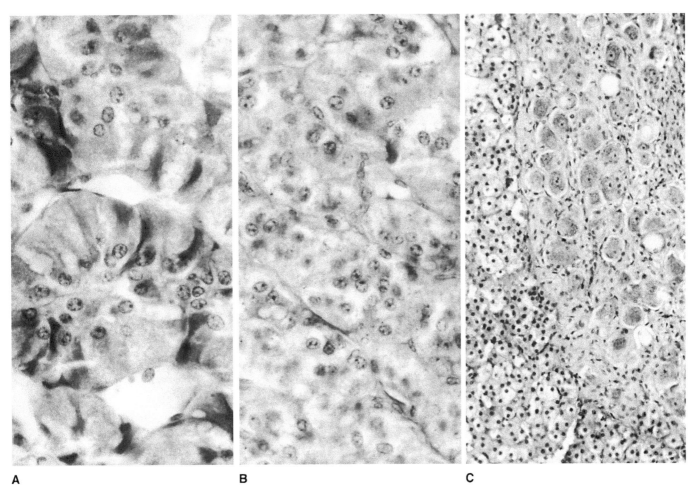

A   **B**   **C**

FIGURE 15-21   Adrenal medulla. In the cow (and some other species) large, columnar, epinephrine-producing cells are located in the "outer zone" of the medulla (**A**) and also next to the sinusoids; the smaller, norepinephrine-producing cells are located in the "inner zone" (**B**), having less direct contact with the venous drainage of the adrenal cortex; parenchymal cells may coexist with clusters of neurons (**C**). Hematoxylin and eosin (**A, B:** ×40; **C:** ×20).

leads to depolarization of the cell membrane, increases calcium influx, and results in exocytosis of catecholamines from the secretory vesicles. Epinephrine and norepinephrine both bind to α- and β-adrenergic receptors, differentially expressed in many tissues of the body. These receptors are members of the GPCR family, and the tissue-specific hormone effect depends on the receptor subtype activated (e.g., activating phospholipase C and PI3-kinase, which increases intracellular calcium concentration; activating adenylate cyclase, leading to increased concentrations of cAMP; or inhibiting [uncoupling] adenylate cyclase and reducing concentrations of cAMP). Epinephrine and norepinephrine are the molecular mediators of the **"fight or flight mechanism,"** the immediate physiologic response to fear and stress, resulting in increased heart rate and the breakdown of glycogen in skeletal muscle and liver.

ENDOCRINE TISSUES AND CELLS

Pancreatic Islets

Endocrine cells of the pancreas form islets within the exocrine pancreatic tissue. These islets vary in size from a few endocrine cells to clusters of a few hundred cells (Fig. 15-22A, B, and C). The exocrine pancreas is derived from endoderm. Some evidence suggests that the islet cells arise from endoderm and then separate from ducts. However, the shared APUD characteristics of islet cells (see Diffuse Neuroendocrine System Cells below) and enteroendocrine cells in the epithelium of the gut are intriguing, suggesting that these cells arise from a common precursor. This question is of clinical importance as it relates to the potential for regeneration of islet cells. The principal cells of the islets include **alpha (α) cells, beta (β) cells,** and **delta (δ) cells;** small numbers of other enteroendocrine cells may also appear in the islets.

Alpha cells synthesize and store **glucagon** and represent 5 to 30% of the islet cell population (Figs. 15-22D and E and 15-23). In the pig, the number of α cells decreases from nearly 50% at birth to 8 to 20% in the adult. In the horse, α cells are located in the center of the islet, but in cattle, they tend to be peripheral. Islets in the ventral area of the right lobe of the canine pancreas lack α cells (perhaps reflecting the different site of origin of this lobe). Glucagon release occurs in response to hypoglycemia (low blood sugar). Glucagon binds its GPCR on hepatocytes, skeletal myocytes, and adipocytes, activating adenylate cyclase and elevating the concentration of cAMP, thus promoting glycogenolysis and gluconeogenesis and opposing hypoglycemia. (This influence is augmented by cortisol, GH, epinephrine, and norepinephrine.)

Beta cells synthesize and store **insulin,** constituting 60 to 80% of the islet cells (98% in sheep) (Figs. 15-22D and E and 15-23). The β cell is signaled by hyperglycemia (elevated blood sugar), the principal signal for insulin release. Glucose is transported by GLUT-2 into the β cell. Within the cell, glucose is utilized to generate ATP, which closes the ATPase-sensitive potassium channel, leading to depolarization of the cell membrane. The depolarization activates calcium channels, resulting

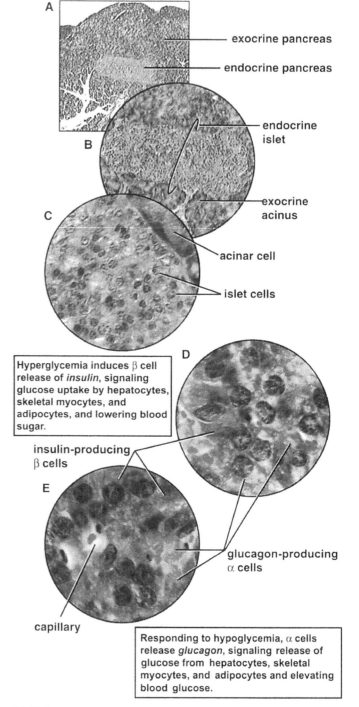

Hyperglycemia induces β cell release of *insulin,* signaling glucose uptake by hepatocytes, skeletal myocytes, and adipocytes, and lowering blood sugar.

insulin-producing β cells

glucagon-producing α cells

capillary

Responding to hypoglycemia, α cells release *glucagon,* signaling release of glucose from hepatocytes, skeletal myocytes, and adipocytes and elevating blood glucose.

FIGURE 15-22 Random sectional plane pancreas of dog. **A.** ×4.5. **B.** Endocrine islet and exocrine acini (×10). **C.** Endocrine islet parenchyma with exocrine acini (×40). **D. E.** Islet parenchyma and blood capillaries (×100). Saffron-modified Masson's trichrome.

in increased intracellular calcium concentration and triggering exocytosis of insulin. Insulin binds to its receptor, a tyrosine kinase on hepatocytes, skeletal myocytes, and adipocytes. The activated receptor autophosphorylates and initiates phosphorylation of the insulin receptor substrate-1 (IRS-1), signaling downstream via protein kinases and phosphatases. Insulin promotes synthesis of enzymes that favor anabolism and oppose hyperglycemia. Insufficient secretion of insulin causes diabetes mellitus, a clini-

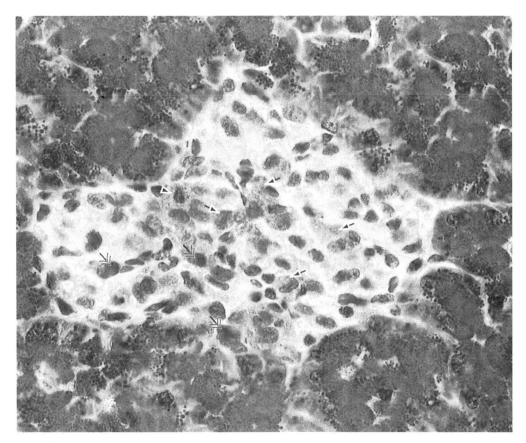

FIGURE 15-23 Pancreatic endocrine islet of dog. An endocrine islet (central and lightly stained) is surrounded by exocrine acini. The acinar cells have dark-staining zymogen granules. The proinsulin granules of β cells (arrows) within the islet stain while other islet cells (e.g. α, δ) are not selectively stained by this dye. The endocrine islet is perfused by blood sinusoids (double arrows). Saffron-modified Masson's trichrome (×100).

cal condition that results in many signs including the production of a large volume of urine with high levels of sugar.

Delta cells synthesize and store **somatostatin** (SST) and represent a relatively small percentage of the islet parenchyma. SST exerts broad endocrine and neural effects. Acting in an autocrine mode, SST inhibits its own secretion; acting in a paracrine mode, SST inhibits secretion of insulin and glucagon within the islet. Furthermore, SST expressed in neurons of the hypothalamus inhibits the release of GH and TSH; SST serves as a neurotransmitter centrally and acts as a paracrine regulator of the enteroendocrine cells peripherally. SST binds its GPCR, uncoupling cAMP, lowering intracellular calcium concentration, and inhibiting release of the relevant hormones. By the same mechanism, SST also downregulates mitogen-activated kinases in target cells and suppresses entry of these cells into the mitotic cycle.

Paraganglia

Small clusters of extraadrenal medullary, catecholaminergic cells are called **paraganglia.** The paraganglia are composed of parenchymal cells, **glomus cells,** nested within a small plexus of sinusoidal capillaries called a **glomus.**

Of the several glomera, the most studied is the **carotid body,** found in the fascia at the bifurcation of the common carotid ar-

tery. The sinusoids provide the glomus cells with a continual sample of arterial blood en route to the brain. Glomus cells have secretory vesicles that store epinephrine, dopamine, and serotonin. Evidence suggests that glomus cells, sensing lowered blood oxygen, stimulate the output from the carotid body via afferent axons of the carotid sinus branch of the glossopharyngeal nerve to the distal (petrosal) ganglion, and then to the brainstem. Parasympathetic and sympathetic axons terminate near the sinusoids; sensory axons project to contact some type I glomus cells, and type II glomus cells serve as support cells. Synaptic contacts exist between some glomus cells and also between them and sensory and sympathetic axons. Functioning as chemoreceptors, the type I glomus cells monitor the concentration of oxygen in the blood. Potassium channels in the sensor cell are oxygen sensitive and hypoxia suppresses their activity, depolarizing the cell membrane and opening voltage-gated calcium channels. The influx of calcium triggers exocytosis of secretory vesicles from the glomus cell. The secretions released as neurotransmitters (epinephrine, dopamine, serotonin) bind to their receptors on the adjacent sensory axons. Depolarization of these sensory axons results in afferent signals traversing to the nuclei of the brainstem, which regulate respiration, increasing respiratory rate and the blood oxygen.

Glomera are also found in the **aortic body** and coccygeal body and along some arteriovenous anastomoses, and have a similar structure to that of the carotid body. The mechanism of the function of these glomera remains unclear.

Diffuse Neuroendocrine System Cells

Diffuse neuroendocrine system (DNES) cells are scattered in the epithelium throughout the respiratory, urinary, reproductive, and digestive systems. More than 30 DNES cell types have been identified. The cytoplasm of these cells contains either peptide hormones (see below) or biogenic amines (e.g., epinephrine, norepinephrine, and serotonin). A subcategory of DNES cells are **amine precursor uptake and decarboxylation (APUD) cells,** which are able to take up and decarboxylate amines. Some DNES cells stain with silver and are therefore called **argentaffin cells.**

About 1% of the epitheliocytes (enterocytes) in the gastrointestinal lining are DNES cells and constitute the **enteroendocrine cells (system).** Some evidence shows that these cells are not derived from endoderm, but from neural crest ectoderm. Enteroendocrine cells are dispersed among the absorptive and secretory enterocytes and adhere to the basal lamina. Most are pyramidal in shape with a narrow projection to the lumen; secretory granules are stored nearer to the base. With specific antibody staining of their secretions, these cells can be identified as producing one of these hormones: gastrin, secretin, motilin, pancreatic polypeptide (PP), glucagon, insulin, vasoactive intestinal polypeptide (VIP), somatostatin, ghrelin, neuropeptide Y (NPY), neurotensin, peptide YY, or cholecystokinin (CCK). Secretions of enteroendocrine cells bind to specific receptors on target cells and signal by paracrine and endocrine modes, effecting epithelial cell secretion, contraction of smooth myocytes, and conduction in enteric and central neurons. Their effects primarily inhibit, or alternatively stimulate, processes affecting food intake, digestion, and absorption of nutrients, and basal metabolism.

Other Endocrine Cells

Adipocytes

Unilocular (white) adipocytes secrete **leptin,** a 16 Kda protein hormone that is an afferent signal to the hypothalamus, regulating energy homeostasis for the organism. Leptin is one of the inputs to the hypothalamic "lipostat," the output of which affects feeding behavior. Leptin binds to its cytokine receptor on neurons of the hypothalamus and inhibits food intake, for example, by inhibiting the release of the food intake–stimulating (orexigenic) hormones **neuropeptide Y** and **agouti-related peptide (AgRP).**

Endocrine Cells of the Heart

In the atrial myocardium, some cardiac myocytes synthesize and store in secretory vesicles a peptide hormone known as **atrial natriuretic peptide (ANP)** (see Chapter 7). When blood volume is increased, the stretch of the atrial myocytes during the filling of the atrium causes membrane calcium channels to open, increasing intracellular calcium concentration and triggering exocytosis of ANP. ANP binds to its receptor on target cells, activating guanylyl cyclase and increasing the concentration of cyclic guano-

sine 3′, 5′-monophosphate (cGMP). cGMP activates a phosphodiesterase that deactivates cAMP, inhibiting cell functions driven by cAMP. In the kidney, ANP acts in the collecting tubule to antagonize the effect of ADH and upon juxtaglomerular cells to inhibit release of renin. In the brain, ANP inhibits ADH release.

Juxtaglomerular Cells of the Kidney

At the vascular pole of the renal corpuscle, the tunica media of the afferent arterioles contain rounded smooth myocytes, called juxtaglomerular (JG) cells (see Chapter 11). These modified smooth myocytes synthesize and store renin granules, which are an important element of the renin–angiotensin–aldosterone system discussed above. JG cells release renin in response to a baroreceptor signal, initiated by lowered blood perfusion pressure. This signal arises from either a mechanical perturbation of the myocyte membrane (in the wall of the arterioles) or a chemoreceptor signal (e.g., elevated [K^+], synthesis of prostaglandin E_2, release of ATP) response by the macula densa cells (in the distal tubule). Renin release triggers a cascade of enzymatic reactions creating angiotensin II that binds the AT1 receptor in the zona glomerulosa of the adrenal cortex, releasing aldosterone. Aldosterone, in turn, increases expression of Na^+-K^+ ATPase transporters and Na^+ channels in distal tubule and collecting duct epitheliocytes, and increases fluid volume and reduction of K^+ levels. Accordingly, the stimulus for renin release is obviated.

Endocrine Cells of the Ovary

The endocrine tissues of the ovary are derived from mesoderm. Oogonia develop from primordial germ cells, which migrate into the gonadal ridge during the genesis of the ovary and are enveloped by a single layer of mesenchymal cells, defining a follicle. As follicles develop, the mesenchymal cells become the **follicular epithelial cells (granulosal cells).** The stromal cells adjacent to the growing follicle, called **internal theca cells,** are transformed from fibroblasts to epithelioid, steroidogenic cells. Upon ovulation, the follicular epithelial cells and the internal thecal cells proliferate, forming the **corpus luteum.**

Follicular epithelial cells express the FSH receptor, a GPCR, and FSH signaling results in follicular cell proliferation and differentiation (see Chapter 13), as well as the expression of aromatase P450 and additional FSH receptors. In larger follicles, FSH also induces the expression of LH receptors on the same follicular epitheliocytes. Follicular epitheliocytes take up androgen, synthesized and released from the adjacent internal theca cells; the aromatase P450 expressed by these cells converts the androgen to **estrogen.** In addition, follicular cells also release a peptide hormone, **inhibin.**

Internal thecal cells express the LH receptor, a GPCR, and via adenylate cyclase and elevated concentrations of cAMP activate transcription of the steroidogenic enzymes and the conversion of cholesterol to androgen. In some species (e.g., rodents doe rabbit, bitch, and queen), the thecal cells of atretic tertiary follicles remain viable as steroidogenic **interstitial endocrine cells (the "stromal organ"),** independent of follicles.

Following ovulation, follicular epithelial cells and thecal cells proliferate, forming a **corpus luteum.** Under the influence of LH, the lutein cells are able to utilize cholesterol to synthesize **progesterone.** Small (theca) lutein cells continue the synthesis of androgen, which then is converted to estrogen by the large (granulosa) lutein cells. With the decline of LH and in the absence of a signal from an implanting trophoblast (i.e., chorionic gonadotropin), the **corpus luteum cyclicum** regresses and progesterone declines. The corpus luteum is also a source of inhibin. With development of a conceptus, cells of the extraembryonic trophoblast synthesize chorionic gonadotropin, which binds the same LH receptors found in the corpus luteum, maintaining its viability and steroidogenesis. This is the **corpus luteum graviditas** (corpus luteum of pregnancy).

The ovarian hormones affect uterine and mammary gland target tissues and exert a negative feedback on GnRH release from hypothalamic neurons and FSH and LH release from the hypophyseal gonadotrophs. Inhibin targets the gonadotroph, effecting a selective inhibition of FSH release.

Endocrine Cells of the Placenta

Like the corpus luteum, the placenta is also a transient endocrine organ (see Chapter 14). Marked species differences of the placental endocrine role are correlated with the intimacy of the fetal–maternal tissue contact (e.g., porcine versus carnivore versus primate), the structure of the trophoblast, and the molecular weight of the hormones. Trophoblast cells of the fetal placenta synthesize estrogen, progesterone, and **equine chorionic gonadotropin** (ECG, pregnant mare's serum gonadotropin [PMSG]), prolactin, and POMC derivatives. In the mare, some trophoblast cells of the foal placental membranes migrate into the endometrium where they proliferate, forming large clusters ("endometrial cups") that synthesize PMSG. Additional targets of placental hormones include the fetal gonads and the maternal uterus, ovary, mammary tissue, and immune system.

Endocrine Cells of the Testis

The endocrine cells of the testis are derived from mesoderm. Spermatogonia arriving at the developing testis are enveloped by mesenchyme that differentiates, forming a simple columnar epithelium of **sustentacular cells** (Sertoli cells). Organized as tubules, they are separated by a basal lamina from the interstitial connecting tissues. Some stromal cells adjacent to the tubules differentiate as the steroidogenic **interstitial cells** (Leydig cells) and other stromal cells provide support for the many blood and lymph capillaries.

The interstitial cells of the testis (see Chapter 12) express the LH receptor and, upon binding the LH (ICSH) ligand, activate transcription of the steroidogenic enzymes and conversion of cholesterol to **androgen.** FSH receptors on the sustentacular cell bind the FSH ligand, resulting in the expression of aromatase P450 and the synthesis of estrogen from androgens released by the interstitial cells; the sustentacular cells also release the peptides inhibin and **androgen-binding protein.**

The testicular hormones target secondary sex tissues (e.g., prostate, skeletal muscle) and also exert a negative feedback on

GnRH release from hypothalamic neurons and FSH and LH release from the hypophyseal gonadotrophs. Inhibin targets the gonadotroph, selectively inhibiting FSH release.

SUGGESTED READINGS

Andreoli TE, Reeves WB, Bichet DG. Endocrine control of water balance. In: Goodman HM, ed. Handbook of Physiology Vol 3. New York: Oxford University Press, 2000.

Bringhurst FR, Demay MB, Kronenberg HM. Hormones and disorders of mineral metabolism. In: Larsen PR, Kronenberg HM, Melmed S, et al., eds. Williams Textbook of Endocrinology. 10th Ed. Philadelphia: Saunders, 2002.

Chester-Jones I, Ingleton PM, Phillips JG. Fundamentals of Comparative Vertebrate Endocrinology. New York: Plenum Press, 1987.

Cone RD. Neuroendocrinology. In: Larsen PR, Kronenberg HM, Melmed S, et al., eds. Williams Textbook of Endocrinology. 10th Ed. Philadelphia: Saunders, 2002.

Constanti A, Bartke A, Khardori R. Basic Endocrinology for Students of Pharmacy and Allied Health Sciences. Amsterdam: Harwood Academic Publishers, 1998.

De Bold AJ, Bruneau BG. Natriuretic peptides. In: Goodman HM, ed. Handbook of Physiology. Vol 3. New York: Oxford University Press, 2000.

Denef C. Autocrine/paracrine intermediates in hormone action and modulation of cellular responses to hormones. In: Goodman HM, ed. Handbook of Physiology. Vol 1. New York: Oxford University Press, 1998.

Ganguly A. Aldosterone. In: Goodman HM, ed. Handbook of Physiology. Vol 3. New York: Oxford University Press, 2000.

Halász B. The hypothalamus as an endocrine organ. In: Conn PM, Freeman ME, eds. Neuroendocrinology in Physiology and Medicine. Totowa, NJ: Humana Press, 2000.

Hullinger RL. The endocrine system. In: Evans HE, ed. Miller's Anatomy of the Dog. 3rd Ed. Philadelphia: W. B. Saunders, 1993.

Kaplan NM. The adrenal glands. In: Griffin JE, Ojeda SR, eds. Textbook of Endocrine Physiology. 4th Ed. New York: Oxford University Press, 2000.

Lavine JE. The hypothalamus as a major integrating center. In: Conn PM, Freeman ME, eds, Neuroendocrinology in Physiology and Medicine. Totowa, NJ: Humana Press, 2000.

Melmed S, Kleinberg D. Anterior pituitary. In: Larsen PR, Kronenberg HM, Melmed S, et al., eds. Williams Textbook of Endocrinology. 10th Ed. Philadelphia: Saunders, 2002.

Mendelson CR. Mechanisms of hormone action. In: Griffin JE, Ojeda SR, eds. Textbook of Endocrine Physiology. 4th Ed. New York: Oxford University Press, 2000.

Robinson AG, Verbalis JG. Posterior pituitary gland. In: Larsen PR, Kronenberg HM, Melmed S, et al., eds. Williams Textbook of Endocrinology. 10th Ed. Philadelphia: Saunders, 2002.

Sehgal A. Molecular Biology of Circadian Rhythms. Hoboken, NJ: John Wiley & Sons, Inc., 2004.

Tucker HA. Neuroendocrine regulation of lactation and milk ejection. In: Conn PM, Freeman ME, eds. Neuroendocrinology in Physiology and Medicine. Totowa, NJ: Humana Press, 2000.

Zeidel ML. Physiologic responses to natriuretic hormones. In: Goodman HM, ed. Handbook of Physiology. Vol 3. New York: Oxford University Press, 2000.

16

Integument

NANCY A. MONTEIRO-RIVIERE

Epidermis
  Epidermal Keratinocytes
  Epidermal Nonkeratinocytes
    Melanocytes
    Tactile epithelioid cells (Merkel cells)
    Intraepidermal macrophages (Langerhans cells)
  Layers of the Epidermis
    Stratum basale
    Stratum spinosum
    Stratum granulosum
    Stratum lucidum
    Stratum corneum
  Keratinization
  Epidermal–Dermal Junction
Dermis
Hypodermis
Skin Appendages
  Hair
  Hair Follicles
    Structure
    Types of hair follicles
    Hair cycle
  Skin Glands
    Sebaceous glands
    Sweat glands
Blood Vessels, Lymph Vessels, and Nerves
Special Structures of the Integument
  External Ear
  Eyelids

Infraorbital Sinus
Nose
Mental Organ
Submental Organ
Carpal Glands
Interdigital Sinus
Inguinal Sinus
Scrotum
Anal Sacs
Circumanal Glands
Supracaudal Gland
Mammary Gland
  Alveoli
  Interstitium
  Ducts
  Teat
  Mammary gland involution
Digital Organs and Horn
  Equine Hoof
    Wall
    Sole
    Frog
  Ruminant and Swine Hoofs
  Claw
  Digital Pads
  Chestnut and Ergot
  Horn
Avian Integument

Skin is a complex, integrated, dynamic organ that has functions far beyond its role as a barrier to the environment (Table 16-1). The skin, or integument (derived from the Latin word meaning "to cover"), is the largest organ system of the body and consists of a superficial epidermis and an underlying dermis (Fig. 16-1).

In general, the basic architecture of the integument is similar in all mammals. However, differences in the thickness of the epidermis and dermis in various regions of the body exist between species and within the same species. Because dermatologic, cutaneous pharmacologic, and toxicologic studies use skin from different animal species and body sites, species differences in cutaneous structure must be taken into consideration.

Usually, the skin is thickest over the dorsal surface of the body and on the lateral surfaces of the limbs. It is thinnest on the ventral surface of the body and medial surfaces of the limbs. The surface of the skin may be smooth in some areas but has ridges or folds in other regions that reflect the contour of the underlying connective tissue layer (Fig. 16-2).

EPIDERMIS

The **epidermis** is a keratinized stratified squamous epithelium derived from ectoderm and is the outermost layer of the skin (Fig. 16-2). In regions with a heavy protective coat of hair, the epidermis is thin; in nonhairy skin, such as that of the mucocutaneous junctions, the epidermis is thicker. Cells of the epidermis undergo an orderly pattern of proliferation, differentiation, and keratinization, the processes of which are not completely understood. During development, the epidermis can become spe-

cialized to form various skin appendages such as hair; sweat and sebaceous glands; digital organs (hoof, claw, digital pads); feathers; horn; and specialized glands.

The cells of the epidermis are categorized into two major groups: keratinocytes and nonkeratinocytes. The epidermal layers can be classified from the basement membrane to the outer surface as follows: stratum basale (basal layer), stratum spinosum (spinous or prickle layer), stratum granulosum (granular layer), stratum lucidum (clear layer), and stratum corneum (horny layer).

Epidermal Keratinocytes

Keratinocytes comprise about 85% of the epidermal cells and are classified into layers based on morphology. They vary in size and shape and differentiate as they migrate upward to form keratin.

Epidermal Nonkeratinocytes

Nonkeratinocytes are scattered throughout the epidermis and include melanocytes, tactile epithelioid cells, and intraepidermal macrophages.

Melanocytes

Melanocytes are derivatives of neural crest ectoderm and are located in the basal layer of the epidermis (Fig. 16-1). They also occur in the external epithelial root sheath and hair matrix of hair follicles, in sweat gland ducts, and in sebaceous glands. Melanocytes have several dendritic processes that either extend between adjacent keratinocytes or run parallel to the basement membrane. The melanocyte has a spherical nucleus and contains typical organelles (ribosomes, endoplasmic reticulum, Golgi, etc.). The cytoplasm is clear except for pigment-containing ovoid granules, which are referred to as **melanosomes.** The melanosomes impart color to skin and hair. Dark brown pigment in skin is called **eumelanin,** while yellowish-red pigment is called **pheomelanin.** The enzyme tyrosinase is needed to produce melanin within the melanocytes, and the reaction involves the following series of steps, in short: tyrosine⟹dopa⟹dopaquinone⟹melanin. Albino animals lack tyrosinase; therefore, they cannot produce melanin, even though they have a normal number of melanocytes. After melanogenesis, the melanosomes migrate to the tips of the dendritic processes of the melanocyte; the tips then become pinched off and are phagocytized by the adjacent keratinocytes. They remain as discrete membrane-bounded organelles or become aggregated and surrounded by a membrane to form a melanosome complex. Melanosomes are randomly distributed within the cytoplasm of the keratinocytes, although they often become localized over the nucleus, thereby forming a caplike structure that presumably protects the nucleus from ultraviolet radiation (Fig. 16-3). Skin color is determined by several factors, such as the number, size, distribution, and degree of melanization of melanosomes.

Tactile Epithelioid Cells (Merkel Cells)

Tactile epithelioid cells, also known as Merkel cells, are located in the basal region of the epidermis in both hairless and hairy

---

TABLE 16-1 Functions of the Skin

Environmental barrier
  Diffusion barrier
  Metabolic barrier
Temperature regulation
  Regulation of blood flow
  Hair and fur
  Sweating
Immunologic affector and effector axis
Mechanical support
Neurosensory reception
Endocrine (e.g., vitamin D)
Apocrine/eccrine/sebaceous glandular secretion
Metabolism
  Keratin
  Collagen
  Melanin
  Lipid
  Carbohydrate
  Respiration
Biotransformation of xenobiotics

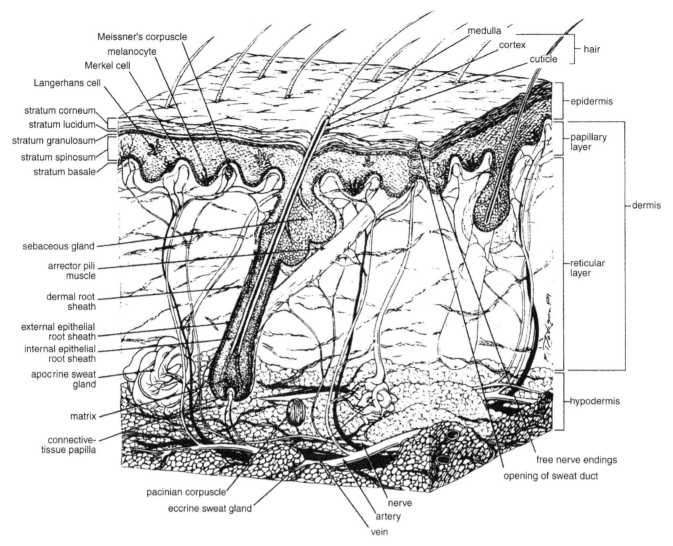

FIGURE 16-1 Schematic drawing representing the structure of the integument found in typical skin in various regions of the body. *(Adapted from Monteiro-Riviere NA. Comparative anatomy, physiology, and biochemistry of mammalian skin. In: Hobson DW, ed. Dermal and Ocular Toxicology: Fundamentals and Methods. Boca Raton, FL: CRC Press, 1991;1:3).*

skin. Their long axis is usually parallel to the surface of the skin and, thus, perpendicular to the columnar basal epithelial cells above (Figs. 16-1 and 16-4). The nucleus is lobulated and irregular, and the cytoplasm is clear and lacks tonofilaments. These cells have a characteristic region of vacuolated cytoplasm near the dermis, which has spherical electron-dense granules containing species-specific chemical mediators (e.g., serotonin, serotoninlike substances, vasoactive intestinal polypeptide, peptide histidine-isoleucine, and substance P). Tactile epithelioid cells are connected to adjacent keratinocytes by desmosomes. When associated with an axon, a tactile epithelioid cell–neurite complex or nonencapsulated tactile corpuscle is formed, and specialized areas of skin containing these complexes are known as **tactile hair discs** (Haarscheiben, hair discs, tactile pads, or tylotrich pads). The axon associated with a tactile epithelioid cell is myelinated, but as it approaches the epidermis, the axon loses its myelin sheath and terminates as a flat meniscus on the basal aspect of the cell (Fig. 16-4). Tactile epithelioid cells can release trophic factors that attract nerve endings into the epidermis and can also stim-

ulate keratinocyte growth. In addition, tactile epithelioid cells can function as slow-adapting mechanoreceptors for touch.

Intraepidermal Macrophages (Langerhans Cells)

The dendritic cells located in the epidermis are called **intraepidermal macrophages** (Langerhans cells). They have been reported in adult pigs, cats, and dogs and are well characterized in rodents and humans. However, the specific phenotype (membrane receptors and antigens related to immune function) can vary between species. Intraepidermal macrophages are most commonly found in the upper spinous layer of the epidermis (Figs. 16-1 and 16-5). These cells have also been identified in the stratified squamous epithelium of the upper digestive tract, female genital tract, and sheep rumen. In addition, the cells are present in dermal lymph vessels (referred to here as "veiled cells"), in lymph nodes (interdigitating cells), and in the dermis. Further, they have been reported in the lung in fibrotic disorders, mycosis fungoides, atopic dermatitis, and the nondermatologic disorder eosinophilic granulomatosis.

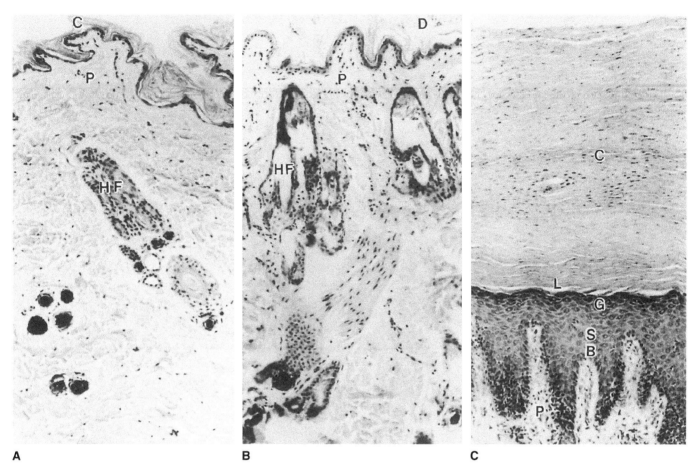

A   **B**   **C**

FIGURE 16-2 Skin (cat). **A.** Thin skin with one to two viable epidermal cell layers, abdomen. **B.** Skin with thin epidermis, lumbar region. **C.** Skin with thick stratum corneum and epidermis, foot pad. Stratum disjunctum (D); stratum corneum (C); stratum lucidum (L); stratum granulosum (G); stratum spinosum (S); stratum basale (B); superficial (papillary) layer of the dermis (P); hair follicle cluster in dermis (HF). Hematoxylin and eosin (×120).

Intraepidermal macrophages usually are not apparent in routine sections but may appear as clear cells in the suprabasal epidermis. They can only be positively identified with special stains. At the ultrastructural level, intraepidermal macrophages have an indented nucleus and the cytoplasm contains typical organelles; they lack tonofilaments and desmosomes. A unique feature of this cell is distinctive rod- or racket-shaped granules in the cytoplasm that are known as intraepidermal macrophage (Birbeck) granules. Depending on the species, these granules can contain Langerin, a Ca^{++}-dependent type II lectin. Intraepidermal macrophages have long dendritic processes that traverse the intercellular space up to the granular cell layer. The cells are derived from bone marrow and are part of the mononuclear phagocyte system (monocyte–macrophage system). They are capable of presenting antigen to lymphocytes and are considered to be the initial receptors for cutaneous immune responses (delayed-type hypersensitivity).

Layers of the Epidermis

Stratum Basale

The **stratum basale** (stratum germinativum) consists of a single layer of columnar or cuboidal cells that rests on the basal lamina (Fig. 16-6). The cells are attached laterally to each other and to the overlying stratum spinosum cells by desmosomes and to the underlying basal lamina by hemidesmosomes. The nucleus is large and ovoid and occupies most of the cell. These basal cells are heterogeneous functionally. Some basal cells can act as stem cells, with the ability to divide and produce new cells, whereas others primarily serve to anchor the epidermis.

Stratum Spinosum

The succeeding outer layer is the **stratum spinosum,** or "prickle cell layer," which consists of several layers of irregular polyhedral cells (Figs. 16-2C and 16-7). Desmosomes connect these cells to adjacent stratum spinosum cells and to the stratum basale cells below. Tonofilaments are more prominent in this layer than in the stratum basale. The large intercellular space usually seen in this layer is a shrinkage artifact, which occurs in preparing the sample for light microscopic study. The uppermost layers of the stratum spinosum contain small membrane-bounded organelles known as **lamellar granules** (Odland bodies, lamellated bodies, or membrane-coating granules).

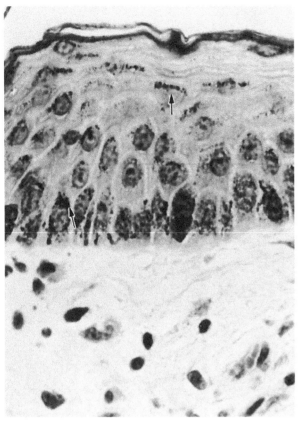

FIGURE 16-3 Melanin granules (arrows) highly concentrated in the stratum basale cell layer and forming apical caps in the upper layers of the horse abdominal skin. Hematoxylin and eosin (×800).

Stratum Granulosum

The third layer is the **stratum granulosum,** which consists of several layers of flattened cells lying parallel to the epidermal–dermal junction (Figs. 16-2C and 16-8). This layer contains irregularly shaped, nonmembrane-bounded, electron-dense **keratohyalin granules.** These granules contain profilaggrin, a structural protein and a precursor of filaggrin, and are believed to play a role in keratinization and barrier function. The stratum granulosum is not present in all stratified squamous epithelia such as in the mucous membranes of the mouth (buccal mucosa). Another characteristic feature of the stratum granulosum is the presence of the **lamellar granules.** These granules are smaller than mitochondria and occur near the Golgi complex and smooth endoplasmic reticulum (sER). Higher in the epidermis, these granules increase in number and size, move toward the cell membrane, and release their lipid contents by exocytosis into the intercellular space between the stratum granulosum and stratum corneum, thereby coating the cell membrane of the stratum corneum cells (Fig. 16-8). As one can now appreciate, the term "membrane-coating granule" is appropriate. The major components of lamellar granules are lipids (ceramides, cholesterol, fatty acids, and small amounts of cholesteryl esters) and hydrolytic enzymes (acid phosphates, proteases, lipases, and glycosidases). The content and mixture of lipids can vary between species.

Stratum Lucidum

The **stratum lucidum** (clear layer) is only found in specific areas of exceptionally thick skin and in hairless regions (e.g., plantar and palmar surfaces, planum nasale) (Fig. 16-2C). It is a thin,

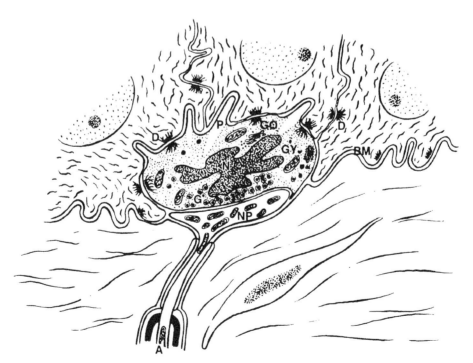

FIGURE 16-4 Schematic drawing of a tactile epithelioid cell–neurite complex from a foot pad of a cat. Irregular nucleus (N); Golgi (GO); desmosomes (D) glycogen (GY); cytoplasmic process (P); basement membrane (BM); Merkel cell dense core granules (G); axon (A); nerve plate or disc (NP).

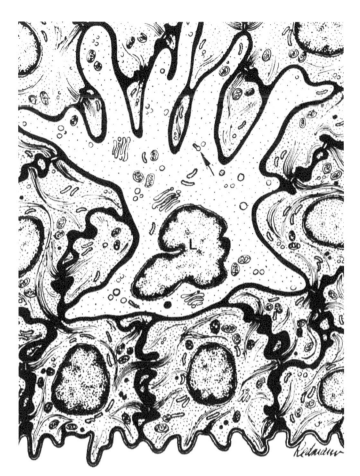

FIGURE 16-5 Schematic of an intraepidermal macrophage (L). Heavy black areas represent the intercellular space. The racket shape granules (arrow) can be found in the dendritic processes. Note the indented nucleus and electron-lucent cytoplasm. *(From Monteiro-Riviere NA. Ultrastructural evaluation of the porcine integument. In: Tumbleson ME, ed. Swine in Biomedical Research. New York: Plenum Press, 1986;1:641.)*

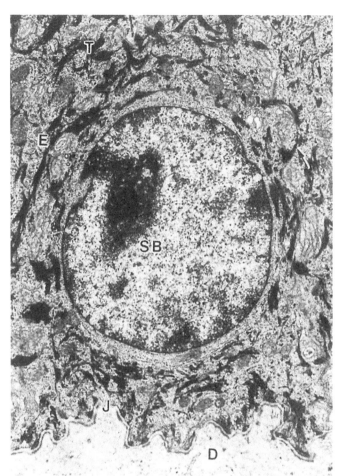

FIGURE 16-6 Transmission electron micrograph of pig skin. Area depicting the epidermis (E); dermis (D); epidermal–dermal junction (J); stratum basale cell (SB); tonofilaments (T); and desmosome attachments (arrow) (×10,700).

translucent, homogeneous line between the stratum granulosum and stratum corneum. This stratum consists of several layers of fully keratinized, closely compacted, dense cells devoid of nuclei and cytoplasmic organelles. The cell cytoplasm contains protein-bound phospholipids and **eleidin,** which is a protein that is similar to keratin but has a different staining affinity.

Stratum Corneum

The **stratum corneum** is the outermost layer of the epidermis and consists of several layers of completely keratinized dead cells, which are constantly being shed. This layer appears clear and contains no nuclei or cytoplasmic organelles (Figs. 16-2 and 16-8). The most superficial layers of the stratum corneum that undergo constant desquamation are referred to as the **stratum disjunctum.** The stratum corneum varies in thickness in different areas (i.e., abdomen versus back) of the body and between species. On the palmar and plantar surfaces, where considerable abrasive action occurs, the stratum corneum is thickest (Fig. 16-2C). The

stratum corneum cells are highly organized and stacked one upon another to form vertical interlocking columns with a flattened tetrakaidecahedron shape. This 14-sided polygonal structure provides a minimum surface:volume ratio, which allows for space to be filled by packing without interstices. This spatial arrangement, typical of hairy skin, helps one to understand that transepidermal water loss is a function of the integrity and permeability of this layer. The intercellular substance derived from the lamellar granules is present between the stratum corneum cells and forms the intercellular lipid component of a complex stratum corneum barrier, which prevents both the penetration of substances from the environment and the loss of body fluids. The keratinized cells are surrounded by a plasma membrane and a thick submembranous layer that contains a protein, **involucrin.** This protein is synthesized in the stratum spinosum and cross-linked in the stratum granulosum by an enzyme that makes it highly stable. Therefore, involucrin provides structural support to the cell, thereby allowing the cell to resist invasion by microorganisms and destruction by environmental agents, but it does not seem to regulate permeability.

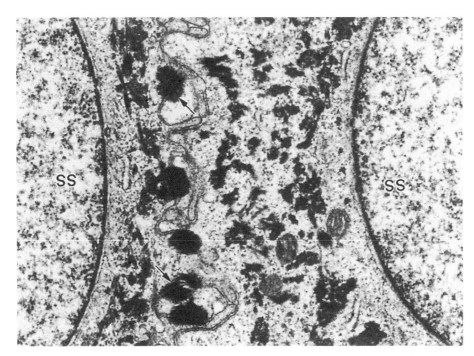

FIGURE 16-7 Transmission electron micrograph of the stratum spinosum of pig skin. Area shows the nuclei of two stratum spinosum (SS) cells attached by desmosomes (arrows) (×23,500).

Keratinization

Keratinization is the process by which epidermal cells (keratinocytes) differentiate. After the basal epithelial cells undergo mitosis, they migrate upward. The volume of the cytoplasm increases and the differentiation products (tonofilaments, keratohyalin granules, and lamellar granules) are formed in large amounts. The tonofilaments and the amorphous material, keratohyalin, form a meshwork. As the cellular contents increase, the nuclei disintegrate and the lamellar granules discharge their contents into the intercellular space, coating the cells. The remaining organelles such as mitochondria and ribosomes disintegrate, and the flattened cells become filled by filaments and keratohyalin, which then form bundles. The final product of this epidermal differentiation and keratinization process is the stratum corneum, which consists of protein-rich cells containing fibrous **keratin** and keratohyalin surrounded by a thicker plasma membrane coated by the exterior lipid matrix. This forms the commonly known "brick and mortar" structure in which the lipid matrix acts as the mortar between the cells, which are the bricks.

Epidermal–Dermal Junction

The **epidermal–dermal junction** (or skin basement membrane zone) is a complex and highly specialized structure recognized with the light microscope (periodic acid-Schiff stain) as a thin, homogeneous band. When viewed with the transmission electron microscope, however, the epidermal–dermal junction consists of four components: (a) the cell membrane of the basal epithelial cell, which includes the hemidesmosomes; (b) the lamina lucida (lamina rara); (c) the lamina densa (basal lamina); and

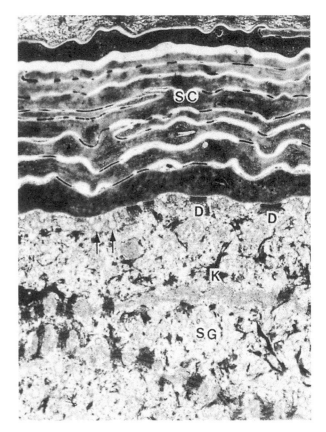

FIGURE 16-8 Transmission electron micrograph of the upper stratum granulosum (SG) and stratum corneum (SC) of pig skin. Membrane-coating granules or lamellar bodies (arrows) are present in the stratum granulosum, with some fusing to the plasma membrane to release their contents. Keratohyalin granules (K) and numerous desmosomes (D) are present (×14,900).

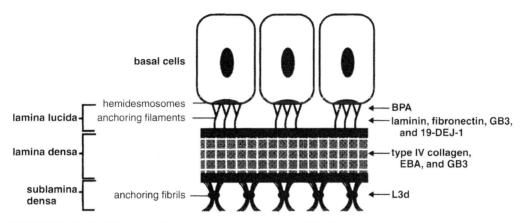

FIGURE 16-9 Schematic of the basement membrane of skin depicting the precise location of the macromolecular components. *(From Monteiro-Riviere NA, Inman AO. Indirect immunohistochemistry and immunoelectron microscopy distribution of eight epidermal-dermal junction epitopes in the pig and in isolated perfused skin treated with bis (2-chloroethyl) sulfide. Toxicol Pathol 1995;23:313–325.)*

(d) the subbasal lamina (sublamina densa or reticular lamina) with a variety of fibrous structures (anchoring fibrils, dermal microfibril bundles, microthreadlike filaments) (Fig. 16-9). The basement membrane has a complex molecular architecture with numerous components that play a key role in adhesion of the epidermis to the dermis. The macromolecules that are ubiquitous components of all basement membranes include type IV collagen, laminin, entactin/nidogen, and heparan sulfate proteoglycans. Other basement membrane components such as bullous pemphigoid antigen (BPA), epidermolysis bullosa acquisita (EBA), fibronectin, GB3, L3d, and 19DEJ-1 are limited in their distribution to the epithelial basement membrane of skin. The basal cell membrane of the epidermal–dermal junction is not always smooth. It may be irregular, forming fingerlike projections into the dermis. The basement membrane (a) plays a role in maintenance of epidermal–dermal adhesion, (b) acts as a selective barrier between the epidermis and dermis by restricting some molecules and permitting the passage of others, (c) influences cell behavior and wound healing, and (d) serves as a target for both immunologic (bullous diseases) and nonimmunologic injury (friction- or chemical-induced blisters).

DERMIS

The **dermis,** or corium, lies beneath the basement membrane and extends to the hypodermis. This layer is of mesodermal origin and consists primarily of dense irregular connective tissue with a feltwork of collagen, elastic, and reticular fibers embedded in amorphous ground substance. Predominant cell types of the dermis are fibrocytes, mast cells, and macrophages. Plasma cells, chromatophores, fat cells, and extravasated leukocytes are often found. The dermis is traversed by blood vessels, lymph vessels, and nerves. Sebaceous and sweat glands are also present, along with hair follicles and arrector pili muscles.

The dermis can be divided into a superficial papillary layer that blends into a deep reticular layer without a clear line of demarcation (Fig. 16-10). The **papillary layer** is the thinnest layer,

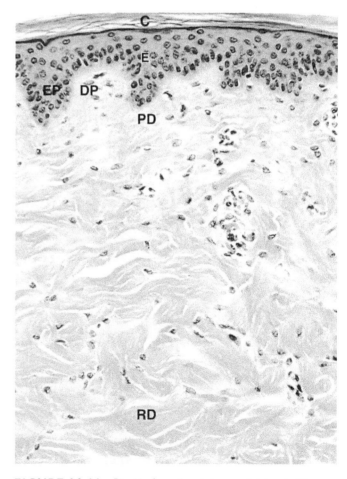

FIGURE 16-10 Pig skin from the abdomen. Epidermis (E); stratum corneum (C); superficial papillary dermis (PD); epidermal peg (EP); dermal papilla (DP); deep reticular dermis (RD). Hematoxylin and eosin (×250).

consists of loose connective tissue, is in contact with the epidermis, and conforms to the contour of the stratum basale. The papillary layer can protrude into the epidermis, thereby giving rise to the **dermal papilla.** When the epidermis invaginates into the dermis, **epidermal pegs** are formed. The **reticular layer** is thicker and consists of dense irregular connective tissue. Connective tissue cells are fewer in the deeper layers of the dermis.

In the dermis, smooth muscle fibers are located near hair follicles and are referred to as **arrector pili muscles.** In addition, dermal smooth muscle fibers are present in specialized areas such as the scrotum, penis, and teat. Skeletal muscle fibers of the cutaneous trunci penetrate the dermis and allow voluntary movement of the skin. Also, skeletal muscle fibers are associated with the large sinus hairs of the facial region.

HYPODERMIS

Beneath the dermis is a layer of loose connective tissue, the **hypodermis** (subcutis), which is not part of the skin but rather the superficial fascia seen in gross anatomic dissections. The hypodermis anchors the dermis to the underlying muscle or bone. The loose arrangement of collagen and elastic fibers allows the skin flexibility and free movement over the underlying structures. Adipose tissue is present in this layer and may form small clusters of cells or large masses that create a cushion or pad of fat called the **panniculus adiposus** (Fig. 16-11). Pork bacon and fatback are derived from the panniculus adiposus. Large fat deposits (structural fat) in the hypodermis are characteristic of the carpal, metacarpal/metatarsal, and digital pads, where they act as shock absorbers.

SKIN APPENDAGES

Hair

In domestic mammals, hair covers the entire body, with the exception of the foot pads, hoofs, glans penis, mucocutaneous junctions, and teats of some species. **Hair** is a flexible, keratinized structure produced by a hair follicle. The distal or free part of the hair above the surface of the skin is the hair **shaft.** The part within the follicle is the hair **root,** which has a terminal, hollow knob called the hair **bulb,** which is attached to a dermal papilla.

The hair shaft is composed of three layers: an outermost cuticle, a cortex of densely packed keratinized cells, and a medulla of loose cuboidal or flattened cells (Fig. 16-12). The **cuticle** is formed by a single layer of flat keratinized cells in which the free edges, which overlap like shingles on a roof, are directed toward the distal end of the shaft. The **cortex** consists of a layer of dense, compact, keratinized cells with their long axes parallel to the hair shaft. Nuclear remnants and pigment granules are present within the cells. Desmosomes hold the cells firmly together. Near the bulb, the cells are shorter and more oval and contain spherical nuclei. The **medulla** forms the center of the hair and is loosely

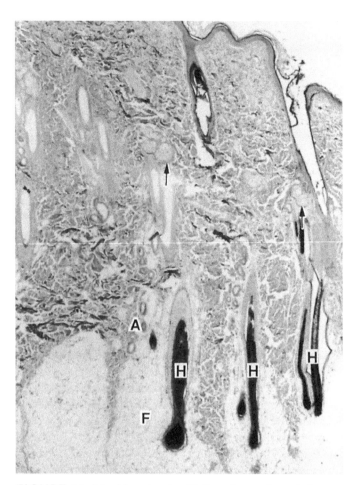

FIGURE 16-11 Hypodermis with three large primary hair follicles (H) extending into the subcutaneous fat (F) (dog). Note the sebaceous glands (arrows) and apocrine gland ducts (A). Hematoxylin and eosin (×35).

filled with cuboidal or flattened cells (Fig. 16-12). In the root, the medulla is solid, whereas in the shaft, it contains air-filled spaces. The pattern of the surface of the cuticular cells, together with the cellular arrangement of the medulla, is characteristic for each species.

The hair or fleece of sheep is referred to as **fibers.** The three types of fibers are (a) wool fibers, tightly crimped fibers of small diameter lacking a medulla; (b) kemp fibers, coarse and with a characteristic medulla; and (c) coarse fibers of intermediate size relative to wool and kemp fibers. The various breeds of sheep produce wools with different characteristics, and these various kinds of fleece are used for different purposes.

Hair Follicles

Structure

The **hair follicle** is formed by growth of the ectoderm into the underlying mesoderm of the embryo. The epithelial downgrowth becomes canalized, and the surrounding cells differentiate into several layers or sheaths that surround the hair root. The follicle is embedded in the dermis, usually at an angle, and the bulb may

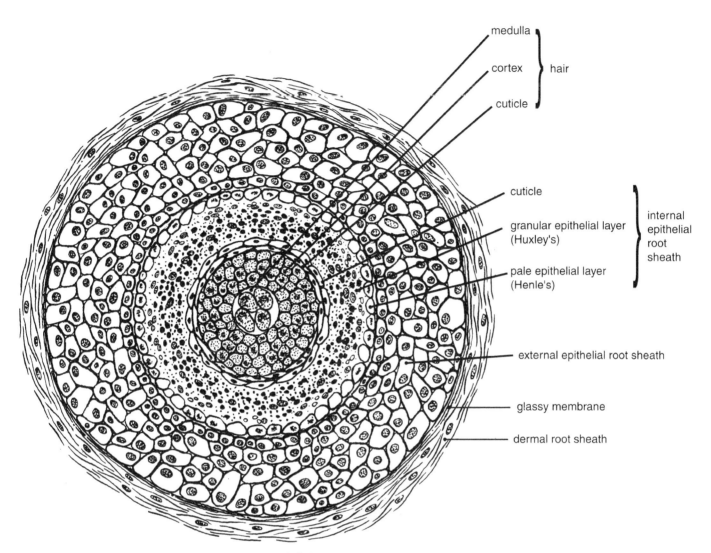

medulla ⎱
cortex ⎰ hair
cuticle

cuticle
granular epithelial layer (Huxley's) ⎱ internal epithelial root sheath
pale epithelial layer (Henle's) ⎰

external epithelial root sheath

glassy membrane

dermal root sheath

FIGURE 16-12 Schematic of a cross section of a hair follicle.

extend as deep as the hypodermis (Figs. 16-11 and 16-13). The hair follicle consists of four major components: (a) internal epithelial root sheath, (b) external epithelial root sheath, (c) dermal papilla, and (d) hair matrix.

The innermost layer, next to the hair root, is the **internal epithelial root sheath,** which is composed of three layers: (a) internal root sheath cuticle, (b) middle granular epithelial layer (Huxley's layer), and (c) outer pale epithelial layer (Henle's layer) (Fig. 16-12). The **cuticle** of the internal epithelial root sheath is formed by overlapping keratinized cells similar to those of the cuticle of the hair, except that the free edges are oriented in the opposite direction or toward the hair bulb. This arrangement results in a solid implantation of the hair root in the hair follicle. The **granular epithelial layer** is composed of one to three layers of cells rich in trichohyalin (keratohyalin in hair) granules. The **pale epithelial layer** is the outermost layer of the internal epithelial root sheath and is composed of a single layer of keratinized cells. Immediately below the opening of the sebaceous glands, the internal epithelial root sheath of the large follicles becomes

corrugated, forming several circular or follicular folds. The sheath then becomes thinner, and the cells fuse, disintegrate, and become part of the sebum.

The **external epithelial root sheath** is composed of several layers of cells similar to the epidermis with which it is continuous in the upper portion of the follicle. External to this layer is a homogeneous glassy membrane corresponding to the basal lamina of the epidermis (Fig. 16-12). The entire epithelial root sheath (internal and external) is enclosed by a **dermal root sheath** composed of collagen and elastic fibers richly supplied by blood vessels and nerves, especially in the dermal papilla.

The **dermal papilla** of the hair follicle is the region of connective tissue directly underneath the hair matrix. The cells covering the dermal papilla and composing most of the hair bulb are the **hair matrix cells.** These are comparable to stratum basale cells of regular epidermis and give rise to the cells that keratinize to form the hair (Fig. 16-13). They differ from the keratinocytes of the surface epidermis with respect to the type of keratin produced. The surface keratinocytes produce a "soft" form of keratin

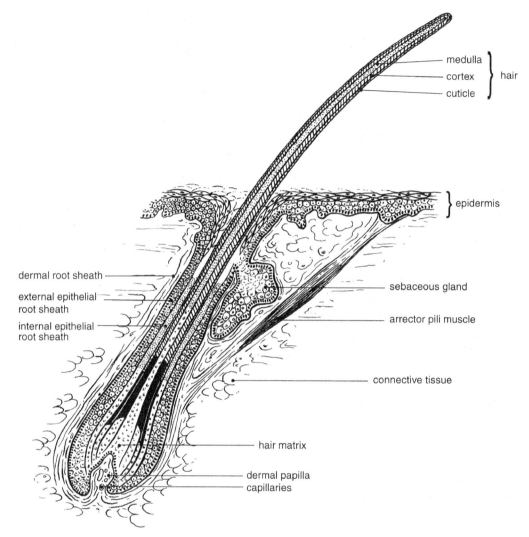

medulla ⎫
cortex ⎬ hair
cuticle ⎭

epidermis

dermal root sheath

external epithelial
root sheath

internal epithelial
root sheath

sebaceous gland

arrector pili muscle

connective tissue

hair matrix

dermal papilla
capillaries

FIGURE 16-13   Schematic of a longitudinal section of a hair follicle.

that passes through a keratohyalin phase. The cells containing "soft" keratin have a high lipid content and a low sulfur content and desquamate when they reach the surface of the epidermis. In contrast, the matrix cells of the hair follicle produce a "hard" keratin, which is also characteristic of horn and feather. The keratinocytes of the follicle do not go through a keratohyalin phase, do not desquamate, and have a low lipid and high sulfur content.

Hair pigment is derived from the epidermal melanocytes located over the dermal papilla. Gray hair results from the inability of melanocytes in the hair bulb to produce tyrosinase. Hair color is determined by the amount and distribution of pigment and by the presence of air, which appears white in reflected light. Silvery white hair is the result when the pigment has faded and the medulla becomes filled with air.

Associated with most hair follicles are bundles of smooth muscle called the **arrector pili muscle.** This muscle attaches to the dermal root sheath of the hair follicle and extends toward the epidermis, where it connects to the papillary layer of the dermis (Fig. 16-14). These muscles are anchored by elastic fibers at their attachments and are innervated by autonomic nerve fibers. The

arrector pili muscles are especially well developed along the back of dogs, where they cause the hair to "bristle" when they contract. The contraction of the arrector pili muscles during cold weather elevates the hairs, thus allowing minute air pockets to form in the coat. This dead-air space provides significant insulation that helps to maintain internal body temperature. The contraction of this muscle not only erects the hairs but also may play a role in emptying the sebaceous glands. In addition to the arrector pili muscle, the **interfollicular muscle,** which spans the triad of hair follicles, has been described in pigs (Figs. 16-15 and 16-16). It is located midway between the level of the sebaceous gland and the apocrine sweat gland. Upon contraction, the interfollicular muscle draws the three follicles close together and rotates the outer follicles of the triad into a new relationship. Adjustment of the hair follicle and hair may play a part in thermoregulation, sensory function, emptying of the skin glands, or self defense.

Types of Hair Follicles

Hair follicles are classified into several types. A **primary hair follicle** has a large diameter, is rooted deep in the dermis, and is usu-

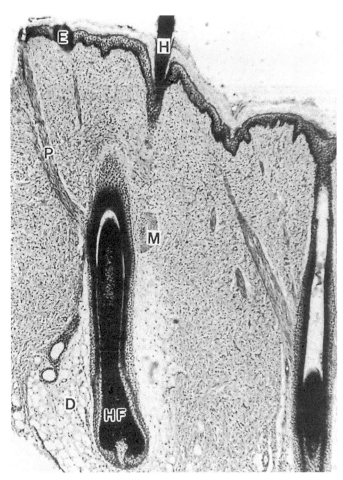

FIGURE 16-14 Longitudinal section of a hair follicle (HF) showing an attached arrector pili muscle (P), cross section of the interfollicular muscle (M), epidermis (E), hair (H), and hypodermis (D) (pig). Hematoxylin and eosin (×50).

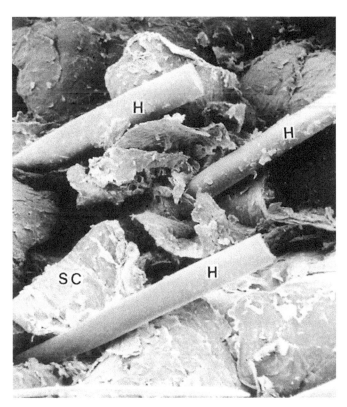

FIGURE 16-16 Scanning electron micrograph of pig skin depicting hairs (H) occurring in groups of three emerging from the stratum corneum. Note the flaky appearance of the stratum corneum (SC) cells (×60). *(From Monteiro-Riviere NA. Comparative anatomy, physiology, and biochemistry of mammalian skin. In: Hobson DW, ed. Dermal and Ocular Toxicology: Fundamentals and Methods. Boca Raton, FL: CRC Press, 1991;1:3)*

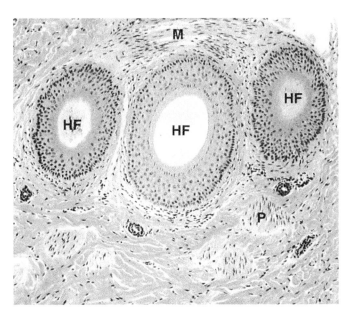

FIGURE 16-15 Hair follicle triad (pig). Note the hair follicles (HF) occurring in groups of three, typical of young pigs. The interfollicular muscle (M) and arrector pili muscle (P) can be seen. Hematoxylin and eosin (×100).

ally associated with sebaceous and sweat glands and an arrector pili muscle (Fig. 16-11). The hair that emerges from such a follicle is called a **primary hair** (guard hair). A **secondary follicle** is smaller in diameter than a primary follicle, and the root is nearer the surface. It may have a sebaceous gland but lacks a sweat gland and an arrector pili muscle. Hairs from these follicles are **secondary hair,** or underhairs. Secondary hairs lack a medulla.

Follicles with only one hair emerging to the surface are called **single** or **simple follicles. Compound follicles** are composed of clusters of several hair follicles located in the dermis. At the level of the sebaceous gland opening, the follicles fuse and the various hairs emerge through one external orifice. Compound hair follicles usually have one primary hair follicle and several secondary hair follicles.

Many differences exist in the arrangement of the hair follicles among the domestic animals. Horses and cattle have single hair follicles that are distributed evenly. Pigs have single follicles grouped in clusters of two to four follicles; clusters of three are most common in young pigs (Figs. 16-15 and 16-16). This cluster is usually surrounded by dense connective tissue. The compound follicle of dogs consists of a single large primary hair and a group of smaller secondary underhairs (Fig. 16-17). A diversity of

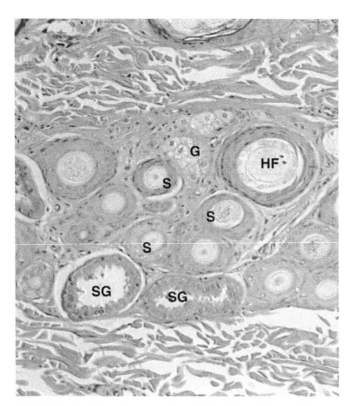

FIGURE 16-17   Compound hair follicle (dog). Primary hair follicle (HF); sebaceous gland (G); sweat glands (SG). The other round structures are all secondary follicles (S). Hematoxylin and eosin (×150).

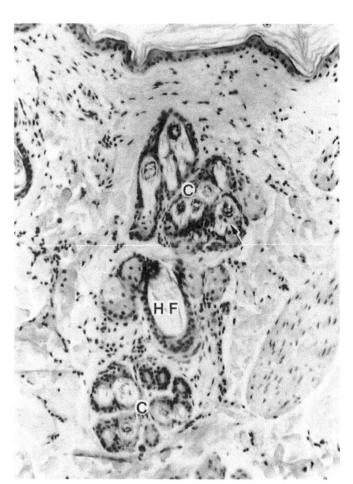

FIGURE 16-18   Hair follicle cluster (cat). Primary hair follicle (HF) surrounded by groups of compound follicle clusters (C) that contain primary and secondary hairs (arrow). Hematoxylin and eosin (×160).

hair types are found in different breeds of dogs. For example, in the German Shepherd, a greater number of secondary hairs exist, whereas in the short-coat breeds such as Rottweilers and terriers, a greater number of primary hairs are present. The arrangement of the follicles in cats consists of a single large primary (guard) hair follicle surrounded by clusters of two to five compound follicles (Fig. 16-18). Each compound follicle has 3 coarse primary hairs and 6 to 12 secondary hairs. The skin of sheep has hair-growing regions, such as the face, the distal part of the limbs, and the pinna of the ear, and has wool-growing regions that cover most of the body. The hair-growing regions contain mostly single follicles, whereas the densely covered wool-growing regions have many compound follicles. The typical follicle cluster contains three single primary hair follicles and several secondary hair follicles. In goats, the single primary hair follicles occur in groups of three; three to six secondary hair follicles are associated with each group.

Sinus or **tactile hair follicles** of the head (e.g., the vibrissae [whiskers] of a cat) are highly specialized for tactile sense. They are very large single follicles characterized by a blood-filled sinus between the inner and outer layers of the dermal root sheath (Fig. 16-19). The sinus is divided into an upper annular sinus (nontrabecular, not separated by connective tissue) and a lower cavernous sinus (trabecular, separated by connective tissue) (Fig. 16-20) except in horses and ruminants, in which the annular sinus

is traversed by fibroelastic trabeculae throughout its length. In pigs and carnivores, in the upper portion of the sinus hair follicles, the inner layer of the dermal root sheath thickens, forming a sinus pad, and this pad is surrounded by an annular sinus free of trabeculae (Fig. 16-19). Skeletal muscles are attached to the outer layer of the dermal root sheath of the follicle, allowing some voluntary control of hair movement. Numerous nerve bundles penetrate the outer layer of the dermal root sheath and ramify in the trabeculae and inner layer of the dermal root sheath.

Hair Cycle

In the surface epidermis, the process of keratinization is continuous because of the uninterrupted production of new keratinocytes, but in the hair follicle, the matrix cells undergo periods of quiescence during which no mitotic activity occurs. When the matrix cell proliferation is reinstituted, a new hair is formed. This cyclic activity of the hair bulb allows for the seasonal change in the hair coat of domestic animals. Hair requires approximately 3 to 4 months to regrow after shaving for normal or short coats and up to 18 months for long coats. The length of time varies, depending on the growth stage of the hair follicle.

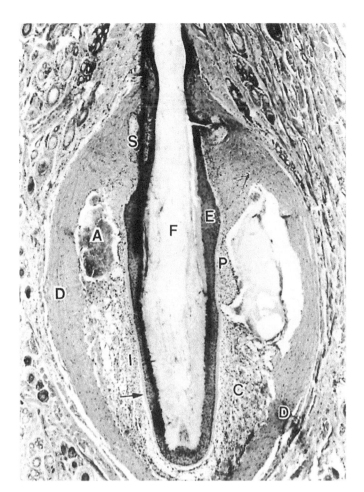

FIGURE 16-19 Sinus hair follicle (cat). Outer layer of the dermal root sheath (D); inner layer of the dermal root sheath (I); upper annular sinus filled with blood (nontrabecular) (A); cavernous blood sinus with trabeculae (C); glassy membrane (arrow); external epithelial root sheath (E); hair (F); sinus pad (P); sebaceous glands (S) opening into the pilosebaceous canal. Hematoxylin and eosin (×50).

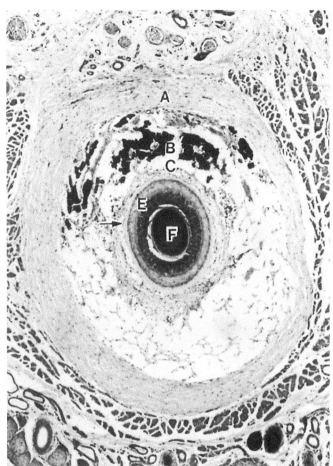

FIGURE 16-20 Cross section of a sinus hair follicle (cat). Outer layer of the dermal root sheath (A); lower cavernous blood sinus with trabeculae (B); inner layer of the dermal root sheath (C); glassy membrane (arrow); external epithelial root sheath (E); hair (F). Hematoxylin and eosin (×60).

The period during which the cells of the hair bulb are mitotically active is called **anagen** (Fig. 16-21). After this growth phase, the hair follicles go through a regressive stage, referred to as **catagen.** During this period, metabolic activity slows down, and the base of the follicle migrates upward in the skin toward the epidermal surface, until all that remains of the bulb is a flimsy, disorganized column of cells, or club hair. The hair follicle then enters **telogen,** a resting or quiescent phase in which growth stops and the base of the bulb is at the level of the sebaceous canal. After the resting phase, mitotic activity and keratinization start again in the renewed anagen phase and a new hair is formed. As the new hair grows beneath the telogen follicle, it gradually pushes the old hair upward toward the surface, where it is eventually shed. This intermittent mitotic activity and keratinization of the hair matrix cells constitute the **hair cycle,** which is controlled by several factors, including length of daily periods of light, ambient temperature, nutrition, and hormones, particularly estrogen, testosterone, adrenal steroids, and thyroid hormone.

Skin Glands

Sebaceous Glands

Sebaceous glands may be simple, branched, or compound alveolar glands that release their secretory product, sebum, by the holocrine mode. **Sebum,** an oily secretion containing a mixture of lipids and disintegrated cells, acts as an antibacterial agent and, in hairy mammals, as a waterproofing agent. The sebaceous glands are most frequently associated with hair follicles, into which their ducts empty to form the pilosebaceous canal of the hair follicle (Fig. 16-19). In certain hairless areas, such as the anal canal, the teat of horses, and the internal layer of the prepuce of some species, sebaceous glands empty directly onto the skin surface through a duct lined with stratified squamous epithelium. The secretory unit consists of a solid mass of epidermal cells, enclosed by a connective-tissue sheath that blends with the surrounding dermis. At the periphery of the glandular mass, a single layer of low cuboidal cells rests on a basal lamina (Fig. 16-22). Most of the mitotic activity takes place in this layer, and as the cells move inward, they enlarge, become polygonal, and accumulate numerous lipid droplets. The

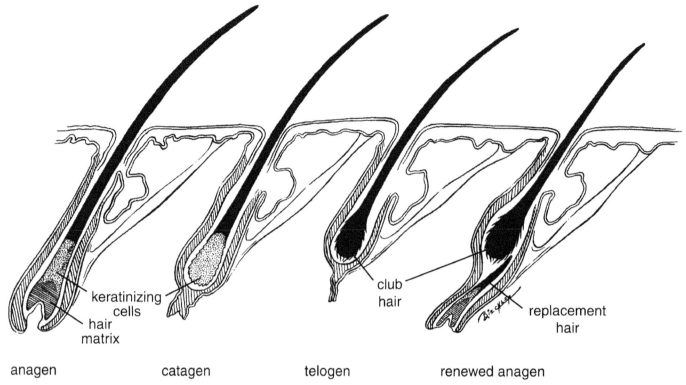

anagen   catagen   telogen   renewed anagen

FIGURE 16-21 Schematic of the three main stages of hair follicle growth and replacement.

cells near the duct contain pyknotic nuclei. The sebum passes into the lumen of the hair follicle through a short duct lined with stratified squamous epithelium. Many areas of the body of certain species have especially well-developed accumulations of sebaceous glands, some of which are associated with sweat glands. These sites include the infraorbital, inguinal, and interdigital regions of sheep,

the base of the horn of goats, anal sacs of cats, and the prepuce and circumanal region of dogs, and are described later in this chapter. Some areas of the skin, such as the foot pads, hoofs, claws, and horn, lack sebaceous glands.

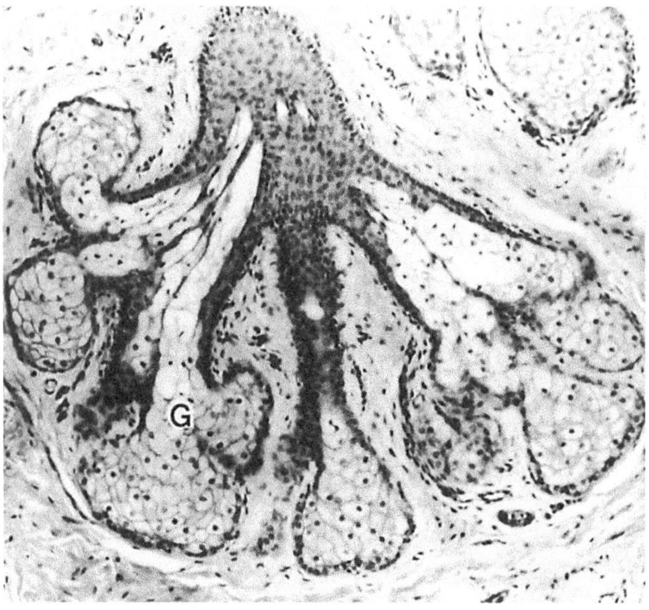

Sweat Glands

Based on their mode of release of the secretory product, sweat (sudoriferous) glands are classified into two types: apocrine and merocrine (eccrine). The apocrine type is the most extensively developed in the domestic mammals. The structure of apocrine sweat glands varies considerably among species, and whether the apocrine mode of secretion occurs in all sweat glands designated as apocrine and in all domestic species is uncertain. Nevertheless, the term apocrine is retained, primarily for didactic reasons.

The **apocrine sweat glands** are simple saccular or tubular glands with a coiled secretory portion and a straight duct (simple coiled tubular glands). The secretory portion has a large lumen lined with flattened cuboidal to low columnar epithelial cells, depending on the stage of their secretory activity (Fig. 16-23). The cytoplasm may contain glycogen, lipid, or pigment granules. The free surface of cells in apocrine sweat glands has varying cytoplasmic protrusions, indicative of secretory activity. Myoepithelial cells are located between the secretory cells and the basal lamina. The duct pursues a straight course toward the upper part of the dermis. It has a narrow lumen and two layers of flattened cuboidal cells. Most frequently, the duct penetrates the epidermis of the hair follicle just before it opens onto the surface of the skin. The apocrine glands in the domestic animals are located throughout most of the skin. This characteristic contrasts with their distribution in

FIGURE 16-22 Multilobular sebaceous glands (G) of the labium (horse). Hematoxylin and eosin (×110).

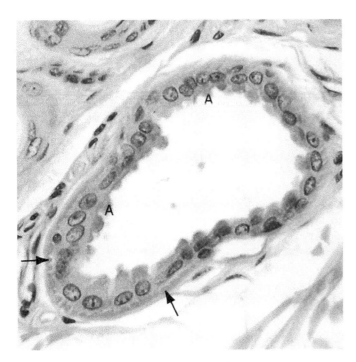

FIGURE 16-23 Apocrine sweat gland from a dog, illustrating myoepithelial cells (arrows) and apical secretory caps (A). Hematoxylin and eosin (×660).

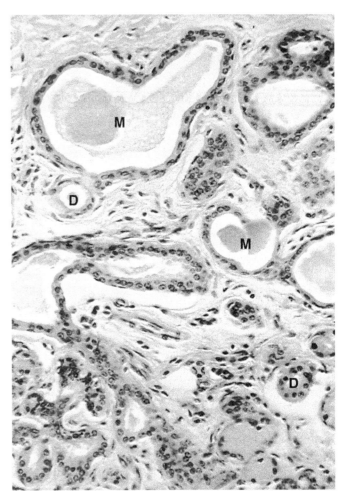

FIGURE 16-24 Merocrine sweat glands (M) and ducts (D) from the nasolabial plane (cow). Hematoxylin and eosin (×300).

humans, in which they are mainly in the axillary, pubic, and perianal regions. In horses, these glands secrete abundantly and produce visible sweat during exercise and at high temperature. In other species, the secretion is scant and rarely perceptible. In dogs and cats, the glands may be tortuous or serpentine, and in ruminants, the lumen is dilated, giving the appearance of large saccules. The apocrine glands are least active in goats and cats. The function of apocrine glands is to produce a viscous secretion that contains a scent that is related to communications between species, probably as a sex attractant or as a territorial marker. Apocrine glands in several areas of the body are specialized in structure and function and are described later in this chapter.

The **merocrine** (eccrine) **sweat glands** are found mainly in special skin areas, such as the foot pads of dogs and cats, the frog of horse hoofs, the planum rostrale of pigs, the carpal glands of swine, and the bovine planum nasolabiale (Fig. 16-24). They are simple tubular glands that open directly onto the skin surface rather than into hair follicles. The secretory portion is composed of cuboidal epithelium with two distinct cell types. **Dark cells** have more ribosomes than the clear cells, and numerous mucin droplets occur in the apical part of the cell. In contrast, **clear cells** lack cytoplasmic basophilia, contain lipid inclusions, and produce aqueous sweat. At the base of these cells, there is an infolding of the plasma membrane, which suggests that they play a role in electrolyte transport. Intercellular canaliculi occur between adjacent clear cells and course from the lumen to the base of the epithelium. Myoepithelial cells surround the secretory units and aid in emptying the gland of secretion. The duct, which is composed of two layers of cuboidal epithelial cells, is relatively straight and opens directly onto the surface of the epidermis.

BLOOD VESSELS, LYMPH VESSELS, AND NERVES

Terminal branches of the cutaneous arteries give rise to three plexuses: (a) the deep or **subcutaneous plexus,** which in turn gives off branches to the (b) middle or **cutaneous plexus,** which provides branches to make up the (c) superficial or **subpapillary plexus** (Fig. 16-1). The reverse applies for venous return to the cutaneous veins. By this arrangement, all components of the skin are ensured an adequate blood supply. The superficial plexus also furnishes the capillary loops that extend into the dermal papillae when present. Lymph capillaries arise in the superficial dermis and form a network that drains into a subcutaneous plexus.

The nerve supply to the skin varies in different parts of the body. Small subcutaneous nerves give rise to a nerve plexus that pervades the dermis and sends small branches to the epidermis. Several kinds of endings are present: free afferent nerve endings in the epidermis and dermis (encircle hair follicles); free efferent endings in the hypodermis (at arrector pili muscles, glands, and blood vessels); nonencapsulated tactile corpuscles (Merkel cells); and encapsulated tactile (Meissner's) corpuscles (see Chapter 6).

Lamellar (pacinian) corpuscles have been observed in the frog of the equine hoof, the digital cushion of the dog and cat, and the anal sac wall of the cat.

SPECIAL STRUCTURES OF THE INTEGUMENT

External Ear

The pinna (auricle) of the ear is covered on both sides by thin skin containing sweat and sebaceous glands and hair follicles (Fig. 16-25). The convex surface of the pinna usually has more hair follicles per unit area than does the concave surface. Blood vessels traverse perforations in the elastic cartilage that forms the core of the pinna. Trauma to or even bending of the cartilage can damage the blood vessels and may cause subcutaneous hematomas in ears of dogs.

The lumen of the external acoustic meatus is irregular in contour, the result of several permanent skin folds. The skin that lines the canal contains small hair follicles, sebaceous glands, and **ceruminous glands.** Ceruminous glands are simple coiled tubular apocrine sweat glands. The ceruminous glands open either into hair follicles or onto the surface. They increase in number in the lower third of the meatus. The combination of sebum, ceruminous gland secretion, and the desquamating stratified squa-

mous epithelium forms the **cerumen** or ear wax. The external acoustic meatus is supported by elastic cartilage in the outer portion and by bone near the tympanic membrane.

Eyelids

The outermost covering of both upper and lower eyelids is typical skin containing sweat and sebaceous glands and hair follicles (Fig. 16-26). The cilia, also known as eyelashes, and their associated sebaceous glands (glands of Zeis) are numerous in the upper lid of all species except cats. In the lower eyelid, the cilia are fewer in number in ruminants and horses and are generally absent in cats, dogs, and pigs. Tactile hairs may be present on or near the eyelids. The inner surface of the eyelids, the palpebral conjunctiva, is a mucous membrane and contains lymphatic tissue at its base (conjunctival fornix). Its epithelial covering varies with the area and species from stratified squamous epithelium near the edge of the eyelid to various combinations of columnar, cuboidal, polyhedral, and squamous cells. As a result, it is variously described as stratified squamous, stratified cuboidal, strat-

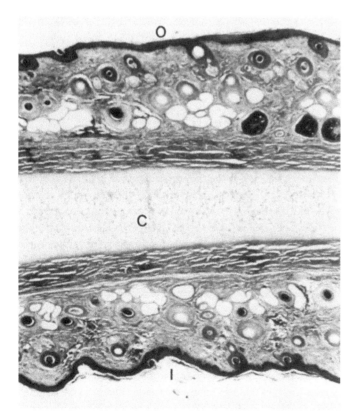

FIGURE 16-25 Auricula of the ear (cow). Outer surface (O); inner surface (I); auricular elastic cartilage (C). Masson's Trichrome (×30)

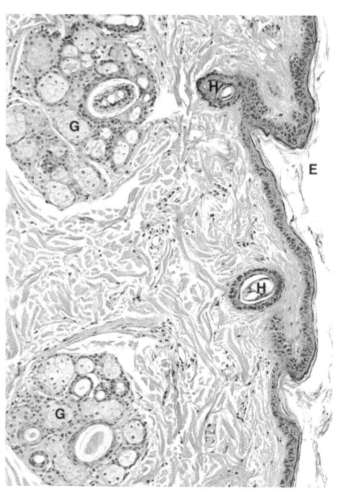

FIGURE 16-26 Upper eyelid (dog), anterior or skin surface (E). Numerous hairs (H) and sebaceous glands (G) are present. Hematoxylin and eosin (×50).

ified columnar, and transitional or pseudostratified. Goblet cells are often present (Fig. 16-27).

The most characteristic feature of the eyelids is the **tarsal glands** (meibomian glands), which are better developed in the upper lid (Fig. 16-28). They are multilobular sebaceous glands with a central duct, which opens at the margin of the eyelid. These glands are most highly developed in the cat and poorly developed in swine. The tarsal glands are surrounded by the **tarsal plate,** a compact layer of collagen and elastic fibers. Skeletal muscle fibers from the orbicular muscle (orbicularis oculi) penetrate the eyelid, and scattered bundles of smooth muscle fibers are also present.

Apocrine sweat glands, referred to as **ciliary glands** (glands of Moll), open rostrally to the tarsal glands and near the cilia or into the follicles of the cilia. Unlike ordinary sweat glands, the terminal portions of ciliary glands are only slightly coiled, and the gland lumina are more dilated. They are lined by typical cylindric secretory and myoepithelial cells. Their structure and location are similar in all domestic animals, but their function is obscure.

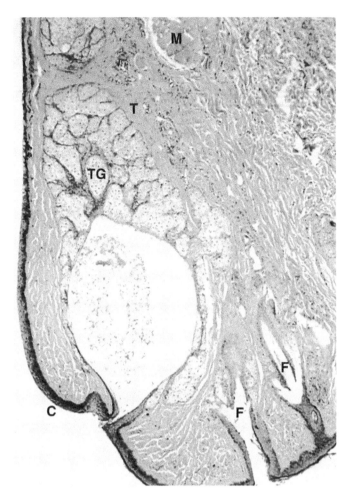

FIGURE 16-28 Tarsal gland in the upper eyelid (dog). Multilobular sebaceous tarsal gland (TG) in longitudinal section surrounded by the tarsal plate (T), skeletal muscle (M), and hair follicles (F). The conjunctival surface (C) is nonkeratinized stratified squamous epithelium. Hematoxylin and eosin (×40).

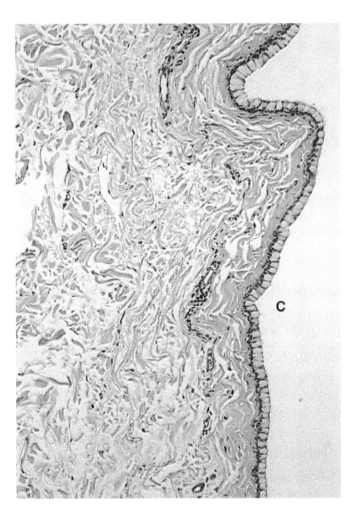

FIGURE 16-27 Upper eyelid (dog). Posterior or conjunctival surface (C) with pseudostratified epithelium with many goblet cells. Hematoxylin and eosin (×150).

Infraorbital Sinus

The infraorbital sinus of sheep, located medially and rostrally to the eye, is lined with thin skin that contains few hairs, large sebaceous glands that form a continuous layer around the sinus, and a few peripherally located apocrine sweat glands. The secretions of these glands are responsible for the sticky, yellow fatty substance on the skin.

Nose

The skin around the external openings (nares) of the nasal cavity is slightly modified in each species. The planum nasolabiale of cattle has a smooth, thick keratinized epidermis (Fig. 16-29), whereas the planum nasale of dogs and cats is composed of a thick, keratinized epidermis with distinct elevations and grooves. These characteristics provide the basis for identification by nose printing, similar to fingerprinting. Neither sweat nor sebaceous glands are associated with the planum nasale. The skin around the nos-

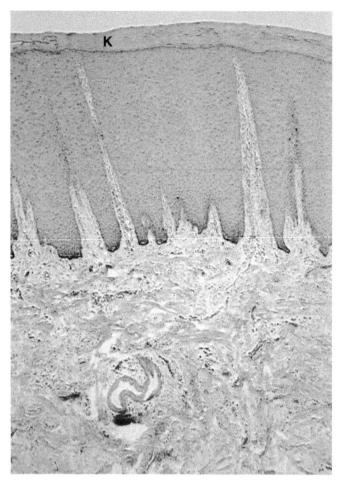

FIGURE 16-29 Planum nasolabiale (cow). Notice the thickened keratinized stratified squamous epithelium (K). Hematoxylin and eosin (×50).

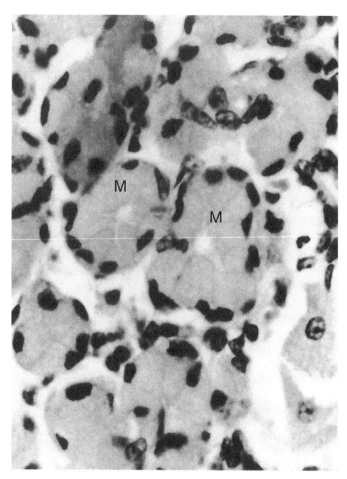

FIGURE 16-30 Merocrine glands (M) of the nasolabial region (cow). Hematoxylin and eosin (×780).

tril of horses is usually thin and contains fine hairs and numerous sebaceous glands. The planum rostrale of pigs has tactile (sinus) hairs distributed over the surface and numerous large merocrine sweat glands. The planum nasale of small ruminants and the planum nasolabiale of large ruminants contain no hair follicles but have large merocrine glands (Fig. 16-30) with the same morphologic characteristics as salivary glands. The secretion from these glands aids in keeping the nasolabial plane moist.

Mental Organ

The **mental organ** of pigs consists of a large spherical mass of apocrine and sebaceous glands with a few tactile hairs located midway between the mandibles behind the angle of the chin. Tactile (Meissner's) corpuscles and nerve fibers are present in the dermis and, therefore, are believed to play a role in transmitting mechanical stimuli.

Submental Organ

The **submental organ** of cats, located in the intermandibular space, is composed of sebaceous gland lobules, each containing a central collecting space. These lobules are surrounded by skeletal muscle. Cats rub this gland on specific items during olfactory marking and the sebaceous scent is transferred to the rubbed object.

Carpal Glands

The **carpal glands** of pigs are accumulations of numerous lobules of densely packed merocrine sweat glands on the medial surface of the carpus. They open to the skin surface through three to five diverticula lined with stratified squamous epithelium. Each lobule is drained by a duct lined with a bilayered cuboidal epithelium, which pursues a tortuous course through the dermis and epidermis and then opens into a diverticulum.

Interdigital Sinus

The **interdigital sinus** of sheep is located between the digits just above the hoofs. The opening of the sinus is at the dorsal tip of the interdigital space. The skin of the sinus contains a few hair follicles, associated sebaceous glands, and numerous large apocrine glands collectively referred to as the **interdigital glands**.

Inguinal Sinus

The **inguinal sinus** of sheep is a cutaneous diverticulum in the inguinal region of both sexes that contains scattered small hair follicles, sebaceous glands, and apocrine glands.

Scrotum

Generally, scrotal skin is thinner than skin on other parts of the body. Sebaceous and apocrine sweat glands are present but differ in size and number in various species. Boars have only a few small apocrine sweat glands in the scrotal skin, whereas stallions have both large sebaceous glands and well-developed apocrine sweat glands. The amount of pigment varies with species and breed. Short, fine hair is characteristic of scrotal skin of all species. The **tunica dartos** is a unique layer of smooth muscle and fibroelastic connective tissue within the subcutaneous tissue of the scrotum. These muscle fibers play an important role in the regulation of testicular temperature.

Anal Sacs

The **anal sacs** (sinus paranales) of domestic carnivores are paired cutaneous diverticula, the ducts of which open into the anal canal at the level of the anocutaneous line (Fig. 16-31). The ducts and sacs are lined by keratinized stratified squamous epithelium. The **glands of the anal sac,** modified sweat glands located beneath the epithelium, empty into the lumen of the anal sac. Both sebaceous and apocrine sweat glands are present in the wall of the anal sac in cats (Fig. 16-32), but dogs have only large apocrine sweat glands. The anal sac duct of dogs is prone to occlusion, which results in anal sac engorgement with secretory material and detritus. The infection that frequently follows this occlusion necessitates either the expression of the content of the sac or the surgical removal of the sac. This problem is rare in cats, probably because the sebaceous glands within the wall of the sac add sufficient amounts of lipid to the secretory material, consequently decreasing the possibility of occlusion of the duct. The secretion of these glands is a brownish and oily fluid that may function in social recognition in dogs and can have a pungent odor with impaction and infection. **Anal glands,** which empty into the anal canal, are discussed in Chapter 10.

Circumanal Glands

The **circumanal glands** of dogs are lobulated, modified sebaceous glands located around the anus in the cutaneous zone (Fig. 16-33). They extend from the mucocutaneous junction peripherally for approximately 1 to 3 cm in all directions. Similar glands have been described in the skin of the prepuce, tail, loin, and groin.

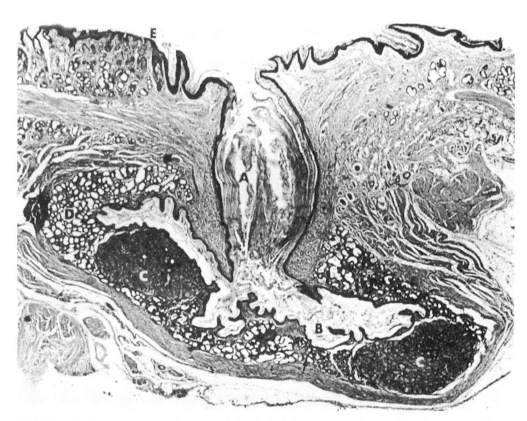

FIGURE 16-31   Anal sac and associated glands (cat). Duct (A) and lumen (B) of the anal sac filled with keratinized epithelial fragments and secretory material. Sebaceous gland masses (C); apocrine anal sac glands (D); linea anocutanea (E). Hematoxylin and eosin (×17). *(From Greer MB, Calhoun ML. The anal sacs of the domestic cat—Felis domesticus. Am J Vet Res 1966;27:773.)*

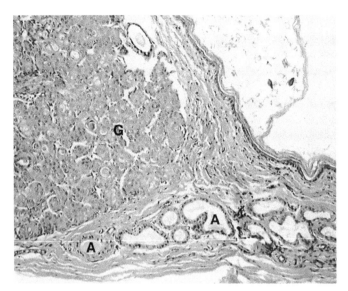

FIGURE 16-32   Higher magnification of the anal sac (cat). Note the large apocrine glands (A) and sebaceous glands (G). Hematoxylin and eosin (×100).

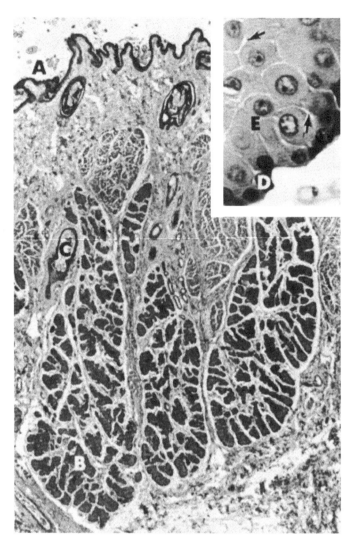

FIGURE 16-33   Circumanal glands (dog). Cutaneous zone (A); hepatoid circumanal gland (B); duct (C). Hematoxylin and eosin (×20). Inset, peripheral cells (D); nonsebaceous gland cells (E); intercellular canaliculi (arrows). Hematoxylin and eosin (×480).

These glands are present shortly after birth, increase in size throughout adult life, and tend to atrophy at senility. The superficial portion of the circumanal glands consists of typical sebaceous glands, whereas the deep portion is ductless and composed of solid, compact masses of polygonal cells arranged in lobules. The cells have granular eosinophilic cytoplasm and intercellular canaliculi (Fig. 16-33). The term **hepatoid** has been used to describe the glandular parenchyma of each lobule because it resembles closely packed liver cells. A precise function for these glands has not been determined; however, they may be involved in the metabolism of a steroid hormone. The circumanal glands are clinically important because they rank third in frequency as a site of canine tumors.

Supracaudal Gland

The **supracaudal gland** (tail gland or preen gland), located in an oval circumscribed area on the dorsum of the tail (3 to 9 cm from base of the tail) in dogs and cats, is an accumulation of large sebaceous glands that empty into single hair follicles (Fig. 16-34). The apocrine sweat glands in this region are rudimentary. Well-developed arrector pili muscles appear as large bundles of smooth muscle. The epidermis above this gland is extremely thin, and the structure of this gland is similar to the superficial portion of the circumanal glands. The secretion may aid in olfactory recognition, and it can cause a matting of the hair of the region, especially if the glands are overactive. This matting can present a problem in show cats, because the appearance of the hair coat of the tail is affected.

Mammary Gland

Knowledge of the microscopic anatomy of the mammary gland is important to the understanding of mastitis in large animals and mammary tumors in small animals. Mastitis is inflammation of this gland and is one of the most common and economically significant clinical diseases in the cow. In response to bacterial infection, inflammatory changes occur in the gland with influx of many bloodborne neutrophils.

The mammary gland is a compound tubuloalveolar gland (Fig. 16-35). Groups of tubuloalveolar secretory units form lobules separated by connective-tissue septa.

Alveoli

Secretory alveoli of the mammary gland are spherical to ovoid in shape with a large lumen (Figs. 16-35 and 16-36). Continuous milk production enlarges the lumen, and adjacent alveoli may fuse partially (Fig. 16-36). Shortly after milking, as the alveolus begins a new secretory cycle, the lumen is partially collapsed and irregular in outline.

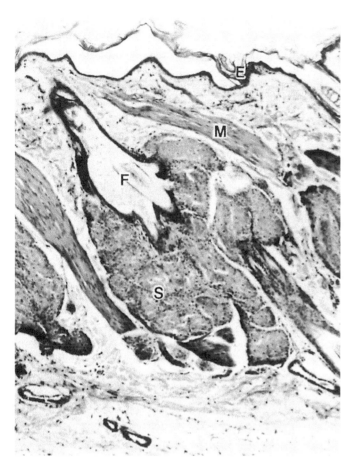

FIGURE 16-34 Supracaudal gland, tail region (cat). Thin epidermis (E), sebaceous glands (S), and ducts opening into hair follicles (F), and large bundles of smooth muscle (M). Hematoxylin and eosin (×80).

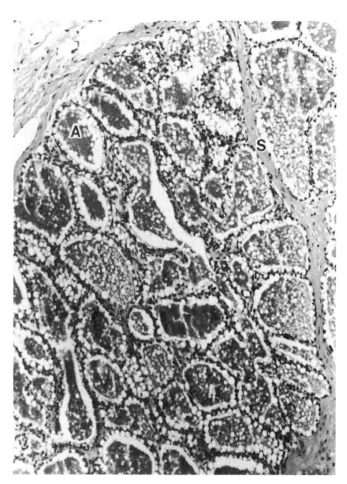

FIGURE 16-36 Lactating mammary gland filled with colostrum (sheep). Alveolus (A); interlobular septum (S). Hematoxylin and eosin (×120)

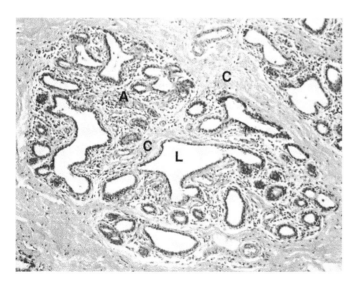

FIGURE 16-35 Nonlactating mammary gland (cow). Gland lobules with alveoli (A); large irregular openings representing intralobular ducts (L); and loose connective tissue (C). Hematoxylin and eosin (×100).

Clusters of alveoli form lobules within the gland. All the lobules are not in the same secretory phase at the same time. Some lobules may complete their secretory cycle and be filled with milk before others begin. Therefore, a single histologic section may contain lobules in various stages of activity. Usually, all of the secretory alveoli within a lobule are in approximately the same secretory phase.

The epithelium of the alveoli varies markedly in height during various stages of secretory activity. During active secretion, the basal portion of the columnar epithelial cells contains a well-developed rough endoplasmic reticulum. The spherical nuclei are located near the center of the cell. Lipid droplets, in close association with mitochondria, and vesicles, filled with micelles of milk protein, occur throughout the cell apex. As the secretory cycle continues, the lipid droplets move toward the cell surface that protrudes into the alveolar lumen. The lipid droplets are released from the cell, surrounded by varying amounts of cytoplasm and the plasmalemma. The protein-filled vesicles also move toward the cell surface, where they are released by exocytosis. Milk is thus produced by both apocrine and merocrine secretion. At the end of the secretory cycle, the epithelial cells are low cuboidal in shape.

Myoepithelial cells, surrounding the alveolar epithelial cells, contract in response to oxytocin released from the neurohypophysis. The contraction forces the milk from the secretory units into the duct system. This phenomenon is called **milk letdown.**

Interstitium

The interstitial tissue of the mammary gland provides important structural support for the secretory units and contains the blood vessels, lymph vessels, and nerves. Each secretory unit is surrounded by loose connective tissue with an extensive plexus of blood and lymph capillaries. Plasma cells and lymphocytes are common, particularly at parturition when the immunoglobulin-rich colostrum is secreted. The interlobular connective tissue is thick and contains the interlobular ducts and larger blood and lymph vessels.

Ducts

The duct system begins with an **intralobular duct** (Fig. 16-35), which drains into an **interlobular duct.** The interlobular duct, in turn, drains into a **lactiferous duct,** which is the primary excretory duct for a lobe. The intralobular duct epithelium is simple cuboidal. Spindle-shaped myoepithelial cells may be associated with these ducts. Interlobular ducts are lined proximally by a simple cuboidal epithelium and, more distally, by two layers of cuboidal cells. Longitudinal smooth muscle fibers become associated with these ducts as they merge with other interlobular ducts to form the large lactiferous ducts. The two-layered cuboidal epithelium continues in these larger ducts, and smooth muscle becomes more prominent. Sacculations result from variations in the diameter of the lumen. The constrictions between these sacculations may have an annular fold containing smooth muscle. Several lactiferous ducts empty into a **lactiferous sinus** (gland sinus) at the base of the teat.

Teat

The **teat,** or nipple, contains the terminal part of the duct system. The lactiferous sinus is continuous with the **teat sinus** (teat cistern, cavity of the teat), which is lined by stratified cuboidal epithelium. The lamina propria of the teat sinus may contain small clusters of mammary gland tissue. Smooth muscle bundles, oriented parallel to the long axis of the teat, are prominent in some species and form the boundary between the teat mucosa and the surrounding dermis of the skin. Numerous blood vessels in the dermis form a vascular stratum, which becomes engorged with blood during the milking or suckling process; thus, the overlying skin of the teat is stretched, resulting in a smooth surface. After milking, when the blood has drained from the teat vessels and the longitudinal smooth muscle has contracted, the teat surface returns to its typical corrugated appearance.

An annular fold of the mucosa extends into the opening between the lactiferous sinus and teat sinus. The size of this opening is somewhat variable from one animal to another. Occasionally, trabeculae of connective tissue may extend across the opening, resulting in reduction of milk flow from the lactiferous sinus to the teat sinus. These trabeculae are called "spiders," and frequently, veterinarians must cut them surgically.

The teat sinus empties into one or more **papillary ducts** (teat canal, streak canal) leading to the external surface of the teat. A single papillary duct is present in ruminants while multiple papillary ducts open separately onto the teat surface of other species. Horses have 2 papillary ducts, pigs have 2 to 3, cats have 4 to 7, and dogs have 7 to 16. The papillary duct is lined with stratified squamous epithelium. Circularly oriented bundles of smooth muscle in the mucosa form a sphincter to hold the milk in the teat sinus above the duct until it is forced out by milking or suckling.

The skin of the teat in cows and sows is composed of a thick, keratinized stratified squamous epithelium and dermis without hair follicles and sweat or sebaceous glands. However, in some domestic species, such as sheep and goats, the teat may contain fine hairs and sweat and sebaceous glands.

Mammary Gland Involution

After the lactation period or sudden arrest of suckling or milking, glandular involution begins. The alveoli are distended by accumulated milk and no further secretion occurs until they are emptied. It was once believed that if the secretory product were not removed for several days, the epithelial cells would degenerate and the residual milk in the lumen would be absorbed gradually. However, recent research has suggested less loss of mammary epithelial cells than previously believed. Characteristically, the involuted mammary gland has more interstitial tissue than glandular elements, and isolated clusters of branched tubules with a few small alveoli are all that remain of the parenchyma (Fig. 16-35). The alveoli are lined by a low cuboidal epithelium with prominent underlying myoepithelial cells. The connective-tissue septa are thicker, and fat cells may occur singly or in clusters. Lymphocytes and plasma cells are present in significant numbers. Small, dark-staining bodies of casein (corpora amylacea) may be found in the alveoli, ducts, or interstitial tissue.

DIGITAL ORGANS AND HORN

The digital organ consists of a keratinized epidermis, underlying dermis, and a hypodermis of variable thickness. Hard keratin, or horn, forms the keratinized portion of the hoofs of horses, ruminants, and pigs and the claws of carnivores. The dermis (corium) contains blood vessels and nerves. The hypodermis is absent in some regions of the digit (hoof wall, sole, claw), but in the ground contact region, the hypodermis is modified to form the digital cushion located deep to the dermis. Bones and their associated ligaments and tendons form the supportive structure of the digit.

Equine Hoof

The epidermis of the skin on the equine limb continues distally as the **periople,** a ring of epidermis that produces soft, nonpigmented tubular and intertubular horn above the coronary border of the hoof. Toward the back of the foot, the periople widens into a broad keratinized layer or **bulb** (heel). From the periople, the epidermis angles internally to line the **coronary groove**. Finally, **epidermal laminae** extend vertically from the coronary groove to the ground surface of the hoof.

The dermis of the hoof is usually referred to as the **corium**. **Perioplic corium** is continuous with **coronary corium**, anchoring epidermal structures (periople and coronary epidermis) to underlying tissues. The **laminar corium** interdigitates with the epidermal laminae and fills the space between the laminae and the distal phalanx. The corium is composed of bundles of coarse collagen fibers and a massive network of large arteries and veins without valves. This vascular bed helps to dampen the compressive forces transmitted from the hard inflexible hoof to the phalanx.

The keratinized portion of the equine hoof is composed of three main parts. The wall (paries) is that portion that is visible when the foot is placed on the ground. The sole (solea) forms the greatest part of the ventral surface of the foot; the frog (cuneus ungulae) is a wedge-shaped structure that projects into the sole.

Wall

The **wall** of the hoof is composed of three layers (Fig. 16-37). From the outside inward, they are the **stratum externum** (tectorium), the **stratum medium**, and the **stratum internum** (lamellatum). Each of these is structurally distinct and is described separately in the following paragraphs.

The **stratum externum** is a thin layer of tubular and intertubular horn, which is a continuation of the stratum corneum of the perioplic epidermis. This layer covers the outer surface of the hoof wall.

The **stratum medium** consists of tubular and intertubular "hard" horn and is the main supportive structure of the wall (Fig. 16-38). The **horny tubules** are solid rods and are oriented parallel to the outer surface of the hoof, and their keratinized cells have a highly ordered arrangement. The cross-sectional profiles of the tubules may be circular, oval, or wedge-shaped and have a central region (**medulla**) of loose keratinized cells similar to the medulla of a hair shaft and a peripheral cortex of more compact keratinized cells. The **cortex** of the tubule has three zones (Fig. 16-39). The **inner zone** contains keratinized cells oriented around the medulla in fairly tight coils; the cells of the **middle zone** form loose spirals; and the cells of the **outer zone** form another layer of tight coils. This coiled, springlike arrangement of the cells of tubular horn helps dampen the compression of the hoof when it strikes a hard surface. The **intertubular horn** fills the spaces between the tubular horn.

The stratum medium is produced by the stratum basale and stratum spinosum of the epidermis lining the coronary groove. This epidermis covers the **coronary corium**, a bed of vascularized connective tissue with long papillae. The germinal cells covering

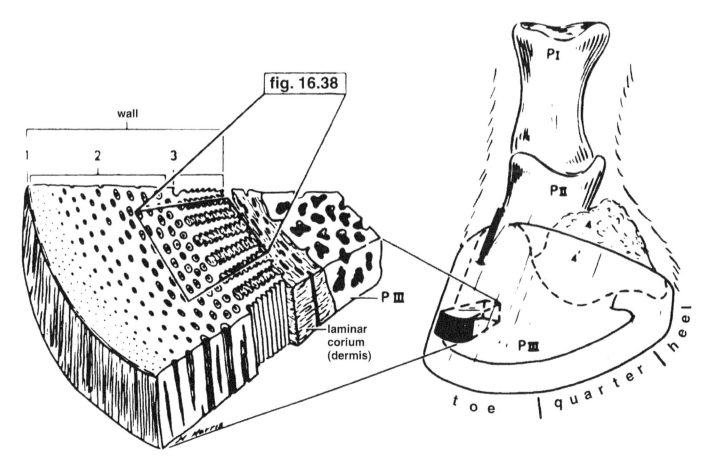

FIGURE 16-37 Equine foot (dorsolateral view). The wall of the hoof is composed of three layers: stratum externum (1), stratum medium (2), stratum internum (3). Proximal (PI), middle (PII), distal (PIII) phalanges; cartilage of the hoof (4) and (4'). (*From Stump JE. Anatomy of the normal equine foot, including microscopic features of the laminar region. J Am Vet Med Assoc 1967;151:1588.*)

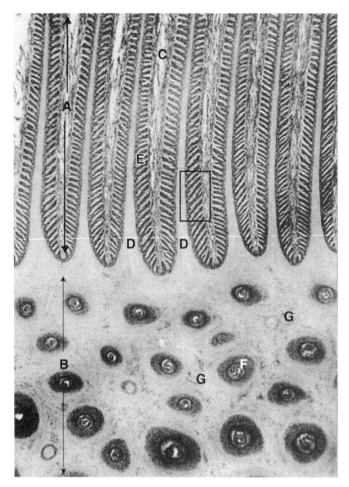

FIGURE 16-38 Wall of hoof (horse) from the area marked in Figure 16-37. Stratum internum (A); stratum medium (B); primary dermal lamina (C); primary epidermal lamina (D); secondary epidermal and dermal laminae (E); tubular horn (F); intertubular horn (G). Area in box is Figure 16-40. Hematoxylin and eosin (×38).

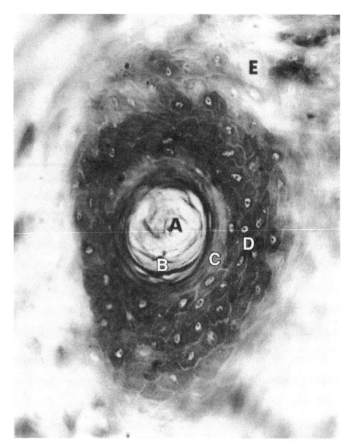

FIGURE 16-39 Stratum medium showing the cellular arrangement of tubular horn, hoof (horse). Medulla (A); inner zone of cortex (B); middle zone of cortex (C); outer zone of cortex (D); intertubular horn (E). Trichrome (×250).

the tips of the papillae give rise to loose cells of the medulla of the tubule, whereas those over the sides and base of the papillae proliferate to form the keratinized cells of the cortex. The germinal cells covering the interpapillary part of the coronary corium give rise to the intertubular horn. The layers of the intertubular horn consist of hard keratin that helps hold the tubules together. The hypodermis deep to the coronary corium is referred to as the coronary cushion. It is composed of dense collagen fibers and numerous large blood vessels.

The **stratum internum** (lamellatum) consists of approximately 600 vertically oriented, keratinized primary epidermal laminae extending inward from the stratum medium, with which they are continuous (Fig. 16-38). One hundred to 200 secondary laminae project at acute angles from each primary lamina (Fig. 16-40). These laminae interdigitate with similar laminae of the lamellar corium and form a complex epidermal–dermal association that anchors the keratinized hoof to the underlying connective tissue. The **primary epidermal laminae** are part of the stratum corneum (hard keratin) produced by the stratum germinativum located between the proximal ends of the dermal lami-

nae at the deep edge of the coronary groove. The cells keratinize as they move downward toward the ground surface of the hoof, accompanying the lengthening stratum medium. The **secondary epidermal laminae** are cellular and are composed of stratum germinativum. The stratum basale of each secondary epidermal lamina rests on the connective tissue of each **secondary dermal lamina,** forming the interdigitation between the two laminae. The central core of each secondary epidermal lamina is composed of stratum spinosum, one to three cell layers in thickness, that attaches to the sides of the keratinized primary epidermal lamina (Fig. 16-40). The germinal cells of the secondary epidermal laminae multiply throughout the length of the laminae only at a rate to keep up with the downward growth of the horny primary laminae. The wall grows in length at the rate of 6.4 mm per month; 9 to 12 months are required for the hoof to grow from the coronary border to the ground at the toe region. Growth is accomplished by the distal sliding of the stratum medium and primary epidermal laminae over the stationary secondary epidermal laminae. The interdigitation between the nonpigmented wall laminae with the pigmented tubular and intertubular horn of the sole is referred to as the **white line.**

Knowledge of the structure of the tissues of the hoof is important to the understanding of the pathophysiology of laminitis,

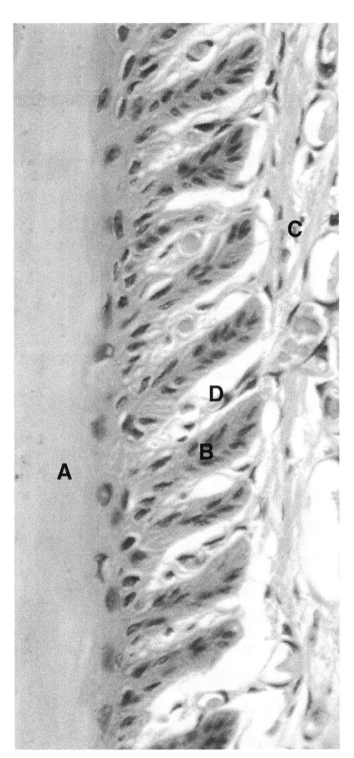

FIGURE 16-40 Secondary laminae, hoof (horse). See area marked in Figure 16-38. Primary epidermal lamina of the wall (A); secondary epidermal lamina (B); primary dermal lamina (C); secondary dermal lamina (D). Hematoxylin and eosin (×435).

the most devastating clinical disease syndrome of the equine hoof. A disturbance in the physical and physiologic (nutritional blood supply) influences on various parts of the hoof results in inflammation of the laminae, often resulting in separation of the hoof from the digit and loss of the horse.

Sole

The epidermis of the **sole** produces tubular and intertubular horn. Its superficial layers are not firmly attached and can be peeled off in the form of small flakes. The corium (dermis) of the sole bears long papillae, the epidermal covering of which gives rise to the tubular horn of the sole. In addition, the corium blends with the periosteum of the ventral surface of the distal phalanx.

Frog

The epidermis of the **frog** produces tubular and intertubular horn that is softer than that of the wall and sole. The corium (dermis) of the frog forms small short papillae. The corium blends with the **digital cushion,** which is a wedge-shaped mass of collagen and elastic fibers among masses of fat that acts as a shock absorber. Branched coiled merocrine sweat glands occur chiefly in the part that overlies the central sulcus of the frog.

Ruminant and Swine Hoofs

The hoofs of ruminants and pigs are similar to those of horses, with a few exceptions. The stratum internum and corresponding laminar corium consists of only primary laminae (Fig. 16-41).

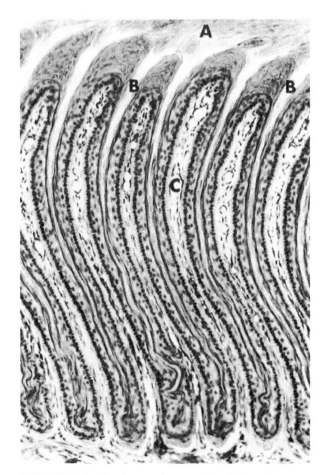

FIGURE 16-41 Stratum internum, hoof (sheep). Stratum medium (A); primary laminae (B); laminar corium with numerous capillaries (C). Hematoxylin and eosin (×120).

The sole consists of a narrow rim next to the angle of inflection of the wall. There is no frog, but a prominent bulb of soft thin horn that is continuous with the skin makes up a large part of the ventral surface of the hoof.

Claw

The **claws,** or nails, of dogs and cats are specialized structures that are continuous with the epidermis and dermis of the skin of the foot. Claws consist of shields of hard keratin that cover the distal phalanges and possess both a wall and a sole (Fig. 16-42).

The **wall** or **claw plate** covers the coronary corium and the wall corium. It is thickest in the area of the dorsal ridge and gradually thins out along the side. Its thin ventral margins extend beyond the junction of the wall with the sole. The epidermis of the dorsal ridge forms a few short laminae that interdigitate with similar dermal laminae.

The epidermis of the **sole** is thick and produces a softer form of keratin than that of the wall. A stratum granulosum and a stratum lucidum are present.

The dermis of the claw is composed of dense irregular connective tissue that forms a thick ridge over the dorsal surface of the distal phalanx. It is rich in blood vessels and prone to hemorrhage if the nail is cut too short.

The **claw fold** is a fold of skin, similar to the periople of the hoof, that covers the claw plate for a short distance on its dorsal and lateral margins. As the plate grows, it carries with it a thin layer of keratinized cells. This layer of cells is produced by the epidermis of the inner surface of the claw fold.

Digital Pads

The **digital pads** of the dog and cat are covered by a thick hairless epidermis that contains all epidermal cell layers, including a stratum lucidum. The surface is smooth in the cat (Fig. 16-43) and roughened by keratinized conical/rounded papillae in the dog (Fig. 16-44). The dermis has prominent papillae that interdigitate with the epidermal pegs and contains coiled merocrine sweat glands that extend into the digital cushion, the hypodermis. Subcutaneous masses of adipose tissue are separated and enclosed by collagen and elastic fibers.

Chestnut and Ergot

The equine **chestnut** and **ergot** have a thick epidermis composed of tubular and intertubular horn interdigitating with long dermal papillae (Fig. 16-45). Arrector pili muscles, glands, and hairs are absent in both of these structures.

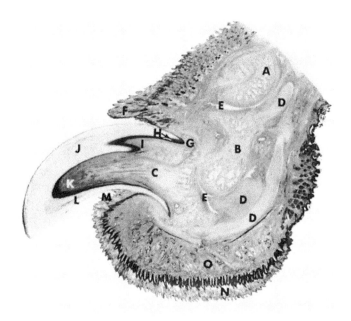

FIGURE 16-42 Claw (dog). Proximal phalanx (A); middle phalanx (B); distal phalanx (C); tendons (D); joint cavities with accompanying joint capsules and articular cartilages (E); fold of skin overlying claw (F); ungual crest (G); nonkeratinized epidermal layers of the claw (H); dorsal ridge (I); stratum corneum of the claw epidermis (J); dermis (K); sole (L); limiting furrow (M) between the sole and digital pad (N); dermis of the digital pad with clusters of coiled merocrine sweat glands and fat (O). Hematoxylin and eosin (×4). *(From Adam WS, Calhoun ML, Smith EM, et al. Microscopic Anatomy of the Dog: A Photographic Atlas. Springfield, IL: Charles C. Thomas, 1970.)*

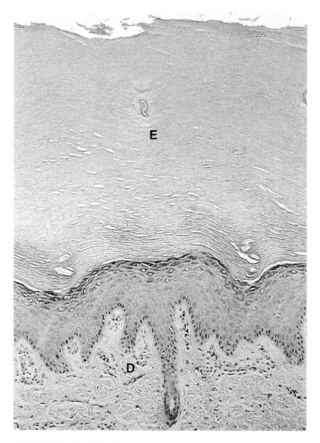

FIGURE 16-43 Foot pad (cat). The keratinized epidermis (E) is smooth and the dermis (D) is papillated. Hematoxylin and eosin (×130).

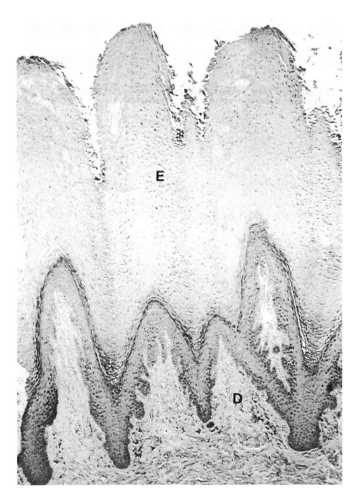

FIGURE 16-44 Foot pad (dog). The keratinized epidermis (E) is rough and the dermis (D) is papillated. Hematoxylin and eosin (×50).

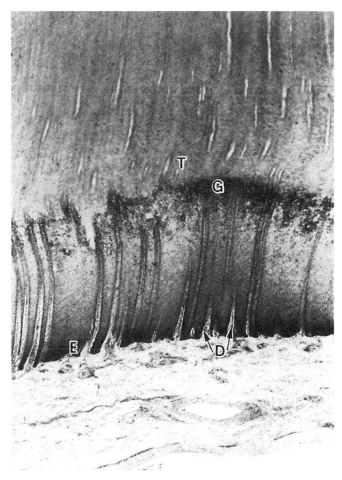

FIGURE 16-45 Chestnut (horse). Epidermal peg (E); stratum granulosum (G); dermal papillae (D); horny tubules (T). Hematoxylin and eosin (×25).

Horn

Horns of the ruminant species are actually coverings of the cornual processes of the frontal bone of the skull. The horns consist of a hard keratinized epidermis, a dermis, and a hypodermis.

The epidermis has a thick stratum corneum composed of hard tubular and intertubular horn. A thin outermost layer of soft keratin, the **epikeras,** forms at the root of the horn and is similar to the epidermis of the periople. It desquamates as keratinized scales, similar to the stratum externum of the hoof. The dermis is papillated and, together with the thin hypodermis, fills the space between the epidermis and the periosteum of the bone.

AVIAN INTEGUMENT

The avian **epidermis** is composed of keratinized stratified squamous epithelium that is similar to but thinner than that of mammals (Fig. 16-46). The epidermis of feathered skin consists of only a few cell layers (Fig. 16-47), whereas unfeathered skin is much thicker. The terminology of the epidermal cell layers is different from that in mammals. The avian layers include a **stratum**

basale, a **stratum intermedium** (actually stratum spinosum), a **stratum transitivum** (actually stratum granulosum but lacks keratohyalin granules), and a **stratum corneum.** The term **stratum germinativum** is also used to represent all the cell layers except for the stratum corneum. The avian integument is sometimes referred to as an organ of lipogenesis because of the extensive amount of lipid found in the epidermal cells in most avian species. The epidermis synthesizes triacylglycerols, phospholipids, wax esters, free fatty acids, monoglycerols, and diacylglycerols.

The skin of birds, unlike that of mammals, is completely aglandular, with the exception of the **uropygial gland** or preen gland (Figs. 16-48 and 16-49). This gland is a bilobed structure (Fig. 16-48) that lies dorsally at the base of the tail and opens through a papilla to the surface of the skin. This gland is considered to be analogous to the sebaceous gland in mammals because it produces a fatty and oily substance that is released by the holocrine mode of secretion and is regulated by hormonal influences (Fig. 16-49). The combination of both the uropygial gland sebum and the lipid from the epidermal cells acts as an antibacterial agent, prevents the feather keratin from drying out, and acts as a waterproofing agent.

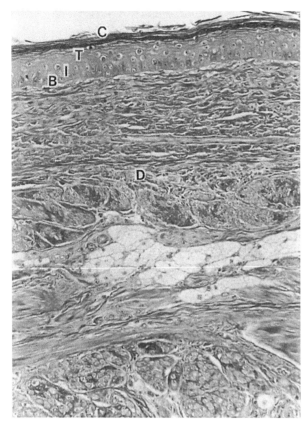

FIGURE 16-46 Unfeathered chicken skin. Note the stratum basale (B), stratum intermedium (I), stratum transitivum (T), and stratum corneum (C) cell layers. The dermis (D) is subdivided into layers, Hematoxylin and eosin (×250).

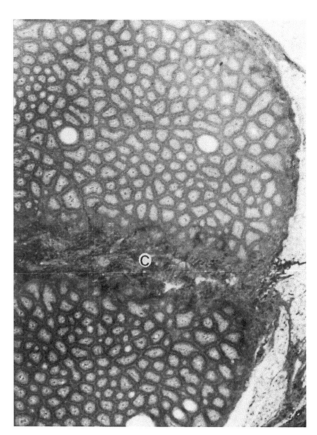

FIGURE 16-48 Uropygial gland. Note the bilobed structure separated by connective tissue (C). Hematoxylin and eosin (×35).

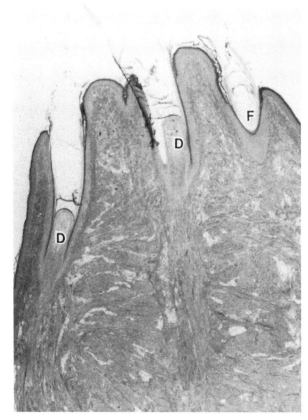

FIGURE 16-47 Feathered chicken skin. Note two developing follicles (D) and a mature follicle (F). Hematoxylin and eosin (×35).

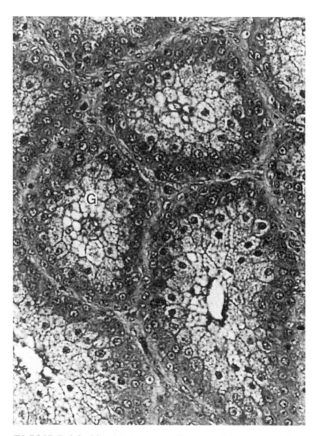

FIGURE 16-49 Higher magnification of the uropygial gland in Figure 16-48. Note the large sebaceous glands (G). Hematoxylin and eosin (×350).

Feathers are structurally similar to hair, are of epidermal origin, and develop within a follicle (Fig. 16-47). The feather consists primarily of keratin and remains in the follicle until it is plucked or molted and then a new feather develops in its place. Interfollicular muscles are common in birds and are believed to play a significant role in governing the radiative heat load by adjusting the angle of the feather.

The dermis is subdivided into the **stratum superficiale** (superficial layer); **stratum profundum** (deep layer), which includes the **stratum compactum** (dense layer) and the **stratum laxum** (loose connective tissue containing fat, large vessels, smooth muscle, and follicles); and **lamina elastica** (elastic lamina of the dermis). In addition, several smooth muscles with elastic tendons are associated with each feather follicle, and cutaneous striated muscles function in voluntary movement of the skin in response to stimuli.

The avian plantar skin does not possess all cell layers like the plantar skin of dogs and cats (Fig. 16-50). Skin from this region lacks a true stratum granulosum and has a thick smooth surface consisting of ridges of keratin.

The comb, paired wattles, and ear lobes consist of a double layer of skin with numerous blood vessels in the dermis. During mating, the vessels become congested, thereby giving a bright red appearance to the comb and wattles.

SUGGESTED READINGS

Anderson RR. Mammary gland. In: Larson BL, ed. Lactation. Ames, IA: Iowa State University Press, 1985:3.

Briggaman RA. Epidermal-dermal junction: structure, composition, function and disease relationships. In: Moshnell AN, ed. Progress in Dermatology, Part II. Evanston, IL: Dermatology Foundation, 1990:1.

Budras KD, Hullinger RL, Sack WO. Light and electron microscopy of keratinization in the laminar epidermis of the equine hoof with reference to laminitis. Am J Vet Res 1989;50:1150.

Elias PE. Epidermal lipids, barrier function, and desquamation. J Invest Dermatol 1983;80:44s.

Hodges RD. The Histology of the Fowl. New York: Academic Press, 1974:1.

Lavker RM, Sunt TT. Heterogeneity in basal keratinocytes: morphological and functional correlations. Science 1982;215:1239.

Lucas AM, Stettenheim PR. Avian Anatomy. Integument. Agricultural Handbook 362, Part II. Washington, DC: U.S. Department of Agriculture, 1972.

Marcarian HQ, Calhoun ML. The microscopic anatomy of the integument of the adult swine. Am J Vet Res 1966;27:765.

Menton DN. A liquid film model of tetrakaidecahedral packing to account for the establishment of epidermal cell columns. J Invest Dermatol 1976;66:283.

Monteiro-Riviere NA. Comparative anatomy, physiology, and biochemistry of mammalian skin. In: Hobson DW, ed. Dermal and Ocular Toxicology: Fundamentals and Methods. Boca Raton, FL: CRC Press, 1991;1:3.

Monteiro-Riviere NA. Integument. In: Pond WG, Mersmann HJ, eds. Biology of the Pig. Ithaca, NY: Cornell University Press, 2001; 14:653.

Monteiro-Riviere NA. Ultrastructural evaluation of the porcine integument. In: Tumbleson ME, ed. Swine in Biomedical Research. New York: Plenum Press, 1986;1:641.

Monteiro-Riviere NA, Bristol DG, Manning TO, et al. Interspecies and interregional analysis of the comparative histologic thickness and laser Doppler blood flow measurements at five cutaneous sites in nine species. J Invest Dermatol 1990;95:582.

Monteiro-Riviere NA, Inman AO. Indirect immunohistochemistry and immunoelectron microscopy distribution of eight epidermal-dermal junction epitopes in the pig and in isolated perfused skin treated with bis (2-chloroethyl) sulfide. Toxicol Pathol 1995;23:313.

Monteiro-Rivere NA, Stromberg MW. Ultrastructure of the integument of the domestic pig (Sus scrofa) from one through fourteen weeks of age. Anat Histol Embryol 1985;14:97.

Smith JL, Calhoun ML. The microscopic anatomy of the integument of the newborn swine. Am J Vet Res 1964;24:165.

Stromberg MW, Hwang YC, Monteiro-Riviere NA. Interfollicular smooth muscle in the skin of the domesticated pig (Sus scrofa). Anat Rec 1981;201:455.

Talukdar AH, Calhoun ML, Stinson AW. Sweat glands of the horse: a histologic study. Am J Vet Res 1970;31:2179.

Webb AJ, Calhoun ML. The microscopic anatomy of the skin of mongrel dogs. Am J Vet Res 1954;15:274.

Wolff-Schreiner EC. Ultrastructural cytochemistry of the epidermis. Int J Dermatol 1977;16:77.

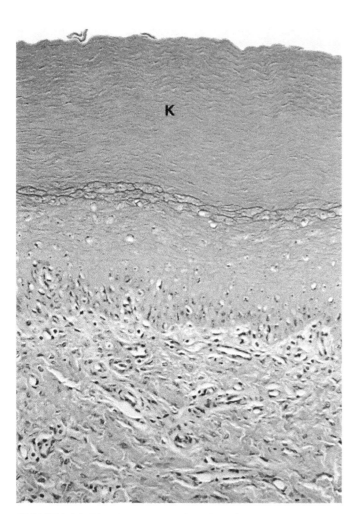

FIGURE 16-50 Avian plantar skin. Note that the thickened keratinized region (K) is smooth. Hematoxylin and eosin (×250).

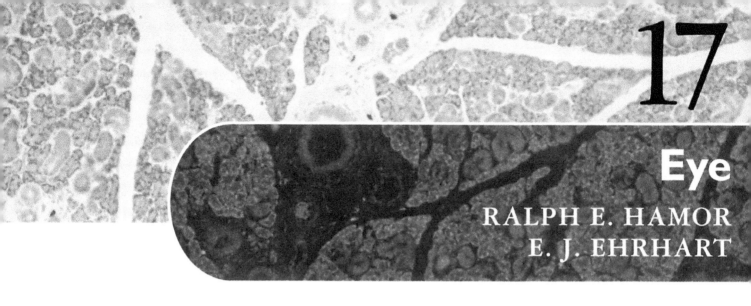

17

Eye

RALPH E. HAMOR
E. J. EHRHART

Fibrous Tunic
  Sclera
  Cornea
    Anterior epithelium
    Subepithelial basement membrane
    Substantia propria (stroma)
    Posterior limiting lamina (Descemet's membrane)
    Posterior epithelium (corneal endothelium)
  Corneoscleral Junction (Limbus)
Vascular Tunic
  Choroid
    Suprachoroid layer
    Vascular layer
    Tapetum lucidum
    Choriocapillary layer
    Basal complex
  Ciliary Body
    Ciliary epithelium
    Vascular layer

    Ciliary muscle
    Aqueous humor
  Iris
    Iridial stroma
    Iridial muscles
    Iridial epithelium
  Iridocorneal Angle
    Pectinate ligament
    Trabecular meshwork
    Venous drainage
Neuroepithelial Tunic—Retina
Refractive Media
  Lens and Zonular Fibers
  Vitreous Body
Accessory Organs
  Eyelids
  Third Eyelid and Conjunctiva
  Lacrimal Apparatus
Species Variations

The eye is located in the bony orbit, along with extraocular muscles, ligaments, adipose tissue, blood vessels, nerves, and glands. The lacrimal apparatus, the eyelids, and the third eyelid provide protection to the eye. The globe consists of three tunics that enclose chambers containing refractive media.

The three tunics of the eye are (Fig. 17-1): (1) the **fibrous**, or outer, tunic (tunica fibrosa bulbi), which is in turn subdivided into (a) the sclera, the white tough posterior portion of the globe, and (b) the cornea, the transparent portion of the fibrous tunic, which bulges slightly in the center of the anterior pole of the eye; (2) the **vascular**, or middle, tunic (tunica vasculosa bulbi), also

referred to as the uvea, composed of (a) the choroid, (b) the ciliary body, and (c) the iris; and (3) the **neuroepithelial**, or inner, tunic (tunica interna bulbi) with (a) an optic portion, the retina (pars optica retinae), containing the sensory receptors, and (b) a blind portion (pars caeca retinae) that is epithelial in nature and covers the ciliary body (pars ciliaris retinae) and the posterior surface of the iris (pars iridica retinae).

The **anterior chamber** (camera anterior bulbi) is located between the cornea and the iris. The **posterior chamber** (camera posterior bulbi) is located between the iris and the vitreous body and contains the lens. Both the anterior and posterior

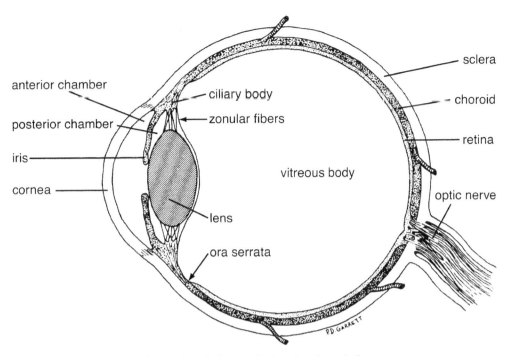

FIGURE 17-1 Schematic drawing of a longitudinal section through the eye.

chambers are filled with aqueous humor. The **vitreous chamber** (camera vitrea bulbi) of the eye, located between the lens and the retina, is filled with the vitreous body.

FIBROUS TUNIC

Sclera

The **sclera** is a layer of dense irregular connective tissue that protects the eye and maintains its form (shape). While the size of the globe can be quite variable in different species, the shape is essentially spherical. Some ungulates, such as the horse and large ruminant, have globes that are slightly compressed in the anteroposterior axis. Thickness of the sclera varies in different parts of the eye and among species. The sclera is thinnest at the equator of the globe. The sclera is thickest at the limbus (junction of the cornea and sclera) in dogs and cats and in the region of the optic nerve in ungulates. The sclera contains primarily collagen fibers but elastic fibers, fibrocytes, and melanocytes (anteriorly) are interlaced among the collagen fibers. These fibers are arranged meridionally, obliquely, and radially in an irregular pattern. In the layer of the sclera adjacent to the choroid, elastic fibers predominate, and fibroblasts and melanocytes are more numerous; this layer is referred to as the **lamina fusca sclerae.**

The orbital fasciae, located outside the sclera, consist of the periorbita (connected to the external or dural sheath of the optic nerve), the bulbar sheath (Tenon's capsule), and the fascial sheaths of the extraocular muscles. A firm attachment to the sclera is provided for the tendons of the extraocular muscles through the interweaving of tendon and scleral fibers. The optic nerve leaves the eye through numerous perforations in a sievelike area of the sclera referred to as the **area cribrosa.**

Cornea

The transparent **cornea** is a convex–concave lens, slightly thicker at the periphery than at the center, and with a smaller radius of curvature centrally than peripherally. Because the cornea also has a radius of curvature smaller than that of the sclera, it is more curved than the sclera. The horizontal corneal diameter is greater than the vertical corneal diameter, resulting in a mildly elliptical shape.

The cornea is composed of five layers: (a) anterior epithelium, (b) subepithelial basement membrane, (c) substantia propria, or stroma, (d) posterior limiting lamina (Descemet's membrane), and (e) posterior epithelium (corneal endothelium).

Anterior Epithelium

The **anterior** (corneal) **epithelium** is nonkeratinized stratified squamous, between 4 and 12 layers in thickness (Fig. 17-2).

In the dog, cat, and bird, the corneal epithelium consists of a single layer of basal cells, two to three layers of polyhedral (wing) cells, and two to three layers of nonkeratinized squamous cells. Large animals have more layers of polyhedral and squamous cells. The epithelial cells are tightly packed, interdigitate profusely, and adhere through numerous desmosomes. The numerous microvilli on the surface of the superficial cells function to retain the tear film on the corneal surface. Numerous free nerve endings are present among the epithelial cells.

The regenerative capability of injured corneal epithelium is pronounced; mitotic divisions, along with cell movements, ensure a rapid return of injured epithelium to normal structure. An intact epithelium is necessary for maintenance of corneal transparency.

Subepithelial Basement Membrane

The **subepithelial basement membrane** consists of a basal lamina and a layer of reticular fibers. The basal cell layer of the epi-

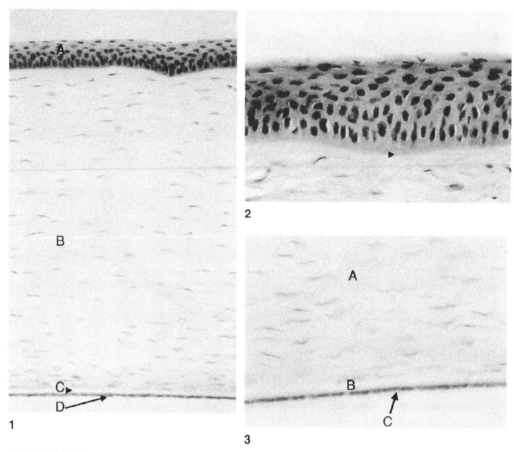

FIGURE 17-2 Cornea (dog). **1.** Corneal epithelium (A); substantia propria (B); posterior limiting lamina (C); posterior epithelium (D). Hematoxylin and eosin (×250). **2.** The corneal nonkeratinized stratified squamous epithelium is separated from the substantia propria by a rather thick basement membrane (arrowhead). Hematoxylin and eosin (×500). **3.** Substantia propria with fibrocytes and collagen fibers (A), posterior limiting lamina (B), and the posterior epithelium (C). Hematoxylin and eosin (×500).

thelium is firmly attached to the basal lamina by numerous hemidesmosomes, collagen fibrils, and laminin (a glycoprotein). Frequently, this layer can be distinguished with the light microscope (Fig. 17-2). It should not be confused with the **anterior limiting lamina** (Bowman's membrane), a modified outermost layer of the substantia propria that is present in primates and avians.

Substantia Propria (Stroma)

The corneal **substantia propria,** or stroma, consists of varying numbers (approximately 100 in the cat) of layers or lamellae and constitutes 90% of the corneal thickness (Fig. 17-2). Within one layer, the collagen fibers are always parallel with the corneal surface and traverse the entire diameter of the cornea; in successive layers, the fibers cross each other at right angles. Adjacent lamellae are held together firmly by fibers that deviate from their parallel course. Occasional elastic fibers are observed at the periphery of the cornea. The precise arrangement (periodicity of 620 to 640 angstroms) of the lamellae in the corneal stroma allows 99% of the light entering the cornea to pass into the globe without scatter. This accounts for the transparency of the cornea.

The predominant cell type of the corneal substantia propria is the fibrocyte (keratocyte), located mainly between the collagen

layers rather than within them. These cells are elongated and branched, with little cytoplasm (Fig. 17-2). If the cornea is injured, the fibrocytes can transform into fibroblasts and form scar tissue.

There are at least five different types of collagen in the stroma, with type I being the most common. The amorphous ground substance stains metachromatically owing to the presence of sulfated glycosaminoglycans (chondroitin sulfate, keratan sulfate). The ground substance plays an essential role in the transparency of the cornea by maintaining an optimal degree of hydration; excessive water content causes opacification of the cornea.

Posterior Limiting Lamina (Descemet's Membrane)

With the light microscope, the **posterior limiting lamina** (Descemet's membrane) appears as a highly refractile, thick amorphous layer that gives a positive periodic acid-Schiff (PAS) reaction (Fig. 17-2). At the fine structural level, the lamina consists of three regions: an anterior unbanded zone, an anterior banded zone, and a posterior unbanded zone. The anterior unbanded zone has types V and VI collagen, the anterior banded zone has types IV and VIII collagen, and the posterior unbanded zone has types III and IV collagen. The posterior limiting lamina is continually produced throughout life by the posterior epithelial cells, resulting in a thicker membrane in aging animals.

Posterior Epithelium (Corneal Endothelium)

A single layer of flat hexagonal cells covers the posterior surface of the cornea as the **posterior epithelium** and is often referred to as the corneal endothelium (Fig. 17-2). The cells interdigitate heavily and contain numerous mitochondria and pinocytotic vesicles. The epithelium functions in the maintenance of the transparency of the cornea. Both the anterior and posterior epithelial cells actively move water out of the stroma by Na$^+$-K$^+$ ATPase (adenosine triphosphatase) and carbonic anhydrase pumps. Defects in the epithelium can cause edema and opacification of the cornea. The regenerative ability of the posterior epithelium is limited and varies with species and age. It is generally accepted that active mitosis only occurs in immature animals.

Corneoscleral Junction (Limbus)

At the **corneoscleral junction** or limbus, the sclera overlaps the cornea. The corneal epithelium gradually changes into conjunctival epithelium, which rests on a lamina propria of loose connective tissue. The characteristically layered collagen fibers of the substantia propria assume a more irregular arrangement, become

associated with elastic fibers, and are continuous with the equatorial bundles of the sclera. The posterior limiting lamina of the posterior epithelium ends at the limbus near the apex of the trabecular meshwork.

The only blood vessels supplying the cornea are located at the level of the limbus; the normal cornea is completely devoid of blood vessels. Corneal nerves originate from a dense, marginal nerve fiber plexus at the same level as the blood vessels or from the ciliary plexus of the vascular tunic.

VASCULAR TUNIC

The **vascular tunic**, or uvea, comprises three portions: the choroid, the ciliary body, and the mesenchymal components of the iris.

Choroid

The **choroid** is a thick, highly vascularized layer that is continuous with the stroma of the ciliary body anteriorly and extends posteriorly around the globe (Figs. 17-3 and 17-4). The external surface of the choroid is connected to the sclera; the internal surface is adjacent and intimately attached to the pigmented epithelium of the retina. The choroid is subdivided into five layers.

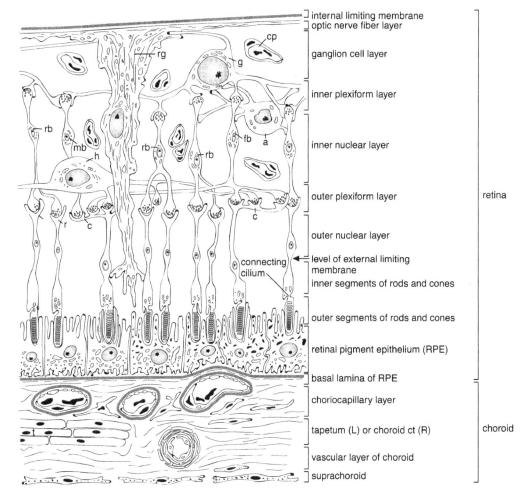

FIGURE 17-3 Schematic drawing of the organization of the retina and choroid. The rod spherules (r) have synaptic contact with rod bipolar cells (rb), which synapse with ganglion cells. The cone pedicles (c) have synaptic contact with midget bipolar cells (mb), which contact a single cone, and flat bipolar cells (fb), the dendrites of which contact several cones and the axon of which then synapses with amacrine (a) and ganglion cells (g). Horizontal cell (h) processes contact rod spherules and cone pedicles. Amacrine cells (a) contact the axons of bipolar cells and dendrites and perikarya of ganglion cells. Radial glial (Müller) cells (rg) provide support to the retina; their cytoplasmic processes extend between and around the other cells, and their foot processes participate in the formation of the internal limiting membrane. Retinal capillaries (cp) are located in the inner nuclear, ganglion cell, and nerve fiber layers. A cellular tapetum lucidum (t) is shown in the left half of the schematic drawing.

Labels in figure:
- internal limiting membrane
- optic nerve fiber layer
- ganglion cell layer
- inner plexiform layer
- inner nuclear layer
- outer plexiform layer
- outer nuclear layer
- level of external limiting membrane
- inner segments of rods and cones
- outer segments of rods and cones
- retinal pigment epithelium (RPE)
- basal lamina of RPE
- choriocapillary layer
- tapetum (L) or choroid ct (R)
- vascular layer of choroid
- suprachoroid
- retina
- choroid

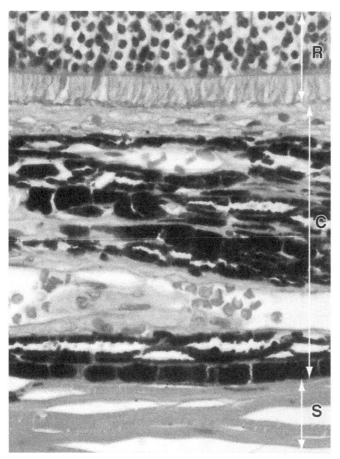

FIGURE 17-4   The choroid layer (C) is located between the retina (R) and sclera (S). The choroid is highly vascularized and many pigmented cells are present.

Suprachoroid Layer

The **suprachoroid layer** is the most external layer (Fig. 17-3) of the choroid and is the transition between the sclera and the choroid. It consists of bundles of collagen and some elastic fibers, fibrocytes, and numerous melanocytes.

Vascular Layer

Numerous large arteries and veins, separated by a stroma similar to that of the suprachoroid layer, make up the **vascular layer** (Fig. 17-3). These vessels provide a major source of oxygen and nutrients to the retina.

Tapetum Lucidum

A layer of medium vessels and connective tissue lies internal to the vascular layer. The dorsal portion of this layer contains the **tapetum lucidum,** which acts as a light-reflecting layer, supposedly increasing light perception under conditions of poor illumination. In herbivores, the tapetum is fibrous (**tapetum fibrosum**), consisting of intermingling collagen fibers and a few fibrocytes. In carnivores, the tapetum consists of a varying number of layers of flat polygonal cells (**tapetum cellulosum**) that appear bricklike in cross section (Figs. 17-3 and 17-5; see also Fig. 17-9). The thickness of the tapetum varies, being multi-

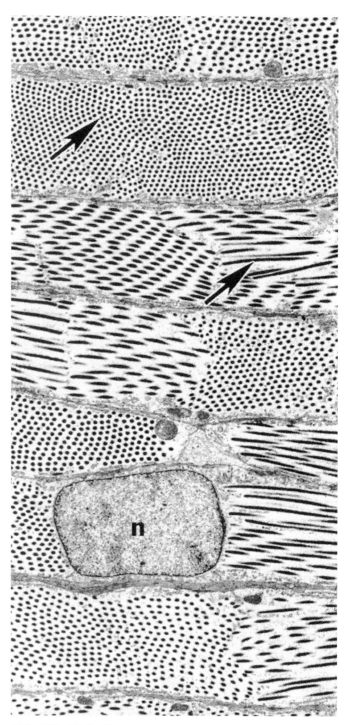

FIGURE 17-5   Electron micrograph of the feline tapetum lucidum illustrating the bricklike arrangement of cells and bundles of parallel rods (arrows) oriented in various directions with their long axes perpendicular to the angle of incident light and a tapetal cell nucleus (n) (×3780). *(Courtesy of E. J. King.)*

layered at its center (up to 15 cell layers thick in dogs and 35 cell layers thick in cats) and thinning to a single cell at its periphery. The tapetal cells are packed with bundles of parallel small rods, all of which are oriented with their long axes parallel to the retinal surface. In cats, the rods in the inner tapetal cells may be modified melanosomes, which are present along with typical melanosomes in the outer tapetal cells near the sclera. Zinc is associated with the rods in dogs and riboflavin with the rods in cats. Diffraction of light as a result of the spatial orientation of the rods (or of the collagen fibrils in herbivores) is probably responsible for producing the light reflection of the tapetum. In swine and camelids, the tapetum is absent.

Choriocapillary Layer

The **choriocapillary layer** (lamina choroidocapillaris) is a dense network of capillaries immediately adjacent to the pigmented epithelium of the retina (Fig. 17-3). Wide capillaries often deeply indent the pigmented epithelial cells. The endothelium is fenestrated, and endothelial nuclei and pericytes are located toward the choroidal side of the capillaries only. The basal laminae of the capillary and pigmented epithelial are fused. Capillaries provide nutrients to the pigmented epithelium and photoreceptors (rods and cones).

Basal Complex

The **basal complex** (complexus basalis) is also referred to as Bruch's membrane. The complex serves as a barrier between the blood in the choriocapillary vessels and the retinal pigmented epithelium. Species variation occurs among domestic animals with respect to the degree of development and thickness of the basal complex. In species without a tapetum, the basal complex has five layers: basal lamina of the retinal pigmented epithelium, two layers of collagen with an intervening band of elastic fibers, and the basal lamina of the choriocapillary endothelium. In species with a tapetum, the complex has three layers: the two basal laminae separated by a layer of collagen.

Ciliary Body

The **ciliary body** is the direct anterior continuation of the choroid (Fig. 17-1). It begins posteriorly at the ora serrata, a sharply outlined dentate border that marks the transition between the optic part (pars optica retinae) and the blind part (pars caeca retinae) of the retina. Anteriorly, the ciliary body is continuous with the iris and participates in the formation of the trabecular meshwork of the iridocorneal angle. All layers of the choroid extend into the ciliary body, except the tapetum lucidum and the choriocapillary layer.

Anteriorly, the ciliary body projects **ciliary processes** into the posterior chamber (Fig. 17-1). Collectively, the ciliary processes form a region of the ciliary body referred to as the **pars plicata** (corona ciliaris). The processes greatly increase the surface area for production of aqueous humor and also serve as the origin for zonular fibers, which attach to the lens. The posterior portion of the ciliary body is flat and smooth and is referred to as the **pars plana** (orbiculus ciliaris). Histologically, the ciliary body consists of ciliary epithelium, a vascular layer, and the ciliary muscle.

Ciliary Epithelium

The ciliary body is covered by two layers of cuboidal epithelial cells of neuroepithelial origin. Cells of the epithelial layers are joined apex to apex by cell junctions, with the basal laminae facing toward the outsides of the fused epithelial layers.

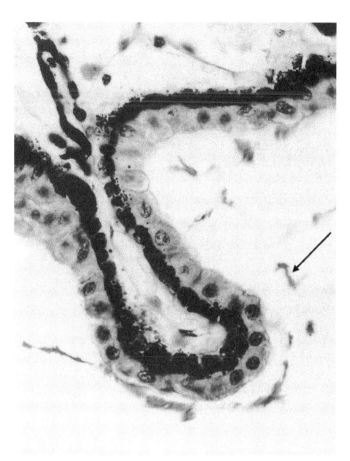

FIGURE 17-6 This canine ciliary process is covered by pigmented and nonpigmented epithelial cells. Remnants of zonular fibers (arrow) are present in the posterior chamber. Masson's trichrome (×600).

The outer **pigmented epithelial layer** is continuous with the pigmented epithelium of the optic part of the retina. It consists of heavily pigmented, simple cuboidal epithelium (Fig. 17-6) on a basal lamina next to the stroma. These cells have deep basal invaginations of the plasma membrane.

The inner **nonpigmented epithelial layer** consists of cuboidal or columnar cells (Fig. 17-6) with a basal lamina, which separates it from the posterior chamber. Nonpigmented epithelium is continuous with the neurosensory layers of the retina and with the pigmented epithelium of the iris. The cells possess numerous deep plasmalemmal invaginations and associated mitochondria. Extensive rough endoplasmic reticulum (rER) and Golgi complexes are present in the cell apices. The lateral surfaces of the epithelial cells are joined by tight junctions, resulting in a blood-aqueous barrier. The pigmented and nonpigmented epithelial layers of the ciliary body form the pars ciliaris retinae. The pars ciliaris retinae and the pars iridica retinae form the blind part of the retina (pars ceca retinae).

Vascular Layer

The ciliary body and the ciliary processes have a core of loose connective tissue permeated by a dense network of capillaries. Blood vessels are derived from the anterior and posterior ciliary arteries, which form the major arterial circle that supplies the ciliary body and processes.

Ciliary Muscle

The **ciliary muscle** is located peripherally in the ciliary body. It consists of smooth muscle fibers, which are primarily oriented meridionally in most species. The meridional fibers originate from the corneal stroma, the connective tissue of the trabecular meshwork of the iridocorneal angle, and the sclera. They are attached by elastic tendons to the basal complex of the choroid. In addition, radiate and circular fibers are present; the latter predominate in the nasal portion of the ciliary body. Contraction of the ciliary muscle during accommodation reduces tension of the zonular fibers of the lens and the lens becomes more convex, whereas relaxation has the opposite effect.

Aqueous Humor

The **aqueous humor** is a thin, clear fluid similar to blood plasma, but it has considerably lower protein content. The aqueous humor is produced in the ciliary processes and is transported via the epithelial layers into the posterior chamber. The enzyme carbonic anhydrase (necessary to the formation of aqueous humor) has been localized to the nonpigmented epithelium of the ciliary processes. The transport of aqueous humor is selective in that certain molecules are excluded from transepithelial passage. The aqueous humor flows from the posterior chamber through the pupil to the anterior chamber, where it drains via the iridocorneal angle (described below).

Iris

The **iris** is located anterior to the lens and separates the anterior and posterior chambers, which communicate through the central opening, the **pupil**. The iris consists of a stroma of pigmented, highly vascularized loose connective tissue, the **sphincter** and **dilator muscles,** and a posterior epithelium.

Iridial Stroma

Epithelium is lacking on the anterior surface of the iris. Toward the anterior chamber, fibrocytes, separated by large intercellular spaces, form an almost continuous covering over dense melanocytes. This layer of fibrocytes and melanocytes is known as the **nonvascular layer** (or anterior border layer) (Fig. 17-7). The layer lacks a basal lamina and blood vessels; however, it is rich in proteoglycans. Channel-like spaces or crypts frequently penetrate deep into the underlying stroma, especially at the pupillary margin. These spaces often communicate with the anterior chamber.

The deep **vascular layer** of the stroma consists of regular, arcuate bundles of collagen fibers and fibrocytes supported by highly vascularized loose connective tissue containing many melanocytes. Spiral collagen fiber bundles derived from several arcuate collagen fiber bundles surround each stromal blood vessel. Through this arrangement, blood vessels change their position in synchrony with the fiber bundles during contraction or dilation of the iris, thereby eluding compression and kinking.

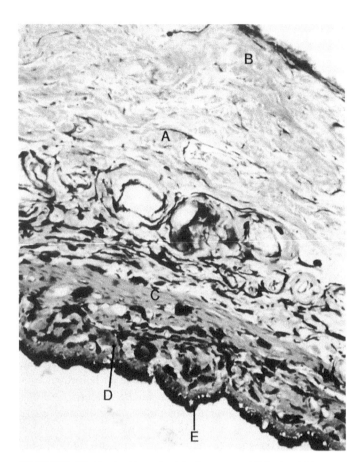

FIGURE 17-7   In this canine iris, the stroma (A) is the thickest layer containing many blood vessels and melanocytes; toward the anterior chamber, a nonvascular layer (B) is present. This section of the iris was taken near the pupillary opening; the fibers of the sphincter muscle (C) were cut longitudinally. Dilator muscle (D); posterior pigmented epithelial cell layer (E). Hematoxylin and eosin (×175).

The arterial blood vessels originate from the **major arterial circle** (circulus arteriosus major) at the periphery of the iris and radiate, spirally wound, into the stroma, forming capillary loops in the vicinity of the pupillary margin. In nonprimates, the major arterial circle is incomplete. The veins have a straighter arrangement than the arteries and return to the base of the iris and the ciliary body.

Eye color is determined by the amount of pigmentation within the pigment-containing cells of the stroma.

Iridial Muscles

Two muscles that regulate the size of the pupil are present in the iris. They are both of neuroepithelial (pigmented epithelium) origin. In domestic animals, these muscles are smooth, while in birds, they are striated.

The **sphincter muscle** (musculus sphincter pupillae) is composed of a network of smooth muscle cells, circularly arranged near the pupillary margin (Fig. 17-7). The fibers encircle the pupil in animals with circular pupils (dogs, pigs, primates, and avians). The muscle fibers are oriented dorsoventrally around the pupil in animals with slitlike pupils (cat) or horizontally around the pupil in ruminants and horses. The arches of the collagen fiber bundles of the iris stroma loop through the muscle network, thus enabling the muscle fibers to act on them. The sphincter muscle receives parasympathetic innervation through the oculomotor nerve (nucleus of Edinger–Westphal; synapses in the ciliary ganglion).

The **dilator muscle** (musculus dilator pupillae) is a partial differentiation of the anterior epithelial layer, a continuation of the pigmented epithelial layer of the ciliary body (Fig. 17-7). Whereas the basal portions of the epithelial cells possess the structural characteristics of smooth muscle cells, the apical portions have retained those of typical pigmented epithelial cells (myopigmentocytes). The dilator muscle is innervated by sympathetic postganglionic neurons located in the cranial cervical ganglion.

Iridial Epithelium

The posterior pigmented **epithelial layer** (Fig. 17-7) of the iris is a continuation of the nonpigmented epithelial layer of the ciliary processes, which gradually becomes pigmented toward the base of the iris. Frequently, the epithelial cells are separated by wide intercellular spaces. On its posterior (inner) surface, the epithelium is covered by a basal lamina.

In ungulates, several dark masses, called **iridial granules** (granulae iridica or corpora nigra) are found at the dorsal and ventral pupillary margins. The granulae originating from the dorsal pupillary margin are much larger than those originating from the ventral margin. Iridial granules are focal proliferations of the two epithelial layers that project into the anterior chamber at the dorsal and ventral pupillary margins.

Iridocorneal Angle

The **iridocorneal angle** (or iris, filtration, or drainage angle) (Fig. 17-8) is a region located at the periphery of the anterior chamber, where the corneoscleral junction, the ciliary body, and the iris converge. Structurally, the iridocorneal angle is a meshwork that comprises the pectinate ligament, trabecular meshwork, and trabecular (aqueous) veins. Aqueous humor from the anterior chamber drains into the blood vessels of the angle.

Pectinate Ligament

The **pectinate ligament** consists of numerous long, thin primary and accessory strands extending between the corneoscleral junction and the base of the iris (Fig. 17-8). Each strand comprises a core of collagen fibrils covered by simple squamous epithelium (continuous with the corneal endothelium). The spaces between the strands of the pectinate ligament are known as the **spaces of Fontana**. It is through these spaces that aqueous humor leaves the anterior chamber.

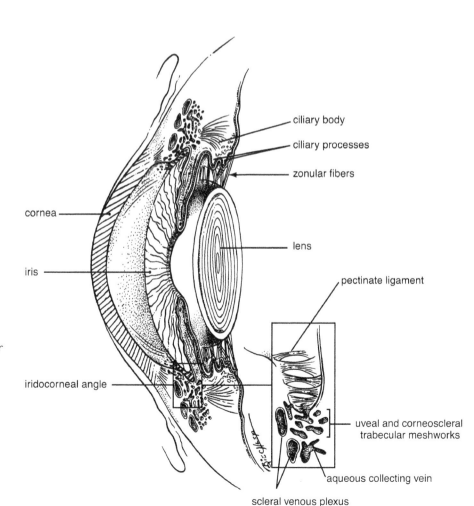

FIGURE 17-8 Schematic of the anterior portion of the eye, illustrating the drainage route of aqueous humor from the anterior chamber of the eye (between cornea and iris), through the strands of the pectinate ligament, into the spaces of the uveal and corneoscleral trabecular meshworks, into aqueous collecting veins and the scleral venous plexus. The inset shows a higher magnification of the rectangular area of the iridocorneal angle.

ciliary body
ciliary processes
zonular fibers
lens
pectinate ligament
uveal and corneoscleral trabecular meshworks
aqueous collecting vein
scleral venous plexus
cornea
iris
iridocorneal angle

Trabecular Meshwork

The **uveal trabecular meshwork** is continuous with the pectinate ligament and is a dense network of simple squamous epithelium-covered collagen fibrils (Fig. 17-8). The uveal trabecular meshwork gradually becomes the structurally identical but tighter-meshed **corneoscleral trabecular meshwork** (adjacent to the cornea and sclera).

Venous Drainage

Aqueous humor is removed from the eye by two methods: conventional or nonconventional (uveoscleral) outflow. In most species, conventional outflow accounts for most of the drainage of aqueous humor. With **conventional outflow,** the aqueous humor drains through the spaces of Fontana of the pectinate ligament into the trabecular meshwork, where it gains access to **aqueous collecting veins.** It then passes into the **scleral venous plexus** (plexus venosus sclerae), two to four large vessels located in the sclera posterior to the limbus (Fig. 17-8). The aqueous humor then passes into the vortex veins and enters the blood circulation. The canal of Schlemm, a circumferential endothelium-lined chan-

nel present in the human eye, is absent in domestic mammals. The **nonconventional outflow** consists of "percolation" of aqueous humor through the uvea into the supraciliary and suprachoroidal space and then into the adjacent sclera.

NEUROEPITHELIAL TUNIC— RETINA

The neuroepithelial tunic, or retina, consists of three parts. The sensory portion (pars optica retinae) contacts the choroid. The nonsensory portion of this tunic, which begins at the ora serrata, covers the ciliary body (pars ciliaris retinae) and the iris (pars iridica retinae) as a double epithelial layer.

Except at the optic disk, the sensory portion of the retina consists of the following layers (Figs. 17-3 and 17-9): (1) retinal pigment epithelium, (2) layer of rods and cones, (3) external limiting membrane, (4) outer nuclear layer, (5) outer plexiform layer, (6) inner nuclear layer, (7) inner plexiform layer, (8) ganglion cell layer, (9) nerve fiber layer, and (10) internal limiting membrane.

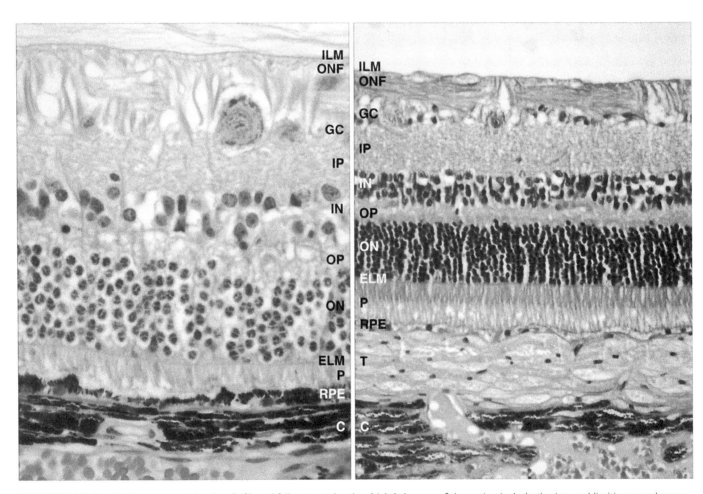

FIGURE 17-9 Canine nontapetal retina (left) and feline tapetal retina (right). Layers of the retina include the internal limiting membrane (ILM); optic nerve fiber layer (ONF); ganglion cell layer (GC); inner plexiform layer (IP); inner nuclear layer (IN); outer plexiform layer (OP); outer nuclear layer (ON); external limiting membrane (ELM); photoreceptors (P); and retinal pigment epithelium (RPE). The RPE is not pigmented in the region of the retina where it overlies the tapetum (T) (right image). Many of the cells of the choroid (C) are heavily pigmented. Hematoxylin and eosin (left, ×950; right, ×500).

The **retinal pigment epithelium (RPE)** is a layer of flat, polygonal cells resting on a basal lamina (Figs. 17-3 and 17-9). Capillaries of the choriocapillary layer frequently deeply indent the cells. The base of the cell is characterized by deep infoldings of the plasma membrane and numerous associated mitochondria. Cell apices are connected by zonulae adherens and occludens. Numerous melanin granules are present, except in the cells overlying the tapetum. Microvillous apical processes partially surround the outer segments of the photoreceptors (Fig. 17-3).

The functions of the RPE are complex. They include transport of nutrients and metabolites from the capillaries in the choriocapillary layer to the rods and cones, phagocytosis, lysosomal degradation and recycling of the shed outer segments of the photoreceptors, and absorption of light by the melanin.

Rods and **cones** are the first neurons of the visual pathway. Each cell has an outer segment connected by a cilium to an inner segment. The cells are so named because the inner segment of rods is long and thin, while the inner segment of cones has a broad base. These photoreceptive cells form the distinct **photosensory layer** adjacent to the RPE (Figs. 17-3 and 17-9).

The **outer segment** of the photoreceptors consists of stacks of **membranous disks,** which are actually flattened membrane spheres. The disks are surrounded by the cell membrane in rods, whereas in cones, the disks are occasionally open to the extracellular space. Molecules of **visual pigments** (rhodopsin in rods, iodopsins in cones) are present in the membranes. Each day, triggered by onset of morning light, short stacks of the oldest disks are shed from the outer ends of the photoreceptors and are subsequently phagocytized and degraded by the RPE cells. New disks are continually added to the inner ends of the outer segments. Each outer segment is connected to its inner segment by a **cilium.**

The **inner segment** includes an outer portion, or **ellipsoid,** and an inner portion, or **myoid.** The ellipsoid is densely packed with mitochondria. A large oil droplet, which is thought to enhance visual acuity, is present in the avian ellipsoid. The myoid contains smooth endoplasmic reticulum, Golgi complex, and microtubules. Myofilaments are present in the myoid of lower vertebrates but are absent in domestic animals.

The rod cells are responsible for vision in dim light, whereas the cone cells function in bright light and are responsible for color vision. Thus, animals that are mainly active at night have retinas with fewer cone cells than those of animals active during the day.

The **external limiting membrane** is formed by zonulae adherens between processes of adjoining radial glial (Müller) and photoreceptor cells. The microvilli of the radial glial cells project peripherally between the inner segments of the rods and cones (Figs. 17-3 and 17-9).

The **outer nuclear layer** contains the perikarya of the rods and cones (Fig. 17-3). The **outer plexiform layer** is composed of the axon terminals of the photoreceptor cells, that is, rod spherules and cone pedicles, forming synapses with the processes of the horizontal cells, and the dendrites of the bipolar cells (Fig. 17-9).

As many as four (in dogs) layers of nuclei make up the **inner nuclear layer** (Figs. 17-3 and 17-9), which comprises bipolar, horizontal, amacrine, and radial glial cells. Most of the nuclei in the center of this layer belong to the **rod** and **cone bipolar cells** (the second neuron of the visual pathway). The dendrite of the rod bipolar cell contacts several rods, and the axon synapses with amacrine and/or ganglion cells (Fig. 17-3). The cone bipolar cells are either midget bipolar cells that contact a single cone or flat bipolar cells in which dendrites contact several cones while their axons synapse with amacrine and ganglion cells. Nuclei located in the outer portion of this layer belong to **horizontal cells,** the processes of which synapse with rod and cone axon terminals in the outer plexiform layer. Nuclei located in the inner portion belong to **amacrine cells.** Their cell processes extend into the inner plexiform layer and establish contact with the dendrites and perikarya of ganglion cells and with the axons of bipolar cells. Amacrine cells also seem to be interconnected (Fig. 17-3). The nuclei of the **radial glial (Müller) cells** are interspersed among the other nuclei. The radial glial cells are elongated, fibrous astrocytes extending between the internal and external limiting membranes (Fig. 17-3). They provide mechanical support and nutrition to the retina.

The **inner plexiform layer** is the region of synaptic contacts between bipolar and ganglion cells, between amacrine and ganglion cells, and between adjacent amacrine cells (Figs. 17-3 and 17-9).

The **ganglion cell layer** (third neuron of the visual pathway) is composed of large neuronal perikarya. Recently, it has been shown that the ganglion cells in rodents and primates contain melanopsin, a photopigment that can sense light. Axons of the ganglion cells form a separate layer, the **nerve fiber layer** (Figs. 17-3 and 17-9). The axons converge and exit at the **optic disk** (papilla) of the retina and form the **optic nerve.** Some of the axons have been traced to the suprachiasmatic nuclei, where they may play a role in regulating circadian rhythm.

The **internal limiting membrane** is formed by the expanded processes of the radial glial cells, which unite to form a continuous layer, analogous to the glial limiting membrane in the central nervous system (Figs. 17-3 and 17-9), and a basal lamina. Occasional astrocytes, microglial cells, and oligodendrocytes are present in the retina in the inner plexiform, ganglion cell, and optic nerve fiber layers.

The **area centralis retinae** is a small round or oval area of the retina located dorsally and laterally to the optic disk. This area differs from the remainder of the retina in that it is characterized by an increased number of cones, a thickening of the inner plexiform layer, an increased number of ganglion cells, thinning of the nerve fiber layer, and absence of large blood vessels. The area centralis retinae is the area of most acute vision and corresponds to the area of the macula and fovea in primates.

The retinal vascular pattern varies greatly among species. In the **holangiotic** pattern (cats, dogs, cattle, pigs, and sheep), blood vessels occur in the optic nerve fiber layer. Wide capillaries are found at the periphery of the retina, and venules and arterioles are present toward the optic disk. Numerous capillaries are present in the inner nuclear, ganglion cell, and nerve fiber layers (Fig. 17-3). In the **paurangiotic** pattern (horses), the vessels radiate only a short distance from the optic disk. In the merangiotic retina (rabbits), the vessels migrate medially and laterally. **Anangiotic** retinas (birds and reptiles) are devoid of blood vessels.

REFRACTIVE MEDIA

Lens and Zonular Fibers

The **lens** is a transparent, biconvex structure that is situated between the iris and the vitreous body and suspended by the zonular fibers from the ciliary body (Fig. 17-8). It consists of the lens capsule, lens epithelium, and lens fibers.

The lens is entirely surrounded by the **lens capsule** (Fig. 17-10), which consists of several layers of collagen fibrils alternating with basal lamina material. It is much thicker on the anterior lens surface than on the posterior surface.

Beneath the anterior lens capsule is the **lens epithelium** (Fig. 17-10), a layer of simple cuboidal epithelial cells. The basal region of the cells faces the lens capsule, while the apical region is toward the lens fibers. At the equator, the cells elongate and differentiate into **lens fibers,** which make up the bulk of the lens (Figs. 17-10 and 17-11). Fully differentiated lens fibers are U-shaped prism-shaped cells that extend toward the anterior and posterior poles of the lens. They lack a nucleus and are virtually devoid of organelles. Lens fibers interdigitate extensively (especially where fibers from opposite sides of the equator meet to form lens sutures [Fig. 17-11]) and are connected through gap junctions and desmosomes. Through continuous differentiation of lens epithelial cells and addition of fibers, the lens grows throughout life.

The **zonular fibers** originate from the basal lamina of the inner layer of the ciliary epithelium (Figs. 17-6 and 17-12). The fibers are composed of noncollagenous glycoproteins similar to

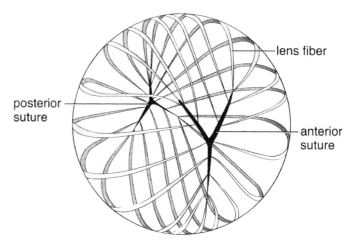

FIGURE 17-11 Three-dimensional schematic of the outer layer of lens fibers. The capsule and lens epithelium have been removed. Lens fibers form Y-shaped sutures where the ends of the fibers meet. The "Y" is upright in the anterior region of the lens and inverted in the posterior region of the lens.

elastic fibers (see Chapter 3) and are attached to the lens capsule by fusion with its outermost layers.

When the ciliary muscle contracts during accommodation, the zonular fibers slacken, the elastic lens fibers then shorten, and the lens assumes a more spherical shape, focusing the image on the retina. During ciliary muscle relaxation, the zonular fibers tense and the lens becomes more discoid with decreased axial thickness.

Vitreous Body

The **vitreous body** occupies the vitreous chamber, the space between the lens and the retina, or about two thirds of the volume of the globe (Fig. 17-1). The primary vitreous forms first and is

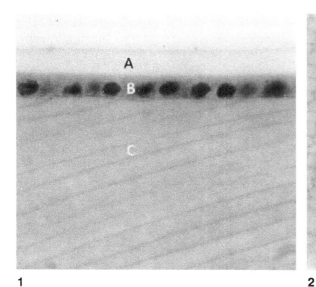

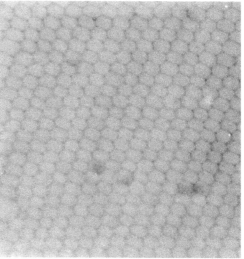

1   2

FIGURE 17-10 Canine lens. **1.,** The lens capsule (A) covers the anterior lens epithelium (B) underneath which are the lens fibers (C). **2.,** Cross section through lens fibers. Hematoxylin and eosin (×660).

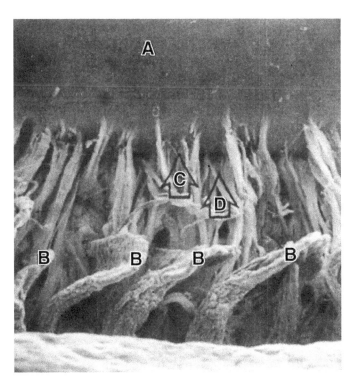

FIGURE 17-12 Scanning electron micrograph illustrating a posterior view of ciliary processes and attachment of zonular fibers to the lens (cat). Posterior lens (A); ciliary process (B); posterior zonular fibers (C); anterior zonular fibers (D). Notice that the zonular fibers extend from between the bases of the ciliary processes and aggregate at their lenticular insertion. *(From Gelatt KM. Textbook of Veterinary Ophthalmology. Philadelphia: Lea & Febiger, 1981.)*

mostly fibrovascular tissue that functions to nourish the developing globe. The primary vitreous regresses (usually completed by birth) and is replaced by secondary vitreous that is seen in normal patients. The zonular fibers are termed the tertiary vitreous, but their exact origin is uncertain. Vitreous is a hydrogel containing 99% water, and the remaining 1% is primarily hyaluronic acid. It adheres tightly to the optic disk (papilla) and the ora serrata; it also attaches to the internal limiting membrane of the retina and the posterior part (pars plana) of the ciliary body. In most domestic mammals, the vitreous body is firmly attached to the posterior lens capsule as well (hyaloideocapsular ligament).

The vitreous body contains a network of sparse collagen fibrils. Fibrils are concentrated peripherally, forming a layer called the **hyaloid membrane** or **cortex.** These collagen fibrils connect to the radial glial (Müller) cells of the retina. In the cortex, a few fibrocytes and macrophages are also present.

ACCESSORY ORGANS

Eyelids

The **eyelids** are movable folds of skin that protect the eyes. Their structure is described in Chapter 16.

Third Eyelid and Conjunctiva

The **third eyelid** (nictitating membrane) is a conjunctival fold fortified by hyaline (ruminants, dogs) or elastic (horses, pigs, cats) cartilage. The conjunctiva consists of a conjunctival epithelium covering a connective-tissue lamina propria. The **conjunctival epithelium** is either a pseudostratified columnar or transitional epithelium that becomes stratified squamous near the eyelid margin (Fig. 17-13-1). Goblet cells are scattered throughout the conjunctiva, with the highest cell densities in the dog found in the lower nasal to middle fornix region of the conjunctiva (Fig. 17-13-2). Goblet cells produce the inner layer of the tear film. The conjunctival epithelium lies over a lamina propria of highly vascularized loose connective tissue rich in fibrocytes, lymphocytes, and plasma cells, with some mast cells and macrophages also present. It also may contain solitary and aggregated lymphatic nodules.

The **superficial gland of the third eyelid** surrounds the base of the shaft of the T-shaped cartilage plate. It is similar in structure to the lacrimal gland and likewise contributes secretion to the tear film; it is serous in horses and cats, seromucous in cattle and dogs and mucous in the pig. Frequently, acinar cells secrete lipid. A **deep gland of the third eyelid** (Harderian gland) is present in cattle and pigs.

Lacrimal Apparatus

The **lacrimal gland** is a compound tubuloacinar or tubuloalveolar gland (Fig. 17-14). It is serous in cats and seromucous in dogs and ungulates. The acinar cells frequently contain lipid inclusions and are surrounded by myoepithelial cells (Fig. 17-14).

The intercalated and secretory ducts are lined with simple and stratified cuboidal epithelia, respectively (Fig. 17-14). The lacrimal ductules are lined with stratified cuboidal epithelium.

The glands of the third eyelid (see above) are likewise included in the lacrimal apparatus. The lacrimal gland and the superficial gland of the third eyelid produce approximately 60% and 35%, respectively, of the aqueous portion of the tear film.

Excess tears accumulate in the lacrimal lake (lacus lacrimalis), a medially located widening of the conjunctiva lined by a stratified squamous and columnar epithelium. They enter the **lacrimal canaliculi,** which are lined with stratified squamous epithelium, through the **lacrimal puncta** to reach the lacrimal sac and its continuation, the nasolacrimal duct.

The **nasolacrimal duct** is lined by a stratified columnar epithelium with goblet cells or by transitional epithelium (pigs). It begins with an ampullar widening, the **lacrimal sac,** the lamina propria of which contains lymphatic tissue. Toward the nasal end of the duct, simple branched tubuloacinar mucous (or seromucous in sheep and goats) glands are present.

SPECIES VARIATIONS

Many ocular anatomic and histologic variations occur among species. In mammals, differences include size and shape of the

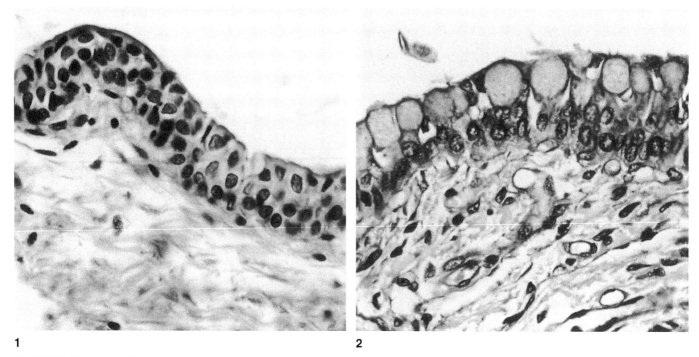

1   **2**

FIGURE 17-13   **1.** Transitional epithelium of the porcine conjunctiva. Hematoxylin and eosin (×540). **2.** Many goblet cells in pseudostratified columnar epithelium of the canine conjunctiva. Hematoxylin and eosin (×540).

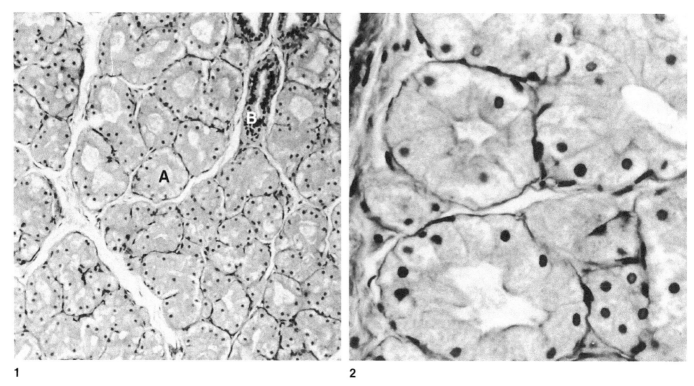

1   **2**

FIGURE 17-14   Porcine lacrimal gland. **1.** Acini (A) and a secretory duct (B). Trichrome (×185). **2.** The light staining of the acinar cells is due to dissolution of lipid inclusions. Trichrome (×600).

globe; size and shape of the cornea; thickness of the cornea and sclera; point of optic nerve exit; shape and orientation of the pupil; shape and distribution of melanin granules; degree of development of the ciliary muscle; shape, relative size, and color of the lens; thickness of various retinal layers; retinal vascular patterns; absence of or location and type of tapetum; thickness of choroid; and types of lacrimal glands.

The differences between mammals and other vertebrates are much more striking. For example, eyes of birds vary greatly in shape, and their scleras contain cartilage and, in many species, ossicles. The avian cornea has an anterior limiting lamina, unlike other domestic animals. In birds and some other vertebrates, such as snakes and lizards, a highly vascular structure called the **pecten** extends from the optic disk into the vitreous body. The pecten is responsible for nourishment of the inner eye and retina. These species also have skeletal muscle within their iris and ciliary body rather than smooth muscle. Several other differences exist between mammalian eyes and those of other vertebrates. In some of these species, the ciliary processes actually attach directly to the lens to allow for more accommodation. For details of the structure of many nonmammalian eyes and of species differences among mammals, the reader is referred to the suggested readings list.

SUGGESTED READINGS

Dowling JA. The Retina: An Approachable Part of the Brain. Cambridge, MA: Harvard University Press, 1987.

Duke-Elder S. The Eye in Evolution. Vol. 1, System of Ophthalmology. London: Henry Kimpton, 1958.

Fine BS, Yanoff M. Ocular Histology, a Text and Atlas. 2nd Ed. Hagerstown, MD: Harper and Row, 1979.

Samuelson DA. Ophthalmic anatomy. In: Gelatt KN, ed. Veterinary Ophthalmology. 3rd Ed. Philadelphia: Lea & Febiger, 1999.

Walls GL. The Vertebrate Eye and its Adaptive Radiation. Bloomfield Hills, MI: The Cranbrook Press, 1942.

18

Ear

JO ANN EURELL

External Ear
Middle Ear
    Tympanic Membrane
    Tympanic Cavity
    Auditory Ossicles and Muscles of the Middle Ear
    Auditory Tube
Internal Ear
    Bony Labyrinth
    Membranous Labyrinth
        Semicircular ducts
        Utricle and saccule
        Cochlear duct

Stria vascularis
Vestibular Apparatus
    Crista ampullaris
    Maculae of the utricle and saccule
    Vestibular mechanism
Auditory Apparatus
    Spiral organ (organ of Corti)
        Sensory cells
        Supporting cells
        Tectorial membrane
    Spiral ganglion
    Auditory mechanism

The ear is composed of three divisions: the external ear, the middle ear, and the internal (inner) ear. Structured for sound collection, the external ear is composed of the auricle and the external acoustic meatus. The middle ear consists of the tympanic membrane, tympanic cavity, and three auditory ossicles plus their associated muscles and ligaments. The air-filled tympanic cavity of the middle ear is connected to the nasopharynx by the auditory tube. Sound conduction is the primary function of the middle ear. The inner ear, consisting of the membranous labyrinth enclosed within the osseous (bony) labyrinth in the petrous temporal bone, plays a role in both hearing and equilibrium.

EXTERNAL EAR

The microscopic description of the auricle, or pinna, and the external acoustic meatus is included in Chapter 16.

MIDDLE EAR

Tympanic Membrane

The thin **tympanic membrane** delimits the external acoustic meatus from the tympanic cavity (Fig. 18-1). It is covered externally by stratified squamous epithelium and internally by simple squamous epithelium continuous with that of the tympanic cavity. Between these two epithelial sheets is a connective-tissue layer composed of a central region of circularly arranged collagen fibers and a peripheral region of radially arranged collagen fibers. Where the manubrium of the malleus attaches to the tympanic membrane, the connective tissue is somewhat thicker and contains blood vessels and nerves that course along the manubrium and spread radially. Collagen fibers are sparse or even absent in the dorsal portion of the membrane, referred to as the **flaccid** part.

Tympanic Cavity

The air-filled tympanic cavity contains small bones, the auditory ossicles, and their muscles and ligaments (Fig. 18-1). The cavity is lined with simple squamous or simple cuboidal epithelium, which covers the ossicles. The epithelium rests on a thin layer of connective tissue. A few epithelial cells are ciliated, particularly those on the floor of the cavity.

Auditory Ossicles and Muscles of the Middle Ear

The three **auditory ossicles** (malleus, incus, and stapes) traverse the middle ear, connecting the tympanic membrane to the membrane of the vestibular (oval) window of the internal ear (Fig. 18-1).

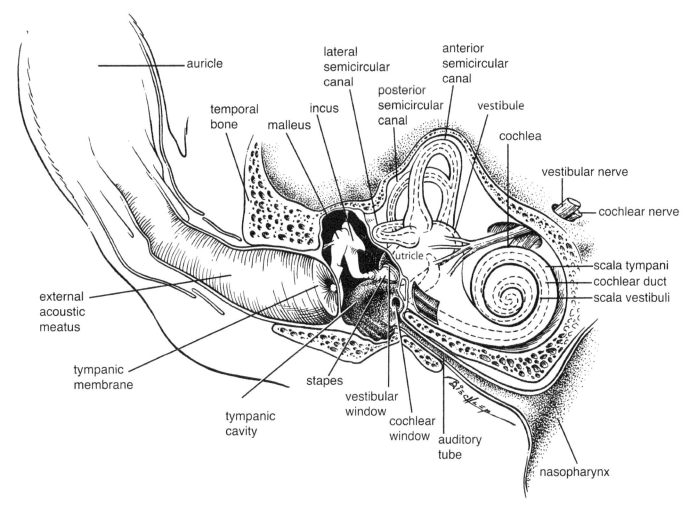

FIGURE 18-1 Schematic drawing of the right ear (dog), rostral aspect, showing the external ear with the auricle and external acoustic meatus; middle ear with the tympanic membrane; auditory ossicles comprising the malleus, incus, and stapes; tympanic cavity; auditory tube with connection to the nasopharynx; cochlear window; vestibular window, where the footplate of the stapes is located; internal ear with the bony labyrinth (bone cut away for easier viewing of the membranous labyrinth) comprising the anterior, lateral, and posterior semicircular canals, each with an osseous ampulla; vestibule; cochlea with the scala vestibule and the scala tympani; membranous labyrinth (dotted lines) comprising the anterior, lateral, and posterior semicircular ducts (each with a membranous ampulla), utricle, saccule, and cochlear duct. Moreover, the vestibulo-cochlear nerve, comprising the vestibular nerve and the cochlear nerve, is depicted entering the cranial cavity through the temporal bone.

These compact bones transmit vibrations across the middle ear cavity. The manubrium of the malleus is firmly attached to the tympanic membrane, and the small hooklike process on the neck of the malleus serves as an attachment for the tendon of the tensor tympani muscle. The head of the malleus articulates with the incus, which, in turn, articulates with the stapes. Ligaments hold these synovial articulations in place.

Muscles of the middle ear (tensor tympani and stapedius) are composed of skeletal muscle and function to dampen ossicle movement, protecting the inner ear structures from excessive vibration. The stapedius muscle attaches to the rostral crus of the stapes, and the footplate (base) of the stapes is attached to the vestibular window by an annular ligament.

Auditory Tube

The **auditory tube** connects the tympanic cavity to the nasopharynx (Fig. 18-1). The tube is lined by ciliated pseudostrati-

fied columnar epithelium (with goblet cells) resting on loose connective tissue. The lamina propria of the tube is thin and lacks glands in the osseous region of the tube; it becomes thicker in the cartilaginous region, containing seromucous glands and lymphatic nodules. Aggregated lymphatic nodules (the tubal tonsil) are present near the pharynx. The auditory tube is surrounded either by bone near the tympanic membrane and or by an incomplete cartilaginous tube toward the pharynx (Fig. 18-1). Hyaline cartilage is present in the proximal portion of the tube near the bone, but the tissue transitions to elastic cartilage toward the pharynx.

In the horse, the auditory tube expands ventrally to form the **guttural pouch.** The pouch has the same histologic features as the pharyngeal portion of the auditory tube but lacks cartilaginous support.

The function of the auditory tube is to ensure equal air pressure on both sides of the tympanic membrane. Usually, the auditory tube is closed, but it opens during yawning and swallowing.

INTERNAL EAR

The structural divisions of the inner ear comprise the bony labyrinth and the membranous labyrinth. The functional divisions of the internal ear are the vestibular apparatus and the auditory apparatus.

Bony Labyrinth

The **bony labyrinth** is a system of canals and cavities within the petrous temporal bone. Bone of the labyrinth is very dense and lamellar.

The cavities of the labyrinth include the vestibule, three semicircular canals, and the cochlea (Fig. 18-1). The **vestibule** is a small oval space connecting the cochlea with the semicircular canals located near the medial wall of the tympanic cavity. Three **semicircular canals** (anterior, posterior, and lateral) lie at right angles to each other and all communicate with the vestibule. The **cochlea** is a bony tube wound in the shape of a spiral. The spi-

ral canal of the cochlea makes several turns around an axis of spongy bone, the **modiolus.** The modiolus is a cone-shaped hollow osseous structure in which the cochlear nerve and its spiral ganglion are located. The number of coils varies from species to species (e.g., dog, $3\frac{1}{4}$; cat, 3; horse, $2\frac{1}{4}$; pig, 4; guinea pig, $4\frac{1}{2}$; cow, $3\frac{1}{2}$; man, $2\frac{3}{4}$). The base of the modiolus forms the rostral part of the internal acoustic meatus, where the cochlear nerve and blood vessels enter the cochlea. The bony canal is partially divided by a hollow bony projection, the osseous **spiral lamina,** which contains the branches of the cochlear nerve coursing to the spiral organ. The width of this lamina is largest at the cochlear window and diminishes toward the apex of the cochlea.

The canals and cavities of the bony labyrinth are lined by periosteum. A clear fluid, **perilymph,** fills the **perilymphatic space** between the periosteum and the membranous labyrinth (Figs. 18-2 and 18-3). Perilymph is similar in ionic composition to cerebrospinal fluid and plasma, with sodium as the main cation. Perilymph flows from the subarachnoid space through the cochlear canaliculus into the cavities of the bony labyrinth. The **vestibular**

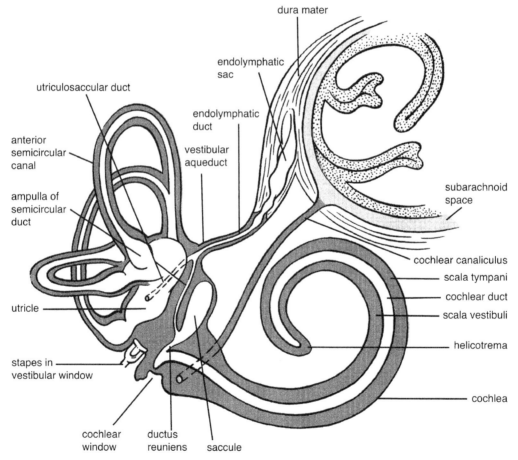

FIGURE 18-2 Schematic drawing of the right internal ear with its connections to the cranial cavity, intradural space, and subarachnoid space (rostral aspect). The cochlea with its contents is drawn uncoiled to show the helicotrema, where there is an open connection between the scala vestibuli and scala tympani. Note especially that the cochlear canaliculus connects with the subarachnoid space, which contains cerebrospinal fluid (light gray), and the scala tympani. Perilymph (dark gray) fills the space between the membranous labyrinth and the bony labyrinth. The other connection to the cranial cavity is the vestibular aqueduct, which houses portions of the endolymphatic duct and endolymphatic sac. Structures of the membranous labyrinth containing endolymph are shown in white. Dura mater, the utriculosaccular duct, ductus reuniens, saccule, utricle, and stapes in the vestibular window are also indicated.

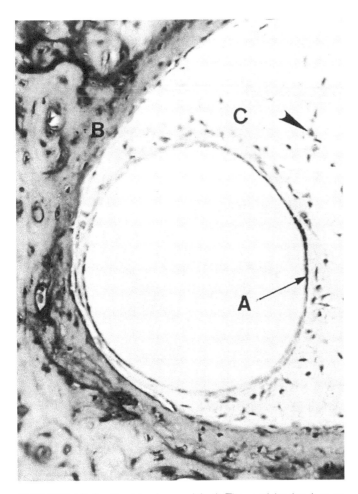

FIGURE 18-3 Semicircular canal (cat). The semicircular duct, an epithelium-lined membranous tube (A), lies within the semicircular canal of the osseous labyrinth (B). The perilymphatic space (C) contains delicate connective tissue trabeculae (arrowhead). The spaces between the trabeculae are lined with mesothelium. Hematoxylin and eosin (×400).

aqueduct, a space surrounding the endolymphatic duct, also contains perilymph.

Membranous Labyrinth

The **membranous labyrinth** comprises the semicircular ducts, utricle, saccule, cochlear duct, endolymphatic duct, and endolymphatic sac (Fig. 18-2). The membranous labyrinth is lined with simple squamous epithelium and filled with a fluid called **endolymph,** which is more viscous than perilymph. Endolymph contains high levels of potassium and low to minimal levels of sodium when compared to perilymph. The protein profile of endolymph is similar to that of perilymph but different from proteins found in plasma. Epithelial cells of the vestibule and the stria vascularis, which is described later in this chapter, are thought to produce endolymph. The connective tissue underlying the epithelium of the membranous labyrinth forms fine trabeculae (Fig. 18-3). The trabeculae span the adjacent perilymphatic space and anchor the suspended membranous labyrinth to the peri-

osteum of the bony wall. The periosteum and the spaces between the trabeculae are lined by flattened mesothelial cells.

Semicircular Ducts

The semicircular ducts lie within the semicircular canals (Fig. 18-1). One end of each duct is enlarged as an **ampulla.** The ducts are lined by simple squamous epithelium. Connection of the ducts with the utricle is shown in Figure 18-2.

Utricle and Saccule

The medial wall of the vestibule has two depressions in which the **utricle** (caudodorsal) and the **saccule** (rostroventral) are housed (Fig. 18-2). Two parts of the **utriculosaccular duct** extend from the utricle and saccule respectively and converge to form the **endolymphatic duct,** which terminates as the **endolymphatic sac.** Part of the endolymphatic duct lies within the vestibular aqueduct. The endolymphatic sac lies partially within the **vestibular aqueduct,** and partially between two laminae of the dura. The function of the sac is to regulate the pressure and volume of endolymph.

Cochlear Duct

The **cochlear duct** is connected to the saccule by a small duct, the **ductus reuniens,** and ends as a blind sac at the apex of the cochlea. The triangular cochlear duct lies between two additional compartments of the cochlea (Fig. 18-4). The dorsal compartment, or **scala vestibuli,** extends from the region of the **vestibular (oval) window** to the apex of the cochlea, where it becomes confluent with the ventral compartment, the **scala tympani,** through an opening called the **helicotrema** (Fig. 18-2). The scala tympani ends at the **cochlear (round) window.** The cochlear duct is separated from the scala vestibuli by the **vestibular membrane** (Reissner's membrane) and from the scala tympani by the **basilar membrane** (Figs. 18-4 and 18-5). Scant collagen fibers form the vestibular membrane, which is covered with simple squamous epithelium on both surfaces. Basement membranes separate the epithelia from the connective tissue. The basilar membrane is attached to the outer osseous cochlea by the **spiral ligament** and extends to the **spiral lamina** of the modiolus. The membrane is composed of collagen fibers embedded in homogeneous ground substance; it increases in thickness as it progresses from the cochlear window to the helicotrema. Width of the basilar membrane increases continuously from the cochlear window, where it is narrowest, to the helicotrema, where it is widest. On the side facing the scala tympani, the basilar membrane is covered with simple squamous epithelium, while the **spiral organ** (organ of Corti) is present on the cochlear duct surface.

Stria Vascularis

The third wall of the triangular-shaped cochlear duct contains the **stria vascularis,** which contributes to the production of endolymph and regulates its unique ion content (Figs. 18-4, 18-5, and 18-6). Stratified cuboidal cells of the stria rest directly on a layer of connective tissue without an intervening basal lamina (Fig. 18-7). Three epithelial cell types (basal, intermediate, and marginal cells) appear similar with electron microscopy. Dark-

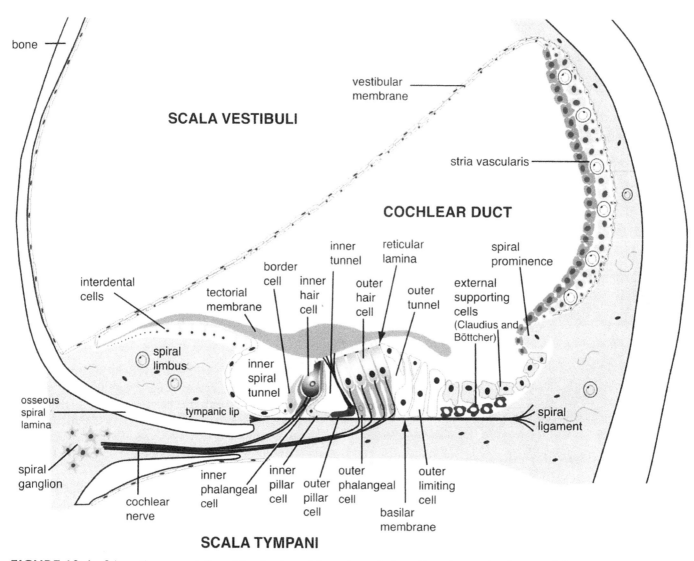

FIGURE 18-4   Schematic representation of the structure of the scala vestibuli, cochlear duct, and scala tympani. Note the structure of the spiral organ, which includes many cell types that lie under the tectorial membrane above the basilar membrane. Other major structures include the stria vascularis, vestibular membrane, spiral ligament, cochlear nerve, and spiral ganglion.

staining **marginal cells** lie adjacent to the cochlear duct lumen and are known to pump Na⁺ out of the endolymph. Light-staining intermediate and basal cells are found between the marginal cells and the spiral ligament. The **intermediate cells** contain melanin and also play a role in the generation of electrical potentials in the inner ear. **Basal cells** are flat cells that form a barrier between the stria vascularis and the spiral ligament. While epithelium in general is considered to be avascular, many capillaries are present between the epithelial cells of the stria vascularis (Fig. 18-6). At the junction of the stria vascularis with the spiral organ, the stratified epithelium changes abruptly to simple cuboidal. This region is called the **spiral prominence** (Fig. 18-4).

Vestibular Apparatus

The **vestibular apparatus** includes the organs of equilibrium, composed of the semicircular ducts, saccule, and utricle. Within

these structures are specialized neuroepithelial areas, the crista ampullaris, macula utriculi, and macula sacculi, which function to detect motion and maintain equilibrium.

Crista Ampullaris

The membranous ampulla of each semicircular duct contains a **crista ampullaris,** which is sensitive to rotary movements (angular acceleration and deceleration) (Figs. 18-8 and 18-9). The crista ampullaris is composed of a ridge of sensory epithelium resting on thickened connective tissue, which projects into the lumen of the ampulla.

Sensory epithelium of the crista ampullaris consists of hair cells and supporting cells (Figs. 18-8 and 18-10). Two types of hair cells are recognized at the ultrastructural level. The **type I hair cell** has a narrow neck and a rounded base that fits into a cup-shaped afferent nerve terminal (nerve chalice). Efferent nerve fibers contact the chalice and may be inhibitory in function. The

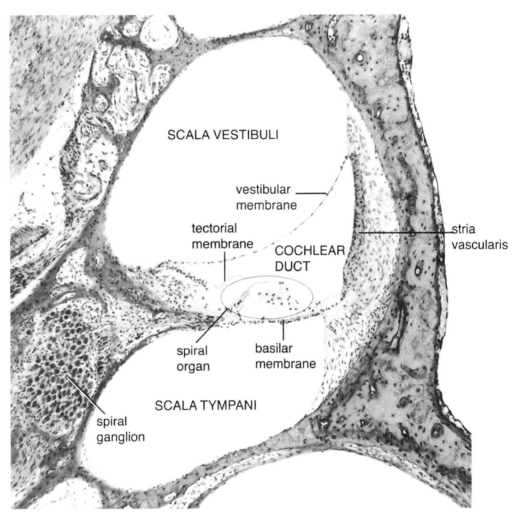

FIGURE 18-5 A section through one turn of the cochlea with the modiolus to the left. The vestibular membrane separates the scala vestibuli from the cochlear duct. The tectorial membrane lies over cells of the spiral organ (circled), which are located above the basilar membrane. Nerve fibers from the spiral ganglion innervate the hair cells of the spiral organ. Hematoxylin and eosin (×75).

type II hair cell is cylindrical and is innervated by both afferent and efferent nerve endings at its base. The nerve endings are branches of the vestibular portion of the vestibulocochlear nerve (cranial nerve VIII).

A single kinocilium and 40 to 80 stereocilia are present on the apical surface of each hair cell. In the crista ampullaris of the lateral semicircular duct, the kinocilium of each hair cell is oriented toward the utricle. In contrast, in the anterior and posterior semicircular ducts, the hair cell kinocilium is oriented away from the utricle. Each kinocilium has the typical ciliary microtubule arrangement of nine peripheral pairs and one central pair; however, the hair cell kinocilium is incapable of independent motion. The stereocilia are arranged in four or five rows and tilt toward the kinocilium, forming a cone-shaped bundle. Stereocilium length increases progressively toward the region of the cell where the kinocilium is located. The tip of each stereocilium is linked to its neighbor in the adjacent row by a fine protein strand called **tip link,** composed of cadherin 23. Within each stereocilium, numerous actin filaments anchor in a complex terminal web called the **cuticular plate.**

The orientation of the stereocilia and the single kinocilium gives each hair cell a functional polarization. Whenever the stereocilia bend toward the kinocilium, the afferent nerve fiber in contact with the cell is excited. Conversely, movement in the opposite direction causes inhibition of neural transmission.

The sensory hair cells of the crista ampullaris project into an overlying gelatinous **cupula.** The cupula contacts the opposite wall of the ampulla and deflects in the direction of endolymph movement, much like an elastic diaphragm. This deflection causes the hair bundles (stereocilia and the kinocilium) to bend, thereby generating neural impulses.

The **supporting cells** of the epithelium are tall and columnar with microvilli. They synthesize the matrix of the cupula and therefore contain numerous secretory vesicles.

Maculae of the Utricle and Saccule

Two receptor organs, the **macula utriculi** and **macula sacculi,** lie perpendicular to each other, located on the lateral wall of the utricle and the floor of the saccule, respectively.

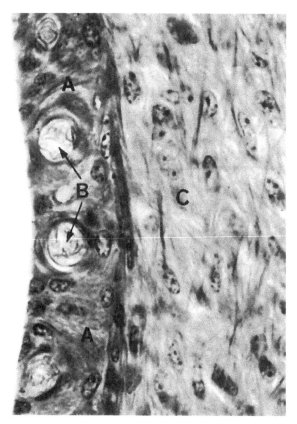

FIGURE 18-6   The epithelium of the stria vascularis (A) is traversed by numerous capillaries (B) and rests on loose connective tissue (C) (guinea pig). Crossmon's trichrome (×600).

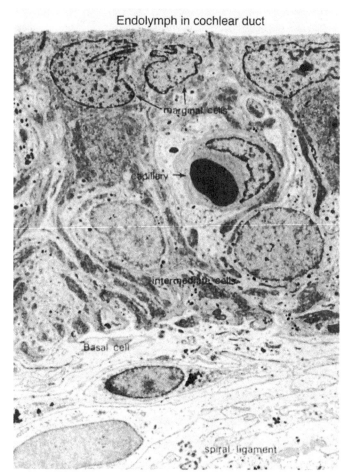

FIGURE 18-7   Three different cell types (marginal, intermediate, and basal) surround a capillary in the stria vascularis epithelium (squirrel monkey). Transmission electron micrograph, (×3752). *(From Schuknecht HF. Anatomy. In: Schuknecht HF, ed. Pathology of the Ear. 2nd Ed. Philadelphia: Lea & Febiger, 1993:31.)*

The sensory epithelium of both maculae rests on loose connective tissue containing blood vessels and nerves (Figs. 18-10 and 18-11). The cells of the sensory epithelium of the maculae are essentially the same as those of the crista ampullaris, that is, type I and II sensory cells and supporting cells (Figs. 18-10 and 18-11). The arrangement of the sensory cells differs between the two maculae. In the macula utriculi, the kinocilium of each cell faces toward a stripe, the **striola,** which divides the sensory cell population into two oppositely polarized groups (Fig. 18-10). In the macula sacculi, the hair cells polarize such that the kinocilium of each cell faces away from the striola.

Hair bundles of the sensory cells of the maculae penetrate an overlying gelatinous mass with calcium carbonate crystals called **statoconia** (otoliths). Together, the hair bundles, gelatinous material, and statoconia form the **statoconial** (otolithic) **membrane.**

Vestibular Mechanism

With rotation of the head, the endolymph flows through the semicircular ducts. In the ampulla of each duct, the movement of the fluid displaces the cupula, which then bends the underlying stereocilia of the hair cells of the crista ampullaris. As the stereocilia bend toward the kinocilium, each hair cell increasingly stimulates neural impulses. The neural stimulus decreases as the stereocilia bend away from the kinocilium.

Linear movements of the head are detected by the maculae. As endolymph moves in the utricle and saccule, the statoconia shift in the gelatinous material over the sensory epithelium, thus stimulating underlying hair cells.

Neural impulses from the hair cells in the crista ampullaris and the maculae are transmitted to the brain via the axons of the vestibular nerve, a branch of cranial nerve VIII (vestibulocochlear nerve)

Auditory Apparatus

The auditory apparatus comprises the organ of hearing, which includes the scala tympani, scala vestibuli, and cochlear duct. Within the cochlear duct is the epithelial spiral organ, which functions in hearing.

Spiral Organ (Organ of Corti)

The sensory portion of the **spiral organ** is a complex structure that rests on the cochlear duct side of the basilar membrane (Figs. 18-4

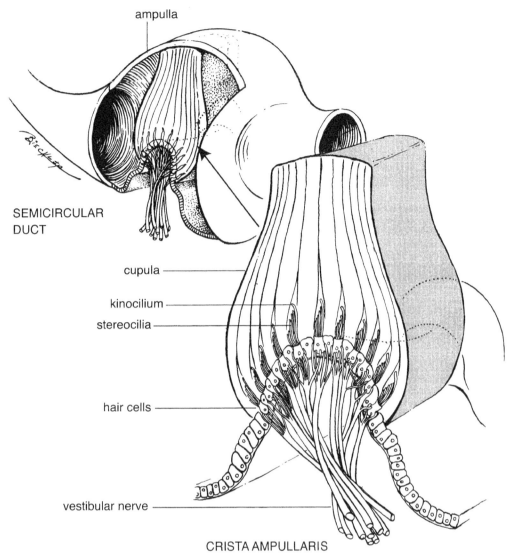

ampulla

SEMICIRCULAR
DUCT

cupula

kinocilium

stereocilia

hair cells

vestibular nerve

CRISTA AMPULLARIS

FIGURE 18-8 Schematic drawing of the ampulla of the semicircular duct, open to show the crista ampullaris within. The enlarged drawing of the crista shows the hair cells beneath the cup-shaped gelatinous cupula. Each hair cell has one kinocilium and several stereocilia of different lengths on the apical surface. Processes of the vestibular nerve contact the basal region of the hair cells.

and 18-5). This receptor organ has three major components: (a) the sensory cells that transform mechanical energy of sound vibrations into electrical energy, (b) a supportive structure for the sensory cells, and (c) the afferent and efferent nerve terminals of the cochlear nerve, a branch of cranial nerve VIII (Fig. 18-4).

Sensory Cells

The sensory cells are arranged in two groups: the outer hair cells that form three to four rows adjacent to the outer pillar cells, and the inner hair cells that form a single row just outside the inner pillar cells.

The cylindrical **outer hair cells** are slanted toward the inner tunnel (Figs. 18-4 and 18-12). From the apex of each cell, a bundle of approximately 100 stereocilia projects in a W pattern (V or U pattern in some mammals). The stereocilia of each cell form four

to five rows of increasing height toward the spiral ligament. Thus, the outer hair cells are morphologically polarized, much like the vestibular hair cells. The longest stereocilia are embedded in the tectorial membrane. The tips of the stereocilia are connected to their adjacent taller neighbors by means of tip link. At the base of the outer hair cells, a few afferent nerve endings and many efferent terminals containing vesicles are present. Both the inner and outer hair cells have synaptic ribbons where afferent synapses occur.

The **inner hair cells** are pear-shaped. Each cell has 50 to 60 stereocilia that form three straight, parallel rows that increase in height toward the inner tunnel. The stereocilia are not embedded in the tectorial membrane; however, the longest stereocilia do touch it. Tip links connect the stereocilia of inner hair cells in a fashion similar to that seen in outer hair cells. In contrast to outer hair cells, many afferent nerve endings and a few efferent terminals are present at the base of the inner hair cells.

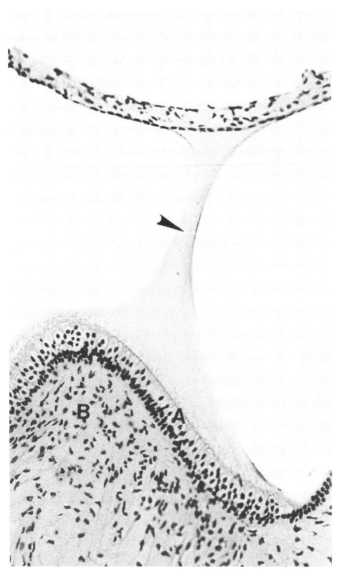

FIGURE 18-9 The sensory and supporting cells (A) and the underlying connective tissue (B) form the crista ampullaris within the ampulla. The gelatinous cupula (arrowhead) on top of the epithelium extends across the lumen of the ampulla to the opposite wall (guinea pig). Hematoxylin and eosin (×400).

Supporting Cells

The supporting cells of the spiral organ include the border cells, inner and outer pillar cells, inner and outer phalangeal cells, outer limiting cells, and external supporting cells (Fig. 18-4).

The columnar **border cells** rest on the **tympanic lip** of the spiral limbus, forming a single row on the inner side of the inner hair cells. The **inner** and **outer pillar cells** line a prominent triangular space, the **inner tunnel** (Corti's tunnel). They have a broad base containing the nucleus and an elongated body packed with tonofilaments that fan out to form the cuticular plate in the cell apex.

The **inner** and **outer phalangeal cells** (outer cells were formerly known as Deiter's cells) are supportive cells that rest on the basilar membrane and extend upward to cradle the base of the hair

cells and then send long cytoplasmic processes toward the surface. Phalangeal cells have a bundle of filaments originating from the basal cell membrane and extending to the apex. The phalangeal processes expand into a flat plate held to the hair cells by junctional complexes. Inner hair cells are almost totally enveloped by inner phalangeal cells, while the outer hair cells are partially surrounded by outer phalangeal cells. The free surface of phalangeal cells and hair cells, with its massive terminal web and intercellular junctions, forms the **reticular lamina,** which holds the apical part of the hair cells rigid.

The outer limiting cells and the external supporting cells complete the cellular component of the spiral organ. The **outer limiting cell** (Hensen's cell) is very tall and the presence of microvilli suggests that these cells may be engaged, to some extent, in fluid absorption. Outer limiting cells are separated from the outer phalangeal cells by a space, the **outer tunnel** (Fig. 18-12).

External supporting cells (Claudius' and Böttcher's cells) are located between the outer limiting cells and the **spiral prominence,** a projection into the cochlear duct. The supporting cells are similar in their cytoplasmic characteristics, although their sizes and shapes vary. Large cuboidal cells (Claudius' cells) overlay smaller basal cells (Böttcher's cells). The function of these cells is unknown.

Tectorial Membrane

Overlying the spiral organ is the **tectorial membrane,** a gelatinous structure containing glycoprotein and extending from the spiral limbus over the hair cells (Figs. 18-4 and 18-5). The lower surface of this membrane rests on the tips of the tallest stereocilia in each bundle of the inner hair cells, whereas the tallest stereocilia of the outer hair cells are embedded in the membrane. **Interdental cells,** located where the tectorial membrane attaches to the spiral limbus, secrete the gel-like substance of the membrane.

Spiral Ganglion

Bipolar neurons in the **spiral ganglion** at the base of the modiolus project to either the inner hair cells (type I spiral ganglion cells) or the outer hair cells (type II spiral ganglion cells) of the spiral organ (Fig. 18-4). The spiral ganglion neurons project in the opposite direction to form the cochlear nerve, a branch of the vestibulocochlear nerve (cranial nerve VIII).

Auditory Mechanism

Sound is composed of vibrations that alternately compress the air and then allow it to expand in successive waves. The simplest sound wave, a pure tone, is characterized by frequency and amplitude. Extrapolated from human hearing, the frequency and amplitude of sound waves correspond to perception of pitch and loudness (intensity).

The ear is constructed as a receptor of sound waves in air. The outer ear captures sound waves with varying efficiency, depending on the size of the auricle. In mammals, sensitivity of hearing also relates to the ability to either raise or close the outer ear (auricle). Animals raise the outer ear in an attempt to sharpen their hearing or cover the ear canal to block sound.

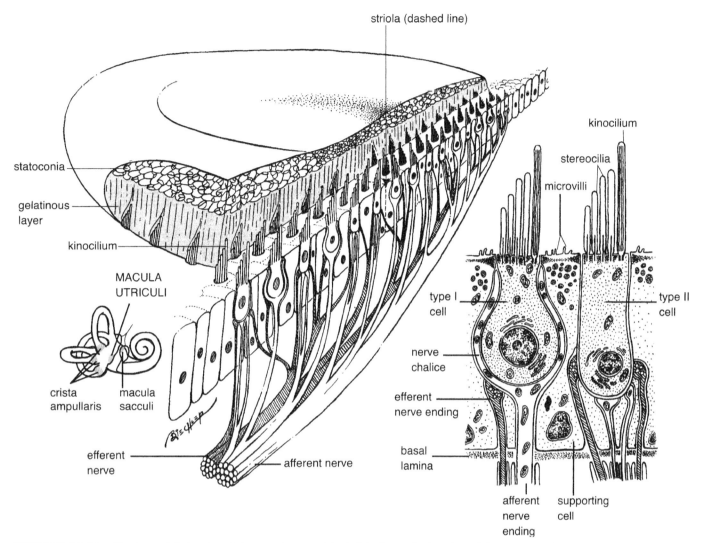

FIGURE 18-10 The lower left drawing of the membranous labyrinth indicates the location of the macula utriculi, macula sacculi, and cristae ampullaris with gray shading. The larger schematic drawing of the macula utriculi illustrates the sensory epithelium. The statoconial membrane has been cut away to better illustrate the underlying cells. The numerous stereocilia and single kinocilium of each sensory cell form a conelike arrangement; each kinocilium faces the striola, represented as a dashed line. Note the change in the morphologic polarization of the sensory cells at the striola. Afferent nerve fibers are white, while efferent nerve fibers are hatched gray. In the lower right corner, a schematic drawing illustrates the general structure of the vestibular sensory epithelium. The type I hair cell has a constricted neck and a rounded base and is almost completely surrounded by a nerve chalice. The more cylindrical type II cell is innervated by two types of bud-shaped nerve endings: sparsely vesiculated afferent (white) and richly vesiculated efferent (hatched). *(Modified and redrawn after Lindemann HH. Anatomy of the otolith organs. Adv Otorhinolaryngol 1973;20:405.)*

The tympanic membrane acts as a transmitter of sound wave–generated vibrations from the air in the external acoustic meatus to the middle ear (Fig. 18-13). The bridge of the malleus, incus, and stapes transports the vibrations across the middle ear to the perilymph on the medial side of the stapes footplate. In addition to transporting vibrations, the middle ear mechanism also protects the inner ear from receiving too much energy by damping excessive vibration.

Sound vibrations in the middle ear are transferred by the stapes footplate through the vestibular window to the perilymph of the scala vestibuli and eventually the scala tympani. Simultaneously, the pressure waves push the vestibular membrane into the endolymph within the cochlear duct. As a result of the pressure, the basilar membrane on the opposite side of the cochlear duct bulges outward into the scala tympani. As the pressure varies within the cochlear duct fluid, regions of the basilar membrane begin to vibrate with different maximum amplitudes along the length of the duct. Vibration of the basilar membrane causes the hair cells of the spiral organ to contact the overlying tectorial membrane. Contact ultimately generates neural impulses that pass via the cochlear branch of the vestibulocochlear nerve (cranial nerve VIII). Residual vibration within the scala tympani is released through the cochlear window.

The variation of width, thickness, and elasticity of the basilar membrane allows **tonotopical localization.** Low-frequency sounds cause the basilar membrane to vibrate in the apical end of

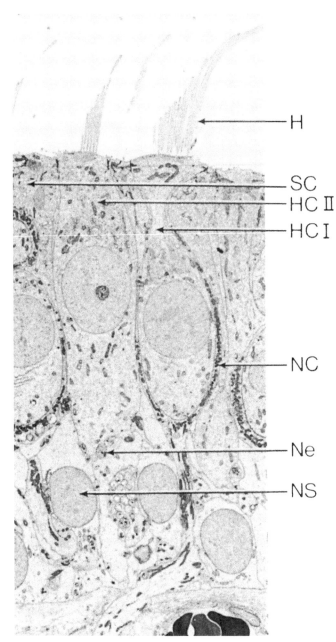

FIGURE 18-11 The type I (HC I) and type II (HC II) sensory hair cells of the epithelium of the macula utriculi are separated by supporting cells (SC). Stereocilia (H) of varying length are present on the surface of the hair cells. The nuclei (NS) of the supporting cells are located in the basal region of the epithelium. An efferent nerve ending (Ne) is located near the basal surface of a type II sensory cell. A type I cell is surrounded by an afferent nerve chalice ending (NC) (cat). Transmission electron micrograph (×2331). *(From Schuknecht HF. Anatomy. In: Schuknecht HF, ed. Pathology of the Ear. 2nd Ed. Philadelphia: Lea & Febiger, 1993:31.)*

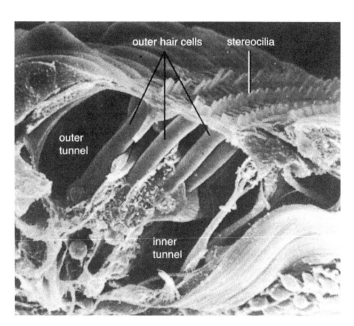

FIGURE 18-12 Outer hair cells with rows of stereocilia on their apical surface are shown in this scanning electron micrograph of a portion of the spiral organ. *(From Weiss L, ed. Cell and Tissue Biology, a Textbook of Histology. 6th Ed. Baltimore: Urban & Schwarzenberg, 1988:1118.)*

The site of transduction of mechanical energy to electrical signals seems to be the tip of the stereocilia of the hair cells, where the receptor current enters the sensory cell in response to displacement of the hair bundle. The tip links and the ionic channels situated in the plasma membrane covering the terminal ends of the stereocilia are believed to be involved in the transduction. When pushed in the excitatory direction, tip links are stretched and ionic channels in the terminal membrane of the stereocilium are in the open state. The channels close when the stereocilium is pushed in the opposite direction. The ionic currents regulate neurotransmitter release at the afferent synapse located at the base of the hair cell. The speed of hair cell response is faster than in any other sensory receptor cells, including neurons. The result is electrical signals that are transferred to the brain via afferent nerve fibers.

The function of the efferent nerve fibers at the base of the hair cells is not yet completely understood. The innervation may have a regulating function in noisy environments, which allows filtering of unwanted sounds to focus on a particular sound. The efferent system is also believed to play a role in **otoacoustic emissions (OAE)**, the recording of a tone that has radiated into the ear canal from the inner ear in response to a sound stimulus. OAE is currently the most important diagnostic test to determine inner ear status in humans, especially in babies and small children. The existence of OAE in animals has been proven in several species, but diagnostic test results do not agree.

Loss of hearing may be related to any condition that interferes with the conduction of sound through the structure of the ear. External or internal ear infections, changes in the bones of the middle ear, or conditions that affect nerve impulse transmission can all affect hearing.

the cochlea, whereas high frequencies cause vibration in the region close to the cochlear window.

At low-vibration amplitudes, only the outer hair cells are stimulated. At greater amplitudes, the inner hair cells are also activated. Stimulation of the outer hair cells results in determination of sound intensity (loudness), whereas stimulation of inner hair cells results in frequency (pitch) determination.

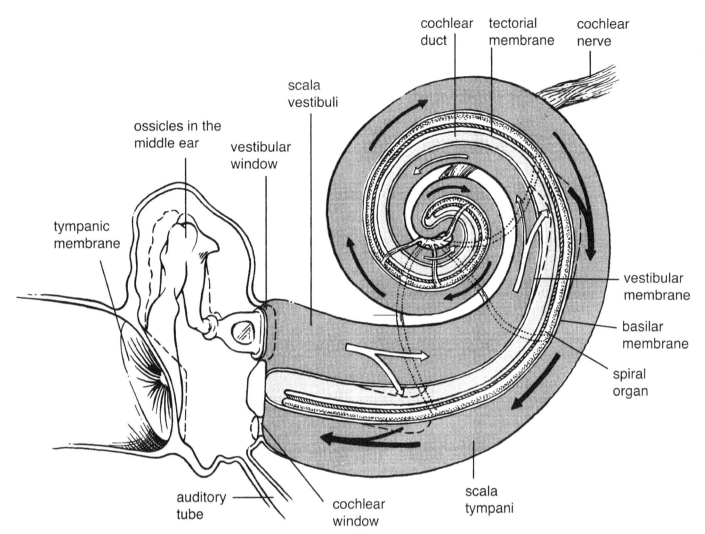

FIGURE 18-13 Schematic diagram of the events of sound transmission in the ear. The cochlea has been uncoiled to more easily visualize the process. Sound waves impinge on the tympanic membrane, causing it to vibrate. The ear ossicles vibrate as a unit; the range of position of ear ossicles is indicated by dashed lines. The footplate of the stapes moves in and out of the vestibular window, causing changes in fluid pressure within the scala vestibuli. Perilymph (dark gray) fills the scala vestibuli and scala tympani while endolymph (light gray) fills the cochlear duct. The thickness of the white arrows in the scala vestibuli and the black arrows in the scala tympani indicates increased (thick arrow) or decreased (thin arrow) fluid pressure. Because fluid is incompressible, pressure changes cause distortion of the vestibular and basilar membranes. Deflection of the basilar membrane pushes the hair cells of the spiral organ into the overlying tectorial membrane, generating neural impulses in the cochlear nerve. Short sound waves (high frequency, high pitch) affect the base of the cochlea, while long waves (low frequency, low pitch) affect the apex of the cochlea. Waves may also travel around the helicotrema at the apex of the cochlea. Impact of the waves on the secondary tympanic membrane covering the cochlear window causes it to move in and out in opposite phases to the vestibular window.

SUGGESTED READINGS

Békésy GV. Zur Theorie des Höhrens; die Schwingungsform der Basilarmembran. Physik Zeits 1928;29:793.

Berry MM, Standring SM, Bannister LH. Auditory and vestibular apparatus. In: Williams PL, ed. Gray's Anatomy. 38th Ed. Edinburgh: Churchill Livingstone, 1995:1367.

Couloigner V, Teixeira M, Sterkers O, et al. The endolymphatic sac: its roles in the inner ear. Med Sci (Paris) 2004;20(3):304.

Erway LC, Mitchell SE. Prevention of otolith defect in pastel mink by manganese supplementation. J Hered 1973;64:111.

Fay RR. Hearing in Vertebrates: A Psychophysics Databook. Winnetka, IL: Hill-Fay Associates, 1988.

Flock Å. The ear. In: Weiss L, ed. Cell and Tissue Biology. A Textbook of Histology. 6th Ed. Baltimore: Urban & Schwarzenberg, Inc., 1988:1107.

Flock Å, Wersäll J, eds. Cellular mechanisms in hearing. Proceedings of Nobel Symposium 63. Hear Res 1986;22:1.

Flottorp G. Pure-tone tinnitus evoked by acoustic stimulation: the idiophonic effect. Acta Otolaryngol (Stockh) 1953;43:396.

Flottorp G, Foss I. Development of hearing in hereditarily deaf white mink (Hedlund) and normal mink (Standard) and the subsequent deterioration of the auditory response in Hedlund mink. Acta Otolaryngol (Stockh) 1979;87:16.

Foss I. Development of hearing and vision, and morphological examination of the inner ear in hereditarily deaf white Norwegian Dunkerhounds and normal dogs (black and dappled Norwegian Dunkerhounds). Master's thesis. Ithaca, NY: Cornell University, 1981.

Foss I, Flottorp G. A comparative study of the development of hearing and vision in various species commonly used in experiments. Acta Otolaryngol (Stockh) 1974;77:202.

Friedmann I, Ballantyne J. Ultrastructural Atlas of the Inner Ear. London: Butterworths & Co., 1984.

Gacek RR. Efferent innervation of the labyrinth. Clinical review. Am J Otolaryngol 1984;5:206.

Hudspeth AJ. How the ear's works work. Review article. Nature 1989; 341:397.

Kemp DT. Stimulated acoustic emissions from within human auditory system. J Acoust Soc Am 1978;64:1386.

Kimura RS. Distribution, structure, and function of dark cells in the vestibular labyrinth. Ann Otol Rhinol Laryngol 1969;48: 542.

Lagardre F, Chaumillon G, Amara R, et al. Examination of otolith morphology and microstructure using laser scanning microscopy. In: Secor DH, Dean JM, Campana SE, eds. Recent Developments in Fish Otolith Research. Columbia, SC: University of South Carolina Press, 1995:7.

Metz O. The acoustic impedance measured on normal and pathological ears. Acta Otolaryngol (Stockh) 1946;(Suppl 63):1.

Osborne MP, Comis SD, Pickles JO. Morphology and cross linkage of stereo-cilia in the guinea-pig labyrinth examined without the use of osmium as a fixative. Cell Tissue Res 1984;237:43.

Pitovski DZ, Kerr TP. Sodium- and potassium-activated ATPase in the mammalian vestibular system. Hearing Research 2002;171(1–2):51.

Probst R. Otoacoustic emissions: an overview. In: Pfaltz CR, ed. New Aspects of Cochlear Mechanics and Inner Ear Pathophysiology. Adv Otorhinolaryngol 1990;44;1.

Rabinowitz J. Les effets physiologiques du bruit. Recherche 1991; 22(229):178.

Raphael Y, Altschuler RA. Structure and innervation of the cochlea. Brain Res Bull 2003;60:397.

Ross MH, Romrell LJ, Kaye GI. Ear. In: Ross MH, Romrell LJ, Kaye GI, eds. Histology: A Text and Atlas. 3rd Ed. Baltimore: Williams & Wilkins, 1995:768.

Schuknecht HF. Anatomy. In: Schuknecht HF, ed. Pathology of the Ear. 2nd Ed. Philadelphia: Lea & Febiger, 1993:31.

Thalmann R, Thalmann, I. Source and role of endolymph macromolecules. Acta Otolaryngol 1999;119(3):293.

Tortora GJ, Grabowski SR. Auditory sensations and equilibrium. In: Tortora GJ, Grabowski SR, eds. Principles of Anatomy and Physiology. 7th Ed. New York: HarperCollins College Publishers, 1993:487.

Zwislocki J. Theorie der Schneckenmechanik. Acta Otolaryngol (Stockh) 1948;(Suppl 72):1.

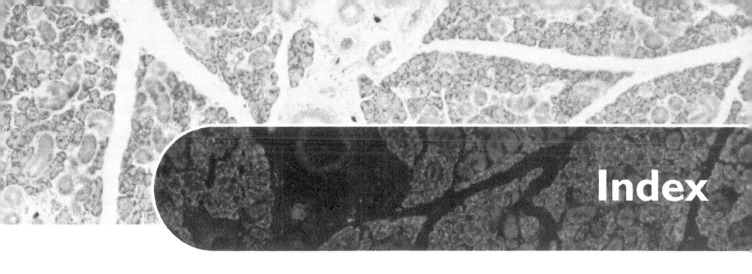

Index

A band, 82
Abomasum, 190, 194
Accessory glands, 248–251, 249f–251f
Accessory pancreatic duct, 208, 209f
Acellular cementum, 178, 178f
Acetylcholine, release of, 84
Acidophil(s), 302
Acidophilic, 2
Acidophilic granular cells, 196, 198f
Acinus, 24, 27f, 161f, 162, 163f
Acrosomal cap, 239
Acrosomal phase, 238–239
Acrosome reaction, 239
ACTH. *See* Adrenocorticotropic hormone (ACTH)
α-Actinin, 84
Activin, 306
Adenohypophysis, 300–303, 301f–304f
    pars distalis of, 301–302, 301f–303f
    parts of, 300–303, 301f–304f
Adenosine triphosphate (ATP), 10
ADH. *See* Antidiuretic hormone (ADH)
Adhesion(s), focal, 16
Adipocyte(s), 33–34, 33f, 34f, 318
    multilocular, 34, 34f
    perisinusoidal, 205
    unilocular, 33–34, 33f
Adipose tissue, 33, 34f, 43
    brown, 43
    white, 43
Adrenal cortex
    inner cortex of, 311
    outer cortex of, 311
Adrenal gland, 311–316, 312f–315f
    adrenal cortex of, 311–315, 312f–314f
Adrenal medulla, 315–316, 315f
Adrenocorticotropic hormone (ACTH), 302, 306
Adventitial cells, 75
Afferent arterioles, 224, 225f
Afferent fibers, 104
Afterbirth, retained, 293
Agglutination, 63
Aggrecan(s), 44

Aggregated lymphatic nodules, 143, 144f
    in distal small intestine, 139–140, 139f
Agouti-related peptide (AgRP), 318
Agranulocyte(s), 63
AgRP. *See* Agouti–related peptide (AgRP)
Air capillaries, avian, 168
Air sacs, avian, 168
Airway(s), intrapulmonary conducting, 161–162, 161f, 162f
Albumen, 277
Aldosterone, 311, 313
Allantoamnion, 280
Allantochorion, 280
Alveolar ducts, 161f, 163, 163f, 164f
Alveolar epithelial cells
    granular, 164, 166f
    squamous, 164, 164f
Alveolar macrophages, 164, 167f
Alveolar sacs, 161f, 163, 163f, 164f
Alveolus, 24, 27f, 177
Alveolus(i), 161f, 163–164, 164f–167f
Amacrine cells, 359
Amine precursor uptake and decarboxylation (APUD) cells, 24, 160, 309, 318
Amnion, 279
Amniotic plaques, 293
Ampulla, 262, 264, 265f, 266f
Anagen, 333, 334f
Anal canal, of large intestine, 201, 201f
Anal glands, 201, 339
Anal sacs, 201, 339, 339f, 340f
    glands of, 339, 340f
Anaphase, of cell cycle, 13, 14f
Anastomosis(es), arteriovenous, 125–126
Androgen(s), 311, 319
Androgen-binding protein, 319
Anestrus, 271, 274, 274f
Angiogenesis, 123
Angiotensin I, 313
Angiotensin II, 227, 313
Angiotensinogen, 313
Anisocytosis, 63
Annulospiral ending, 109, 109f

Annulus fibrosus, 58, 58f
Anorectal line, 201
ANP. *See* Atrial natriuretic peptide (ANP)
Anterior epithelium, of cornea, 351, 352f
Anterior lamina, 352
Antidiuretic hormone (ADH), 229, 303, 304f
Antigen(s), 135
Antigen receptors, 135, 135f
Antigen-presenting cells, 136–137, 136f
Antiparamesonephric hormone, 236
Antrum, 257f, 258, 259f, 260f
Apocrine mode of secretion, 29, 29f
Apocrine sweat glands, 334–335, 335f
Apoptosis, 14
Apoptotic bodies, 14
Appositional growth, 46
APUD cells, 24, 160, 309, 318
APUD (amine precursor uptake and decarboxylation) cells, 24, 160, 309, 318
Aquaporin(s), 228, 229
Aqueous humor, 356
Arachnoid, 113
Arachnoid trabeculae, 113–114, 114f
Arachnoid villi, 114, 114f
Arcuate arteries, 224, 225f
Area centralis retinae, 359
Area cribrosa, 351
Areola-gland complexes, 281f, 286, 287f
Argentaffin cells, 189, 318
Argentaffin fibers, 39, 39f
Arginine vasopressin (AVP), 303
Argyrophilic cells, 189
Argyrophilic fibers, 39, 39f
Arrector pili muscles, 328, 330, 331f
Arteriole(s), 118, 122, 122f, 123f
   afferent, 224, 225f
   efferent, 224, 225f
   interlobular hepatic, 202f, 204
   pulp, 150
Arteriovenous anastomoses, 125–126
Artery(ies), 120–121, 121f, 122f
   arcuate, 224, 225f
   bronchial, 166
   elastic, 118, 120, 122f
   interlobar, 224, 225f
   interlobular, 224, 225f
   muscular, 118, 119f, 120–121, 122f
   penicillar, 150
   pulmonary, 165–166
   trabecular, of spleen, 149–150, 150f
Artery of the white pulp, 149, 150f
Articular cartilage, 48, 58, 59f, 60f
Ascending vasa recta, 225, 226f
A-spermatogonia, 237, 238f, 239f
Astrocyte(s), 98–99, 99f
   fibrous, 98, 99f
   protoplasmic, 98, 99f
ATP. *See* Adenosine triphosphate (ATP)
Atresia, 261, 261f
   cystic, 261, 261f
   follicular, 261, 261f, 262f

Atrial granules, 130
Atrial natriuretic peptide (ANP), 88–89, 130, 318
Atrioventricular bundle, 130
Atrioventricular node, 130
Atrioventricular valves, 129, 129f
Atrium(a), 163
   avian, 168, 168f
Atrophy, of skeletal muscle, 86
Auditory apparatus, of internal ear, 370–374, 374f, 375f
Auditory mechanism, of internal ear, 372–374, 375f
Auditory ossicles, 364–365, 365f
Auditory tube, 365, 365f
Autocrine signaling, 16
Autonomic ganglia, 101f, 106
Autonomic nervous system, 104
Autonomic neurons
   postganglionic, 106
   preganglionic, 106
Autophagosome(s), 9
Alveolus(i), of mammary gland, 340–342, 341f
Avian. *See* Bird(s)
AVP. *See* Arginine vasopressin (AVP)
Axodendritic synapse, 93, 93f
Axon(s), 94, 96
   efferent, 104
Axonal reaction, 93, 93f
Axoplasm, 94

B cells, 135, 135f, 136f, 137
   effector, 135
B lymphocytes, 75
BALT. *See* Bronchus-associated lymphatic tissue (BALT)
Band neutrophil, 64
Barr body, 5, 92
Basal cells, 20, 155, 156
Basal complex, of choroid, 355
Basal lamina, 18
Basal zone, of endothelium, 265
Basilar membrane, 367, 368f, 369f
Basophil(s), 65, 72, 302
Basophilic, 2
Basophilic rubricyte, 72
Bile canaliculi, 203, 204f
Bile ducts, 203, 204f
Binucleate cells, 292
Binucleate trophoblast cell, 285
Bird(s)
   cloacal bursa of, 140, 140f
   digestive system of, 208–210, 209f, 210f
   female reproductive system of, 275–277, 276f
   integument of, 347–349, 348f, 349f
   respiratory system of, 167–168, 168f
Bitch(es)
   cyclic changes in endometrium in, 272
   cyclic changes of vaginal epithelium in, 274–275, 274f, 275f
   placentation in, 294–296, 294f, 295f
Bladder, urinary, 230–231, 231f
Blastocyst(s), 279
Blood, 61–66, 62f–66f
   before and after sedimentation, 61–62, 62f
   basophils, 65

composition of, 61–66, 62f–66f
    eosinophils, 64–65, 64f
    erythrocytes, 62–63, 62f
    functions of, 61
    leukocytes, 63–66, 63f–66f
    lymphocytes, 66, 66f
    monocytes, 65, 65f
    neutrophils, 63–64, 63f
    plasma, 61–62, 62f
    platelets, 66, 67f
Blood pressure, regulation of, kidneys in, 227, 227f
Blood supply
    to liver, 203–205, 204f, 205f
    to small intestine, 199
    to testis, 244–245
Blood vascular system, 117
Blood vessels, 114–115, 115f, 117–129. *See also Vein(s); specific types,*
    e.g., Artery(ies)
    arterioles, 122, 122f, 123f
    arteriovenous anastomoses, 125–126
    capillaries, 122–125, 123f–127f
    cardiac, 131
    general structural organization of, 118, 119f, 120f
    of immune system, 141–142
    of integument, 335–336
    of lung, 165–166
    of lymph nodes, 146, 147f
    microvasculature, 122–126, 122f–127f
    of ovary, 262
    specialized, 128, 128f
    of spleen, 149–150, 150f
    structure–function relationships of, 117–118
    of uterine tube, 265
    of uterus, 266f, 267–268, 267f
    vascular endothelium, 119–120, 121f
    veins, 126–128, 128f
    venules, 125, 127f
Blood–air barrier, 165
Blood–brain barrier, 115
Blood–CSF barrier, 115
Blood–nerve barrier, 105
Blood–testis barrier, 236
Blood–thymus barrier, 142
Body stalk, 280
Bone(s), 46–58, 47f, 49f–57f
    cells of, 46–48, 47f
    classification of, 50, 53f
    compact, 48
    entoglossal, 208
    fracture of, repair of, 57–58
    function of, characteristics of, 48–50, 49f–53f
    histologic preparation of, 48, 49f, 53f
    lamellar, 49f, 50
    modeling of, 56, 56f
    osteogenesis, 50–58, 53f–57f. *See also* Osteogenesis
    remodeling of, 56–57, 57f
    spongy, 48
    structure of
        characteristics of, 48–50, 49f–53f
        macroscopic, 48, 50f–52f
        microscopic, 49–50, 49f, 51f
    woven, 50, 53f

Bone cells, 46–48, 47f
Bone lining cells, 47
Bone marrow, 66–74, 67f, 68f, 70f–74f, 138
    cells in, 66–74, 67f, 68f, 70f–74f
    cellular compartments of, 67–68, 67f
    function of, 67–68, 68f
    granulopoiesis in, 70–72, 71f
    HSCs in, 69–70, 70f
    lymphopoiesis of, 75
    microcirculation of, 68, 68f
    monocytopoiesis of, 72
    red, 76
    structure of, 66–68, 67f, 68f
    thrombopoiesis of, 75, 75f
    vascular compartments of, 67–68, 67f
    yellow, 76
Bone marrow smears, 76, 76f
Bone matrix, 48
Bony labyrinth, of internal ear, 366–367, 366f, 367f
Böttcher's cells, 372
Bowman's capsule, 216f–218f, 217–218
Bowman's membrane, 352
Bowman's space, 216f, 217, 217f
Brachydont teeth, 177, 177f
Bronchial arteries, 166
Bronchial glands, 162
Bronchiolar exocrine cells, 162
Bronchiole(s), 161f, 162, 162f
    respiratory, 162–163, 163f, 164f
    terminal, 162–163, 163f, 164f
Bronchus(i), 161–162, 161f
    avian, 168, 168f
    extrapulmonary, 160, 161f
    primary, 160
Bronchus-associated lymphatic tissue (BALT), 143
Brown adipose tissue, 43
Brunner's glands, 197, 198f
Brush cells, 155
B-spermatogonia, 237, 238f, 239f
Buccal glands, 173
Buccal papillae, 173, 173f
Bud(s), periosteal, 51
Bulb, 342
Bulbourethral glands, 251, 251f
Bulbous corpuscles, 108, 108f
Bulbous vestibuli, 270
Bursa, cloacal, of birds, 140, 140f

C protein, 83
Ca-ATPase, 229
Cadherin(s), 15
Calcitonin, 309
Call-Exner bodies, 258f, 259
Callus(i)
    external, 57
    internal, 57
Calmodulin, 80
Camera anterior bulbi, 350
Camera posterior bulbi, 350
Camera vitrea bulbi, 351
cAMP. *See* Cyclic adenosine monophosphate (cAMP)

Canaliculus(i)
  bile, 203, 204f
  intracellular, 188
  lacrimal, 361
Cap phase, 238
Capillary(ies), 118, 122–125, 123f–127f
  air, avian, 168
  continuous, 123f–125f, 124
  fenestrated, 123f, 124, 125f
    peritubular capillary networks of, 224–225
  glomerular, 215–216, 216f, 217f
  lymph, 131–132, 131f, 132f
  sheathed, 150, 150f
  terminal, 150, 150f
Capillary beds, 123
Capitance vessels, 155
Capsule(s), 27
  of liver, 201–202, 202f
  splenic, 147–148
Cardiac conduction fibers, 130
Cardiac conduction system, 130–131
Cardiac glands, 187, 189f
Cardiac muscle, 86–90, 87f–90f
  contraction of, 89
  fine structure of, 87–89, 88f–90f
  hypertrophy of, 89–90
  light microscopic structure of, 86–87, 87f, 88f
  myogenesis of, 89–90
  regeneration of, 89–90
  T tubules of, 87, 88f
Cardiac nodes, 89, 90f
Cardiac skeleton, 130
Cardiac sphincter muscle, 185
Cardiac valves, 129, 129f
Cardiovascular system, 117–133
  blood vessels of, 117–129. *See also* Blood vessels
Carotid body, 128, 128f, 317
Carotid sinus, 128–129
Carpal glands, 338
Carrier proteins, 228
Cartilage, 43–46, 44f–46f
  articular, 48, 58, 59f, 60f
  cells of, 43–44, 44f
  classification of, 44–45, 44f
  development of, 45–46
  elastic, 45, 45f
  hyaline, 44–45, 44f
  nutrition of, 46
  vomeronasal, 158
  zones of, 58, 59f
Cartilage canals, 53, 54f
Cartilage cells, 43–44, 44f
Cartilage matrix, 40f, 44
Cartilaginous joints, 58, 58f
Caruncle(s), 267, 267f, 282, 289, 292f
Caruncular crypts, 282
Catagen, 333, 334f
Cavernous stratum, 155, 157f
CDKs. *See* Cyclin-dependent kinases (CDKs)
Cecum, of large intestine, 200
Cell(s)

adventitial, 75
amacrine, 359
antigen-presenting, 136–137, 136f
APUD, 24, 160, 309, 318
argentaffin, 189, 318
argyrophilic, 189
B, 135, 135f, 136f, 137
  effector, 135
basal, 155, 156
binucleate, 292
bone, 46–48, 47f
bone lining, 47
in bone marrow, 66–74, 67f, 68f, 70f–74f
Böttcher's, 372
brush, 155
cartilage, 43–44, 44f
centroacinar, 207, 208f
chemoreceptor, 176
chief, 188, 188f, 310, 311f
chromaffin, 315, 315f
ciliated, 154
Claudius', 372
clear, 335
columnar, undifferentiated, 196
cone bipolar, 359
cytotoxic, T, 135
dark, 335
Deiter's, 372
dendritic. *See* Dendritic cells
described, 1, 17. *See also specific component of, e.g.,* Nucleus(i)
  basal, 20
  cell membrane, 2–4, 3f
  cytoskeleton of, 10–12, 11f, 12f
  cytosol in, 6
  epithelial, nonciliated, 20
  goblet, 20, 21f
  inclusions of, 12
  nucleus of, 4–6, 4f, 5f
  organelles of, 6–10, 6f–9f
  organization of, 1, 2f
  prokaryotic, 1
  tissues from, 14–16, 15f, 16f
DNES, 318
endocrine. *See* Endocrine cells
enterochromaffin, 189
enteroendocrine, 189, 196, 198f, 318
ependymal cells, 99–100, 100f
epithelial. *See* Epithelial cells
epithelioid, 35
  perineural, 105
  tactile, 321–322, 324f
exocrine, bronchiolar, 162
follicular, 257, 257f, 258f
germ, primordial, 257
giant, multinucleated, 35, 36f
glomus, 317
goblet, 24, 154, 160, 196, 197f
granular, 226, 227f
  acidophilic, 196, 198f
granule, 111
granulosa, 258, 318

hair. *See* Hair cells
hair matrix, 329, 330f
 Hensen's, 372
 horizontal, 359
 of immune system, 134–137, 135f, 136f. *See also specific cells and*
   Immune system, cells of
 intercalated, 223
 internal thecal, 306
 interstitial, 306, 319
 juxtaglomerular, 226, 227f
   of kidney, 318
 Kupffer, 204, 204f
 Langerhans, 322–323, 325f
 Leydig, 306, 319
 of loose connective tissue, 37
 M, 143, 144f
 macrolecithal, telolecithal, 275
 mast, 34–35, 34f
   connective tissue, 34–35
   mucosal, 34
 memory, 135
 Merkel, 108, 321–322, 324f
 mesangial, extraglomerular, 226, 227f
 mesenchymal, 32, 32f
 migratory, 160
 mononuclear, 292
 mucous neck, 188, 188f
 Müller, 359
 myoepithelial, 29, 29f
 neuroendocrine, 160
 NK, 135
 olfactory, neurosensory, 156
 osteoprogenitor, 47
 oxyniticopeptic, 209, 209f
 parafollicular, 307f, 309
 parietal, 188, 188f
 peripolar, 217, 218f
 peritubular, 235
 phalangeal, of internal ear, 372, 374f
 pigment, 36–37, 37f
 of placenta, 295
 plasma, 36, 36f, 135
 principal, 223, 310, 311f
 Purkinje, 111, 112f
 radial glial, 359
 reticular. *See* Reticular cells
 rod bipolar, 359
 satellite, 82
 Schwann, 100–101, 101f, 102f
 secretory, 154
 sensory, of internal ear, 368f, 371, 374f
 Sertoli, 236–237, 236f, 237f, 319
 SIF, 106
 spermatogenic, 237
 stromal, 136
 supporting, of internal ear, 368f, 372, 374f
 sustentacular, 128, 156, 236–237, 236f, 237f, 306, 319
 T, 135, 135f, 136f
   effector, 135, 136f
 T helper, 135
 theca, 258
   internal, 318

 trophoblast, binucleate, 285
   veiled, 137
Cell body, 96
   of neuron, 92–93, 92f, 93f
Cell body cytoplasm, of neuron, 93f, 93–94
Cell communication, 16
Cell cycle, 13–14, 14f
Cell division, 13–14, 14f
Cell membrane, 1, 2–4, 3f
   organization of, 3, 3f
   proteins associated with, 3, 3f
   size of, 2–3, 3f
Cell nests, 45
Cell surface, modifications of, 12–13, 12f
Cell-mediated immune response, 135
Cellular cementum, 178, 178f
Cement lines, 49f, 55
Cementoalveolar (Sharpey's) fibers, 178
Cementoblast(s), 178
Cementum, 178, 178f
Central canal, 49, 49f, 112, 114f
Central channel, 125
Central gliocytes, 303, 306, 309
Central nervous system (CNS)
   gliocytes of, 98–100, 99f, 100f
   tissue of, 109–112, 110f–114f
     cerebellum, 111–112, 111f–113f
     cerebral cortex, 110–111, 110f, 111f
     spinal cord, 112, 114f
Centriole(s), 10
Centroacinar cells, 207, 208f
Centromere(s), 13, 14f
Cerebellar cortex, 111, 111f
Cerebellum, 111–112, 111f–113f
Cerebral cortex, 110–111, 110f, 111f
Cerebrospinal fluid (CSF), 115–116
Ceruminous glands, 336
Cervix, 268–269, 269f
   histologic structure of, 268–269
CFU–GEMM. *See* Colony-forming unit–granulocyte, erythrocyte,
   monocyte/macrophage, and megakaryocyte (CFU–GEMM)
CFU–L. *See* Colony-forming unit–lymphoid (CFU–L)
CGP. *See* Circulating granulocyte pool (CGP)
Channel proteins, 228
Cheeks, 172–173, 173f
Chemoreceptor(s), 108
Chemoreceptor (taste) cells, 176
Chestnut, 346, 347f
Chief cells, 188, 188f, 310, 311f
Cholecystokinin, 207
Chondroblast(s), 43, 44f
Chondrocyte(s), 43–44, 44f, 45
Chondroitin-4-sulfate, 40, 40f
Chordae tendineae, 129
Chorioallantoic placenta, 280, 280f
Chorion
   frondose, 281
   smooth, 281
Chorionic girdle, 289
Choriovitelline placenta, 280, 280f

Choroid, 350, 351f, 353–355, 353f, 354f
  basal complex of, 355
  choriocapillary layer of, 353f, 355
  suprachoroid layer of, 353f, 354
  tapetum lucidum of, 353f, 354–355, 354f
  vascular layer of, 353f, 354
Choroid plexus epithelium, 100, 115
Chromaffin cells, 315, 315f
Chromatid(s), 13, 14f
Chromatin(s), 4–5, 4f
  sex, 5, 5f
Chromatin fibers, 5
Chromatolysis, 93
Chromophobe(s), 302
Chrondroitin-6-sulfate, 40, 40f
Ciliary body, 350, 351f, 355–356, 355f
  aqueous humor of, 356
  vascular layer of, 355–356
Ciliary epithelium, 355, 355f
Ciliary glands, 337, 337f
Ciliary muscle, 356
Ciliary processes, 351f, 355
Ciliated cells, 154
Circulating granulocyte pool (CGP), 71
Circulation, in placenta, 284–285, 284f
Circulus arteriosus major, 356
Circumanal glands, 339–340, 340f
Cisterna(ae), terminal, 84
Citric acid cycle, 10
Clathrin, 7
Claudin, 15
Claudius' cells, 372
Claw, 346, 346f
Claw fold, 346
Claw plate, 346
Clear cells, 335
Cleavage furrow, 13
Cleft(s), synaptic, 93, 97
Clitoris, 270
Cloaca, of birds, 277
Cloacal bursa, of birds, 140, 140f
"Closed" theory, 150, 150f
Closing cone, 57, 57f
CNS. *See* Central nervous system (CNS)
Coated pits, 8, 8f
Cochlear duct, of internal ear, 366f, 367, 368f, 369f
Cochlear window, 367
Collagen(s)
  anchoring, 38
  connecting, 38
  FACIT, 37
  fibril-forming, 37, 38f
  sheet-forming, 37
  transmembrane, 38
Collagen fibers, 37–38, 38f
Collagen fibrils, 37, 38f
Collagenous ligaments, 42
Collagenous tendons, 38f, 42
Collateral branches, 94
Collecting ducts, 132, 132f, 219t, 222–224, 223f–225f
  renal, 229
Collecting venules, 125, 127f

Colon, of large intestine, 200, 200f
Colony-forming unit–granulocyte, erythrocyte, monocyte/macrophage, and megakaryocyte (CFU–GEMM), 69, 70f
Colony-forming unit–lymphoid (CFU–L), 69
Colony-stimulating factor (CSF), 70
Columnae rectales, 201
Columnar cell, undifferentiated, 196
Communication
  cell, 16
  neuronal, 96–98
Complement system, 135
Compound follicles, 331
Compound glands, 24, 24t, 25–27, 28f
Compound tubular glands, 24t, 26, 28f
Compound tubuloacinar gland, 24t, 26, 28f
Conceptus, 279
Conduction, saltatory, 103
Conduction fibers, impulse, 89, 90f
Cone(s), 359
Cone bipolar cells, 359
Conical papillae, 174
Conjunctiva, 361, 362f
Conjunctival epithelium, 361
Connecting and anchoring collagen, 38
Connecting segment, 219t, 220
Connective tissue(s), 32–43
  adult, 41–43, 42f
  cells of, 32–37, 32f–37f. *See also* Connective tissue cells
  dense, 41–43, 42f
  embryonic, 41, 41f
  fibers of, 37–40, 38f–40f. *See also* Connective tissue fibers
  interstitial, 164
  irregular, dense, 42, 42f
  loose, 41, 42f
    cells of, 37
  mucous, 41, 41f
  regular, dense, 42–43, 42f
  reticular, 39f, 43
Connective tissue cells, 32–37, 32f–37f
  adipocytes, 33–34, 33f, 34f
  fibroblasts, 32–33, 33f
  fibrocytes, 32, 33f
  macrophages, 35–36, 35f, 36f
  mesenchymal, 32, 32f
  pericytes, 34
  pigment cells, 36–37, 37f
  plasma cells, 36, 36f
  reticular cells, 33, 33f
Connective tissue fibers, 37–40, 38f–40f
  collagen fibers, 37–38, 38f
  elastic fibers, 39, 39f, 40f
  reticular fibers, 38–39, 39f
Connective tissue mast cell (MC$_{TC}$), 34–35
Connexon(s), 16
Constitutive secretion, 8
Continuous capillaries, 123f–125f, 124
Contraction
  of cardiac muscle, 89
  of skeletal muscle, 84, 86
  of smooth muscle, 80

Convoluted semniferous tubules, 235–243, 236f–242f
   lamina propria of, 235–236
   meiosis of, 237–238
   spermatocytogenesis of, 237, 238f, 239f
   spermatogenic cells of, 237
   spermatozoa of, 239–240, 241f
   spermiogenesis of, 238–239, 240f
   sustentacular cells of, 236–237236f, 237f
Corium, 327–328, 327f, 343
   coronary, 343–344
Cornea, 350, 351–353, 351f, 352f
   anterior epithelium of, 351, 352f
   Descemet's membrane of, 352–353, 352f
   posterior epithelium of, 352f, 353
   posterior limiting lamina of, 352–353, 352f
   stroma of, 352, 352f
   subepithelial basement membrane of, 351–352, 352f
   substantia propria of, 352, 352f
Corneal endothelium, 352f, 353
Corneoscleral junction, 353
Corneoscleral trabecular meshwork, 358
Corona ciliaris, 355
Corona radiata, 259, 259f
Coronary corium, 343–344
Corpora arenacea, 306
Corpora cavernosa penis, 252, 253f
Corpora lutea, 257, 257f
Corpora nigra, 357
Corpus albicans, 262
Corpus hemorrhagicum, 261
Corpus luteum, 261–262, 263f, 264f, 318, 319
Corpus luteum cyclicum, 319
Corpus luteum graviditatis, 319
Corpus luteum of pregnancy, 319
Corpuscle(s)
   bulbous, 108, 108f
   Hassall's, 140, 142f
   lamellar, 108, 108f
   Pacini's, 208
   renal, 214–218, 216f–218f
   salivary, 142–143, 143f
   tactile
      encapsulated, 108, 108f
      nonencapsulated, 108, 108f
   thymic, 140, 142f
Cortex, 140, 141f, 361
   adrenal, outer cortex of, 311
   of kidney, 213, 214f, 215f
   of lymph nodes, 145, 145f
   of ovaries, 257–262, 258f–264f
   of tubule, 343, 344f
Cortical labyrinth, 213, 214f
Cortical remodeling units, 56, 57f
Cortical sinuses, 145, 145f
Corticosterone, 311, 313
Corticotroph(s), 302
Corticotropin-releasing hormone (CRH), 306
Corti's tunnel, 372
Cortisol, 311
Cortisone, 311
Costamere(s), 84

Cotyledon(s), 281f, 282, 289, 292f
Cotyledonary placenta, 282
Countercurrent system, 228
Cow(s)
   cyclic changes in endometrium in, 272, 273f
   cyclic changes of vaginal epithelium in, 273–274
   placentation in, 289, 292–293, 292f, 293f
Cranial dura mater, 113, 114f
Creatine phosphokinase, 83
Crenated RBCs, 63
CRH. *See* Corticotropin-releasing hormone (CRH)
Crista ampullaris, of internal ear, 368–369, 371f–373f
Cristae, 9, 9f
Crop, 208
Crown, 177
Crypt(s), caruncular, 282
Crypts of Lieberkühn, 195, 195f, 196
CSF. *See* Cerebrospinal fluid (CSF); Colony-stimulating factor (CSF)
Cumulus oophorus, 259, 259f
Cupula, 369
Cutaneous plexus, 335
Cuticular plate, 369
Cutting cone, 56, 57f
Cyclic adenosine monophosphate (cAMP), 80
Cyclin(s), 13
Cyclin-dependent kinases (CDKs), 13
Cystic atresia, 261, 261f
Cytocrine mode of secretion, 29
Cytokeratin, 17
Cytokeratin filaments, 22
Cytokinases, of cell cycle, 13, 14f
Cytokine(s), 135
   of hematopoiesis, 69–70, 70f
Cytology, 1–16
Cytoplasm, 1
   cell body, of neuron, 93f, 93–94
Cytoskeleton, 10–12, 11f, 12f
   intermediate filaments in, 12
   microfilaments in, 11–12, 12f
   microtubules in, 10–11, 11f
Cytosol, 1, 6
Cytotoxic cells, T, 135
Cytotrophoblast(s), 283f, 285

Dark cells, 335
Dark zones, 137, 138f
DCT. *See* Distal convoluted tubule (DCT)
Deciduate placenta, 282
Deiter's cells, 372
Demilune(s), serous, 28f, 29
Dendrite(s), 93–94, 93f, 94f
Dendritic bulb, 156
Dendritic cells, 136–137, 136f
   follicular, 136, 137
   integrating, 136f, 137
   interdigitating, 136f, 137
   interstitial, 136f, 137
Dendritic spines, 94, 94f
Dendritic zone, 96
Dense bodies, of smooth muscle, 80, 81f
Dense connective tissue, 41–43, 42f

Dense irregular connective tissue, 42, 42f
Dense regular connective tissue, 42–43, 42f
Dense tubular system (DTS), 66
Dental lamina, 179, 179f
Dental papilla, 180, 180f
Dental pulp, 179
Dental sac, 180f, 181
Denticulate ligament, 114, 114f
Dentin, 178
    interglobular, 178, 179f
    intertubular, 178
    peritubular, 178
Dentinal tubules, 178
Dermal laminae, secondary, 344, 345f
Dermal papilla, 328
    of hair follicle, 329, 330f
Dermal root sheath, of hair follicle, 329, 329f, 330f
Dermatan sulfate, 40
Dermis, 327–328, 327f
Descemet's membrane, 352–353, 352f
Descending vasa recta, 225, 226f
Desmin filaments, 84
Diakinesis, 238
Diaphragm, slit, 217, 217f
Diaphysis, 48, 50f
Diestrus, 271, 272, 272f
Diffuse lymphatic tissues, 137
Diffuse neuroendocrine system (DNES), 189
Diffuse neuroendocrine system (DNES) cells, 318
Diffuse placenta, 281–282
Digestive system, 170–211
    avian, 208–210, 209f, 210f
    bile canaliculi, 203, 204f
    esophagus, 184–186, 184t, 185f
    gallbladder, 206, 206f
    large intestine, 199–201, 199f–201f
    liver, 201–206, 202f–207f
    oral cavity, 172–181, 172f–181f
    pancreas, 206–208, 207f–209f
    pharynx, 184
    salivary glands, 181–183, 182f–184f
    small intestine, 194–199, 195f–199f
    stomach, 186–194, 186f–194f
    tubular organs, 171–172, 171f
Digestive tract, cross sections through portions of, 171f
Digital cushion, 345
Digital organs, 342–347, 343f–347f
Digital pads, 346, 346f, 347f
Diiodotyrosine, 308–309
Dilator muscle, 356f, 357
Diplotene phase, 238
Discoid placenta, 281f, 282
Disk(s), intercalated, 87, 88f
Disse, perisinusoidal space of, 204
Distal convoluted tubule (DCT), 219t, 220f, 222, 224f, 229
Distal small intestine, aggregated lymphatic nodules in, 139–140, 139f
Diverticulum(a), suburethral, 231
Diverticulum ventriculi, 187, 187f
DNES. *See* Diffuse neuroendocrine system (DNES)
DNES cells. *See* Diffuse neuroendocrine system (DNES) cells

Dohle bodies, 64
Dorsal funiculus, 112, 114f
Dorsal gray column, 112
Dorsal median septum, 112, 114f
DTS. *See* Dense tubular system (DTS)
Duct(s)
    alveolar, 161f, 163, 163f, 164f
    bile, 203, 204f
    cochlear, of internal ear, 366f, 367, 368f, 369f
    collecting, 132, 132f, 219t, 222–224, 223f–225f
        renal, 229
    excretory, 26–27, 28f
    intercalated, 26, 28f, 207, 208f
    interlobular, 26, 28f, 208, 209f
    intralobular, 26, 28f, 208, 209f
    lobar, 26, 28f
    of mammary gland, 342
    nasolacrimal, 361
    pancreatic, 208, 209f
        accessory, 208, 209f
    secretory, 26, 28f
    semicircular, of internal ear, 365f, 366f, 367
    striated, 26, 28f
    utriculosaccular, 367
    vomeronasal, 157–158, 158f
Ductuli efferentes, 245, 245f
Ductus deferens, 247–248, 247f, 248f
Ductus epididymidis, 245–247, 246f
Duodenum, 194, 195f
Dura mater, 113, 114f
    cranial, 113, 114f
    spinal, 113
Dural venous sinuses, 113
Dynein, 13
Dystrophin, 84

Ear(s), 364–376
    components of, 364
    external, 336, 336f, 364
    internal, 366–374, 366f–375f
        auditory apparatus of, 370–374, 374f, 375f
        auditory mechanism of, 372–374, 375f
        bony labyrinth of, 366–367, 366f, 367f
        cochlear duct of, 366f, 367, 368f, 369f
        crista ampullaris of, 368–369, 371f–373f
        hair cells of, 371, 374f
        macula sacculi of, 369–370, 373f, 374f
        macula utriculi of, 369–370, 373f, 374f
        membranous labyrinth of, 367–368, 367f
        phalangeal cells of, 372, 374f
        saccule of, 366f, 367
        semicircular ducts of, 365f, 366f, 367
        sensory cells of, 368f, 371, 374f
        spiral ganglion of, 368f, 372
        stria vascularis of, 367–368, 368f–370f
        supporting cells of, 368f, 372, 374f
        tectorial membrane of, 368f, 369f, 372
        utricle of, 366f, 367
        vestibular apparatus of, 368–370, 371f–374f
        vestibular mechanism of, 370

middle, 364–365, 365f
  auditory ossicles of, 364–365, 365f
  auditory tube of, 365, 365f
  muscles of, 364–365, 365f
  spiral organ of, 368f, 369f, 370–372, 374f
  tympanic cavity of, 364, 365f
  tympanic membrane of, 364, 365f
  sound transmission in, schematic diagram of events of, 375f
Early endosomes, 8
Eccrine mode of secretion, 29, 29f
ECM. *See* Extracellular matrix (ECM)
Ectoderm, 18, 19f, 279
Edema, endometrial, 267
Effector B cells, 135
Effector T cells, 135, 136f
Efferent arterioles, 224, 225f
Efferent axons, 104
Efferent neurons, 106–108, 107f
Elastic arteries, 118
Elastic cartilage, 45, 45f
Elastic fibers, 39, 39f, 40f
Elastic ligaments, 39f, 43
Elastic membrane, external, 118, 119f
Elastin, 39
Elaunin, 39
Electron-dense granules, 66, 67f
Eleidin, 22
Ellipsoid, 150, 150f, 359
Embryo, nourishment of, 281f, 282, 284, 284f
Embryology, 279–280, 280f
Embryonic connective tissues, 41, 41f
Embryotroph, 282
EMH. *See* Extramedullary hematopoiesis (EMH)
Enamel
  interrod, 177, 177f
  tooth, 177–178,178f
Enamel crests, 179
Enamel epithelium, 180, 180f
  outer, 180, 180f
Enamel organ, 180, 180f
Enamel plicae, 179
Enamel prisms, 177
Encapsulated tactile corpuscles, 108, 108f
End feet, 98
Endocardium, 129, 129f
Endochondral ossification, 51–53, 53f
  primary center of, 51–52, 53f
  secondary centers of, 53, 54f
Endocrine cellos, of heart, 318
Endocrine cells, 189, 299, 316–319, 316f, 317f
  granular, 128
  interstitial, 234–235, 235f, 261, 262f, 318
  of ovary, 318–319
  of placenta, 319
  of testis, 319
Endocrine glands, 24, 24t
Endocrine organs, 299–316. *See also specific organ and* Endocrine
  system
  epiphysis cerebri, 306–307, 307f
  hypothalamus, 299–300, 299f, 300t
  neurohypophysis, 301f, 303–306, 304f, 305f
  pars intermedia of, 302–303, 305f

pars tuberalis of, 301f, 303, 304f
  thyroid gland, 307–309, 307f–310f
  types of, 298
Endocrine signaling, 16
Endocrine system, 298–319. *See also specific organ and* Endocrine
  organs
  adenohypophysis, 300–303, 301f–304f
  described, 298
  endocrine cells, 316–319, 316f, 317f
  endocrine organs, 299–316. *See also* Endocrine organs
  endocrine tissues, 316–319, 316f, 317f
  neurohypophysis, 301f, 303–306, 304f, 305f
Endocrine tissues, 298–299, 316–319, 316f, 317f
Endocytosis, 8, 8f
Endoderm, 279, 280f
Endogenous agents, 135
Endolymphatic sac, 366f, 367
Endometrial cups, 267, 289, 290f
Endometrial edema, 267
Endometrium, 265–267, 266f–268f
  cyclic changes of, 271–273, 272f, 273f
  degenerative phase of, 272–273
  regenerative phase of, 272
Endomitosis, 75
Endomysium, 83
Endoneurium, 105
Endosome(s)
  early, 8
  late, 8
Endosteum, 50
Endotendineum, 38f, 42
Endothelial venules, high, 125, 135
Endotheliochorial placenta, 282
Endothelium(a), 118
  corneal, 352f, 353
  of uterus, 265–267, 266f–268f
  vascular, 119–120, 121f
Enteroceptor(s), 108
Enterochromaffin cells, 189
Enteroendocrine cells, 189, 196, 198f, 318
Entoglossal bone, 208
Eosinophil(s), 64–65, 64f
Ependymal cells, 99–100, 100f
Epicardium, 130
Epidermal laminae
  primary, 344, 345f
  secondary, 344, 345f
Epidermal pegs, 328
Epidermal–dermal junction, 326–327, 327f
Epidermis, 321–327, 322f–327f
  described, 321, 323f
  keratinization of, 326
  keratinocytes of, 321
  Langerhans cells of, 322–323, 325f
  layers of, 323–325, 325f, 326f
  melanocytes of, 321, 322f, 324f
  nonkeratinocytes of, 321–323, 324f
  tactile epithelioid cells of, 321–322, 324f
Epididymis, 245–247, 245f, 246f
  ductuli efferentes, 245, 245f
  ductus epididymidis, 245–247, 246f

Epikeras, 347
Epimysium, 83, 84f
Epinephrine, 315, 315f
Epineurium, 105
Epiphysis(es), 48, 50f
Epiphysis cerebri (pineal gland), 306–307, 307f
Epitendineum, 42
Epithelial cells
    alveolar
        granular, 164, 166f
        squamous, 164, 164f
    follicular, 307f, 308, 308f, 318
    mucous, 154
    nonciliated, 20
    serous, 155
Epithelial reticular cells, 136, 140, 141f
Epithelial sheath of Hertwig, 180–181
Epithelial tissue, classification of, 18, 19f
Epitheliochorial placenta, 282
Epithelioid cells, 35
    perineural, 105
    tactile, 321–322, 324f
Epithelium(a), 17–30
    anterior, of cornea, 351, 352f
    characteristics of, 17–18, 18t, 19f
    choroid plexus, 100, 115
    ciliary, 355, 355f
    columnar
        pseudostratified, 19f–21f, 20
        simple, 19, 19f–21f
        stratified, 20f, 23, 23f
    conjunctival, 361
    cuboidal
        simple, 19, 19f–21f
        stratified, 20f, 23, 23f
    enamel, 180, 180f
        outer, 180, 180f
    glandular, 23–29, 24t, 25f–29f. See also Gland(s)
    iridial, 356f, 357
    lens, 360, 360f
    olfactory, 156, 157f
    parietal, 217–218
    posterior, of cornea, 352f, 353
    pseudostratified, 19–22, 19f–22f
    respiratory, 154, 155f, 156f
    retinal pigment, 358f, 359
    sensory, 23
    simple, 18
    spermatogenic, 235
    squamous
        simple, 18–19, 19f–21f
        stratified, 19f, 20f, 22–23, 22f
            keratinized, 22–23, 22f
            nonkeratinized, 22–23, 22f
    structure of, microscopic, 18–23, 19f–23f
    surface, 18–23, 19f–23f
    transitional, 19f, 20–22, 20f, 22f
    vaginal, cyclic changes of, 273–275, 274f, 275f
Equine hoof, 342–345, 343f–345f
Erection, penile, 254–255
Ergot, 346, 347f

Erythrocyte(s), 62–63, 62f
    size of, 62, 63
Erythroid precursors, 72–73, 72f
Erythropoiesis, 72–73, 72f
Erythropoietin, 72
Esophagus, 184–186, 184t, 185f
    characteristics of, 184, 184t
Esophagus–stomach junction, 185–186, 185f
Estrogen(s), 306, 318
    in estrous cycle, 270
Estrous cycle, 270–275, 272f–275f
    cyclic changes of endometrium in, 271–273, 272f, 273f
    estrogens in, 270
    gonadotropins in, 270
    phases of, 271
    progesterone in, 270
Estrus, 271, 272, 272f, 274, 274f
Eukaryotic organisms, 1
Ewe(s), placentation in, 293–294, 293f
Excretory ducts, 26–27, 28f
Exocoelom, 279, 280f
Exocrine cells, bronchiolar, 162
Exocrine glands, 24, 24t
    simple, 24, 24t, 25f, 26f
Exocytosis, 7
Exogenous agents, 135
External callus, 57
External ear, 336, 336f, 364
External elastic membrane, 118, 119f
External epithelial root sheath, of hair follicle, 329, 329f, 330f
External limiting membrane, 359
Exteroceptor(s), 108
Extracellular matrix (ECM), 1
Extraepithelial glands, 24, 24t
Extraglomerular mesangial cells, 226, 227f
Extramedullary hematopoiesis (EMH), 69
Extrapulmonary bronchi, 160, 161f
Eye(s), 350–363
    accessory organs of, 361, 362f
    choroid of, 351f, 353–355, 353f, 354f
    ciliary body of, 351f, 355–356, 355f
    conjunctiva of, 361, 362f
    cornea of, 351–353, 351f, 352f
    corneoscleral junction of, 353
    eyelids of, 361
    fibrous tunic of, 351–353, 352f
    iridocorneal angle of, 357–358, 357f
    iris of, 351f, 356–357, 356f
    lacrimal apparatus of, 361, 362f
    lens of, 360, 360f
    neuroepithelial tunic of, 351f, 358–360, 358f
    refractive media of, 360–361, 360f, 361f
    sclera of, 351, 351f
    species variations, 361, 363
    third eyelid of, 361, 362f
    tunics of, 350–360
    vascular tunic of, 353–358, 353f–357f
    vitreous body of, 351f, 360–361
    zonular fibers of, 360, 360f
Eyelid(s), 336–337, 336f, 337f, 361
    third, 361, 362f

FACIT collagens, 37
Fascia adherens, 88, 90f
Fascicle(s), nerve, 105, 105f
Fast muscle fibers, 86
Fenestrated capillaries, 123f, 124, 125f
  peritubular capillary networks of, 224–225
Fetal membranes, diagram of, 280f
Fetal tissues, three-dimensional structure of interface between fetal
      tissues and, in placentation, 281f, 282
Fetal–maternal anchoring, fate of maternal tissues at birth due to,
      281f, 282
Fetal–maternal interhemal barrier, tissue layers of, in placentation,
      282, 283f
Fiber(s)
  afferent, 104
  argentaffin, 39, 39f
  argyrophilic, 39, 39f
  cardiac conduction, 130
  cementoalveolar, 178
  chromatin, 5
  collagen, 37–38, 38f
  conduction, impulse, 89, 90f
  connective tissue, 37–40, 38f–40f. See also Connective tissue fibers
  elastic, 39, 39f, 40f
  hair, 328
  lens, 360, 360f
  nerve, 104
  nuclear bag, 109, 109f
  nuclear chain, 109, 109f
  perforating, 42, 50, 51f
  Purkinje, 130
  reticular, 27, 38–39, 39f
  Sharpey's, 42, 50, 51f, 178
  skeletal muscle, classification of, 86
  somatic, 104
  visceral, 104
  zonular, 360, 360f
    of eyes, 360, 360f
Fibril(s)
  collagen, 37, 38f
  glial, 98
Fibril-forming collagen, 37, 38f
Fibrillin, 39
Fibroblast(s), 32–33, 33f
Fibrocartilage, 45, 46f
Fibrocyte(s), 32, 33f
Fibronectin, 39
Fibrous adhesive proteins, 39–40
Fibrous astrocytes, 98, 99f
Fibrous joints, 58
Fibrous pericardium, 130
Fibrous perineurium, 105
Fibrous rings, cardiac, 130, 130f
Fibrous triangles, cardiac, 130, 130f
Fight or flight mechanism, 316
Filament(s)
  cytokeratin, 22
  desmin, 84
  glial, 98
  intermediate, in cytoskeleton, 12
Filiform papillae, 174, 174f, 175f

Filopodia, 11
Filtration slits, 217, 217f
Fimbriae, 265
Fissure(s), ventral median, 112, 114f
Fluid(s), synovial, 59
Focal adhesions, 16
Folded placenta, 282
Foliate papillae, 175, 175f, 176f
Follicle(s)
  Graafian, 257f, 258–260, 259f, 260f
  hair, 328–333, 330f–334f. See also Hair follicles
  mature, 258, 260f
  ovarian, development of, 257–260, 258f–260f
  primary, 257f, 258, 258f
  primordial, 257, 258f
  secondary, 257f, 258, 258f
  tertiary, 257f, 258–260, 259f, 260f
  thyroid, 308, 308f
Follicle-stimulating hormone (FSH), 302, 306
Follicular atresia, 261, 261f, 262f
Follicular cells, 257, 257f, 258f
Follicular dendritic cells, 136f, 137
Follicular epithelial cells, 306, 307f, 308, 308f, 318
Folliculus(i), liquor, 258, 260f
Foot processes, 217
Fracture(s), repair of, 57–58
Free nerve endings, 108, 108f
Frog, 345
Frondose chorion, 281
FSH. See Follicle-stimulating hormone (FSH)
Functional zone, of endothelium, 265
Fundic gland region, of stomach, 187–189
Fundus, 187
Fungiform papillae, 174, 175f
Funiculus
  lateral, 112, 114f
  ventral, 112, 114f
Fusimotor motor neuron, 106

G protein–coupled receptor (GPCR), 305
GAGs, 58, 59
Gallbladder, 206, 206f
GALT. See Gut-associated lymphatic tissue (GALT)
Ganglion(a), 100f, 106
  autonomic, 101f, 106
  sensory, 100f, 106
  spiral, of internal ear, 368f, 372
Ganglionic gliocytes, 100, 101f, 102f
Gap junctions, 16
Gas exchange area of lung, 162–165, 163f–167f
GBM. See Glomerular basement membrane (GBM)
Germ cells, primordial, 257
GH. See Growth hormone (GH)
GHRH. See Growth hormone–releasing hormone (GHRH)
Giant cells, multinucleated, 35, 36f
Gizzard, 210, 210f
Gland(s), 23–29, 24t, 25f–29f
  accessory, 248–251, 249f–251f
  acinar
    branched, simple, 24–25, 24t, 25f
    simple, 24, 24t, 25f, 27f

Gland(s) *(continued)*
  adrenal, 311–316, 312f–315f
  alveolar
    branched, simple, 24–25, 24t, 25f
      simple, 24, 24t, 25f, 27f
  anal, 201, 339
  of anal sac, 339, 340f
  bronchial, 162
  Brunner's, 197, 198f
  buccal, 173
  bulbourethral, 251, 251f
  cardiac, 187, 189f
  carpal, 338
  ceruminous, 336
  ciliary, 337, 337f
  circumanal, 339–340, 340f
  classification of, 24–29, 24t, 25f–29f
  compound, 24, 24t, 25–27, 28f
  endocrine, 24, 24t
  exocrine, 24, 24t
  extraepithelial, 24, 24t
  gustatory, 175, 175f, 183
  Harderian, 361
  intestinal, 195, 195f, 196
    submucosal, 189
  intraepithelial, 24, 24t
  labial, 172
  lacrimal, 361, 362f
  lingual, 183
  mammary, 340–342, 341f
  morphologic characteristics of, 24–27, 24t, 25f–28f
  mucous, 27, 28f
  multicellular, 24, 24t
  olfactory, 156–157
  palatine, 173, 174
  parathyroid, 309–311, 311f
  pineal, 306–307, 307f
  pituitary, 300–306, 301f–305f
  proventricular, 209, 209f
  pyloric, 189, 190f
  salivary, 181–183, 182f–184f. *See also* Salivary glands
  sebaceous, 333–334, 334f
  serous, 27, 28f
  shell, 277
  simple, 24–25, 24t, 25f–27f
  skin, 333–335, 334f, 335f
  sperm-host, 277
  submucosal, 172, 197, 198f
  supracaudal, 340, 341f
  sweat, 334–335, 335f
  tarsal, 337, 337f
  tracheal, 160
  tubular
    branched, simple, 24, 24t, 25f, 27f
    coiled, simple, 24, 24t, 25f, 26f
    compound, 24t, 26, 28f
    straight, simple, 24, 24t, 25f, 26f
  tubuloacinar
    compound, 24t, 26, 28f
    simple, 24t, 25
  tubuloalveolar, simple, 24t, 25
  unicellular, 24, 24t

  uropygial, 347, 348f
  vesicular, 248–249, 249f
  vestibular
    major, 270
    minor, 270
  vomeronasal, 158
Glandular epithelium, 23–29, 24t, 25f–29f
Glans penis, 253, 254f
Glassy membrane, 261, 261f
Glial fibrillar acidic protein, 12
Glial fibrils, 98
Glial filaments, 98
Glial-limiting membrane, 98
Gliocyte(s)
  central, 303, 306, 309
  CNS, 98–100, 99f, 100f
  ganglionic, 100, 101f, 102f
  PNS, 100–101, 100f–102f
Globule leukocytes, 37, 160, 196
Glomerular basement membrane (GBM), 216
Glomerular capillaries, 215–216, 216f, 217f
Glomerular capillary tuft, 215, 216f
Glomerular capsule, 216f–218f, 217–218
Glomerulus(i), 112, 215
Glomus, 317
Glomus cells, 317
Glucagon, 316, 316f
Glucocorticoid(s), 311
Glycogen deposits, 12
Glycosaminoglycan(s), 40
GnRH. *See* Gonadotropin-releasing hormone (GnRH)
Goat(s), placentation in, 293–294, 293f
Goblet cells, 20, 21f, 24, 154, 160, 196, 197f
Golgi complex, 259
  in vesicular transport, 7–9, 7f–9f
Golgi phase, 238
Gonadotroph(s), 302
Gonadotropin(s), in estrous cycle, 270
Gonadotropin-releasing hormone (GnRH), 306
GPCR. *See* G protein–coupled receptor (GPCR)
Graafian follicles, 257f, 258–260, 259f, 260f
Granulae iridica, 357
Granular alveolar epithelial cells, 164, 166f
Granular cells, 226, 227f
Granular endocrine cells, 128
Granular epithelial layer, of hair follicle, 329, 329f, 330f
Granule(s)
  α, 66
  atrial, 130
  electron-dense, 66, 67f
  iridial, 357
  keratohyalin, 22, 23f, 324
  lamellar, 22, 23, 323, 324
  lipofusion, 93
  matrix, 45
  membrane-coating, 23
  primary, 63, 63f, 64
  secondary, 63, 63f, 64
  secretory, 7, 8f
  zymogen, 27, 181
α-Granule(s), 66

Granule cells, 111
Granulocyte(s)
    basophilic, 71–72
    eosinophilic, 71–72
Granulopoiesis, 70–72, 71f
    mast cells in, 72
    neutrophilic precursors to, 71
Granulosa cells, 258, 318
Ground substance, 40–41, 40f
Growth
    appositional, 46
    interstitial, 46
Growth hormone (GH), 305
Growth hormone–releasing hormone (GHRH), 305
Guard hair, 328f, 331
Gustatory glands, 175, 175f, 183
Gut-associated lymphatic tissue (GALT), 143, 144f
Guttural pouch, 365

H band, 83
Hair, 328, 328f
    primary, 328f, 331
    secondary, 331
Hair cells
    inner, of internal ear, 371
    outer, of internal ear, 371, 374f
    type I, 368
    type II, 369
Hair cycle, 332–333, 335f
Hair follicle(s), 328–333, 330f–334f
    compound, 331
    differences among species, 331–332, 331f, 332f
    formation of, 328–329
    primary, 328f, 330
    secondary, 331
    simple, 331
    single, 331
    sinus, 332, 333f
    structures of, 328–330, 330f, 331f
    tactile, 332, 333f
    types of, 328f, 330–332, 332f, 333f
Hair follicle terminals, 108
Hair matrix cells, 329, 330f
Hard palate, 173, 173f
Harderian gland, 361
Hassall's corpuscles, 140, 142f
H-ATPase, 229
Haversian canal, 49, 49f
Haversian systems, 49, 49f
Heart, 129–131, 129f, 130f. *See also under* Cardiac
    blood vessels of, 131
    collecting ducts of, 132, 132f
    endocardium of, 129, 129f
    endocrine cells of, 318
    epicardium of, 130
    lymph capillaries, 131–132, 131f, 132f
    myocardium of, 129–130, 130f
    pericardium of, 130
Heel, 342–343
Helicotrema, 366f, 367
Hemal nodes, 151, 151f

Hematoma(s)
    marginal, 294, 295f
    placental, 284
Hematopoiesis, 67, 69–70, 70f
    cytokines of, 69–70, 70f
    extramedullary, 69
    granulocytes in, 71–72
    regulation of, 69–70, 70f
Hematopoietic stem cells (HSCs), 69–70, 70f
    in bone marrow, 69–70, 70f
Hemidesmosome(s), 15–16, 15f
Hemochorial placenta, 282
Hemoglobin, 62
Hemosiderin, 12
Hemotroph, 282
Hensen's cell, 372
Heparan sulfate, 40
Heparin, 34, 40
Hepatic lobules, 205, 205f
Hepatic sinusoids, 204, 205f
Hepatic veins, 205
Hepatoid, defined, 340
Heterophil(s), 63
High endothelial venules, 125, 135
Hilus, 143, 145f
Hippomane(s), 289
Histamine, 34
Histiocyte(s), 35
Histology, 1
Histotroph, 282
H,K-ATPase, 229
Holangiotic pattern, 359
Holocrine mode of secretion, 29, 29f
Homeostasis, defined, 298
Hoof(s)
    equine, 342–345, 343f–345f
    ruminant, 345–346, 345f
    swine, 345–346, 345f
    wall of, 343–345, 343f–345f
Horizontal cells, 359
Hormone(s)
    adrenocorticotropic, 306
    antiparamesonephric, 236
    follicle-stimulating, 302
    growth, 305
    β-lipotropin, 302
    of ovary, 270–271
    releasing, 305
    thyroid-stimulating, 302, 306
Horn(s), 112, 347
Horny tubules, 343, 344f
Howell-Jolly bodies, 62
HSCs. *See* Hematopoietic stem cells (HSCs)
Humoral immune response, 135
Hyaline cartilage, 44–45, 44f
Hyaloid membrane, 361
Hyaluronan, 40, 40f
Hypertrophy
    of cardiac muscle, 89–90
    of skeletal muscle, 86
    of smooth muscle, 80
    zone of, 54

Hypodermis, 328, 328f
Hypophyseal cavity, 301, 301f
Hypophysis cerebri (pituitary gland), 300–306, 301f–305f
Hypothalamo-adenohypophyseal axis, 305–306
Hypothalamo-hypophyseal portal system, 305
Hypothalamo-neurohypophyseal tract, 301f, 303–305, 304f, 305f
Hypothalamus, 299–300, 299f, 300t
Hypsodont teeth, 177, 177f

I band, 82
Ileal Peyer's patch, 139–140, 139f
Ileum, 194
ILs. *See* Interleukin(s) (ILs)
Immune response
    cell-mediated, 135
    humoral, 135
Immune system, 134–152
    BALT, 143
    blood vessels of, 141–142, 146, 147f
    bone marrow, 138
    cells of, 134–137, 135f, 136f
        antigen-presenting cells, 136–137, 136f
        dendritic cells, 136–137, 136f
        lymphocytes, 135–136, 135f, 136f
        organization of, to form lymphatic tissues and organs, 137, 138f
        stromal cells, 136
    cloacal bursa of birds, 140, 140f
    cortex, 140, 141f, 145, 145f
    GALT, 143, 144f
    hemal nodes, 151, 151f
    lymph vessels of, 141–142, 143, 145, 145f
    lymphatic organs of
        primary, 137–142, 139f–142f
        secondary, 142–151, 154f–151f
    MALT, 142–143, 143f, 144f
    medulla, 140–141, 142f, 145f, 146, 146f
    "milk spots," 151
    nerves of, 141–142, 146, 147f
    sinuses, 143, 145, 145f
    spleen, 147–151, 148f–150f
    thymus, 140–142, 141f, 142f
    tonsils, 142–143, 143f
Impulse conduction fibers, 89, 90f
Infraorbital sinus, 337
Infundibulum(a), 179, 262, 264, 265f, 301, 301f
    of birds, 275, 276f, 277
Inguinal sinus, 339
Inhibin, 306, 318
Inner cell mass, 279
Inner hair cells, of internal ear, 371
Inner medulla, 213
Inner mesaxon, 101
Inotropic membrane receptors, 97
Integral proteins, in cell membrane, 3, 3f
Integrating dendritic cells, 136f, 137
Integument, 320–349. *See also* Skin
    anal sacs, 339, 339f, 340f
    avian, 347–349, 348f, 349f
    blood vessels of, 335–336
    carpal glands, 338
    chestnut, 346, 347f

circumanal glands, 339–340, 340f
claw, 346, 346f
digital organs, 342–347, 343f–347f
digital pads, 346, 346f, 347f
equine hoof, 342–345, 343f–345f
ergot, 346, 347f
external ear, 336, 336f
eyelids, 336–337, 336f, 337f
hair, 328, 328f
horns, 347
infraorbital sinus, 337
inguinal sinus, 339
interdigital sinus, 338
lymph vessels of, 335–336
mammary gland, 340–342, 341f
mental organ, 338
nerves of, 335–336
nose, 337–338, 338f
ruminant hoofs, 345–346, 345f
scrotum, 339
skin glands, 333–335, 334f, 335f
special structures of, 336–342, 336f–341f
submental organ, 338
supracaudal gland, 340, 341f
swine hoofs, 345–346, 345f
Interalveolar septa, 164, 164f
Interatrial septa, avian, 168, 168f
Intercalated cells, 223
Intercalated disks, 87, 88f
Intercalated ducts, 26, 28f, 181, 207, 208f
Intercellular junctions, 15–16, 15f, 16f
Interdigital sinus, 338
Interdigitating dendritic cells, 136f, 137
Interferon-gamma, 70
Interfollicular muscle, 330, 331f
Interglobular dentin, 178, 179f
Interleukin(s) (ILs), 70
Interlobar arteries, 224, 225f
Interlobular arteries, 224, 225f
Interlobular ducts, 26, 28f, 181, 208, 209f
Interlobular hepatic arteriole, 202f, 204
Interlobular portal venule, 202f, 204
Interlobular septa, 162
Intermediate filaments, of smooth muscle, 80
Intermembrane space, 9, 9f
Internal callus, 57
Internal ear. *See* Ear(s), internal
Internal elastic membrane, 118, 119f
Internal epithelial root sheath, of hair follicle, 329, 329f, 330f
Internal parathyroids, 309–310, 311f
Internal theca cells, 306, 318
Interneuronal chemical synapses, 97
Internode, 103
Interrod enamel, 177, 177f
Interstitial cells, 306, 319
Interstitial connective tissue, 164
Interstitial dendritic cells, 136f, 137
Interstitial endocrine cells, 261, 262f, 318
    of testis, 234–235, 235f
Interstitial growth, 46
Interstitial lamellae, 49f, 55

Interstitium
    of kidney, 226
    of mammary gland, 342
    of testis, 233–235
Interterritorial matrix, 45
Intertubular dentin, 178
Intertubular horn, 343
Interventricular septum, fibrous part of, 130
Intestinal glands, 195, 195f, 196
Intestinal villi, 195, 196f, 198f
Intestine(s)
    large, 199–201, 199f–201f. *See also* Large intestine
    small, 194–199, 195f–199f. *See also* Small intestine
Intracellular canaliculus, 188
Intraepidermal macrophages, 136f, 137, 322–323, 325f
Intraepithelial glands, 24, 24t
Intralobular ducts, 26, 28f, 208, 209f
    of mammary gland, 341f, 342
Intramembranous ossification, 51, 53f
Intraperiod line, 101
Intrapulmonary conducting airways, of lungs, 161–162, 161f, 162f
Inverted yolk sac placenta, 280
Iridial epithelium, 356f, 357
Iridial granules, 357
Iridial muscles, 356f, 367–367
Iridial stroma, 356, 356f
Iridocorneal angle, 357–358, 357f
    pectinate ligament of, 357, 357f
    trabecular meshwork of, 357f, 358
    venous drainage from, 358
Iris, 350, 351f, 356–357, 356f
Isogenous cell groups, 45
Isthmus, 264, 266f
    of birds, 276f, 277

Jejunum, 194
Joint(s), 58–59, 58f–60f
    cartilaginous, 58, 58f
    described, 58
    fibrous, 58
    function of, 58
    phalangeal, 60f
    synovial, 58–59, 59f, 60f
Juxtaglomerular apparatus, 226, 227f
Juxtaglomerular cells, 226, 227f
    of kidney, 318

Karyorrhexis, 14
Keratan sulfate, 40, 40f
Keratin(s), 12, 326
Keratinization
    described, 22–23
    of epidermis, 326
Keratinized stratified squamous epithelium, 22–23, 22f
Keratinocyte(s), 321
Keratohyalin granules, 22, 23f, 324
Keratohyalin phase, 330
Kidney(s), 212–229
    anatomic features of, 212–213, 213f
    in blood pressure regulation, 227, 227f
    collecting duct of, 229

    cortex of, 213, 214f, 215f
    distal convoluted tubule of, 229
    filtration of, 227, 227f
    function of, 226–227
    general organization of, 212–215
    interstitium of, 226
    juxtaglomerular cells of, 318
    juxtaglomerular apparatus of, 226, 227f
    loop of Henle, thick ascending limb of, 228–229
    lymphatics of, 226
    medulla of, 213, 214f, 215f
    multilobar, 213, 213f
    nephron of, 215, 215f
    nerves of, 226
    renal corpuscle of, 214–215
    renal corpuscles, 215–218, 216f–218f
    renal tubules, 214–215, 218–224, 218f, 219t, 220f–225f
    structure–function relationships in, 226–229
    thin limbs of, 228–229
    tubule function of, 227–228
    unilobar, 213, 213f
    unipapillary, 212–213, 213f
    vasculature of, 224–226, 225f, 226f
Kinase(s), cyclin-dependent, 13
Kinetochore, 13
Koilin membrane, 210
Kupffer cells, 204, 204f

Labial glands, 172
Labyrinth, cortical, 213, 214f
Lacrimal apparatus, 361, 362f
Lacrimal canaliculi, 361
Lacrimal gland, 361, 362f
Lacrimal puncta, 361
Lacrimal sac, 361
Lacteal, 196, 196f
Lactiferous sinus, 342
Lactotroph(s), 302
Lamella(ae), 294
    circumferential
        inner, 49, 49f
        outer, 49, 49f
    interstitial, 49f, 55
Lamellar bodies, 164
Lamellar bone, 49f, 50
Lamellar corpuscles, 108, 108f, 208
Lamellar granules, 22, 23f, 323, 324
Lamellar placentation, 282
Lamellipodia, 11
Lamina(ae), 12, 193, 194f
    anterior, of cornea, 352
    basal, 18
    dermal, secondary, 344, 345f
    epidermal
        primary, 344, 345f
        secondary, 344, 345f
    posterior limiting, of cornea, 352–353, 352f
    reticular, 372
    spiral, 367
    subbasal, 18
Lamina basalis, 18

Lamina choroidocapillaris, 353f, 355
Lamina densa, 18, 216
Lamina fibroreticularis, 18
Lamina fusca sclerae, 351
Lamina lucida, 18
Lamina muscularis, 172
Lamina propria, 172, 235–236
Lamina rara externa, 216
Lamina rara interna, 216
Laminar corium, 343
Laminin(s), 39
Langerhans cells, 322–323, 325f
Large granular lymphocytes (LGLs), 75
Large intestine, 199–201, 199f–201f
    anal canal of, 201, 201f
    cecum of, 200
    colon of, 200, 200f
    rectum of, 200–201
Large motor units, 106
Laryngopharynx, 184
Larynx, 159–160, 159f, 160f
Late endosomes, 8
Lateral funiculus, 112, 114f
Lens, 360, 360f
Lens capsule, 360, 360f
Lens epithelium, 360, 360f
Lens fibers, 360, 360f
Lenticular papillae, 174
Leptin, 318
Leptomeninges, 113
Leptotene stage, 238
Leukocyte(s), 63–66, 63f–66f
    basophils, 65
    eosinophils, 64–65, 64f
    globule, 37, 160, 196
    lymphocytes, 66, 66f
    monocytes, 65, 65f
    neutrophils, 63–64, 63f
Leydig cells, 306, 319
LGLs. *See* Large granular lymphocytes (LGLs)
LH. *See* Luteinizing hormone (LH)
Ligament(s)
    collagenous, 42
    denticulate, 114, 114f
    elastic, 39f, 43
    pectinate, of iridocorneal angle, 357, 357f
    periodontal, 178
    spiral, 367
Limbus, 353
Lingual glands, 183
Lingual papillae, 174
Link proteins, 44
Lip(s), 172, 172f
Lipid droplets, 6f, 12
Lipofuscin, 12
Lipofusion granules, 93
β-Lipotropin hormone (ß–LPH), 302
Liquor folliculi, 258, 260f
Liver, 201–206, 202f–207f
    anatomic unit of, 205, 205f
    bile ducts of, 203, 204f

blood supply to, 203–205, 204f, 205f
    capsule of, 201–202, 202f
    functional units of, 205–206, 205f
    lobules of, 205, 205f
        portal, 205–206, 205f
    lymph in, 205
    lymph vessels of, 205
    parenchyma of, 202–203, 203f
    portal lobule of, 205–206, 205f
    stroma of, 201–202, 202f
Liver acinus, 205f, 206
Lobar ducts, 26, 28f
Lobar lactiferous duct, of mammary gland, 341f, 342
Lobe(s), 26, 28f
    neural, 301, 301f
Lobular duct, of mammary gland, 341f, 342
Lobule(s), 26, 28f, 162
    liver, 205, 205f
    portal, of liver, 205–206, 205f
Loop of Henle, 219t, 220–222, 221f–223f
    thick ascending limb of, 221–222, 223f, 228–229
    thin limbs of, 219t, 220–221, 222f
Loose connective tissue, 41, 42f
-β-LPH. *See* β-Lipotropin hormone (β-LPH)
Lung(s), 160–167, 161f–167f
    alveolar ducts of, 161f, 163, 163f, 164f
    alveolar sacs of, 161f, 163, 163f, 164f
    alveoli of, 161f, 163–164, 164f–167f
    blood vessels of, 165–166
    bronchi of, 161–162, 161f
    gas exchange area of, 162–165, 163f–167f
    innervation of, 166–167
    intrapulmonary conducting airways of, 161–162, 161f, 162f
    lymphatics of, 165–166
    pleura of, 165
    respiratory bronchioles of, 162–163, 163f, 164f
Luteinization, 262
Luteinizing hormone (LH), 302, 306
LVP. *See* Lysine vasopressin (LVP)
Lymph, in liver, 205
Lymph capillaries, 131–132, 131f, 132f
Lymph nodes, 143, 145–147, 145f–147f
    differences among species, 146–147, 147f
Lymph vascular system, 117
Lymph vessels, 131–132, 131f, 132f
    of immune system, 141–142
    of integument, 335–336
    of liver, 205
    of lymph nodes, 143, 145, 145f
    of spleen, 150
Lymphatic(s)
    of kidney, 226
    of ovary, 262
    pulmonary, 165–166
    of uterine tube, 265
    of uterus, 266f, 267–268, 267f
Lymphatic nodules, 137, 138f
    aggregated, 143, 144f
        in distal small intestine, 139–140, 139f
    primary, 137, 138f
    secondary, 137, 138f
    solitary, 197, 198f, 199f

Lymphatic organs
    primary, 137–142, 139f–142f
    secondary, 142–151, 151f–154f
Lymphatic tissues
    bronchus-associated, 143
    diffuse, 137
    gut-associated, 143, 144f
    mucosa-associated, 142–143, 143f, 144f
    organized, 137
Lymphoblast(s), 75
Lymphocyte(s), 66, 66f, 135–136, 135f, 136f
    B, 75
    mature, 75
    T, 75
Lymphocyte recirculation, 135
"Lymphoepithelial organ," 140
Lymphoid precursors, 75
Lymphopoiesis, 75
Lysine vasopressin (LVP), 303
Lysosome(s)
    primary, 9
    secondary, 8, 9
Lysozyme(s), 106
Lyssa, of tongue, 176, 176f

M cells, 143, 144f
M line, 83
Macrolecithal, telolecithal cells, 275
Macrophage(s), 35–36, 35f, 36f, 136f, 137
    alveolar, 164, 167f
    intraepidermal, 136f, 137
    intraepithelial, 322–323, 325f
    stellate, 204–205, 204f, 205f
    tingible body, 140, 141f
Macrovasculature, blood vessels of, 117
Macula densa, 226
Macula sacculi, of internal ear, 369–370, 373f, 374f
Macula utriculi, of internal ear, 369–370, 373f, 374f
Maculae adherens, 15, 16f
Magnum, avian, 276f, 277
Major arterial circle, 356
Major salivary glands, 181
Major vestibular glands, 270
MALT (mucosa-associated lymphatic tissue), 142–143, 143f, 144f
Mammary gland, 340–342, 341f
    alveoli of, 340–342, 341f
    described, 340, 341f
    ducts of, 342
    interstitium of, 342
    involution of, 342
    teat of, 342
Mandibular salivary gland, 181–182, 182f
Mantle, 137, 138f
Mare(s), placentation in, 286t, 289, 290f, 291f
Marginal granulocytic pool (MGP), 71
Marginal hematomas, 294, 295f
Marginal sinus, 149, 150f
Marginal zone of spleen, 149, 149f, 150f
Margo plicatus, 189
Mast cells, 34–35, 34f, 72
    connective tissue, 34–35
    mucosal, 34

Maternal tissues
    fate at birth of, fetal–maternal anchoring effects on, in placentation, 281f, 282
    three-dimensional structure of interface between fetal tissues and, in placentation, 281f, 282
Matrix granules, 45
Matrix vesicles, 50
Maturation phase, 239
Mature follicles, 258, 260f
Mature neutrophil, 64
MC$_T$. *See* Mucosal mast cell (MC$_T$)
MC$_{TC}$. *See* Connective tissue mast cell (MC$_{TC}$)
Mechanoreceptor(s), 108
Median eminence, 301, 301f
Mediastinum testis, 234, 235f
Medulla, 140–141, 142f
    adrenal, 315–316, 315f
    inner, 213
    of kidney, 213, 214f, 215f
    of lymph nodes, 145f, 146, 146f
    outer, 213, 215f
    of ovary, 257f, 262
Medullary cords, 145f, 146
Medullary rays, 213, 214f
Medullary sinuses, 145, 145f
Megakaryoblast(s), 75, 75f
Megakaryocyte(s), 75
Meiosis, 237–238
Meissner's plexus, 172
Melanin, 12
Melanocyte(s), 321, 322f, 324f
α-Melanocyte stimulating hormone (α-MSH), 302
Melanosome(s), 321
Melanotroph(s), 302
Melatonin, 307
Membrane-coating granules, 23
Membranous disks, 359
Membranous labyrinth, of internal ear, 367–368, 367f
Memory cells, 135
Meninges, 112–114, 114f
Meniscus(i), 59, 59f
Mental organ, 338
Merkel cells, 108, 321–322, 324f
Merocrine mode of secretion, 29, 29f
Merocrine sweat glands, 335, 335f
Mesangial cells, extraglomerular, 226, 227f
Mesangium, 216–217, 216f
Mesaxon(s), 101, 102f
    inner, 101
    outer, 101
Mesenchymal cells, 32, 32f
Mesenchyme, 41
Mesobronchus(i), avian, 168
Mesoderm, 279, 280f
Mesotendineum, 42
Messenger ribonucleic acids (mRNAs), 7
Metabotropic receptors, 97
Metamyelocyte(s), 71, 71f
Metaphase, of cell cycle, 13, 14f
Metaphysis, 48, 52f
Metarteriole(s), 125

Metarubricyte(s), 72

Metestrus, 271, 272, 272f

Metestrus–diestrus, 274, 274f

Metorrhagia, 272

MGP. *See* Marginal granulocytic pool (MGP)

Microcotyledon(s), 289

Microfilament(s), in cytoskeleton, 11–12, 12f

Microglia, 99, 99f

Microplacentome(s), 289, 291f

Microtubule(s), in cytoskeleton, 10–11, 11f

Microtubule organizing center (MTOC), 10

Microvasculature, 122–126, 122f–127f

   blood vessels of, 117

Micturition, 232

Middle ear. *See* Ear(s), middle

Migratory cells, 160

Milk letdown, 342

"Milk spots," 151

Mineralocorticoid(s), 311

Mink(s), placentation in, 294–296, 294f, 295f

Minor salivary glands, 181, 183, 184f

Minor vestibular glands, 270

Mitochondria, 9–10, 9f

Mitosis, 13, 14f

Modeling, bone, 56, 56f

Molar salivary gland, 183

Molecule(s)

   procollagen, 37

   tropomyosin, 83

Monestrous, defined, 271

Monoblast(s), 72

Monocyte(s), 65, 65f

Monocytopoiesis, 72

Mononuclear cells, 292

Mononuclear phagocyte system (MPS), 35, 65

Motor end plate, 84, 106

Motor neuron, fusimotor, 106

Motor unit, 84, 106

MPS. *See* Mononuclear phagocyte system (MPS)

mRNAs. *See* Messenger ribonucleic acids (mRNAs)

α-MSH. *See* α-Melanocyte stimulating hormone (α-MSH)

MTOC. *See* Microtubule organizing center (MTOC)

Mucin, 27, 172

Mucinogen, 27, 196

Mucocutaneous junction, 172

Mucosa-associated lymphatic tissue (MALT), 142–143, 143f, 144f

Mucosal mast cell (MC$_T$), 34

Mucous connective tissue, 41, 41f

Mucous epithelial cells, 154

Mucous glands, 27, 28f

Mucous neck cells, 188, 188f

Mucus, 24

Müller cells, 359

Multicellular glands, 24, 24t

Multilobar kidney, 213, 213f

Multilocular adipocytes, 34, 34f

Multinucleated giant cells, 36f, 235

Multiplexin(s), 37

Multiunit smooth muscle, 80

Multivesicular bodies (MVBs), 8

Muscle(s), 79–90. *See also specific types, e.g.,* Smooth muscle

   arrector pili, 328, 330, 331f

   cardiac, 86–90, 87f–90f

   ciliary, 356

   dilator, 356f, 357

   interfollicular, 330, 331

   iridial, 356f, 367–367

   of middle ear, 364–365, 365f

   skeletal, 80, 82–86, 82f–87f. *See also* Skeletal muscle

   smooth, 79–80, 80f–82f. *See also* Smooth muscle

   sphincter, 356f, 367–367

      cardiac, 185

      pyloric, 189, 190f

   trachealis, 160

Muscular arteries, 118, 119f, 120–121, 122f

Muscular tissues, 79

Muscular venules, 125, 127f

MVBs. *See* Multivesicular bodies (MVBs)

Myelin sheath, 101–104, 102f–105f

Myeloblast(s), 71, 71f

Myelocyte(s), 71, 71f

Myoblast(s), of skeletal muscle, 86

Myocardium, 129–130, 130f

Myocyte(s), 79

Myoepithelial cells, 29, 29f

Myofiber(s), 79

Myofibril(s), of skeletal muscle, 82, 83f

Myofibroblast(s), 32–33

Myofilament(s)

   intermediate, of smooth muscle, 80

   of skeletal muscle, 82

   thick

      of skeletal muscle, 83, 86f

      of smooth muscle, 80, 81f

   thin

      of skeletal muscle, 83, 85f

      of smooth muscle, 80, 81f

Myogenesis

   of cardiac muscle, 89–90

   of skeletal muscle, 86

Myoid, 359

Myomesin, 83

Myometrium, 267

Myosin-II, 80

Myotube(s), of skeletal muscle, 86

NaCl cotransporter, 229

Na$^+$–K$^+$ ATPase, 229

NaK2Cl cotransporter, 229

Nasal cavity, 153–157, 154f–158f

   cutaneous region of, 153–154, 154f

   olfactory region of, 156–157, 157f, 158f

   respiratory region of, 154–155, 155f

Nasolacrimal duct, 361

Nasopharynx, 159, 184

Natural killer (NK) cells, 135

Nephron(s), 215, 215f

   long-looped, 215, 215f

   short-looped, 215, 215f

Nerve(s)

   of immune system, 141–142

   of integument, 335–336

   of lymph nodes, 146, 147f

of ovary, 262
   peripheral, 105–106, 105f
      described, 105
   renal, 226
   of spleen, 150
   of uterine tube, 265
   of uterus, 266f, 267–268, 267f
Nerve endings, free, 108, 108f
Nerve fascicle, 105, 105f
Nerve fiber(s), 104
Nervi vasorum, 118, 120f
Nervous tissue, 91–116. *See also* Neuroglia; Neuron(s)
Neural lobe, 301, 301f
Neurocrine signaling, 16
Neuroendocrine cells, 160
Neurofilament(s), 93
Neuroglia, 98–104
   astrocytes in, 98–99, 99f
   described, 98
   ependymal cells in, 99–100, 100f
   gliocytes in
      CNS, 98–100, 99f, 100f
      ganglionic, 100, 101f, 102f
      PNS, 100–101, 100f–102f
   microglia in, 99, 99f
   neurolemmocytes in, 100–101, 101f, 102f
   oligodendrocytes in, 99, 99f
Neurohypophysis, 300, 301f, 303–306, 304f, 305f
   hypothalamo-adenohypophyseal axis of, 305–306
Neurolemmocyte(s), 100–101, 101f, 102f, 106, 107f
Neuromuscular spindles, 109, 109f
Neuromuscular synapse, 106, 107f
Neuron(s), 91–98
   autonomic
      postganglionic, 106
      preganglionic, 106
   bipolar, 95, 96f
   cell body cytoplasm of, 93f, 93–94
   cell body of, 92–93, 92f, 93f
   classification of, 95–96, 96f
   communication among, 96–98
   defined, 91
   efferent, 106–108, 107f
   morphology of, 92, 92f
   motor, fusimotor, 106
   multipolar, 96, 96f
   myelin sheath in, 101–104, 102f–105f
   nucleus of, 92
   piriform, 111, 112f
   processes of, 92f–95f, 93–95
   regions of, 92f, 96
   structure of, 92–95, 92f–95f
   unipolar, 95, 96f
Neuropeptide Y, 318
Neurosensory olfactory cells, 156
Neurotendinous spindles, 108–190, 108f
Neurotransmitter(s), 97
Neutrophil(s), 63–64, 63f
   band, 64
   mature, 64
   segmented, 64
NK cells. *See* Natural killer (NK) cells

Node(s)
   atrioventricular, 130
   cardiac, 89, 90f
   hemal, 151, 151f
   lymph, 143, 145–147, 145f–147f
      differences among species, 146–147, 147f
   sinatrial, 130
Node of Ranvier, 103
Nodule(s), lymphatic. *See* Lymphatic nodules
Nonciliated epithelial cells, 20
Nondeciduate placenta, 282
Nonencapsulated tactile corpuscles, 108, 108f
Nonkeratinized stratified squamous epithelium, 22–23, 22f
Nonkeratinocyte(s), 321–323, 324f
Norepinephrine, 315, 315f
NORs. *See* Nucleolar organizing regions (NORs)
Nose, 337–338, 338f
Nuclear bag fibers, 109, 109f
Nuclear chain fibers, 109, 109f
Nuclear envelope, 4, 4f
Nuclear matrix, 5
Nuclear pulposus, 58, 58f
Nucleation theory, 50
Nucleolar organizing regions (NORs), 5–6
Nucleolus(i), 5–6, 5f
Nucleoplasm, 4–5, 5f
Nucleus(i), 4–6, 4f, 5f
   of neuron, 92
   pyknotic, 14
Nutrition, of cartilage, 46

OAE. *See* Otoacoustic emissions (OAE)
Occludin, 15
OCS. *See* Open canicular system (OCS)
Odontoblast(s), 178
Odontoblast processes, 178
Olfactory cells, neurosensory, 156
Olfactory epithelium, 156, 157f
Olfactory glands, 156–157
Olfactory region, of respiratory system, 156–157, 157f, 158f
Oligodendrocyte(s), 99, 99f
Omasal papillae, 193
Omasum, 193–194, 194f
Oocyte(s), 258
   primary, 257f, 258, 258f
Oogonium, 257
Open canicular system (OCS), 66
"Open" theory, 150, 150f
Oral cavity, 172–181, 172f–181f
   cheeks, 172–173, 173f
   hard palate, 173, 173f
   lips, 172, 172f
   soft palate, 174
   teeth, 177–181, 177f–181f
   tongue, 174–177, 174f–176f
Orbiculus ciliaris, 355
Organ(s), 17, 18f
Organ of Corti, 368f, 369f, 370–372, 374f
Organelle(s), 1, 6–10, 6f–9f
   Golgi complex, 7–9, 7f–9f
   mitochondria, 9–10, 9f
   peroxisomes, 10

Organelle(s) *(continued)*
  ribosomes, 6–7
  rough and smooth endoplasmic reticulum, 6–7, 6f
Organized lymphatic tissues, 137
Oropharynx, 184
Ossification
  endochondral, 51–53, 53f. *See also* Endochondral ossification
  intramembranous, 51, 53f
  zone of, 52f, 54, 56f
Osteoblast(s), 46–47, 47f, 76, 76f
Osteoclast(s), 47–48, 47f, 76, 76f
Osteocyte(s), 47, 47f
Osteocytic osteolysis, 47
Osteogenesis, 50–58, 53f–57f
  bone modeling in, 56, 56f
  bone remodeling in, 56–57, 57f
  endochondral ossification in, 51–53, 53f
  fracture repair in, 57–58
  growth in length in, 54–55, 54f, 55f
  growth in width and circumference in, 55–56
  intramembranous ossification, 51, 53f
Osteolysis, osteocytic, 47
Osteon(s), 49, 49f
  primary, 55
  secondary, 55
Osteoprogenitor cells, 47
Otoacoustic emissions (OAE), 374
Outer enamel epithelium, 180, 180f
Outer hair cells, of internal ear, 371, 374f
Outer medulla, 213, 215f
Outer mesaxon, 101
Ovarian follicle, development of, 257–260, 258f–260f
Ovary(ies), 256–262, 257f–264f
  of birds, 275–277, 276f
  blood vessels of, 262
  cortex of, 257–262, 258f–264f
    corpus luteum and, 261–262, 263f, 264f
    follicular atresia and, 261, 261f, 262f
    follicular development of, 257–260, 258f–260f
    interstitial endocrine cells and, 261, 262f
  endocrine cells of, 318–319
  hormones of, 270–271
  lymphatics of, 262
  medulla of, 257f, 262
  nerves of, 262
  in ovulation, 260–261
  structure of, 256–257, 257f
Oviduct(s), 262, 264–265, 265f, 266f. *See also* Uterine tube (oviduct)
  of birds, 275–277, 276f
Ovulation, 260–261
Oxidative phosphorylation, 10
Oxyniticopeptic cells, 209, 209f
Oxytalan, 39
Oxytocin, 303

Pachymeninx, 113
Pachytene phase, 238
Pacini's corpuscles, 108, 108f, 208
Packed cell volume (PCV), 62
Palate(s)
  hard, 173, 173f
  soft, 174

Palatine gland, 173, 174
Pale epithelial layer, of hair follicle, 329, 329f, 330f
PALS. *See* Periarterial lymphatic sheaths (PALS)
Pancreas, 206–208, 207f–209f
Pancreatic duct, 208, 209f
  accessory, 208, 209f
Pancreatic islets, 316–317, 316f, 317f
Pannicular adiposus, 328, 328f
Papilla(ae)
  conical, 174
  dental, 180, 180f
  dermal, 328
    of hair follicle, 329, 330f
  filiform, 174, 174f, 175f
  foliate, 175, 175f, 176f
  fungiform, 174, 175f
  lenticular, 174
  lingual, 174
  omasal, 193
  reticular, 192
  rumen, 190, 191f
  tonsillar, 174
  vallate, 175, 175f
Paracellular pathway, 228
Parachonchus(i), avian, 168
Paracrine secretion, 16
Parafollicular cells, 307f, 309
Paraganglia, 317–318
Paranasal sinuses, 158–159, 159f, 201
Paranode, 103, 104f
Parathyroid(s), internal, 309–310, 311f
Parathyroid gland, 309–311, 311f
Parathyroid hormone (PTH), 310
Parenchyma, 26–27, 28f
  of liver, 202–203, 203f
Parietal cells, 188, 188f
Parietal epithelium, 217–218
Parietal serous pericardium, 130
Parotid salivary gland, 181, 182f
Pars caeca retinae, 350
Pars ciliaris retinae, 350
Pars distalis, 301–302, 301f–303f
Pars fetalis, 279
Pars intermedia, 302–303, 305f
Pars iridica retinae, 350
Pars optica retinae, 350
Pars plana, 355
Pars plicata, 355
Pars tuberalis, 301f, 303, 304f
Paurangiotic pattern, 359–360
PCT. *See* Proximal convoluted tubule (PCT)
PCV. *See* Packed cell volume (PCV)
Pecten, 363
Pectinate ligament, of iridocorneal angle, 357, 357f
Pedicels, 217
Pelvis, renal, 230, 230f
Pendrin, 229
Penicillar artery, 150
Penis, 252–255, 253f, 254f
  corpora cavernosa, 252, 253f

erection of, mechanisms of, 254–255
  glans, 253, 254f
Peptidase(s), 106
Perforating canals, 49, 49f
Perforating fibers, 42, 50, 51f
Periarterial lymphatic sheaths (PALS), 148–149, 149f, 150f
Pericapillary macrophage sheath, 150, 150f
Pericardial cavity, 130
Pericardium, 130
  fibrous, 130
  parietal serous, 130
Pericellular matrix, 45
Perichondrium, 44f, 45
Pericyte(s), 34, 122–123
Pericytic venules, 125, 127f
Perilymph, 366
Perilymphatic space, 366
Perimetrium, 267
Perimysium, 83, 84f
Perineural epithelioid cells, 105
Perineurium, 105
  fibrous, 105
Periodontal ligament, 178
Periople, 342–343
Perioplic corium, 343
Periosteal bud, 51
Periosteum, 48, 49f, 51f
Peripheral nerves, 105–106, 105f
Peripheral nervous system (PNS), gliocytes of, 100–101, 100f–102f
Peripheral nervous tissue, 104–109, 105f, 107f–109f
  efferent neurons of, 106–108, 107f
  ganglia of, 100f, 106
  nerves of, 105–106, 105f
Peripheral proteins, in cell membrane, 3, 3f
Peripolar cells, 217, 218f
Perisinusoidal adipocytes, 205
Perisinusoidal space (of Disse), 204
Periosteum, 49, 49f, 51f
Peritendineum, 38f, 42
Peritubular capillary networks, of fenestrated capillaries, 224–225
Peritubular cells, 235
Peritubular dentin, 178
Perivascular space, 114, 115f
Peroxisome(s), 10
Peyer's patches, 143, 144f, 197, 198f, 199f
  ileal, 139–140, 139f
PGCs. *See* Primordial germ cells (PGCs)
Phagocytosis, 8
Phagolysosome(s), 9
Phalangeal cells, of internal ear, 372, 374f
Phalangeal joint, 60f
Pharyngoesophageal limen, 184
Pharynx, 184
Phenomelanin(s), 321
Phospholipid(s), in cell membrane, 3, 4f
Phosphorylation, oxidative, 10
Physeal–metaphyseal region, 48, 52f
Physis, 48, 52f
Pia mater, 113
Pigment cells, 36–37, 37f
Pineal gland, 306–307, 307f

Pinealocyte(s), 306
Piriform neurons, 111, 112f
Pituitary gland, 300–306, 301f–305f
Placenta, 279
  chorioallantoic, 280, 280f
  choriovitelline, 280, 280f
  circulation in, 284–285, 284f
  cotyledonary, 282
  deciduate, 282
  diffuse, 281–282
  discoid, 281f, 282
  endocrine cells of, 319
  endotheliochorial, 282
  epitheliochorial, 282
  folded, 282
  hemochorial, 282
  macroscopic structure of, 281–282, 281f
  nondeciduate, 282
  specialized cells of, 295
  vascularity of, 284–285, 284f
  villous, 282
  yolk sac, 280, 280f
    inverted, 280
  zonary, 281f, 282
Placenta endotheliochorialis, 282
Placenta hemochorialis, 282
Placenta zonaria, 281f, 282
Placental hematomas, 284
Placentation, 279–297
  in bitches, 294–296, 294f, 295f
  changes during, 285
  choriovitelline placenta in, 280, 280f
  classification in, 280–282, 280f, 281f
  in cows, 289, 292–293, 292f, 293f
  defined, 279
  embryology, 279–280, 280f
  in ewes, 293–294, 293f
  fate of maternal tissues at birth due to fetal–maternal anchoring in, 281f, 282
  fetal extraembryonic membrane contributions to, 280, 280f, 281f
  fetal–maternal interhemal barrier, tissue layers of, 282, 283f
  function–structure relationships in, 285–286
  in goats, 293–294, 293f
  lamellar, 282
  in mares, 286t, 289, 290f, 291f
  in minks, 294–296, 294f, 295f
  nourishment of embryo in, 281f, 282, 284, 284f
  placental vascularity and circulation in, 284–285, 284f
  in queens, 294–296, 294f, 295f
  in sows, 286–288, 286f–288f, 286t
  species differences in, 286–296, 286f–288f, 286t, 290f–295f
  three-dimensional structure of interface between maternal and fetal tissues in, 281f, 282
Placentome(s), 281f, 282, 289, 292f
Plaque(s), amniotic, 293
Plasma, 61–62, 62f
Plasma cells, 36, 36f, 135
Platelet(s), 66, 67f, 75
  precursors to, 75
  size of, 66
  structure of, 66, 67f

Pleura, 165
  visceral, 161
PNS. *See* Peripheral nervous system (PNS)
Podocyte(s), 217, 217f, 218f
Poikilocytosis, 63
Polychromatophilic RBCs, 63
Polychromatophilic rubricyte, 72
Polyestrous, defined, 272
POMC. *See* Proopiomelanocortin (POMC)
Pore(s), septal, 165, 165f, 167f
Portal lobule, of liver, 205–206, 205f
Postcapillary venules, 125, 127f
Posterior epithelium, of cornea, 352f, 353
Posterior limiting lamina, of cornea, 352–353, 352f
Postganglionic autonomic neurons, 106
Postsynaptic density, 97
Postsynaptic somatodendritic membrane, 97
Precapillary sphincter, 125
Predentin, 178
Preganglionic autonomic neurons, 106
Pregnancy, corpus luteum of, 319
Preleptotene primary spermatocytes, 237
Prepuce, 255, 255f
Presynaptic element, 93f, 97
PRF. *See* Prolactin-releasing factor (PRF)
Primary bronchi, 160
Primary ending, 109, 109f
Primary epidermal laminae, 344, 345f
Primary follicles, 257f, 258, 258f
Primary granules, 63, 63f, 64
Primary hair, 328f, 331
Primary hair follicle, 328f, 330
Primary lymphatic nodules, 137, 138f
Primary lysosomes, 9
Primary oocytes, 257f, 258, 258f, 260
Primary osteons, 55
Primary spongiosa, 52f, 54, 56f
Primate(s), cyclic changes in endometrium in, 272–273
Primordial follicles, 257, 258f
Primordial germ cells (PGCs), 257
Principal cells, 223, 310, 311f
PRL. *See* Prolactin (PRL)
Procollagen molecules, 37
Proestrus, 271, 272, 272f, 274, 274f
Progesterone, 306, 319
  in estrous cycle, 270
Prokaryotic cells, 1
Prolactin (PRL), 302, 305, 306
Prolactin-releasing factor (PRF), 305, 306
Proliferation, zone of, 54, 55f
Prolymphocyte(s), 75
Promoncyte(s), 72
Promyelocyte(s), 71, 71f
Proopiomelanocortin (POMC), 302
Proper gastric gland region, of stomach, 187–189
Prophase, of cell cycle, 13, 14f
Proplatelet(s), 66
Proprioceptor(s), 108
Prorubricyte(s), 72, 72f
Prostate, 249–251, 249f, 250f
Protein(s)
  androgen-binding, 319

C, 83
  carrier, 228
  in cell membrane, 3, 3f
  channel, 228
  fibrous adhesive, 39–40
  glial fibrillar acidic, 12
  integral, in cell membrane, 3, 3f
  link, 44
  peripheral, in cell membrane, 3, 3f
  transmembrane, in cell membrane, 3, 3f
  transport, 228
Proteoglycan(s), 40–41, 40f
Protoplasm, 1
Protoplasmic astrocytes, 98, 99f
Proventricular glands, 209, 209f
Proventriculus, 209, 209f
Proximal convoluted tubule (PCT), 219, 219t, 220f, 221f
Proximal straight tubule (PST), 219, 219t, 220f, 221f
Proximal tubule, 218–219, 218f, 219t, 228
Pseudo–H zone, 83
Pseudostratified columnar epithelium, 19f–21f, 20
Pseudostratified epithelium, 19–22, 19f–22f
PST. *See* Proximal straight tubule (PST)
PTH. *See* Parathyroid hormone (PTH)
Pulmonary arteries, 165–166
Pulmonary lymphatics, 165–166
Pulmonary surfactant, 165
Pulmonary veins, 166
Pulp, dental, 179
Pulp arteriole, 150
Pulp cavity, 178
Pulvinus dentalis, 173
Pupil(s), 356
Purkinje cells, 111, 112f
Purkinje fibers, 130
Pyknotic, 14
Pyloric gland(s), 189, 190f
Pyloric gland region, of stomach, 187f, 189, 190f
Pyloric sphincter muscle, 189, 190f

Queen(s), placentation in, 294–296, 294f, 295f

Radial glial cells, 359
RBCs. *See* Red blood cells (RBCs)
Receptor(s), 97, 108–190, 108f, 109f
  antigen, 135, 135f
  encapsulated, 108–190, 108f, 109f
  inotropic membrane, 97
  metabotropic, 97
  nonencapsulated, 108, 108f
  sensory, 128–129, 128f
  SRP, 7
Recirculation, lymphocyte, 135
Rectal columns, 201
Rectal pits, 201
Rectum, of large intestine, 200–201
Red blood cells (RBCs), 62–63, 62f
Red marrow, 76
Red pulp, 148, 148f, 149f
Red skeletal muscle fibers, 86
Refractive media of eye, 360–361, 360f, 361f

Regeneration
  of cardiac muscle, 89–90
  of skeletal muscle, 86
  of smooth muscle, 80
Regulated secretion, 7
Reissner's membrane, 367
Releasing hormones, 305
Remodeling, bone, 56–57, 57f
Renal corpuscles, 214–218, 216f–218f
  glomerular capsule of, 216f–218f, 217–218
  mesangium, 216–217, 216f
  structure of, 215, 216f
Renal pelvis, 230, 230f
Renal tubules, 214–215, 218–224, 218f, 219t, 220f–225f
  collecting ducts, 219t, 222–224, 223f–225f
  connecting segment, 219t, 220
  distal convoluted tubule, 219t, 220f, 222, 224f
  function of, 227–228
  loop of Henle, 219t, 220–222, 221f–223f
  proximal tubule, 218–219, 218f, 219t, 228
Renewed anagen phase, 333, 334f
Renin, 313
Reproductive system
  female, 256–278
    of birds, 275–277, 276f
    cervix, 268–269, 269f
    clitoris, 270
    estrous cycle, 270–275, 272f–275f
    ovaries, 256–262, 257f–264f
    uterine tube, 262, 264–265, 265f, 266f
    uterus, 265–268, 266f–268f
    vagina, 269, 270f
    vestibule, 269–270
    vulva, 270
  male, 233–255
    accessory glands, 248–251, 249f–251f
    bulbourethral glands, 251, 251f
    convoluted seminiferous tubules, 235–243, 236f–242f
    ductus deferens, 247–248, 247f, 248f
    epididymis, 245–247, 245f, 246f
    penis, 252–255, 253f, 254f
    prepuce, 255, 255f
    prostate, 249–251, 249f, 250f
    straight testicular tubules, 243, 243f, 244f
    testis, 233–245
    urethra, 252, 252f
    vesicular gland, 248–249, 249f
  neurohypophysis of, 301f, 303–306, 304f, 305f
rER. See Rough endoplasmic reticulum (rER)
Reserve zone, 54, 55f
Residual body, 8f, 9
Resorption, zone of, 52f, 54, 55f
Respiratory bronchioles, 162–163, 163f, 164f
Respiratory epithelium, 154, 155f, 156f
Respiratory system, 153–169
  avian, 167–168, 168f
  extrapulmonary bronchi, 160, 161f
  larynx, 159–160, 159f, 160f
  lungs, 160–167, 161f–167f
  nasopharynx, 159
  paranasal sinuses, 158–159, 159f

trachea, 160, 161f
  vomeronasal organ of, 157–158, 158f
Retained afterbirth, 293
Rete ovarii, 257
Rete testis, 243, 244t
Reticular fibers, 38–39, 39f
Reticular cells, 33, 33f, 75–76, 136, 146f, 192
  epithelial, 136, 140, 141f
Reticular crests, 192, 193f
Reticular fibers, 27
Reticular lamina, 372
Reticular layer, of dermis, 328
Reticular papillae, 192
Reticular sulcus, 193, 194f
Reticulocyte(s), 63, 72, 72f
Reticulum, 192–193, 193f, 194f
  rough endoplasmic, 6–7, 6f
  smooth endoplasmic, 6–7, 6f
  stellate, 180, 180f
Retina, 350, 351f, 358–360, 358f
Retinal pigment epithelium (RPE), 358f, 359
Reversal zone, 56, 57f
Ribosomal RNA (rRNA), 5
Ribosome(s), 6–7
Rod(s), 359
Rod bipolar cells, 359
Rough endoplasmic reticulum (rER), 6–7, 6f
Rouleau formation, 63
RPE. See Retinal pigment epithelium (RPE)
rRNA. See Ribosomal RNA (rRNA)
Rubriblast(s), 72, 72f
Rubricyte(s)
  basophilic, 72
  polychromatophilic, 72
Rugae, 173
Rumen, 190–192, 191f, 192f
Ruminant(s)
  hoofs of, 345–346, 345f
  stomach of, 189–194, 191f–194f
    abomasum, 194
    omasum, 193–194, 194f
    reticular sulcus, 193, 194f
    reticulum, 192–193, 193f, 194f
    rumen, 190–192, 191f, 192f
Russell bodies, 36, 36f

Saccule(s)
  of internal ear, 366f, 367
    macula of, 369–370, 373f, 374f
Sensory receptors, 128–129, 128f
Salivary corpuscles, 142–143, 143f
Salivary duct, 181
Salivary glands, 181–183, 182f–184f
  general characteristics of, 191
  Mandibular, 181–182, 182f
  major, 181
  minor, 181, 183, 184f
  molar, 183
  parotid, 181, 182f
  sublingual, 182–183, 183f
  zygomatic, 183, 184f
Saltatory conduction, 103

Sarcomere(s), 84
Satellite cells, 82
Scala tympani, 367
Scala vestibuli, 367
Schwann cells, 100–101, 101f, 102f
Sclera, 350, 351, 351f
Scleral venous plexus, 357f, 358
Scrotum, 339
Sebaceous glands, 333–334, 334f
Sebum, 333
Second maturation division, 238
Second messengers, 4
Secondary capillary plexus, 301, 301f, 305
Secondary dermal laminae, 344, 345f
Secondary ending, 109, 109f
Secondary epidermal laminae, 344, 345f
Secondary follicles, 257f, 258, 258f, 331
Secondary granules, 63, 63f, 64
Secondary hair, 331
Secondary lymphatic nodules, 137, 138f
Secondary lysosomes, 8, 9
Secondary osteons, 55
Secondary spermatocytes, 238
Secondary spongiosa, 55
Secretin, 207–208
Secretion
    constitutive, 8
    modes of, 29, 29f
    paracrine, 16
    regulated, 7
Secretory cells, 154
Secretory ducts, 26, 28f
Secretory granules, 7, 8f
Secretory product
    nature of, 27, 28f, 29
    release of, mode of, 29, 29f
Secretory units, 26, 28f
    types of, 27f–29f
Secretory vesicles, 93
Segmented neutrophil, 64
Semicircular ducts, of internal ear, 365f, 366f, 367
Seminiferous tubules
    convoluted, 235–243, 236f–242f
    cyclic events in, 240, 242f, 243
Sensory cells, of internal ear, 368f, 371, 374f
Sensory epithelium, 23
Sensory ganglia, 100f, 106
Septa, 27
Septal pores, 165, 165f, 167f
Septula testis, 234, 234f
Septum(a)
    dorsal median, 112, 114f
    interalveolar, 164, 164f
    interatrial, avian, 168, 168f
    interlobular, 162
sER. See Smooth endoplasmic reticulum (sER)
Serous demilunes, 28f, 29
Serous epithelial cells, 155
Serous glands, 27, 28f
Sertoli cells, 236–237, 236f, 237f, 319
Sex chromatin, 5, 5f, 92

Sharpey's fibers, 42, 50, 51f, 178
Sheathed capillary, 150, 150f
Sheet-forming collagen, 37
Shell gland, 277
Shell membrane, 277
SIF cells. See Small intensely fluorescent (SIF) cells
Signal peptide sequence, 7
Signal recognition particle (SRP), 7
Signal recognition particle (SRP) receptor, 7
Signaling
    autocrine, 16
    endocrine, 16
    neurocrine, 16
Simple acinar glands, 24, 24t, 25f, 27f
Simple alveolar glands, 24, 24t, 25f, 27f
Simple branched acinar glands, 24–25, 24t, 25f
Simple branched alveolar glands, 24–25, 24t, 25f
Simple branched tubular glands, 24, 24t, 25f, 27f
Simple coiled tubular glands, 24, 24t, 25f, 26f
Simple columnar epithelium, 19, 19f–21f
Simple cuboidal epithelium, 19, 19f–21f
Simple follicle, 331
Simple glands, 24–25, 24t, 25f–27f
Simple squamous epithelium, 18–19, 19f–21f
Simple straight tubular glands, 24, 24t, 25f, 26f
Simple tubuloacinar glands, 24t, 25
Simple tubuloalveolar glands, 24t, 25
Single follicle, 331
Sinoatrial node, 130
Sinus(es), 143, 145, 145f
    carotid, 128–129
    cortical, 145, 145f
    infraorbital, 337
    inguinal, 339
    interdigital, 338
    lactiferous, 342
    marginal, 149, 150f
    medullary, 145, 145f
    paranasal, 158–159, 159f, 201
    trabecular, 145, 145f
    venous, dural, 113
Sinus hair follicles, 332, 333f
Sinusoid(s), 118, 123f, 124–125, 127f
    hepatic, 204, 205f
Sister-chromatids, 13, 14f
Skeletal muscle, 80, 82–86, 82f–87f
    atrophy of, 86
    contraction of, 84, 86
    fine structure of, 83–84, 85f–87f
    hypertrophy of, 86
    light microscopic structure of, 80, 82–83, 82f–84f
    myogenesis of, 86
    regeneration of, 86
Skeletal muscle fibers
    classification of, 86
    fast, 86
    slow, 86
    red, 86
Skin, 320–349. See also specific layers, e.g., Epidermis
    anal sacs, 339, 339f, 340f
    appendages, 328–335, 329f–335f

blood vessels, 335–336
carpal glands, 338
chestnut, 346, 347f
circumanal glands, 339–340, 340f
claw, 346, 346f
dermis, 327–328, 327f
digital organs, 342–347, 343f–347f
digital pads, 346, 346f, 347f
epidermis, 321–327, 322f–327f
equine hoof, 342–345, 343f–345f
ergot, 346, 347f
external ear, 336, 336f
eyelids, 336–337, 336f, 337f
functions of, 321t
glands, 333–335, 334f, 335f
hair, 328, 328f
horns, 347
hypodermis, 328, 328f
infraorbital sinus, 337
inguinal sinus, 339
interdigital sinus, 338
lymph vessels, 335–336
mammary gland, 340–342, 341f
mental organ, 338
nerves, 335–336
nose, 337–338, 338f
ruminant hoofs, 345–346, 345f
scrotum, 339
special structures of, 336–342, 336f–341f
submental organ, 338
supracaudal gland, 340, 341f
swine hoofs, 345–346, 345f
Slit diaphragm, 217, 217f
Slow muscle fibers, 86
Small intensely fluorescent (SIF) cells, 106
Small intestine, 194–199, 195–199f
blood supply to, 199
distal, aggregated lymphatic nodules in, 139–140, 139f
tela submucosa of, 197, 198f, 199f
tunica mucosa of, 195–196, 195f, 197f–199f
tunica muscularis of, 198
tunica serosa of, 198
Smooth chorion, 281
Smooth endoplasmic reticulum (sER), 6–7, 6f
Smooth muscle, 79–80, 80f–82f
contraction of, 80
fine structure of, 80, 81f, 82f
hypertrophy of, 80
light microscopic structure of, 79–80, 80f
multiunit, 80
myogenesis of, 80
regeneration of, 80
unitary, 80
SNARE (Soluble N-ethylmaleimide-sensitive fusion protein Attachment protein REceptors), 7
Sodium iodide symporter, 308
Soft palate, 174
Sole, 345
Sole plate, 106
Solitary (isolated) lymphatic nodules, 197, 198f, 199f
Somatic fibers, 104

Somatopleure, 280
Somatostatin (SST), 317
Sound transmission, in ear, schematic diagram of events of, 375f
Sow(s), placentation in, 286–288, 286f–288f, 286t
Spaces of Fontana, 357
Spermatocyte(s)
preleptotene primary, 237
secondary, 238
Spermatocytogenesis, 237, 238f, 239f
Spermatogenic cells, 237
Spermatogenic cycle, stages of, 242f
Spermatogenic epithelium, 235
Spermatogenic segments, 243
Spermatogenic wave, 243
Spermatozoon(a), 239–240, 241f
Sperm-host glands, 277
Spermiation, 236
Spermiogenesis, 237, 238–239, 240f
Sphincter(s), precapillary, 125
Sphincter muscle, 356f, 367–367
cardiac, 185
pyloric, 189, 190f
Spinal cord, 112, 114f
Spinal dura mater, 113
Spindle(s)
neuromuscular, 109, 109f
neurotendinous, 108–190, 108f
Spine, dendritic, 94, 94f
Spine apparatus, 94
Spiral ganglion, of internal ear, 368f, 372
Spiral lamina, 367
Spiral ligament, 367
Spiral organ, of internal ear, 368f, 369f, 370–372, 374f
Spiral prominence, 368, 368f
Splanchnopleure, 280
Spleen, 147–151, 148f–150f
blood vessels of, 149–150, 150f
capsules of, 147–148
differences among species, 151
lymph vessels of, 150
marginal zone of, 149, 149f, 150f
nerves of, 150
red pulp of, 148, 148f, 149f
supportive tissue of, 147–148
white pulp of, 148–149, 149f, 150f
Spongiosa
primary, 52f, 54, 56f
secondary, 55
Squamous alveolar epithelial cell, 164, 164f
SRP. See Signal recognition particle (SRP)
SST. See Somatostatin (SST)
Statoconial membrane, 370, 373f
Stellate macrophages, 204–205, 204f, 205f
Stellate reticulum, 180, 180f
Stomach, 186–194, 186f–194f
cardiac gland region of, 187, 189f
fundic gland region of, 187–189
proper gastric gland region of, 187–189
pyloric gland region of, 187f, 189, 190f
ruminant, 189–194, 191f–194f
species differences, 187f, 189

Stomach *(continued)*
tunica mucosa of
glandular region of, 187–189, 188f–190f
nonglandular region of, 186, 187f
Straight testicular tubules, 243, 243f, 244f
Stratified columnar epithelium, 20f, 23, 23f
Stratified cuboidal epithelium, 20f, 23, 23f
Stratified squamous epithelium, 19f, 20f, 22–23, 22f
Stratum basale, 20f, 22, 22f, 191, 323, 325f
Stratum cerneum, 323f, 325, 326f
Stratum compactum, 196
Stratum corneum, 22, 22f, 190
Stratum disjunctum, 23, 323f, 324f, 325
Stratum externum, 343
Stratum granulosum, 22, 22f, 190, 192f, 259, 259f, 324, 326f
Stratum internum, 343, 344, 345f
Stratum lucidum, 22, 22f, 323f, 324–325, 324f
Stratum medium, 343
Stratum spinosum, 22, 22f, 190–191, 192f, 323, 326f
Stratum spongiosum, 129, 129f
Stria vascularis, of internal ear, 367–368, 368f–370f
Striated ducts, 26, 28f
Striola, 370, 373f
Stroma, 26, 27, 352, 352f
iridial, 356, 356f
of liver, 201–202, 202f
of testis, 233–235, 234f, 235f
Stromal cells, 136
Stromal organ, 318
Subarachnoid space, 113, 114f
Subbasal lamina, 18
Subcutaneous plexus, 335
Subendothelial layer, 118
Subepithelial basement membrane of cornea, 351–352, 352f
Sublingual salivary gland, 182–183, 183f
Sublobular veins, 205
Submental organ, 338
Submucosal glands, 172, 197, 198f
Submucosal intestinal glands, 189
Submucosal plexus, 172
Subpapillary plexus, 335
Substantia propria, 352, 352f, 361
Suburethral diverticulum, 231
Sulcus(i), reticular, 193, 194f
Supporting cells, of internal ear, 368f, 372, 374f
Supportive tissue(s), 43–58
adult, 43–58
bones, 46–58, 47f, 49f–57f
cartilage, 43–46, 44f–46f
joints, 58–59, 58f–60f
splenic, 147–148
Supracaudal gland, 340, 341f
Surface epithelium, 18–23, 19f–23f
Surfactant(s), pulmonary, 165
Sustentacular cell(s), 128, 156, 236–237, 236f, 237f, 306, 319
Sustentacular cell cycle, 236, 237f
Sweat glands, 334–335, 335f
Swine hoofs, 345–346, 345f
Synapse(s)
axodendritic, 93, 93f
chemical, interneuronal, 97
function of, 97–98

neuromuscular, 106, 107f
ultrastructure of, 97–98
Synaptic cleft, 93, 97
Synaptic vesicles, 93
Synchondrosis(es), 58
Syncytiotrophoblast(s), 282, 283f, 285
Synepitheliochorial, 282
Synovial fluid, 59
Synovial joints, 58–59, 59f, 60f
Synovial membrane, 59, 59f, 60f
Syrinx, avian, 168

T cells, 135, 135f, 136f
effector, 135, 136f
T cytotoxic cells, 135
T helper cells, 135
T lymphocytes, 75
T tubules, 84, 87f
of cardiac muscle, 87, 88f
Tactile corpuscles
encapsulated, 108, 108f
nonencapsulated, 108, 108f
Tactile epithelioid cells, 321–322, 324f
Tactile hair discs, 322
Tactile hair follicles, 332, 333f
Taenia ceci, 200
Taenia coli, 200
Tancyte(s), 100
Tapetum fibrosum, 354
Tapetum cellulosum, 354
Tapetum lucidum, 353f, 354–355, 354f
Target membrane SNAREs (tSNAREs), 8
Tarsal glands, 337, 337f
Tarsal plate, 337, 337f
Taste buds, 175–176, 176f
Taste cells, 176
Teat, of mammary gland, 342
Tectorial membrane, of internal ear, 368f, 369f, 372
Teeth. *See* Tooth (teeth)
Tela choroidea, 115
Tela submucosa
of small intestine, 197, 198f, 199f
structure of, 171f, 172
Telodendrite(s), 92f, 93f, 94–95, 95f
Telodendritic (axon terminal) zone, 96
Telogen, 333, 334f
Telophase, of cell cycle, 13, 14f
Tendon(s), collagenous, 38f, 42
Tendon sheath, 38f, 42
Terminal branches, of neuron, 92f, 93f, 94–95, 95f
Terminal bronchioles, 162–163, 163f, 164f
Terminal capillary, 150, 150f
Terminal cisternae, 84
Terminal synaptic bulb, 94
Territorial matrix, 45
Tertiary follicles, 257f, 258–260, 259f, 260f
Testicular tubules, straight, 243, 243f, 244f
Testis(es), 233–245
blood supply to, 244–245
endocrine cells of, 319
innervation of, 244–245

interstitial endocrine cells of, 234–235, 235f
interstitium of, 233–235, 234f, 235f
lamina propria of, 235–236
mediastinum, 234, 235f
meiosis of, 237–238
rete, 243, 244t
septula, 234, 234f
spermatocytogenesis of, 237, 238f, 239f
spermatogenic cells of, 237
spermatozoa of, 239–240, 241f
spermiogenesis of, 238–239, 240f
stroma of, 233–235, 234f, 235f
sustentacular cells of, 236–237236f, 237f
tunica albuginea of, 234, 234f
tunica vaginalis of, 233–234
Testosterone, 306
Tetraiodothyronine, 308–309
TGF-β. *See* Transforming growth factor-β (TGF-β)
TGN. *See* Trans-Golgi network (TGN)
Theca cells, 258
internal, 318
Theca externa, 260, 260f
Theca interna, 260, 260f
Thermogenin, 10
Thermoreceptor(s), 108
Third eyelid, 361, 362f
Thrombocyte(s), 66
Thrombopoiesis, 75, 75f
Thrombopoietin, 75
Thymic corpuscles, 140, 142f
Thymus, 140–142, 141f, 142f
Thyroglobulin, 308
biosynthesis of, 308, 309f
synthesis, iodination, and proteolysis of, 308, 310f
Thyroid follicle, 308, 308f
Thyroid gland, 307–309, 307f–310f
Thyroid peroxidase, 308
Thyroid-stimulating hormone (TSH), 302, 306
Thyrotroph(s), 302
Thyrotropin-releasing hormone (TRH), 306
Thyroxin, 308
Tidemark, 58
Tingible body macrophages, 140, 141f
Tip link, 369
Tissue(s), 17, 18f, 18t. *See also specific type, e.g.,* Central nervous system (CNS), tissue of
adipose, 33, 34f, 43
brown, 43
white, 43
cells to, 14–16, 15f, 16f
CNS, 109–112, 110f–114f
connective, 32–43. *See also* Connective tissue(s)
endocrine, 298–299, 316–319, 316f, 317f
epithelial, classification of, 18, 19f
fetal, three-dimensional structure of interface between fetal tissues and, in placentation, 281f, 282
lymphatic
diffuse, 137
organized, 137
maternal
fate at birth of, fetal–maternal anchoring effects on, in placentation, 281f, 282

three-dimensional structure of interface between fetal tissues and, in placentation, 281f, 282
muscular, 79
PNS, 104–109, 105f, 107f–109f. *See also* Peripheral nervous tissue
supportive, 43–58. *See also* Supportive tissue(s)
types of, 18t
TNF-α. *See* Tumor necrosis factor-α (TNF-α)
Tongue, 174–177, 174f–176f
lyssa of, 176, 176f
Tonofibril(s), 23
Tonofilament(s), 22, 23
Tonsil(s), 142–143, 143f
Tonsillar papillae, 174
Tooth (teeth), 177–181, 177f–181f
brachydont, 177, 177f
development of, 179–181, 179f–181f
hypsodont, 177, 177f
structure of, 177–179, 178f, 179f
Torus linguae, 174
Trabecula(ae), 27
arachnoid, 113–114, 114f
Trabecular arteries, of spleen, 149–150, 150f
Trabecular meshwork
corneoscleral, 358
of iridocorneal angle, 357f, 358
Trabecular sinuses, 145, 145f
Trachea, 160, 161f
Tracheal glands, 160
Trachealis muscle, 160
Transcellular pathway, 227
Transcytosis, 8, 9f
Transfer RNA (tRNA), 7
Transforming growth factor-β (TGF-β), 70
Trans-Golgi network (TGN), 7, 8f
Transition zone, 162
Transitional epithelium, 19f, 20–22, 20f, 22f
Transmembrane collagens, 38
Transmembrane proteins, in cell membrane, 3, 3f
Transport proteins, 228
TRH. *See* Thyrotropin-releasing hormone (TRH)
Triad, 84
Trilaminar plasma membrane, 3f
tRNA. *See* Transfer RNA (tRNA)
Trophoblast(s), 279
Trophoblast cell, binucleate, 285
Tropomyosin molecules, 83
Troponin, 83
TSH. *See* Thyroid-stimulating hormone (TSH)
Tubular organs, structure of, 171–172, 171f
Tubule(s)
cortex of, 343, 344f
dentinal, 178
distal convoluted, 219t, 220f, 222, 224f, 229
horny, 343, 344f
proximal, 218–219, 218f, 219t, 228
proximal convoluted, 218–219, 218f, 219t
proximal straight, 219, 219t, 220f, 221f
renal, 214–215, 218–224, 218f, 219t, 220f–225f
function of, 227–228
seminiferous
convoluted, 235–243, 236f–242f
cyclic events in, 240, 242f, 243

Tubule(s) *(continued)*
  T, 84, 87f
    of cardiac muscle, 87, 88f
  testicular, straight, 243, 243f, 244f
Tumor necrosis factor-α (TNF-α), 70
Tunica adventitia, structure of, 171f, 172
Tunica albuginea, 234, 234f, 257, 257f
Tunica dartos, 339
Tunica externa, 118, 119f
Tunica fibrosa bulbi, 350
Tunica interna, 118, 119f
Tunica interna bulbi, 350
Tunica media, 118, 119f
Tunica mucosa
  glandular region of, 187–189, 188f–190f
  nonglandular region of, 186, 187f
  of small intestine, 195–196, 195f, 197f–199f
  structure of, 171f, 172
Tunica muscularis, 198
  structure of, 171f, 172
Tunica serosa
  of small intestine, 198
  structure of, 171f, 172
Tunica vaginalis, 233–234
Tunica vasculosa bulbi, 350
Tympanic cavity, 364, 365f
Tympanic membrane, 364, 365f
Type I hair cells, 368
Type II hair cells, 369

Umbilical cord, 280
Undifferentiated columnar cell, 196
Unicellular glands, 24, 24t
Unilobar kidneys, 213, 213f
Unilocular adipocytes, 33–34, 33f
Unipapillary kidney, 212–213, 213f
Unitary smooth muscle, 80
Ureter, 230, 231f
Urethra, 231, 231f
  male, 252, 252f
Urinary bladder, 230–231, 231f
Urinary passages, 229–232, 230f, 231f
Urinary pole, 215
Urinary space, 216f, 217, 217f
Urinary system, 212–232
  kidneys, 212–229
Uropygial gland, 347, 348f
Uterine tube (oviduct), 262, 264–265, 265f, 266f
  blood vessels of, 265
  histologic structure of, 264–265, 265f, 266f
  histophysiology of, 265
  lymphatics of, 265
  nerves of, 265
Uteroferrin, 288
Uterus, 265–268, 266f–268f
  avian, 276f, 277
  blood vessels of, 266f, 267–268, 267f
  described, 265
  endometrium of, 265–267, 266f–268f
  endothelium of, 265–267, 266f–268f
  histologic structure of, 265–267, 266f–268f
  lymphatics of, 266f, 267–268, 267f

  myometrium of, 267
  nerves of, 266f, 267–268, 267f
  perimetrium of, 267
Utricle(s)
  of internal ear, 366f, 367
  macula of, 369–370, 373f, 374f
Utriculosaccular duct, 367
Uvea, 350

Vagina, 269, 270f
  histologic structure of, 269, 270f
Vagina(s), avian, 276f, 277
Vaginal epithelium, cyclic changes of, 273–275, 274f, 275f
Vallate papillae, 175, 175f
Valve(s), 118, 126, 128f
  atrioventricular, 129, 129f
  cardiac, 129, 129f
Vasa nervorum, 105
Vasa recta, ascending, 225, 226f
Vasa recta descending, 225, 226f
Vasa vasorum, 118, 120f
Vascular endothelium, 119–120, 121f
Vascular pole, 215
Vascular system
  blood, 117
  lymph, 117
Vasculogenesis, 122–123
Veiled cells, 137
Vein(s), 118, 126–128, 128f
  hepatic, 205
  large, 127–128, 128f
  medium, 126–127
  pulmonary, 166
  small, 126
  sublobular, 205
Venous sinuses, dural, 113
Ventral funiculus, 112, 114f
Ventral gray column, 112
Ventral median fissure, 112, 114f
Ventriculum(i), diverticulum, 187, 187f
Ventriculus, 210, 210f
Venule(s), 125, 127f
  collecting, 125, 127f
  endothelial, high, 125, 135
  interlobular portal, 202f, 204
  muscular, 125, 127f
  pericytic, 125, 127f
  postcapillary, 125, 127f
Vesicle(s)
  matrix, 50
  secretory, 93
  synaptic, 93
Vesicle SNAREs (vSNAREs), 7–8
Vesicular gland, 248–249, 249f
Vesicular transport, Golgi complex in, 7–9, 7f–9f
Vestibular apparatus, of internal ear, 368–370, 371f–374f
Vestibular aqueduct, 365f, 367
Vestibular glands
  major, 270
  minor, 270

Vestibular mechanism, of internal ear, 370
Vestibular membrane, 367
Vestibule, 269–270
Villous placenta, 282
Villus(i)
    arachnoid, 114, 114f
    intestinal, 195, 196f, 198f
Vimentin, 12
Visceral fibers, 104
Visceral pleura, 161
Visual pigments, 359
Vitelline membrane, 275
Vitreous body, 351f, 360–361
Vitreous chamber, 351
Volkmann's canals, 49, 49f
Vomeronasal cartilage, 158
Vomeronasal duct, 157–158, 158f
Vomeronasal glands, 158
Vomeronasal organ, 157–158, 158f
Vulva, 270

Wall of hoof, 343–345, 343f–345f
Weibel-Palade bodies, 120, 121f
White adipose tissue, 43
White line, 344
White pulp, 148–149, 149f, 150f
    artery of, 149, 150f

Yellow marrow, 76
Yolk sac, 279, 280f

Yolk sac placenta, 280, 280f
    inverted, 280

Z line, 84
Zona arcuata, 311, 312f
Zona fasciculata, 311, 312f
Zona glomerulosa, 311, 312f
Zona intermedia, 311, 312f
Zona pellucida, 258, 258f
Zonary placenta, 281f, 282
Zone(s)
    of cartilage, 58, 59f
    dark, 137, 138f
    dendritic, 96
    marginal, of spleen, 149, 149f, 150f
    reserve, 54, 55f
    reversal, 56, 57f
    telodendritic (axon terminal), 96
    transition, 162
Zone of hypertrophy, 54
Zone of ossification, 52f, 54, 56f
Zone of proliferation, 54, 55f
Zone of resorption, 52f, 54, 55f
Zonula adherens, 15, 15f
Zonula occludens, 15, 15f
Zonular fibers, 360, 360f
Zygomatic salivary gland, 183, 184f
Zygote(s), 260, 265, 279
Zygotene stage, 238
Zymogen granules, 27, 181